ARTICULAR CARTILAGE

SECOND EDITION

ARTICULAR CARTILAGE

SECOND EDITION

KYRIACOS A. ATHANASIOU
ERIC M. DARLING
GRAYSON D. DURAINE
JERRY C. HU
A. HARI REDDI

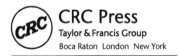

CRC Press
Taylor & Francis Group
Boca Raton London New York

CRC Press is an imprint of the
Taylor & Francis Group, an **informa** business

CRC Press
Taylor & Francis Group
6000 Broken Sound Parkway NW, Suite 300
Boca Raton, FL 33487-2742

First issued in paperback 2019

ISBN-13: 978-1-4987-0622-3 (hbk)
ISBN-13: 978-0-367-87180-2 (pbk)

Library of Congress Cataloging-in-Publication Data

Names: Athanasiou, K. A. (Kyriacos A.), author. | Darling, Eric M., author. | Hu, Jerry C., author. | DuRaine, Grayson D., author. | Reddi, A. H., 1942- author.
Title: Articular cartilage / Kyriacos A. Athanasiou, Eric M. Darling, Jerry C. Hu, Grayson D. DuRaine, and A. Hari Reddi.
Description: Second edition. | Boca Raton : Taylor & Francis, 2016. | Preceded by Articular cartilage / Kyriacos A. Athanasiou ... [et al.]. 2013. | Includes bibliographical references and index.
Identifiers: LCCN 2016021888 | ISBN 9781498706223 (alk. paper)
Subjects: | MESH: Cartilage, Articular
Classification: LCC QM142 | NLM WE 300 | DDC 612.7/517--dc23
LC record available at https://lccn.loc.gov/2016021888

Visit the Taylor & Francis Web site at
http://www.taylorandfrancis.com

and the CRC Press Web site at
http://www.crcpress.com

To Thasos and Aristos, please remember that *pursuit of excellence* is the virtuous objective.

Αφιερωμένο στους Θάσο και Άριστο. Αίεν αριστεύειν. —KAA

To my past and present mentors, who have contributed to my professional success, and to my friends and family, who have contributed to my success in everything else. —EMD

To Irene, Demitri, and Donovan, who make this all worthwhile. —GDD

To my family, my friends, and our past and current students; I think of everyone on my treks, and wish that you could see what I see. —JCH

I dedicate this to Professor Kyriacos Athanasiou, a pioneer in articular cartilage biomechanics and tissue engineering. —AHR

This page intentionally left blank.

CONTENTS

Contents

Foreword to Second Edition

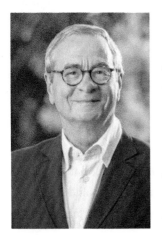

In 1892, the American Poet Walt Whitman celebrated the remarkable design and function of synovial joints: "the narrowest hinge in my hand puts to scorn all machinery" ("Song of Myself," *Leaves of Grass*, Walt Whitman Complete Poetry and Collected Prose 1891-1892, New York, Library of America, 1982, p. 217). Over the last half century, dramatic advances in prosthetic joint replacement have made it possible to restore mobility and relieve pain for millions of people with advanced joint damage. Continuing translational research, technological and procedural advances have made the current practice of synthetic joint replacement one of the most noteworthy successes in the annals of surgery.

Yet, Whitman's observation stands unchallenged; no current artificial joint comes close to replicating the function and durability of synovial joints. These complex structures developed and progressively evolved over millions of years. Formed from multiple self-renewing tissues, including joint capsule, ligament, in some cases meniscus, subchondral bone, synovium, and hyaline articular cartilage, they provide stable pain-free movement with a level of friction less than that achieved by any artificial bearing surface. The tissue central to these extraordinary functional capabilities is hyaline articular cartilage. Although it varies in thickness, cell density, and to some extent composition and mechanical properties among joints and among mammalian species, all articular cartilages share the same general structure and perform the same functions. These include lubricating the joint surface and minimizing peak stresses on subchondral bone by distributing loads. Perhaps the most extraordinary property of articular cartilage is durability; for most people, it provides normal joint function for more than 80 years.

Deterioration of synovial joints due to multiple causes, most commonly osteoarthritis, is the leading cause of pain and impairment in middle-aged and older people. Osteoarthritis can occur in any synovial joint and develops in every human population. Although osteoarthritis increases with aging, it is not a direct or inevitable result of aging changes alone. In addition to increasing age, excessive cumulative joint loading and joint injury are universal risk factors for osteoarthritis in all joints and all populations; yet, despite the recognition of these risk factors, the pathogenesis of the joint destruction that leads to the clinical syndrome of osteoarthritis remains obscure. No current treatments have been shown to prevent the onset or progression of osteoarthritis, although recent findings suggest that interventions to decrease the risk of osteoarthritis following joint injury may be possible.

In a concise cogent fashion, this second edition of *Articular Cartilage* summarizes current understanding of articular cartilage structure, function, development, maintenance, and degradation. Furthermore, exciting new information included in this volume lays the foundation for fresh approaches to preventing loss of articular cartilage and even restoring lost or diseased cartilage.

The book consists of seven chapters. Chapter 1 deals with the structure, composition, and function of articular cartilage, including lucid explanations of how the structure and organization of articular cartilage provide its unrivaled biomechanical properties, including lubrication of the joint surface. Chapter 2 covers articular cartilage embryogenesis, growth and maturation, and signaling pathways that have roles in these changes. Because articular cartilage lacks nerves and blood vessels, it was initially thought to be relatively inert; the identification of signaling pathways that control its formation, growth, and maintenance proves that this early impression was mistaken. Progress in understanding these pathways is likely to help explain the onset and progression of osteoarthritis and may lead to methods of detecting changes in tissue homeostasis before the cartilage begins to deteriorate. Chapter 3, "Articular Cartilage Pathology and Therapies," deals with the various forms of arthritis that lead to loss of articular cartilage and joint function, cartilage injuries and the response to injury, and contemporary and emerging methods for cartilage repair and restoration. Chapter 4 is devoted to tissue engineering of articular cartilage and explores the potential of *in vitro* tissue engineering for the restoration of articular surfaces. This chapter then goes on to summarize the sources of cells, biomaterials, and the use of scaffolds and bioreactors to promote formation of functional articular cartilage. As Chapter 4 clearly shows, tissue engineering has great promise for biologic restoration of synovial joints. In advancing understanding of the disorders of articular cartilage and their treatment or prevention, it is critical to have methods of evaluating articular cartilage quality. Chapter 5 discusses the imaging techniques and the quantitative assessment of cartilage components and methods of measuring mechanical properties to assess cartilage composition, structure, and function. It also includes a summary of the uses of large and small animal models to test the safety and efficacy of cartilage repair or restoration therapies. Breakthroughs in treatment of damaged or degenerated joints will depend on translating advances in basic cartilage research into clinical practice. Chapter 6 summarizes the challenges and opportunities in basic investigations of articular cartilage biology and regeneration and covers the business and regulatory aspects of potential methods of re-creating biologic articular surfaces. Chapter 7 presents detailed explanations of experimental protocols for generating and evaluating articular cartilage, including tissue and cell culture, tissue and matrix molecule analysis, RNA extraction, and testing mechanical properties, as well as animal protocols.

This well-organized, readable, and comprehensive second edition of *Articular Cartilage* is an important milestone in the understanding of one of nature's singular creations. It will serve as an essential resource for those who wish to contribute new insights into articular cartilage biology, as well as those who pursue clinically applicable technologies with the potential to reconstruct damaged or diseased joint surfaces. Although prosthetic joint replacement for people with advanced, essentially complete, destruction of hip, knee, and shoulder joints is effective, these procedures have limitations and in some instances devastating complications. Discovering ways to prevent the onset or progression of synovial joint destruction and to rebuild biologic articular surfaces would be among the most important developments in the history of medicine. This book gives encouragement and direction to those who seek to make these discoveries.

Joseph A. Buckwalter, MS, MD

Professor and Arthur Steindler Chair

University of Iowa Department of Orthopaedics and Rehabilitation

Iowa City Veterans Administration Medical Center

Iowa City, Iowa

This page intentionally left blank.

FOREWORD TO FIRST EDITION

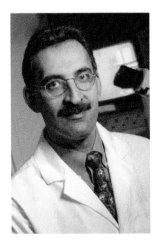

The synovial joint is truly one of nature's marvels, providing our skeleton with a nearly frictionless bearing surface that can withstand forces of several times body weight for millions of loading cycles throughout life. To date, no man-made joint has been able to approach these capabilities. While the mammalian joint is clearly a highly complex biological and biomechanical organ that includes multiple structures, tissues, and cells, it is the articular cartilage—the tissue that lines the surfaces of synovial joints—that is fundamentally responsible for these unparalleled biomechanical properties.

Over the past century, our understanding of articular cartilage has grown exponentially. Building upon early studies that characterized the anatomy and histology of cartilage, scientists recognized its unique mechanical properties and function. By the mid-twentieth century, investigators had begun to develop new methods to quantify the elastic and tribological properties of the tissue. The 1960s and the 1970s were characterized by significant advances in the characterization of the biochemical composition of cartilage, primarily the proteoglycan and collagen components. With the development of the biphasic theory for modeling cartilage mechanics in 1980, the next two decades saw major breakthroughs in the understanding of the highly complex multiphasic, viscoelastic, anisotropic, inhomogeneous, and nonlinear properties of the tissue. Simultaneously, the study of cartilage development was revolutionized by the ongoing breakthroughs occurring in molecular biology and genetics in the 1990s. By the beginning of the twenty-first century, scientists and engineers had made tremendous strides in understanding how the incredibly complex composition and structure of cartilage were responsible for its load-bearing properties.

However, as with any other precision machine, even slight imbalances of the biological or biomechanical processes responsible for maintaining the tissue can lead to cumulative and progressive changes over decades of use, ultimately causing osteoarthritic failure of the joint. With the new depth of understanding of cartilage development, mechanics, and biology, the fields of tissue engineering and regenerative medicine have exploded in the effort to develop new therapies for preventing or treating cartilage damage by combining cells, biomaterials, bioactive molecules, and physical signals. While there are currently no disease-modifying therapies available for treating osteoarthritis, such tissue engineering approaches hold tremendous promise for the near future.

For the first time, the wealth of new knowledge in these areas is brought together in a single volume. *Articular Cartilage* represents the most comprehensive text to date focusing on this tissue and provides a unique and interdisciplinary approach that encompasses the breadth of basic science, bioengineering, translational science, and detailed methodologic approaches.

Chapter 1 broadly reviews the current state of knowledge on the structure and composition of different types of cartilage as well as the chondrocytes. In addition to presenting the molecular components of the tissue, this chapter provides overviews of the biomechanical function and properties of cartilage, as well as the structure-function relationships of the primary constituents of the tissue and cells.

A critical step in understanding cartilage physiology, pathophysiology, and regeneration is an understanding of the fundamental processes involved in cartilage development, maturation, and aging. In Chapter 2, the current state of knowledge of cartilage development is summarized, including the sequences of growth and transcription factors necessary for proper cell-cell and cell-matrix interactions required during the formation of the limb bud and the subsequent formation of the synovial joint. This chapter also reviews the changes that occur in the extracellular matrix and chondrocytes with maturation and aging, under normal or pathologic conditions.

Chapter 3 focuses on the epidemiology, etiopathogenesis, and therapeutic approaches for the major arthritides that affect cartilage and the synovial joints, namely, cartilage injury, osteoarthritis, rheumatoid arthritis, and gout. While these represent distinct disease processes, they are all characterized by degeneration of the articular cartilage and, eventually, loss of joint function. In particular, significant emphasis is placed on the role of biomechanical factors in the onset and progression of osteoarthritis. Furthermore, a review of the (lack of) current therapeutic approaches for osteoarthritis or cartilage injury clearly reveals a substantial unmet need for disease-modifying approaches to diseases that affect articular cartilage.

With recent evidence suggesting that over 10% of osteoarthritis may arise due to joint injury, it is clear that the development of new tissue engineering approaches for cartilage repair or regeneration can have a significant impact on this disease. Chapter 4 provides an up-to-date overview of the field of tissue engineering as applied to articular cartilage repair. Different sections provide highlights of recent advances in the classical "three pillars" of tissue engineering: cell source, scaffold design, and external stimulation through the use of bioactive molecules and mechanical bioreactors. The chapter also includes important discussion of the relative advantages and potential limitations of different cell types, biomaterial scaffolds, bioactive molecules, and bioreactors.

One of the primary hindrances to the development of new therapies for joint disease has been the lack of surrogate measures that provide valid, reliable, and responsive readouts of disease severity or progression. Such biological markers, or "biomarkers," may include proteins, genes, noninvasive or invasive imaging, or even biomechanical measures that reflect certain events in the disease process. In other fields such as cardiology and infectious diseases, biomarkers such as cholesterol levels, blood pressure, or antibody levels have served critical diagnostic and therapeutic roles. Chapter 5 overviews a number of methods that are used to assess the structure, composition, biology, and biomechanical function of articular cartilage. In addition to novel imaging methods such as MRI, such assessments may include histologic or immunohistochemical measures of joint tissues, or direct measures of tissue function through biomechanical testing. Due to the highly complex nature of cartilage, the proper determination of tissue material-level properties often involves the use of mathematical modeling that simulates the precise testing condition in tension, compression, shear, or contact (i.e., tribological testing). Finally, this chapter also provides a summary of different animal models and scoring systems that are often used for modeling and assessing disease or repair processes, with a critical review of their relative advantages and disadvantages.

With these issues in mind, Chapter 6 provides important discussion and perspectives on many of the remaining challenges and opportunities in the development and translation of new approaches for treating diseases of articular cartilage. A variety of issues are discussed, including some of the intrinsic characteristics of cartilage that appear to make repair of cartilage insuperable. In this light, alternative factors are discussed that may influence the success of regenerative therapies for cartilage, such as potential immunogenic responses. The ultimate success of such cell-based or biologic therapies, however, is highly dependent on practical issues such as regulatory pathways, intellectual property concerns, the pathway to market, and potential reimbursement. This chapter provides an important snapshot of the ever-changing landscape of regulatory and commercial affairs for medical products for cartilage repair.

The final chapter of the text provides detailed working protocols for many of the methods used to study articular cartilage. Beginning with standard cell and tissue harvest and culture methods, the chapter also details several culture methods, such as the use of 3D gels, that are commonly used for chondrocyte culture or cartilage tissue engineering. Methods for cartilage assessment via histology and immunohistochemistry are also provided. Importantly, detailed methods are provided for protein and RNA extraction from cartilage, which is generally more complex than other cells due to the presence of significant amounts of extracellular matrix. Finally, detailed protocols for mechanical testing of cartilage are provided.

This thorough and comprehensive text seamlessly integrates concepts of basic science, bioengineering, translational medicine, and clinical care of articular cartilage. By revealing the wealth of knowledge we have accumulated in this area, as well as exposing the tremendous opportunities for advancement, *Articular Cartilage* provides a critical template for those seeking to study one of the most complex tissues of the human body. Only through this level of understanding will we eventually be able to develop new methods to diagnose, prevent, or treat diseases of articular cartilage.

Farshid Guilak, PhD

Professor of Orthopaedic Surgery and Research Director

Shriners Hospital, St. Louis

Co-Director of the Washington University Center of Regenerative Medicine

Washington University

St. Louis, Missouri

MATLAB® is a registered trademark of The MathWorks, Inc. For product information, please contact:

The MathWorks, Inc.
3 Apple Hill Drive
Natick, MA 01760-2098 USA
Tel: 508-647-7000
Fax: 508-647-7001
E-mail: info@mathworks.com
Web: www.mathworks.com

This page intentionally left blank.

Authors

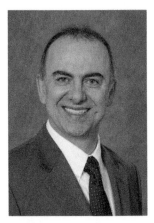

Kyriacos A. Athanasiou is a distinguished professor and the Child Family Professor in the Department of Biomedical Engineering and the Department of Orthopaedic Surgery at the University of California, Davis. He earned a PhD in mechanical engineering (bio-engineering) from Columbia University. He has also served as a faculty member at the University of Texas, and then at Rice University.

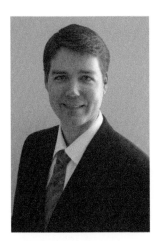

Eric M. Darling is an associate professor of medical science, orthopedics, and engineering in the Department of Molecular Pharmacology, Physiology, and Biotechnology at Brown University. He earned a BS in engineering from Harvey Mudd College, and a PhD in bioengineering from Rice University. He did postdoctoral training at Duke University.

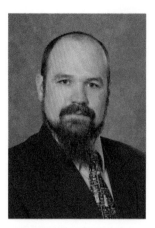

Grayson D. DuRaine is a senior research associate in the Department of Molecular Microbiology and Immunology at Oregon Health & Science University. He earned a BS in biology from California State University of Sacramento and a PhD in cell and developmental biology from the University of California, Davis.

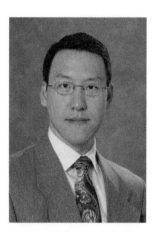

Jerry C. Hu is the director of the Clinical Translational Program in the Department of Biomedical Engineering at the University of California, Davis. He earned a BS in chemical engineering from the University of Texas at Austin and a PhD in bioengineering from Rice University.

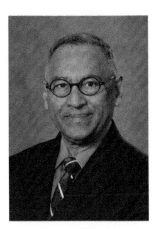

A. Hari Reddi is a student of bone and cartilage biology. He is currently at the University of California, Davis as a distinguished professor and the Lawrence Ellison Chair in Musculoskeletal Molecular Biology. He was previously on the faculty of Johns Hopkins University School of Medicine, National Institutes of Health, and University of Chicago.

This page intentionally left blank.

LIST OF ABBREVIATIONS

ABBREVIATION	NAME
2D	two-dimensional
3D	three-dimensional
AAOS	American Academy of Orthopaedic Surgeons
ACI	autologous chondrocyte implantation
ACL	anterior cruciate ligament
ADAMTS	A Disintegrin and Metalloproteinase with Thrombospondin motifs
ADC	apparent diffusion coefficient
AER	apical ectodermal ridge
AERS	Adverse Event Reporting System
AGE	advanced glycation endproduct
alpha-gal	gal alpha(1,3)gal antigen
Alx4	aristaless-like homeobox
APC	antigen-presenting cell
ASTM	American Society for Testing and Materials
BCA	bicinchoninic acid
BCP	basic calcium phosphate hydroxy-apatite
bFGF	basic fibroblast growth factor
BLA	biologics license application
BME	beta-mercaptaethanol
BMP	bone morphogenetic protein
BSA	bovine serum albumin
C-ABC	chondroitinase ABC
CACP	camptodactyly-arthropathy-coxa vara-pericarditis
cadherin	calcium-dependent adhesion
CAIS	cartilage autograft implantation system
CBER	Center for Biologics Evaluation and Research
CDC	Centers for Disease Control and Prevention
CDER	Center for Drug Evaluation and Research
CDMP	cartilage-derived morphogenetic protein
cDNA	complementary DNA
CDRH	Center for Devices and Radiological Health

CFKH-1	chicken winged-helix-loop/forkhead transcription factor 1
CFR	Code of Federal Regulations
CFSAN	Center for Food Safety and Applied Nutrition
cGMP	current good manufacturing practices
CILP	cartilage intermediate-layer protein
cmd	cartilage matrix deficiency
COMP	cartilage oligomeric matrix protein
COX2	cyclooxygenase 2
CPM	continuous passive motion
CPP	calcium pyrophosphate
CS	chondroitin sulfate
C_t	cycle threshold
CT	computed tomography
Da	dalton
DAB	3,3′-diaminobenzidine
dGEMRIC	delayed gadolinium-enhanced MRI of the cartilage
Dhh	desert hedgehog
DLX	distal-less homeobox
DMEM	Dulbecco's modified Eagle's medium
DMMB	1,9-dimethyl methylene blue
DMOAD	disease-modifying osteoarthritis drug
DMSO	dimethyl sulfoxide
DNA	deoxyribonucleic acid
Dsh	Dishevelled
ECL	enhanced chemiluminescence
ECM	extracellular matrix
EDTA	ethylenediaminetetraacetic acid
EGTA	ethyleneglycoltetraacetic acid
ELISA	enzyme-linked immunosorbent assay
ELP	elastin-like polypeptide
ER	endoplasmic reticulum
ESC	embryonic stem cell
EULAR	European League Against Rheumatism
FACE	fluorophore-assisted carbohydrate electrophoresis

FAOOS	Foot and Ankle Osteoarthritis Outcome Score
FBN1	fibrillin 1 gene
FBS	fetal bovine serum
FDA	Food and Drug Administration
FGF	fibroblast growth factor
Fra2	FOS-like antigen
GAG	glycosaminoglycan
GAIT	Glucosamine/Chondroitin Arthritis Intervention Trial
GAP	GTPase activating protein
GAPDH	glyceraldehyde-3-phosphate dehydrogenase
GDF10	growth/differentiation factor 10
GEF	guanine nucleotide exchange factor
GSK3	glycogen synthase kinase 3
H&E	hematoxylin and eosin
HA	hyaluronan or hyaluronic acid
HCT/P	human cells, tissues, and cell- and tissue-based product
HDE	humanitarian device exemption
HFB	hydrodynamic focusing bioreactor
HGF	hepatocyte growth factor
HH	hedgehog protein
HIF-1α	hypoxia-inducible factor 1α
HMG	High-Mobility Group
HOOS	Hip Osteoarthritis Outcome Score
HOX	homeobox
HRP	horseradish peroxidase
IACUC	Institutional Animal Care and Use Committee
IDE	investigational device exemption
IFN	interferon
IGF	insulin-like growth factor
IHC	immunohistochemistry
Ihh	Indian hedgehog
IKDC	International Knee Documentation Committee
IL	interleukin

IND	investigational new drug
iPSC	induced pluripotent stem cell
IRB	institutional review board
IRS	insulin receptor substrate
JNK (a.k.a. SAPK)	c-jun n-terminal kinase
kDa	kilodalton
KI	knock-in
KO	knockout
KOOS	Knee injury and Osteoarthritis Outcome Score
kPa	kilopascal
KS	keratan sulfate
LCL	lateral cruciate ligament
LEF	lymphoid enhancer factor
LVDT	linear variable differential transformer
MAPK	mitogen-activated protein kinase
MCL	medial cruciate ligament
MDa	megadalton
MFH	mesenchyme forkhead
MHC	major histocompatibility complex
MMP	matrix metalloproteinase
MPa	megapascal
MRI	magnetic resonance imaging
mRNA	messenger RNA
MSC	mesenchymal stem cell
MSU	monosodium urate
MSX	muscle segment homeobox
N-cadherin	neural cadherin
N-CAM	neural cell adhesion molecule
NDA	new drug application
NHIS	National Health Interview Survey
NSAID	nonsteroidal anti-inflammatory drug
OA	osteoarthritis
OARSI	Osteoarthritis Research Society International
OOCHAS	OARSI Osteoarthritis Cartilage Histopathology Assessment System

OP-1	osteogenic protein 1
PAI-1	plasminogen activator inhibitor 1
PAX	paired-box transcription factor
PBS	phosphate-buffered saline
PCL	poly-caprolactone
PCL	posterior cruciate ligament
PCNA	proliferating cell nuclear antigen
PCR	polymerase chain reaction
PDGF	platelet-derived growth factor
PDP	product development protocol
PEG	poly-ethylene glycol
PET	positron emission tomography
PGA	poly-glycolic acid
PGE2	prostaglandin E2
pH	potential hydrogen
PI-3K	phosphoinositide 3-kinase
Pitx	paired-like homeodomain
pKa	acid dissociation constant
PLA	poly-lactic acid
PLGA	poly-lactic-co-glycolic acid
PMA	premarket approval application
PRG4	proteoglycan 4 (analogous to SZP)
PRX	paired-box homeodomain
PSF	penicillin-streptomycin-fungizone
PTC	patched
qRT-PCR	quantitative reverse transcription PCR
QSR	quality system regulation
RA	rheumatoid arthritis
RAOS	Rheumatoid and Arthritis Outcome Score
RGD	Arg-Gly-Asp
rhBMP	recombinant human BMP
RNA	ribonucleic acid
R-Smad	receptor-activated Smad
RT-PCR	reverse transcription polymerase chain reaction
Runx2	runt-domain transcription factor

SA-CAT	stretch-activated cation channel
SCID	severe combined immunodeficiency
SDS	sodium dodecyl sulfate
SEM	scanning electron microscopy
SHG	second harmonic generation
Shh	sonic hedgehog
SLRP	small leucine-rich repeat proteoglycan
SRY	sex-determining region Y
SZP	superficial zone protein (analogous to PRG4)
TBx	T-box
TEM	transmission electron microscopy
TGF-β	transforming growth factor β
TIMP	tissue inhibitor of metalloproteinase
TnBP	tributyl phosphate
TNF-α	tumor necrosis factor α
TNF-β	tumor necrosis factor β
TUNEL	terminal deoxynucleotidyl transferase-mediated dUTP nick end labeling
VEGF	vascular endothelial growth factor
VSCC	voltage-sensitive calcium channel
Wnt	wingless and int-related protein
ZPA	zone of polarizing activity

SYMBOL	NAME
E_R	relaxed modulus
E_Y or E	Young's modulus
F_f	friction force
G	shear modulus
G^*	complex shear modulus
H_A	aggregate modulus
k	permeability
N	normal force
γ	shear strain
ε	normal strain
η	viscosity coefficient

xxxiv

μ	coefficient of friction
σ	normal stress
τ	shear stress
τ_ε	relaxation time for constant strain
τ_σ	relaxation time for constant stress

This page intentionally left blank.

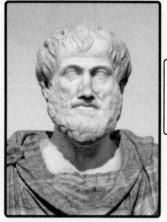

"Cartilage and bone are indeed fundamentally the same thing, the differences between them being merely matters of degree. Thus neither cartilage nor bone, when once cut off, grows again."
Aristotle (384-322 BCE), Greek philosopher and scientist

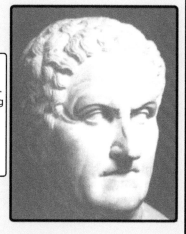

"Spread on some parts of them [bones], such as the joints, to make them smooth, and nature also uses cartilages occasionally as moderately yielding bodies.... Cartilage serves as a grease for the joints … first covering each member of the joint with cartilage and then pouring over the cartilages themselves a sort of oily substance, a greasy, glutinous fluid, which gives every joint an easy movement and protection against wear."
Galen (130-215 CE), Greek physician

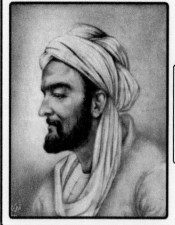

Cartilage is "flexible, but second to bone in hardness."
"It was made for the purpose of providing a cushion between hard bone and the soft members, so that the latter should not be injured when exposed to a blow or fall, or compression…. In the case of joints, it prevents the tissues from being torn by the hard bone."
Avicenna (980-1037 CE), Persian physician

Structure and Function of Cartilage

1

- Cartilage in the body
- Chondrocytes
- Cartilage matrix
- Cartilage biomechanics

This book focuses on articular cartilage—the usual cartilage type found in diarthrodial joints (Huey et al. 2012). Though there is mention of other types of cartilage, the main focus is on hyaline articular cartilage. We know that, in general, the cartilages of the body can be classified into three different types based on biochemical properties: hyaline, elastic, and fibrous cartilage. While all of these cartilages share general features, they differ by histomorphology, biochemical composition, and biomechanical properties. There is an intrinsic and strong relationship between the different functions that these cartilages perform within the body and tissue characteristics—in other words, function dictates tissue properties. In terms of articular cartilage, its function as a load-bearing and stress-dissipating tissue has a direct effect on its biochemical composition, structure, and biomechanical behavior, as manifested by its tensile, shear, and compressive properties. This chapter covers the structure, composition, and function of articular cartilage, at the cell and extracellular matrix levels.

1.1 CARTILAGE IN THE BODY

1.1.1 Hyaline

Hyaline, from Greek *hyalos* (ὕαλος), meaning "glass"

The use of hyaline as a descriptor of cartilage derives from the appearance of articular cartilage, which ranges from a glossy slightly translucent white or bluish-white to a slightly yellowish-off-white tissue depending on its age (Figures 1.1 and 1.2). Hyaline cartilage is the most abundant type of cartilage.

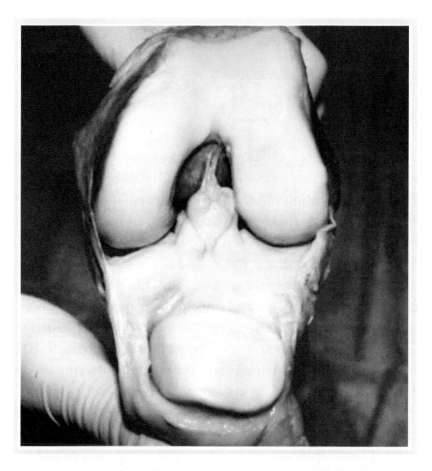

Figure 1.1 Human articular cartilage of the knee, showing the femoral condyles and the patellar groove at the top, as well as the articulating surface of the patella at the bottom.

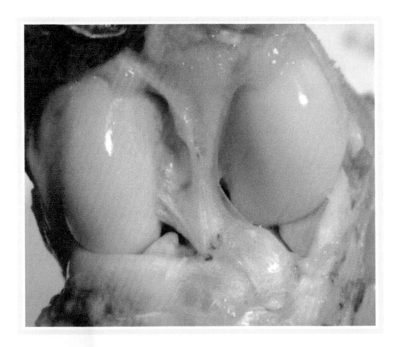

Figure 1.2 Articular cartilage of the juvenile bovine femoral condyles, demonstrating the glistening nature of the hyaline cartilage. Note the close resemblance to that of Figure 1.1 of the human knee.

Hyaline articular cartilage is found at the ends of bones where it acts to provide a low friction bearing surface for movement. It also cushions and distributes forces generated during locomotion. In adult humans, this layer is usually only on the order of 1-2 mm thick, with the thickness varying across different areas of the joint (Koo and Andriacchi 2007). Hyaline articular cartilage is composed of specialized proteins and macromolecules that allow the tissue to function in the rigorous biomechanical environments of articulating joints, such as the knee, hip, and shoulder. Key biochemical features include the predominant presence of type II collagen and large amounts of proteoglycans (discussed in more detail in Sections 1.3.3 and 1.3.4, respectively). Collagens and proteoglycans interact with a charged fluid environment to give articular cartilage its unique biomechanical properties.

Hyaline cartilage is also found in the ends of the ribs, larynx, tracheal rings, bronchi, ears, sclera of the eye, and nose, where it is covered by perichondrium. Another hyaline cartilage structure is the the epiphyseal (growth) plate, in the metaphysis (wider region at the end of the long bones), responsible for the elongational growth of bones. The growth plate organizes into multiple zones of differentiating chondrocytes in columns. These zones include undifferentiated cartilage cells (resting zone), proliferating cells (responsible for volume increases), hypertrophic cells (cells enlarged and aligned in columns, and beginning to undergo apoptosis), and calcified cells (where cartilage is replaced by bone). As skeletal development and maturation proceed, chondrocytes undergo terminal differentiation into hypertrophic chondrocytes, and the growth plates calcify and are eventually replaced by bone, at which point the bone stops elongating (Johnston 1997). Defects or injuries to the growth plate commonly result in shortening of the affected bone, as longitudinal growth is impaired. Long bone growth defects may lead to growth disorders such as achondroplasia, the most common cause of dwarfism.

1.1.2 Elastic

Elastic, from ancient Greek *elastēs* (ἐλαστής), meaning "springy" or "flexible," derived from *elaunein* (ἐλαύνειν), meaning "to drive, set in motion, push, strike, beat out"

Elastic cartilage differs from other cartilage types by having a matrix containing large amounts of elastin, which exists as a highly branched fiber (Figure 1.3). The insoluble elastin fiber complex is formed from cross-linking lysines through a desmosine cross-link of the soluble 65 kDa tropoelastin protein. Other than cartilage, elastin and elastin fibers are found in tissues and organs requiring flexibility, such as arteries, skin, heart, lungs, and bladder. The chondrocytes of elastic cartilage are more numerous than in other cartilages, and lie oriented between the fibers of elastin. Elastic cartilage derives its name from the high amount of flexibility present in the tissue due to the elastin content, but develops in the fetus from a hyaline cartilage precursor (Sucheston and Cannon 1969). Elastin fibers can often be in high enough concentrations to not only impart a yellowish color to elastic cartilage, but also act as

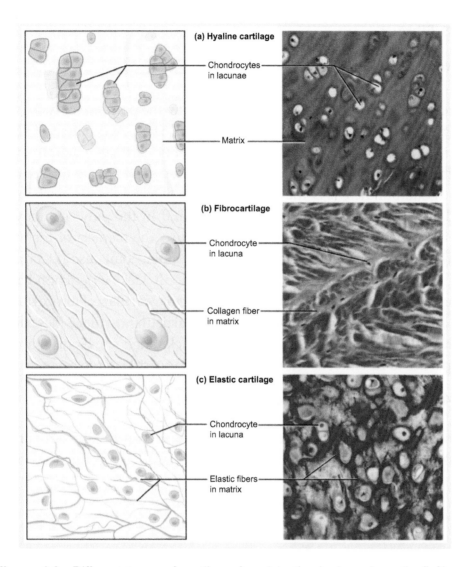

Figure 1.3 Different types of cartilage found in the body: schematic (left) and histology (right). (Image used with a Creative Commons Attribution License 3.0. Canine cartilage micrographs provided by the Regents of the University of Michigan Medical School © 2012. From http://cnx.org/contents/14fb4ad7-39a1-4eee-ab6e -3ef2482e3e22@6.27.)

an impediment to staining of other components of the elastic cartilage matrix (e.g., type II collagen and glycosaminoglycans [GAGs]). Within the body, elastic cartilage is present in several locations, including the outer ear (auricle), pharyngotympanic (Eustachian) tube, larynx, and epiglottis, and is covered by perichondrium (Singh 2006).

1.1.3 Fibrous

Fibrous, from Latin *fibra*, meaning "filament-like"

Fibrocartilage differs from hyaline cartilage by the presence of type I collagen and, to a lesser degree, type II collagen. The GAG content of fibrocartilage is often much lower than that of hyaline cartilage. Chondrocytes in fibrocartilage (fibrochondrocytes) are interspersed among the connective tissue bundles; it is these bundles that help to absorb mechanical loads. Within the body, fibrocartilage is found in the pubic symphysis, the annulus fibrosus of the intervertebral disc, the menisci of the knee (Makris et al. 2011), and the temporomandibular joint disc (Detamore and Athanasiou 2003). Fibrocartilage commonly lacks a perichondrium covering, a feature it shares with hyaline articular cartilage. Fibrocartilage can also form as a repair tissue of damaged articular cartilage (described in more detail in Section 3.2.1), although it lacks adequate biomechanical properties to function as a long-term articular cartilage replacement.

1.1.4 Cartilage's Role in the Joints

Although joints vary by structure and function (Figure 1.4), they can be classified by the range of movement and the tissue connecting the bones

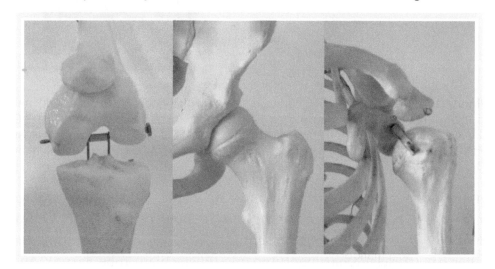

Figure 1.4   The knee, hip, and shoulder joints shown in a model skeleton.

(Figure 1.5). Structurally, joints can be classified by the type of connective tissue present, either fibrous connective tissue, cartilage, or no direct connection. Joints connected by fibrous connective tissue (fibrous joints) include the sutures of the bones of the skull, the syndesmosis of the radius/ulna and fibula/tibia, and the gomphosis of the tooth and socket. Except for the syndesmosis, which permits movement, the fibrous joints

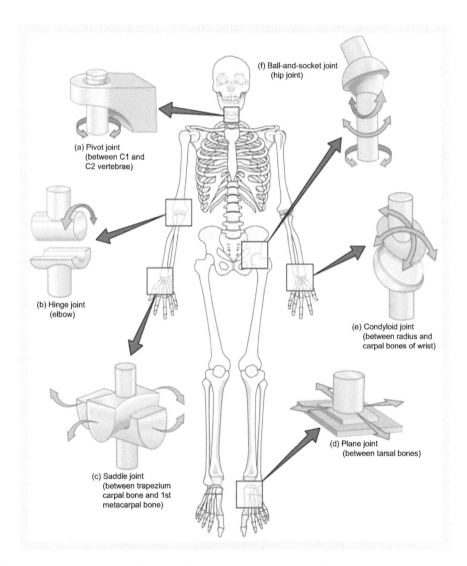

Figure 1.5   Schematic of types of joints found in the body. (Image used with a Creative Commons Attribution License Unported 3.0. From http://cnx.org/contents/14fb4ad7 -39a1-4eee-ab6e-3ef2482e3e22@6.27.)

permit little to no movement and functionally are classified as synarthrosis joint types. Joints connected by cartilaginous tissues (hyaline or fibrocartilage) may be further subdivided into synchondrosis and symphysis joints. Synchondrosis joints (with the exception of the joint of the first rib and sternum) are present during skeletal maturation as growth plates. This offers minimal movement and is later replaced with bone. Symphysis joints, such as the intervertebral discs and the pubic symphysis, generally allow some movement (amphiarthrosis) and are permanent structures. Anatomically, these are composed of hyaline cartilage separated by a fibrocartilage disc (Gray et al. 1980).

The most commonly studied joint is the synovial joint, which is the most mobile joint type. The term *synovial joint* is synonymous with diarthroses or diarthrodial joints. In the synovial joint, a fibrous capsule contiguous with periosteum surrounds the joint forming the synovial capsule and is lined with synovial membrane (Figure 1.6). Within the capsule, the articular cartilage is bathed in a lubricating ultrafiltrate of blood

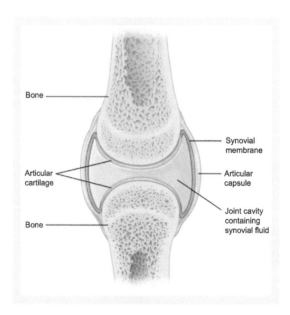

Figure 1.6 Schematic of the simple synovial joint. (Image used with a Creative Commons Attribution License Unported 3.0. From http://cnx.org/contents/14fb4ad7 -39a1-4eee-ab6e-3ef2482e3e22@6.27.)

known as the synovial fluid (discussed in more detail in Section 1.3.1) (Ropes et al. 1939). Furthermore, joints can be classified based on the number of bones and articulating surfaces, and other anatomical structures, as simple (two surfaces, hip joint), complex (more than two surfaces, the wrist), or compound (two or more surfaces and a fibrocartilage disc, the knee and meniscus) (Gray et al. 1980) (Figure 1.5).

1.2 CHONDROCYTES AND THEIR CELLULAR CHARACTERISTICS

When compared with other tissues in the body, articular cartilage is sparsely populated by cells. The cells in cartilage, termed chondrocytes, occupy less than 5% of the tissue volume in humans but are essential for maintaining the extracellular matrix. The chondrocyte, which is the basic metabolic unit of cartilage, is responsible for limited matrix remodeling (Mankin and Lippiello 1969). As the sole cell type resident within hyaline cartilage, the chondrocyte is pivotal for the maintenance of the tissue. Since articular cartilage is avascular and chondrocytes are isolated within the dense extracellular matrix, the primary source of nutrients is through diffusion from the synovial fluid, which is facilitated by joint movement (Archer et al. 1990). Though the phenotype of articular chondrocytes varies as a function of zonal depth, all cartilage cells differentiate from mesenchymal progenitor cells. In healthy adult tissues, chondrocytes have slow to no proliferation.

1.2.1 Genetic, Synthetic, and Mechanical Phenotype

All chondrocytes within articular cartilage share common traits with respect to gene and protein expressions, surface markers, and cell metabolism. A grouping of predominantly expressed genes, namely, type II collagen and aggrecan, uniquely identify articular cartilage and represent the matrix components described in the proceeding chapters. The main cartilage-specific transcription factor is sex-determining region Y (SRY)-box-9 (Sox9), pivotal in initiation and maintenance of phenotypes during differentiation of mesenchymal stem cells to chondrocytes.

Though chondrocytes have been categorized as all belonging to the same phenotype, differences exist in the genetic, synthetic, and mechanical characteristics of cells with respect to their zone of origin in the tissue (Aydelotte and Kuettner 1988; Darling et al. 2004, 2006; Darling and Athanasiou 2005). For instance, superficial zone chondrocytes express the protein proteoglycan 4 (PRG4), also termed lubricin or superficial zone protein (SZP), while middle zone chondrocytes express cartilage intermediate-layer protein (CILP). Superficial zone chondrocytes were also found to attach to tissue culture plastic slower than those from the deeper zones (Siczkowski and Watt 1990). Deep zone cells display a higher level of vimentin (Durrant et al. 1999), which has been hypothesized to resist compression of the cell (Ghadially 1983; Ralphs et al. 1992). Keratan sulfate synthesis has also been observed to gradually increase through cartilage depth (Zanetti et al. 1985; Aydelotte et al. 1988; Aydelotte and Kuettner 1988; Archer et al. 1990; Siczkowski and Watt 1990). The characteristic gene and protein expressions of chondrocytes are closely associated with the matrix constituents of articular cartilage.

There are also transient metabolic differences among chondrocytes of different sizes (Trippel et al. 1980), especially as they relate to zonal origin (Zanetti et al. 1985; Aydelotte et al. 1988; Aydelotte and Kuettner 1988; Archer et al. 1990; Siczkowski and Watt 1990). Articular chondrocytes from the superficial, middle, and deep zones have morphologies and expression profiles specific to their regions within the tissue (see Section 1.3.2). Cell diameters range from 10 to 13 μm, with superficial zone cells being smaller than middle and deep zone cells (Aydelotte and Kuettner 1988). The morphology for cells near the surface of the tissue is flattened and discoidal, whereas in the middle zone the cells are more rounded; in the deep zone, the cells are ellipsoidal and organized in columns perpendicular to the surface (Youn et al. 2006) (Figure 1.7).

In general, middle and deep zone cells possess greater synthetic capabilities for the major molecular constituents of cartilage than superficial zone cells when cultured *in vitro* (Aydelotte and Kuettner 1988;

12

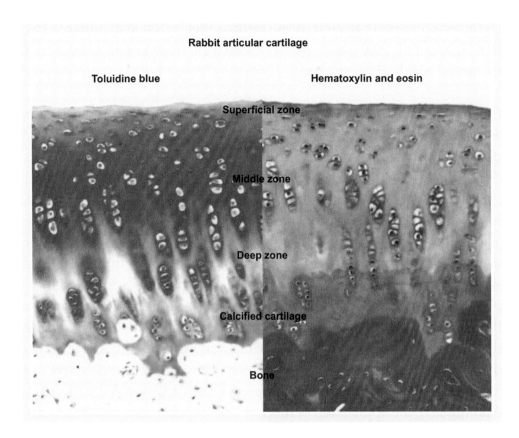

Figure 1.7 Zonal structure of articular cartilage. Histology of full-thickness (~1 mm) adult rabbit articular cartilage from the knee (10×), indicating changes in cell morphology with depth. The histological section is of a slice taken perpendicular to the cartilage surface, with toluidine blue staining proteoglycans (purplish), hematoxylin staining nuclei (blue), and eosin staining protein structures (pink/red).

Archer et al. 1990; Darling and Athanasiou 2005). Chondrocytes from superficial and middle and deep zones also have different biomechanical properties. The Young's modulus of superficial zone chondrocytes is approximately twice that of the middle and deep zone chondrocytes (E_Y = 460 vs. 260 Pa, respectively) (Darling et al. 2006). A similar relationship is seen for other elastic and viscoelastic properties as well. These variations are likely caused by the different strain levels that cells experience within the zones of cartilage. Surface zone chondrocytes secrete SZP (analogous to PRG4), and the cells in this layer are densely packed and oriented along the collagen fibers in a tangential direction (Stockwell 1971; Eggli et al. 1988). Tissue near the surface is compressed more than that in the bulk of the cartilage (Schinagl et al. 1997; Choi et al. 2007), and, hence, those cells might need to be stiffer to survive the higher strains.

Chondrocytes are known to lose their phenotypic markers *in vitro*, as evidenced by a temporal loss of morphologic characteristics and changes in metabolic activities of cells when cultured in monolayers (Siczkowski and Watt 1990; Darling and Athanasiou 2005). However, chondrocytes encapsulated in a three-dimensional gel, like agarose, retain their native morphological and proteoglycan synthesis characteristics (Aydelotte et al. 1988; Aydelotte and Kuettner 1988; Archer et al. 1990; Darling and Athanasiou 2005). This is likely due to the constrained three-dimensional environment, which forces a rounded morphology on the cells. Alternatively, chondrocytes cultured in monolayer flatten over the course of days and begin to proliferate, rapidly losing their characteristic expressions (Darling and Athanasiou 2005). Three-dimensional culture in a hydrogel or similarly constraining material is hypothesized to facilitate the synthesis of cartilage-specific molecules. Additionally, the application of mechanical stimuli such as stress, strain, and pressurization can affect their phenotypic expressions through a phenomenon termed mechanotransduction (Mow et al. 1994).

Immediately surrounding the chondrocyte is the pericellular matrix, which differs in composition from the bulk, extracellular matrix. Until recently, it was thought that the pericellular matrix isolated the chondrocytes and that they lacked cell-to-cell connections. However, the presence of gap junctions has been documented in articular cartilage (Mayan et al. 2015) (Figure 1.8). Within the pericellular matrix, higher levels of decorin and aggrecan and a network of type VI collagen are found (Johnston 1997). The chondrocytes are anchored to this extracellular matrix through the CD44 receptor to hyaluronan-proteoglycan aggregates and by integrins. Chondrocytes express many different α (1, 3, 5, 10, V) and β (1, 3, 5) subunits as integrin heterodimers ($\alpha_1\beta_1$, $\alpha_2\beta_1$, $\alpha_3\beta_1$, $\alpha_5\beta_1$, $\alpha_{10}\beta_1$, $\alpha_V\beta_3$, $\alpha_V\beta_5$). These integrins can serve as receptors for extracellular matrix proteins, such as collagens type II and IV ($\alpha_1\beta_1$, $\alpha_2\beta_1$, $\alpha_{10}\beta_1$),

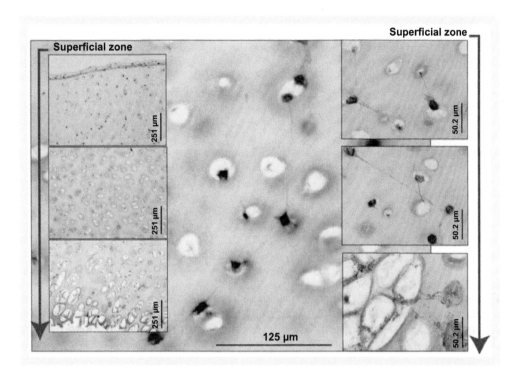

Figure 1.8 Histology of gap junctions present in human articular cartilage indicating cell-to-cell connections between chondrocytes. Junctions are present in all zones. (From Mayan, M. D. et al., *Ann Rheum Dis* 74(1): 275-284, 2015. With permission.)

laminin ($\alpha_6\beta_1$), fibronectin ($\alpha_5\beta_1$), and vitronectin ($\alpha_V\beta_5$), and likely play a role in mechanotransduction (Knudson and Loeser 2002). These molecules are described in more detail in Section 2.1.1.

1.2.2 Cytoskeletal Structure

In eukaryotic cells, the cytoskeleton is comprised of three different filament types that can polymerize from soluble protein monomers into a three-dimensional network that couples intracellular components to extracellular stimuli (Figure 1.9). These cytoskeletal protein monomers consist of the actin microfilaments, intermediate filaments, and tubulin microtubules. The cytoskeleton has been implicated in a variety of cell processes, such as mitosis, migration, cell shape, endocytosis, exocytosis, and mechanotransduction.

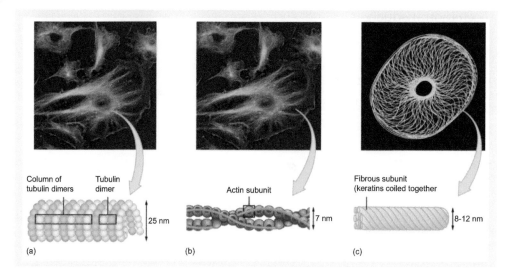

Figure 1.9 Cytoskeletal proteins and their structure. (a-c) Microtubules (green), actin (red), and intermediate filaments (yellow). (Image used with a Creative Commons Attribution License Unported 3.0. From http://cnx.org/contents/14fb4ad7-39a1 -4eee-ab6e-3ef2482e3e22@6.27.)

1.2.2.1 Microfilaments

Depending on cell type, actin can be the most abundant protein present in the cytoplasm of eukaryotic cells. Structurally, actin is the smallest of the cytoskeletal components at 6 nm in diameter (microfilaments). It exists as a 43 kDa globular monomer with ATPase activity (G-actin), which can assemble into a polarized filamentous form (F-actin). Assembly of this filament is coupled to hydrolysis of ATP; the ATP-bound G-actin polymerizes on the growing, barbed end, and the ADP-bound form is released from the pointed end. This filament assembly and disassembly result in a "treadmilling" action, which drives movement (Pollard and Borisy 2003). Actin, primarily responsible for cell migration as well as wound closure and tissue contraction in a tensile network, interacts with myosin to induce contraction. Actin has also been linked to the assembly of extracellular matrix components (Hayes et al. 1999). The actin cytoskeleton is linked to the extracellular matrix through integrins at sites of focal adhesions. These interactions are mediated by members of the Rho family of small GTPases (see Section 2.3.2). This interaction and regulatory pathway is crucial in mechanotransduction, from the extracellular matrix, through integrins, to the focal adhesions, resulting in Rho signaling events (Schwartz 2010).

Chondrocytes are unique compared with many other cells in that, with the exception of the uppermost superficial zone, they maintain a rounded cell shape with minimal actin cytoskeletal stress fibers. This rounded cell shape and actin cytoskeletal organization have been shown to be critical for maintaining the chondrocyte phenotype (Glowacki et al. 1983; Brown and Benya 1988; Daniels and Solursh 1991). With monolayer culture, chondrocytes flatten out and increase actin stress fiber formation (Vinall and Reddi 2001). This results in concomitant changes in Rho signaling (Woods et al. 2005) and decreased synthesis of cartilage-specific matrix components (Siczkowski and Watt 1990; Darling and Athanasiou 2005).

1.2.2.2 Intermediate Filaments

Structurally, intermediate filaments are 10 nm in diameter and "intermediate" in size, being smaller than microtubules but wider than actin microfilaments. Like actin, they play a similar role in resisting tensile forces and have also been indicated to play roles in cell-cell interactions, cell-matrix junctions, and mechanotransduction (Lazarides 1980; Wang et al. 1993). Unlike actin, the three-dimensional network of intermediate filaments helps to organize the internal arrangement of the organelles. Several different proteins make up the intermediate filaments based on cell type. In skin, the intermediate filament is keratin, whereas in neural cells it is lamin, although lamin is also a major component of the nuclear membrane in all cells. In contrast, in chondrocytes and most other cells, vimentin is the most common intermediate filament. The vimentin cytoskeleton has been implicated to play a role in chondrocyte homeostasis (Blain et al. 2006; Haudenschild et al. 2011).

1.2.2.3 Microtubules

Microtubules differ from actin and intermediate filaments in terms of both size and filament construction. Tubulin is a heterodimer composed of α/β monomers 55 kDa in size. It self-assembles into hollow 23 nm diameter "tubes" forming the microtubules, with an internal lumen diameter on the order of 15 nm. GTP binding is required for this assembly, and tubulin has GTPase activity, with GTP hydrolysis driving microtubule assembly. Microtubules also differ in their role in resisting force, acting to resist compression more than tension. The cilia and flagella (including the primary cilium) are composed of a microtubule arrangement described as 9 + 2, featuring an outer circle of nine microtubule doublets interconnected with dynein and with an inner arrangement of two microtubules. In addition to resisting compressive force, microtubules are also critically important in intracellular transport of organelles or vesicles through the actions of the dynein and kinesin motor proteins. The role of microtubules in intracellular transport is elegantly demonstrated in the assembly of the mitotic spindle, a structure that results in the intracellular movement and segregation of the replicated DNA into two daughter cells during mitosis.

1.2.3 Mechanotransduction and Homeostasis in Cartilage Tissue

Mechanotransduction is the process by which cells convert physical forces into biochemical signals. Classically, one of the earliest descriptions of mechanotransduction is the work of Julius Wolff during the nineteenth century, in which he proposed the eponymous law, which states that bone remodeling results from the physical forces applied to the bone. Specifically, sites of increased loading will have more bone deposited, while sites of disuse will resorb bone during remodeling. This would later be refined as the mechanostat by Frost in the 1960s, reviewed elsewhere (Frost 2000). Articular cartilage may also follow Wolff's law, with anatomical regions of increased loading exhibiting thicker cartilage (Shepherd and Seedhom 1999).

The ability of cartilage cells and tissues to respond to mechanical signals such as shear stress, compressive loading, tension, hydrostatic pressure, and fluid flow has functional implications during development and adult life (Figure 1.10). Since chondrocytes are the sole cell

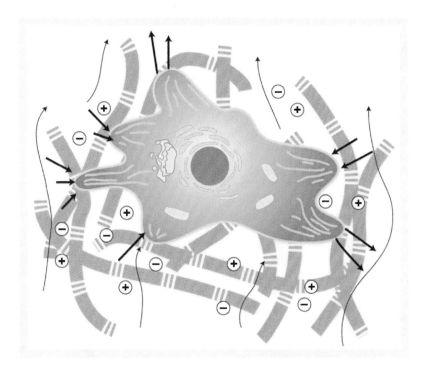

Figure 1.10 Mechanotransduction can occur via pulling, compressing, and shearing the cells (bold arrows). Other stimuli can include streaming potentials (fine arrows).

type within cartilage, and are mostly isolated individually, interactions with the environment are primarily limited to extracellular matrix-cell interactions. Mechanical signals are transduced in all organisms, from prokaryotes to man (Martinac 2004). Mechanisms of mechanotransduction have been investigated with special reference to musculoskeletal tissues, including articular cartilage.

Several groups of molecules have been identified as mechanosensitive, including cell adhesion receptors (such as integrins and cadherins), cytoskeletal components, ion channels, primary cilium, tyrosine kinase receptors, and growth factor receptors (Tschumperlin et al. 2004; Wang et al. 2009) (Figure 1.11). Mechanotransduction can induce changes in gene expression, extracellular matrix remodeling, and proliferation (Jaalouk and Lammerding 2009). Other than biochemical interactions with the extracellular matrix through integrin-mediated adhesions, these adhesions also allow cells to sense the structural environment

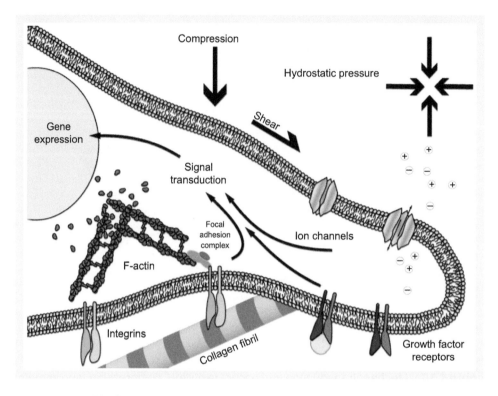

Figure 1.11 Mechanotransduction, such as compression, shear, or hydrostatic pressure, can alter the cell cytoskeleton and actin polymerization to induce gene expression. This can be initiated by activation or conformation change of multiple mediators, including ion channels, integrins, and growth factor receptors.

of the extracellular matrix, and generate and respond to forces produced internally and externally (Wang et al. 2009). Much of the focus of research into mechanosensing has been on focal adhesions, which bring together a large assortment of regulatory and enzymatic molecules into one complex. Arrangements and interactions of the components of focal adhesions are complex and can be regulated by signaling events, such as phosphorylation. The general paradigm of signal sensing in the integrin is one of recruitment of interacting molecules, which then recruit enzymes and substrates capable of transducing or inhibiting signals. Mechanical transduction through these adhesions has been demonstrated to initiate a variety of downstream molecules, including small GTPases and focal adhesion kinase (Katsumi et al. 2004). These adhesions also represent an interacting site with components of the cytoskeleton, such as actin-integrin β domains and numerous anchoring proteins. Other cell adhesion receptors, such as cadherins, may act as adaptors for force transmission, since cadherins are known to interact with integrins and tyrosine kinase receptors (Wang et al. 2009). However, this may not require a secondary signaling cascade, as the nucleus can act as a mechanosensing organelle in the cell. Mechanical pertubations of receptors at the cell membrane (e.g., integrins and cadherins) may propagate signals through the cytoskeletal components to the nucleocytoskeletal components and nuclear surface, directly affecting nuclear signaling or gene transcription (Dahl et al. 2008; Alam et al. 2014; Fedorchak et al. 2014; Driscoll et al. 2015). Ultimately, this cytoskeletal link can tie into the extracellular matrix through adhesion, allowing for forces generated internally to be translated into the external environment and vice versa.

Maintenance of articular cartilage is dependent on correct mechanical loading, and inappropriate loading can affect the matrix properties of articular cartilage (Buckwalter et al. 2006). Chondrocyte gene expression and translation can be altered by deformation of the pericellular matrix and surrounding extracellular matrix, changes in the volume of intracellular organelles, and osmotic pressure due to loading (Szafranski et al. 2004). Likely, this involves mechanosensing by matrix receptors such as CD44 and integrin-mediated adhesions to the extracellular matrix, which can activate stretch-activated ion channels (Knudson and Loeser 2002). See Figure 1.11.

Changes in membrane tension cause stretch-activated ion channels to undergo conformational changes. Interactions between integrins and stretch-activated ion channels can induce multiple intracellular responses either directly or indirectly by raising cytosolic levels of cations such as Ca^{2+}, Na^+, and K^+ within the cell (Martinac 2004).

Interestingly, hydrostatic pressure also induces stretch-activated ion channels in chondrocytes (Mizuno 2005), even though it does not apply a macroscopic strain to the cell (see Section 4.5). However, at the molecular level, void spaces exist in the molecular packing of amino acids in many proteins. As hydrostatic pressure increases, water can fill these spaces, changing the electrostatic interactions of the protein with the surrounding solution. This change in electrostatic conditions facilitates (1) conformational changes to a lower energy state of the protein or (2) changes in how substrates occupy the enzyme active site, altering protein function (Kornblatt and Kornblatt 2002) or, in the case of ion channels, allowing activation.

In chondrocytes, these ion channels can also be activated by shear and fluid flow and can lead to downstream signaling through Indian hedgehog (Ihh) and bone morphogenetic proteins (BMPs) (Wu et al. 2001). As first identified in bone, mechanosensing of fluid flow can be transduced through a rise in cytosolic Ca^{2+} levels through both the release of cytosolic stores and influxes triggered by the L-type voltage-sensitive calcium channel (VSCC) and the stretch-activated cation channel (SA-CAT) (Pavalko et al. 2003). This mediates multiple downstream signaling events, such as phosphorylation and activation of ERK1/2 (Jessop et al. 2002) and p130Cas, the upregulation of the c-fos transcription factor, and the release of prostaglandin E2 (PGE2) (Young et al. 2009).

Recently, primary cilium has come into focus as a mechanosensor of fluid flow. The primary cilium is a small membrane protrusion containing microtubules present on almost all vertebrate cells that can act as an "extracellular antenna" for detection of the external environment (Marshall and Nonaka 2006; Singla and Reiter 2006) (Figure 1.12). It also acts as a signaling center for sonic hedgehog (Shh), patched (PTC), and other molecules that can regulate cell survival, growth and differentiation, and tissue homeostasis (Christensen et al. 2008; Veland et al. 2009). For instance, in bone the primary cilium has been demonstrated to deflect under flow and to be independent of Ca^{2+} flux and stretch-activated ion channels in fluid flow-induced PGE2 release (Malone et al. 2007). Interestingly, in the endothelium of the kidney (Yoder 2007) or vascular system, the primary cilium appears to transduce fluid flow through an increase in intracellular

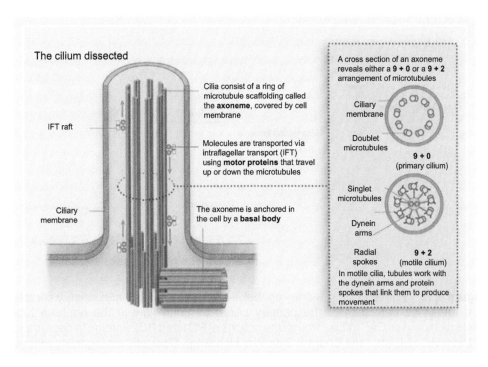

The cilium dissected

Cilia consist of a ring of microtubule scaffolding called the **axoneme**, covered by cell membrane

IFT raft

Molecules are transported via intraflagellar transport (IFT) using **motor proteins** that travel up or down the microtubules

Ciliary membrane

The axoneme is anchored in the cell by a **basal body**

A cross section of an axoneme reveals either a **9 + 0** or a **9 + 2** arrangement of microtubules

Ciliary membrane

Doublet microtubules

9 + 0
(primary cilium)

Singlet microtubules

Dynein arms

Radial spokes

9 + 2
(motile cilium)

In motile cilia, tubules work with the dynein arms and protein spokes that link them to produce movement

Figure 1.12 Schematic of the cilium indicating microtubule and dynein structure. (From Ainsworth, C., *Nature* 448(7154): 638-641, 2007. With permission.)

Ca^{2+} (Van der Heiden et al. 2006). In the kidney, this has been linked to interactions between the primary cilium and polycystins 1 and 2 to form a mechanosensitive ion channel (Forman et al. 2005) (Figure 1.13). In chondrocytes, the length of the primary cilium may be regulated by mechanical loading (McGlashan et al. 2010).

Growth factor receptors have also been implicated as mechanosensors. During tissue loading, the space surrounding the cells is reduced, resulting in a local relative increase in the concentration of growth (Tschumperlin et al. 2004). The rate of growth factor release into the extracellular space, independent of cellular production, may also be enhanced by mechanical loading.

Changes in matrix composition also produce changes in the biomechanical properties of the tissue, which may result in altered mechanical loading, and, therefore, signaling to chondrocytes. The signaling

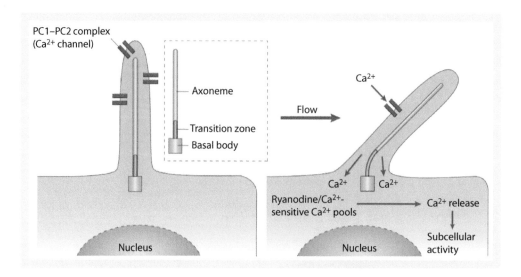

Figure 1.13 Primary cilia of kidney epithelial cells act as a mechanosensory complex that translates deflection of the primary cilium by urine flow in the nephron tube. Deflection causes Ca^{2+} influx through the actions of PC1 and PC2 leading to degradation of Dishevelled (Dsh) (see Chapter 2 on Wnt signaling). Downstream signaling induced by flow ultimately acts to regulate cell proliferation of the kidney epithelium. (From Fliegauf, M. et al., *Nat Rev Mol Cell Biol* 8(11): 880-893, 2007. With permission.)

pathways responsible for these responses are similar to those described above and likely involve interactions between multiple mechanosensory molecules and intracellular signaling pathways, including multiple mitogen-activated protein kinase (MAPK) pathways such as ERK1/2, JNK1, and P38 (Li et al. 2003; Papachristou et al. 2005; Fitzgerald et al. 2008; Ryan et al. 2009). Aggrecan (Fitzgerald et al. 2008), SZP/PRG4 (Grad et al. 2006a,b), cartilage oligomeric matrix protein (COMP) (Giannoni et al. 2003), and many other extracellular matrix components are upregulated by dynamic loading through either shear or compression and decreased by static compression. Mechanical loading alters articular cartilage metabolism, with static compression generally inhibiting protein and proteoglycan synthesis and dynamic compression increasing protein and proteoglycan synthesis. For aggrecan, the response to dynamic loading involves $\alpha_5\beta_1$ integrin and CD47 adaptor protein (Holledge et al. 2008; Orazizadeh et al. 2008), the K^+ stretch-activated ion channels, signaling through the actin cytoskeleton, Fak phosphorylation, and autocrine/paracrine interleukin 4 (IL-4) signaling (Figure 1.11)

24

(Millward-Sadler et al. 2000). Autocrine-paracrine induction of transforming growth factor β (TGF-β) has also been observed in fluid shear-induced proliferation of chondrocytes in monolayer (Malaviya and Nerem 2002). For SZP, shear loading of articular cartilage has demonstrated an increase in SZP protein production mediated through the type I TGF-β receptor (Neu et al. 2007).

1.2.4 Pericellular Matrix Structure

In addition to the zonal organization associated with cartilage extracellular matrix, the tissue also has a microscale structure oriented with respect to distance from the chondrocyte cell membrane. As noted previously, the region immediately surrounding a chondrocyte is termed the pericellular matrix and is characterized by having fine collagen fibers (10-15 nm in diameter); high concentrations of proteoglycans and hyaluronan (Mason 1981); and the presence of fibronectin (Glant et al. 1985), type VI and IX collagen, link protein, biglycan, decorin, and laminin (Hunziker et al. 1983; Poole et al. 1988a; Durr et al. 1996). However, the components that assemble into the aggrecan macromolecule (see Section 1.3.4) remain separate, suggesting that the pericellular matrix may play a role in the assembly of the macromolecule. Type IX collagen regulates type II fiber diameter (Wotton et al. 1988) and likely enables the formation of the fine collagen fibers found in the pericellular matrix. Type VI collagen, a key component of the pericellular matrix, has high pericellular concentrations compared with the bulk extracellular matrix and directly interacts with the chondrocyte. The exact function of the pericellular matrix is not fully understood, although strong evidence indicates that it helps to protect the physical integrity of articular chondrocytes during compressive loading (Poole et al. 1987) and provides a confined location for the assembly of matrix components. The combination of the chondrocyte and this pericellular matrix has been termed the *chondron* and represents a specific, separable, metabolic, and anatomical unit of articular cartilage (Poole et al. 1988b) with morphological differences that vary by zonal collagen architecture (Youn et al. 2006).

25

The pericellular matrix is in turn surrounded by the territorial and inter-territorial matrices (Figure 1.14). These outer regions are also termed, more generally, the extracellular matrix. The region immediately surrounding the pericellular matrix (the territorial matrix) is composed of similar molecular constituents as the surrounding extracellular matrix, namely, type II collagen and higher concentrations of chondroitin sulfate-rich proteoglycans.

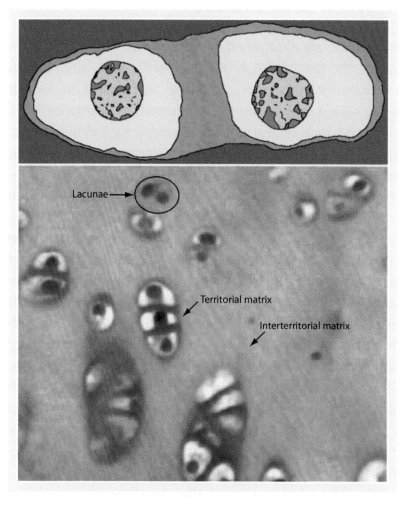

Figure 1.14 Top image: Chondrocytes (light gray) reside in a chondron (medium gray), surrounded by territorial matrix (dark gray). Beyond the territorial matrix are the interterritorial regions that make up the rest of the cartilage (Poole et al. 1987). Collectively, the territorial and interterritorial regions are termed extracellular matrix. Bottom image: Histological image of extracellular matrix.

In normal cartilage, type VI collagen has also been shown to be localized to this region (Youn et al. 2006). The territorial matrix exhibits a higher concentration of proteoglycans than the surrounding extracellular matrix, as well as having a finer collagen structure (Hunziker et al. 1997).

The interterritorial matrix comprises the bulk of articular cartilage, providing the tissue with its biomechanical properties. The interterritorial matrix contains higher concentrations of keratan sulfate-rich proteoglycans and collagen fibrils of larger diameter (50 nm or greater) (Poole et al. 1982). Loading of articular cartilage involves force transmission through the interterritorial, territorial, and pericellular matrices before reaching the chondrocytes. These regions likely assist in modulating strains seen at the cellular level (Choi et al. 2007). The interterritorial regions are representative of bulk extracellular matrix tissue and contain varying concentrations of type II collagen fibers and proteoglycans, dependent on depth from the surface.

1.3 CARTILAGE MATRIX CHARACTERISTICS AND ORGANIZATION

Though articular cartilage is a metabolically active tissue that maintains its extracellular matrix in a state of constant turnover (Guilak et al. 2000), not all molecular components are reconstituted at the same rate, and variations exist based on the spatial location within the tissue. Maintenance of the surrounding matrix requires synthesis of proteoglycans and collagens, as well as other small molecules. Disease and injury can alter cartilage physiology, as well as tissue turnover, which can progressively accelerate tissue breakdown (discussed in more detail in Chapter 3). Compounding the problem is the sparse cell population's inability to repair the cartilage to any extent (Poole et al. 1993). Degradation and synthesis are concentrated in the regions immediately surrounding chondrocytes rather than in the territorial and interterritorial regions of the tissue (Wu et al. 2002). This is likely due to the sparse nature of chondrocytes within the tissue and the need for diffusion-based mechanisms originating from the chondrocytes to spread newly synthesized matrix or matrix remodeling enzymes. The turnover of collagen is estimated to be very slow (>100 years), whereas aggrecan turnover is more rapid, with a half-life of 8-300 days in rabbits (Mankin and Lippiello 1969; Maroudas 1975). Misregulation of this aggrecan turnover can, therefore, lead to the initiation of reduced biomechanical properties of the tissue and eventual failure. The biochemical structure of the matrix, both the fluid and solid fractions, is intimately linked to the mechanical function of cartilage.

1.3.1 Fluid Components

Water is the main liquid component in articular cartilage, as well as in the synovial fluid present in the joint capsule. Synovial fluid is a viscous liquid within the joint possessing non-Newtonian properties. Synovial fluid, which as we discussed earlier is derived from interstitial fluid as a blood ultrafiltrate, provides nourishment and waste product removal, and has a critical function in lubrication. Synovial fluid contains large amounts of hyaluronic acid (~3 mg/ml) (Decker et al. 1959) and other lubricating molecules (such as SZP/lubricin/PRG4) secreted by specialized tissues lining the joint. Synovial fluid also functions to provide a smooth layer to the articular cartilage by filling in valleys between asperities on the cartilage surface. This layer is replenished not only from the reserve fluid in the joint space but also from fluid exuded from the cartilage matrix. These actions maintain a layer of fluid at the articulating surface, enabling "weeping lubrication" to produce the low-friction surface necessary for cartilage function. The non-Newtonian properties of synovial fluid (provided mostly by the viscosity enhancement of hyaluronic acid) allow for absorption of shock as the fluid viscosity increases at the moment shear is applied. However, synovial fluid then immediately decreases in viscosity and thins with prolonged stress.

Inorganic salts such as sodium, potassium, calcium, and chloride are also present in synovial fluid in appreciable amounts. Most of the water in articular cartilage is contained in the molecular pore space of the extracellular matrix, but it also permeates throughout the entire tissue.

Since articular cartilage has no vascularity, the chondrocytes obtain nutrients through diffusion from the joint space. As the primary carrier, interstitial fluid plays an important role in transporting both nutrient and waste within the tissue (Linn and Sokoloff 1965; O'Hara et al. 1990).

Fluid permeating the cartilage matrix also plays an important mechanical role. Compressive loading is a constant stressor of articular cartilage; without a high water fraction, the tissue would break down much more quickly under constant use. Compressive loads can force the fluid from the tissue and, over the course of a day, effectively decrease the total water fraction. However, for short periods of loading, and unloading on the order of 100 seconds, the frictional resistance between the water and solid matrix requires high pressures to cause interstitial fluid flow (Ateshian et al. 1994; Soltz and Ateshian 1998). Functionally, mechanical compression of cartilage causes rapid pressurization of the fluid in the tissue, which, in turn, supports the load (Figure 1.15). This load redistribution as a factor of time is dependent on the permeability of the cartilage and is primarily mediated by pore size of the material and the presence of the large charge density of the aggrecan macromolecular

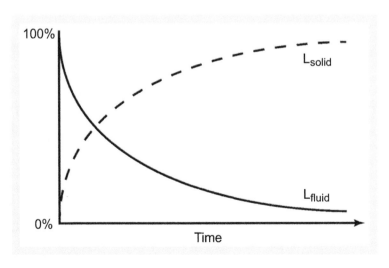

Figure 1.15 Initially, load applied onto cartilage is borne almost exclusively by the fluid phase (L_{fluid}). As the fluid exudes from cartilage, the solid matrix begins to bear more of the load (represented by L_{solid}). As time goes on, load borne by the fluid phase approaches zero.

aggregates. This mechanism allows for the longevity of cartilage under repeated compression since loading is borne by fluid instead of a solid-solid interaction (Mow et al. 1989; Ateshian et al. 1994), resulting in cyclic hydrostatic pressures within the cartilage.

1.3.2 Zonal Variation within Cartilage

The zones of articular cartilage, from the articulating surface down to the subchondral bone, are depicted in Figure 1.16. Zonal variations exist in cell morphology, collagen fiber orientation, and biochemical composition. The zones (superficial/tangential, middle/transitional, deep/radial, calcified) can be identified by extracellular matrix structure and composition, as well as cell shape and arrangement within the tissue. This characteristic zonal architecture is intimately linked to biological and mechanical function; in turn, the changing composition results in the zone-specific biomechanical properties of articular cartilage. Differences in the types and patterns of compression, shear, and hydrostatic pressure result in changes in the distribution, organization, synthesis, and turnover rates of various matrix components. These forces and the biomechanics of articular cartilage are discussed in Section 1.4.

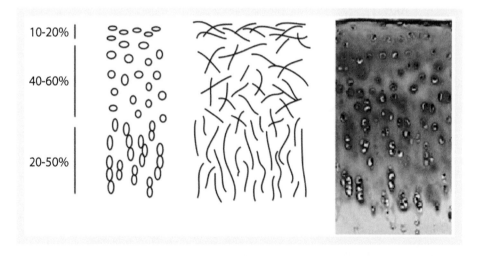

Figure 1.16 Both cells (left) and collagen fibers (middle) are organized within cartilage (right) into superficial, middle, and deep zones, consisting of 10-20%, 40-60%, and 20-50% of the overall tissue depth, respectively.

The composition of articular cartilage changes as the tissue develops. However, mature articular cartilage is composed primarily of water, approximately 70-80% by weight. The solid fraction of the tissue is primarily collagens (50-75%) and proteoglycans (15-30%) (Figure 1.16), with the remaining balance including minor protein molecules and chondrocytes (Guilak et al. 2000; Darling and Athanasiou 2003). This mix of collagens and proteoglycans forms an integrated network that provides the basis for the biomechanical properties observed in articular cartilage.

1.3.2.1 Articulating Surface

The surface of articular cartilage is covered by a very thin, proteinaceous layer termed the lamina splendens (Mac 1951) (Figure 1.17). This acellular, primarily nonfibrous region has a thickness ranging from hundreds of nanometers to a few microns. Several studies using different techniques (confocal microscopy, with scanning electron microscopy [SEM], and atomic force microscopy [AFM]) have confirmed the existence of the lamina splendens (Kumar et al. 2001; Teeple et al. 2007; Wu et al. 2008), and researchers are now trying to understand how it forms and what its function might be. Hypotheses include: (1) the layer exists to facilitate low friction and to protect wear of the cartilage surface, or

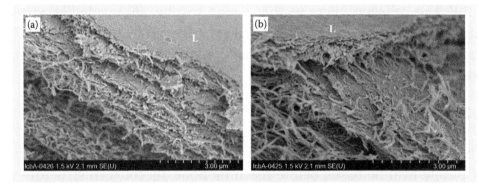

Figure 1.17 SEM of fixed and fractured mouse articular cartilage superficial zone (a and b), including lamina splendens (L) and underlying collagen fibril network. (Modified from Hughes, L. C. et al., *Eur Cell Mater* 9: 68-84, 2005. With permission.)

(2) it forms due to gradual accumulation of proteins and molecules from the synovial fluid.

1.3.2.2 Superficial/Tangential Zone

The superficial, or tangential, zone of articular cartilage comprises the upper 10-20% of the tissue. It is characterized by having small-diameter, densely packed collagen fibers that are oriented parallel to the cartilage surface (Meachim and Sheffield 1969). The matrix has a relatively low proteoglycan content, as well as low permeability (Muir et al. 1970; Maroudas 1979), allowing compressive forces to redistribute radially across the cartilage (Little et al. 1958; Stockwell 1990). This zone of articular cartilage is responsible for appositional growth and appears to contain progenitor cells (Dowthwaite et al. 2004). Superficial zone cells secrete specialized proteins (such as SZP) that are hypothesized to improve the wear and frictional properties of the tissue (Flannery et al. 1999). Fluid exudation and compressive strains align with shear, and this directly relates to the distribution of collagen fibrils within the zone.

1.3.2.3 Middle/Transitional Zone

The middle, or transitional, zone occupies approximately 40-60% of the total tissue thickness. The middle zone consists of randomly arranged spherical cells and is characterized by type II collagen, aggrecan, and CILP. The collagen fibers in this region exhibit an arcade-like structure interspersed with randomly oriented fibers (Hunziker et al. 1997). Proteoglycan content reaches its maximum in the middle zone (Venn and Maroudas 1977) (Figure 1.18).

1.3.2.4 Deep/Radial Zone

The deep zone, comprising 20-50% of total thickness, is the last region of purely hyaline tissue before reaching bone. Its collagen structure is characterized by large fibers that form bundles oriented perpendicular to the articular surface and are anchored in the underlying subchondral bone (Muir et al. 1970). Although fluid flow within this zone is relatively

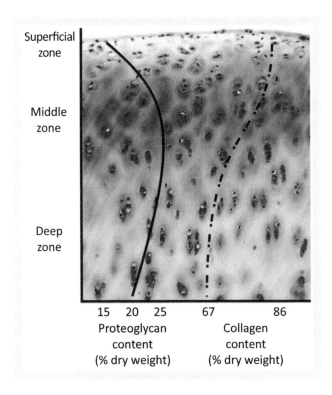

Superficial zone

Middle zone

Deep zone

15 20 25 67 86
Proteoglycan content (% dry weight) Collagen content (% dry weight)

Figure 1.18 Proteoglycan and collagen contents vary throughout the zones of articular cartilage.

low, significant shear forces are experienced between the adjacent tissue types during joint articulation as the cartilage is unable to expand against the bony tissue. Proteoglycan content is much lower than in the middle zone (Venn and Maroudas 1977), and the cell density is also the lowest of the three cartilaginous zones (Stockwell 1971). Cells in the deep zone often group together in a columnar organization. They are slightly elongated and oriented in the direction of collagen fibers, perpendicular to the articular surface (Eggli et al. 1988).

1.3.2.5 Tidemark and Calcified Zone

A thin line termed the *tidemark* is present between the deep zone and calcified zone of articular cartilage (Redler et al. 1975). The calcified zone is a region of the tissue that transitions into the subchondral bone, minimizing the stiffness gradient between the rigid bone and more pliable cartilage (Radin and Rose 1986). Underlying this region of the cartilage is the subchondral bone, which is the ultimate anchorage point for cartilage as a whole.

1.3.3 Collagens in Cartilage

Collagens represent the most abundant proteins of the body by weight. More than 28 types of collagen have been identified in mammals, many with tissue-specific localizations. Generally, collagens serve a primary role in the structure of connective tissues throughout the body as both fibril and nonfibril/globular types.

Fibril collagens represent the most prevalent types of collagen with types I, II, and XI being the predominant members. Fibril collagens have unique nonhelical N- and C-terminal domains per type, but share a characteristic central core of approximately 300 nm in length, comprised of a repeating amino acid sequence G-X-Y, with glycine, proline, and hydroxyproline being the most common constituents (van der Rest and Garrone 1991). This amino acid sequence helps the procollagen monomer exhibit a characteristic left-handed helix structure that can then assemble into a right-handed triple helix in the final trimer. Trimer assembly occurs in the lumen of the endoplasmic reticulum and is mediated by molecular chaperones and the C-propeptides. Hydroxylation of the proline in the Y position is required for the necessary folding and stabilization of the helix through a stereoelectronic effect (Kotch et al. 2008) and is dependent on the presence of ascorbic acid as a cofactor for prolyl-4-hydroxylase to convert proline to hydroxyproline. As primates (and guinea pigs) lack the ability to synthesize ascorbic acid, the lack of dietary ascorbic acid results in the disease state of scurvy. Without ascorbic acid, the hydroxyproline cannot be formed, resulting in procollagen being unable to exit the endoplasmic reticulum, and, thus, the lack of new collagen fibrils being synthesized.

Collagens are initially synthesized by the cells as soluble procollagen trimers and secreted into the surrounding matrix (Table 1.1). These

Table 1.1 Types of collagen found in articular cartilage

Collagen	Genes	Structure	Localization
Collagen I	COL1A1, COL1A2	Fiber forming	Superficial zone, fibrocartilages
Collagen II	COL2A1	Fiber forming	Hyaline cartilage matrix
Collagen VI	COL6A1, COL6A2, COL6A3	Fiber associated	Pericellular matrix
Collagen IX	COL9A1, COL9A2, COL9A3	Fiber associated	Associated with type II, provides cross-linking to type II, regulates type II fiber diameter
Collagen X	COL10A1	Nonfibrillar	Tidemark, calcified cartilage
Collagen XI	COL11A1, COL11A2	Fiber associated	Associated with type II, cross-links other XI molecules, acts as a template for fibrillogenesis

procollagens lack the ability to efficiently self-aggregate into fibrils and require processing by extracellular enzymes (N- and C-procollagen proteinases, members of the metalloproteinases), which cleave the globular N- and C-terminal propeptides, allowing for fibril formation (Leung et al. 1979) (Figure 1.19). It is especially the removal of the C-propeptide that reduces the critical concentration needed for assembly. These fibrils then assemble into much larger fibers in a hierarchical organization, increasing both the fiber diameter and length by both end-to-end fusion and lateral bundling (Graham et al. 2000; Hulmes 2002). By electron microscopy, this macromolecular fiber assembly takes on a characteristic 67 nm repeat banding due to staggering of the collagen fibers (Hulmes and Miller 1979) (Figures 1.20 and 1.21). The assembly of the larger macromolecule collagen fibrils is regulated by multiple collagens, small leucine-rich repeat proteoglycans (SLRPs), collagenases, and other molecules.

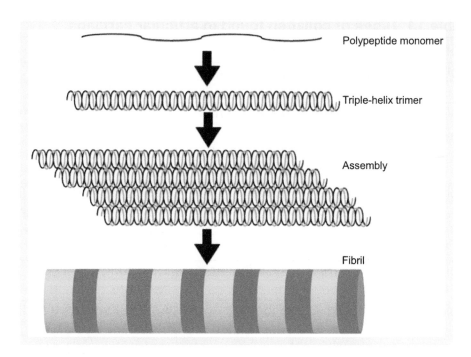

Figure 1.19 Hierarchical organization of collagen fibril assembly from polypeptide monomer to triple-helix trimer, to fiber, and finally to fibril assembly.

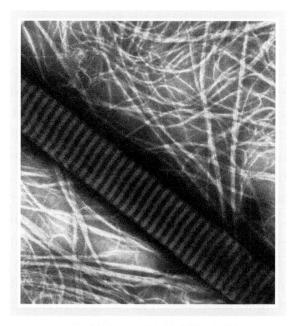

Figure 1.20 Transmission electron micrograph of D-banding of type II collagen fibril. (Image by Rob Young, Wellcome Images. Used under CC BY 4.0.)

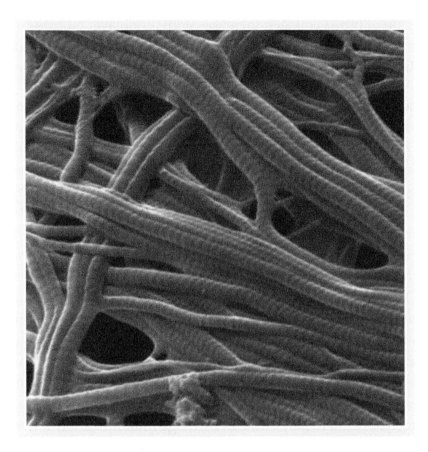

Figure 1.21 Helium ion scanning electron micrograph of collagen from mouse knee articular cartilage. (From Dr. Claus Burkhardt, Natural and Medical Sciences Institute, Reutlingen, Germany. With permission.)

Type II collagen is the predominant collagen type (~90%) in articular cartilage, comprising more than half the dry weight of the tissue (Deshmukh and Nimni 1973) and complexes with type IX and XI collagens. Type II collagen forms an extracellular framework to resist both imparted tensile forces from articulation and the swelling pressures due to proteoglycans. This collagen serves as a marker for articular cartilage differentiation because it is only localized to the hyaline and fibrous cartilages and the vitreous humor of the eye. The presence of type I collagen with type II helps to distinguish between hyaline and fibrocartilages. Except for small amounts of collagen type I in its superficial zone, collagen type I is not found in hyaline articular cartilage. Since the expression of type I collagen increases with monolayer culture-induced dedifferentiation of chondrocytes, the ratio of type I to type II cartilage is further used to track chondrocyte differentiation.

Hyaline cartilage also contains other fibrillar and globular collagen types, such as types VI, IX, X, and XI (Eyre and Wu 1995). While the definitive roles of these other collagen types are not fully known, they are believed to play a role in intermolecular interactions, as well as modulating the structure of type II collagen (Guilak et al. 2000). Nonfibril collagens have secondary structural functions and can be further divided into fibril associated, network forming, and short and long chain. Common fibril-associated collagens, such as type IX, serve to covalently link other collagen fibers, increasing mechanical strength. For example, type VI collagen is found primarily in the pericellular matrix and may contribute to the mechanical function of the chondron (the combined cell-pericellular matrix structure) or regulate interactions between the chondrocyte and extracellular matrix as it directly interacts with chondrocyte receptors (McDevitt et al. 1991; Choi et al. 2007). Collagen X is localized to the tidemark mostly in the calcified cartilage region. Type X collagen appears to play a role in cartilage mineralization at the interface between cartilage and the underlying bone (Aigner et al. 1993).

1.3.3.1 Tissue-Level Organization

On a microscopic scale, the water and collagen contents in the tissue decrease with depth from the articulating surface, while the collagen fibril size increases. Collagen fibrils in the superficial region are oriented tangential to the surface to resist shear and tension, while the organization of collagen fibrils in the middle of the tissue is more random. Fibrils near the tidemark are arranged perpendicular to the surface and penetrate into the underlying bone to resist shear.

Benninghoff in 1925 first described the orientation of collagen with articular cartilage by proposing the "arcades" model (Figure 1.22). In the Benninghoff model, collagen fibrils project perpendicularly from

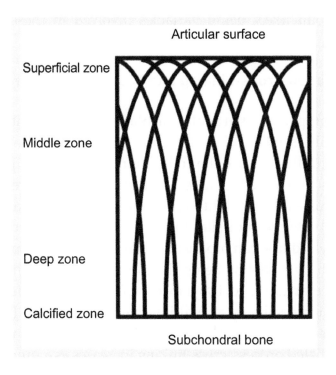

Figure 1.22 Benninghoff arcades model of collagen fibril organization in articular cartilage.

the tidemark up through the tissue to arc over and interweave with each other in the middle and adjacent superficial zones. This model agrees with SEM observations of cartilage ultrastructure wherein zonal collagen fiber orientation varies through the depth of articular cartilage, with the superficial zone containing tangentially arranged fibrils, the deep zone containing radially oriented fibers, and the middle zone having both an arcade-like structure and randomly oriented fibers for the transition between the other zones (Clark 1990). This orientation of fibrils underlies the collagen structure-function relationship, in which different forces are experienced at different depths of the tissue, resulting in an isotropic organization of collagen fibrils to resist these forces. However, although the Benninghoff model describes the majority of findings of collagen ultrastructure, multiple variations in zonal collagen orientation have been described, with age, joint type, and location within the joint likely being variables involved in these differences (Rieppo et al. 2009).

1.3.3.2 Collagen Cross-Linking and Biomechanical Properties

The tensile properties of articular cartilage are dependent on collagen amount, fibril assembly, orientation, and cross-linking. Covalent cross-links dramatically improve the collagen-imparted tensile properties of the tissue, as well as reduce access to proteases and decrease collagen solubility. Cross-links form through hydroxylysyl pyridinoline residues at the N- and C-telopeptide sites through the action of the enzyme lysyl oxidase. Lysyl oxidase can produce several sites available for cross-links to form, with pyridinoline being the more prevalent form over ketoimine in articular cartilage. Lysyl oxidase functions by oxidizing lysine residues, which results in several intermediate products (Figure 1.23). However, the formation of the pyridinoline cross-link is not a directly enzyme-mediated process; cross-linking increases as a function of time, with adult cartilage having more cross-links than juvenile. This increase in cross-linking, along with increasing collagen content with maturation, directly correlates with increased tensile properties (Williamson et al. 2003a,b), while pharmacological inhibition of lysyl oxidase by β-aminopropionitrile results in decreased tissue tensile properties (Fry et al. 1962; Asanbaeva et al. 2008). As the tensile properties of articular cartilage are necessary for its function, formation of cross-links remains a major goal in tissue engineering of cartilage replacements (Makris et al. 2014).

Other types of cross-links also form due to the actions of sugars on collagen amines to produce advanced glycation endproducts (AGEs). These also increase as a function of time and have the unusual characteristic of imparting a slight yellowish hue to the hyaline cartilage. However, increased AGE formation results in articular cartilage that is not only stiffer but also more brittle; in turn, this may lead to degeneration and osteoarthritis (Chen et al. 2002). This is of special importance for patients suffering from diabetes.

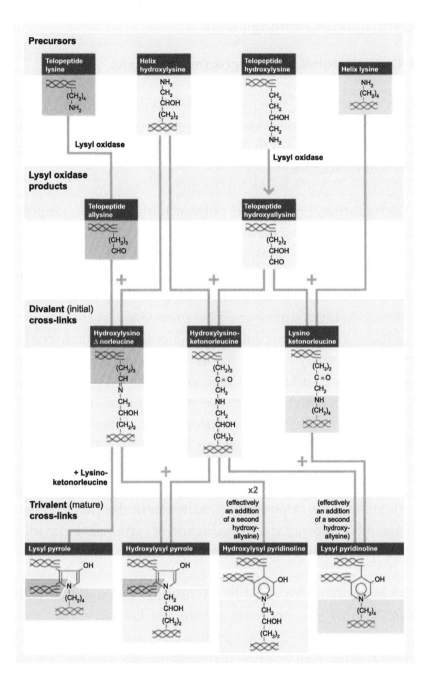

Figure 1.23 Schematic of formation of collagen cross-links in musculoskeletal tissue. This process follows a pathway of chemical changes to various precursor molecules that results in divalent and eventually trivalent cross-links between collagen molecules. Of these cross-links, articular cartilage only contains pyridinolines, while bone contains both pyridinolines and pyrroles. (From Eyre, D. R. et al., *Methods* 45(1): 65-74, 2008. With permission.)

41

1.3.4 Cartilaginous Proteoglycans

1.3.4.1 Core Proteins and Glycosaminoglycans

Proteoglycans are large macromolecules comprised of a protein core with many attached GAGs. Proteoglycan networks in articular cartilage can be thought of as a mesh that is interlaced throughout the more organized collagen structure.

GAGs are repeating, unbranched polysaccharide chains composed of a repeating unit made of six-carbon sugars (hexose or as a hexuronic acid) linked to a nitrogen containing a six-carbon sugar (hexosamine). The common GAGs present in articular cartilage are chondroitin sulfate, keratan sulfate, dermatan sulfate, and hyaluronan. Of these GAGs, chondroitin sulfate and keratan sulfate are most prevalent and are usually found bound to the aggrecan core protein. The chondroitin sulfate chains exist in several differentially sulfated forms and are predominantly sulfated at the 4-O-hydroxyl in fetal cartilage and at the 6-O-hydroxyl in adult cartilage, although both types are present at all times (Plaas et al. 1997). Hyaluronan, also referred to as hyaluronic acid, differs from these other GAGs as it is not sulfated and contains alternating β-1,4 and β-1,3 glycosidic bonds of D-glucuronic acid and D-*N*-acetylglucosamine; also, it is formed by the actions of three separate hyaluronic acid synthases at the plasma membrane, as opposed to production in the Golgi. This unique form of assembly allows for the production of extremely large molecular chains with molecular weights exceeding 1 MDa.

Aggrecan exists as a large, highly glycosylated proteoglycan with long, linear GAG chains of chondroitin sulfate and keratan sulfate molecules radiating from a central ~230 kDa protein core, resulting in a bottle brush structure (Table 1.2). Aggrecan is posttranslationally modified by glycosylation in the late endoplasmic reticulum (specifically an initial xylosylation); the molecular mass of a single proteoglycan can reach more than 2 MDa (Watanabe et al. 1998). The protein core contains several distinct globular domains (G1, G2, and G3), an interglobular domain, and two extended

Table 1.2 Disaccharide units of common GAGs present in articular cartilage

Structure	Name	Sugar composition
	Dermatan sulfate	Commonly sulfated L-iduronate + GalNAc-4 α-1,3 glycosidic bond
	Chondroitin sulfate	D-Glucuronate and GalNAc-4- or 6-sulfate β-1,3 glycosidic bond
	Keratan sulfate	Galactose + GlcNAc-6-sulfate β-1,4 glycosidic bond
	Hyaluronan Widely distributed in the body	D-Glucuronate + GlcNAc Nonsulfated β-1,3 glycosidic bond

domains where GAGs attach, the keratan sulfate (KS) and chondroitin sulfate (CS) domains (Figure 1.24). The globular domains are involved in aggregate formation, while the interglobular domain contains sites available for proteolytic cleavage and is likely involved in the turnover of aggrecan. The KS domain is absent in rodents (Kiani et al. 2002). The CS domain represents the largest domain in aggrecan and is encoded by a single exon

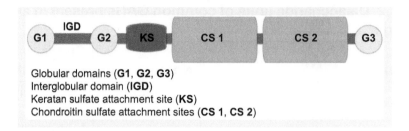

Globular domains (**G1, G2, G3**)
Interglobular domain (**IGD**)
Keratan sulfate attachment site (**KS**)
Chondroitin sulfate attachment sites (**CS 1, CS 2**)

Figure 1.24   The molecular domains of aggrecan proteoglycan in articular cartilage consist of three globular domains (G1, G2, G3), an interglobular domain, a keratan attachment site (KS), and two chondroitin sulfate attachment sites (CS 1, CS 2).

(exon 12) representing a 120-repeat serine-glycine sequence. The carboxyl (COO^-) and sulfate $\left(SO_3^-\right)$ groups present on these attached GAGs produce a strong negative charge that in turn gives cartilage extracellular matrix a net negative charge known as a "fixed charge density," with a charge spacing of 1-2 nm per GAG (Maroudas et al. 1969).

Aggrecan molecules are noncovalently linked to a single long chain of hyaluronan to form large proteoglycan aggregates, which result in an overall molecular weight of 50-100 MDa (Roughley and Lee 1994; Watanabe et al. 1998). Link protein is a small glycoprotein that serves to stabilize noncovalent association of the proteoglycan subunits with hyaluronic acid in aggregates, allowing for aggrecan to self-assemble into a macromolecular structure bound to a hyaluronic acid backbone. Link protein, which is homologous to the G1 globular region of the aggrecan protein core, binds noncovalently to both hyaluronan and the aggrecan core protein (Hardingham et al. 1994), producing a nonsoluble complex fixed within the matrix.

The aggregation of many proteoglycans (Figure 1.25) into large macromolecules is critical for proper functionality of cartilage tissue (Figure 1.26). The large size of this polymer mesh acts to immobilize and restrain it within the collagen network. Because of the strong negative charge, the matrix imbibes fluid, swelling the tissue to maintain equilibrium, also known as the Donnan effect. The swelling is balanced against the mechanical restraint of the collagen network (Maroudas

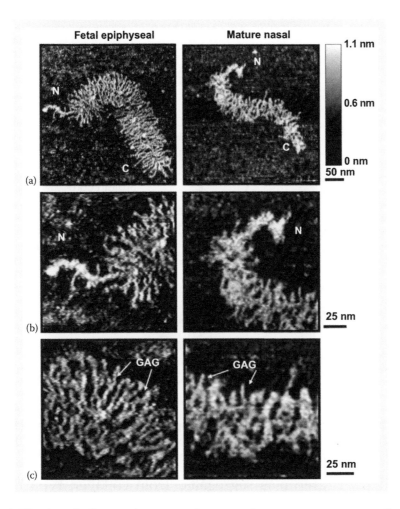

Figure 1.25 Atomic force microscopy images of aggrecan monomers from both (a) fetal epiphysis (left) and mature nasal cartilage (right). (b) Core protein (N) and (c) chondroitin sulfate chains (GAG). (From Ng, L. et al., *J Struct Biol* 143(3): 242-257, 2003. With permission.)

1976). While aggrecan is also located in other tissues, such as heart, brain, tendon, and intervertebral disc, production of aggrecan in the matrix is considered an important marker of chondrogenesis and is directly regulated by Sox9 (Sekiya et al. 2000). Autosomal recessive diseases of aggrecan, including spondyloepimetaphyseal dysplasia in humans (Tompson et al. 2009), nanomelia in chickens, and cartilage matrix deficiency in mice, result in chondrodysplasias.

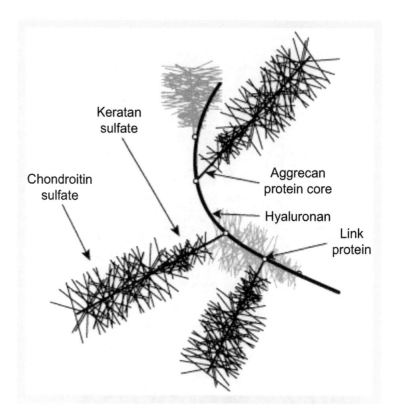

Keratan
sulfate

Chondroitin
sulfate

Aggrecan
protein core

Hyaluronan

Link
protein

Figure 1.26 Aggrecan macromolecule complex. The negatively charged keratan and chondroitin sulfate on the aggrecan protein core repel each other and flare like tube brushes. The overall size of this structure is on the order of microns.

Interestingly, aggrecan is segregated from collagen type II in the endoplasmic reticulum (Vertel et al. 1989), possibly to prevent unwanted interactions between both proteins. However, unlike the century-long half-life of collagen, aggrecan has a much quicker turnover (weeks to months). This indicates that chondrocyte synthesis of aggrecan and its regulation are fundamentally important for continued functionality of the cartilage. Increased aggrecan degradation may play a role in osteoarthritis. Loss of hydration due to loss of aggrecan complexes marks an early and detrimental change in disease progression.

As mentioned in Section 1.3.1, the functional properties of cartilage under compression are highly dependent on fluid pressurization within the tissue. Since the presence of proteoglycans assists in the imbibition of water, it is apparent that a loss of proteoglycans can result in a lack of fluid pressurization, and, therefore, improper mechanical function. This breakdown in functionality is seen in advanced stages of diseases like osteoarthritis.

1.3.4.2 Aggrecan's Role in Articular Cartilage Compressive Properties

Compressive loading is one of the main forces encountered by articular cartilage (see Section 1.4). The movement of the interstitial fluid trapped by the aggrecan network through the matrix dissipates the compressive load due to frictional drag, which is dependent on the hydraulic permeability of the tissue. As the permeability of healthy cartilage is low, this results in high interstitial fluid pressures during load. Over time, the interstitial fluid pressure decreases as a function of the permeability, resulting in the load being transferred to the solid portion of the extracellular matrix, demonstrating the viscoelastic nature of cartilage. As this fluid is exuded from the joint during loading, it also serves as a hydrodynamic lubricant to reduce friction (Ateshian 2009). Both the crucial role of regulation of proteoglycan expression within the tissue and a need for a nonsoluble aggregate relate to the need to maintain this low fluid permeability.

1.3.4.3 Minor Proteoglycans

Other proteoglycans expressed in cartilage or during chondrogenesis include syndecan, glypican (cell surface localized and indicated in signal transduction through binding growth factors and extracellular matrix), and perlecan (localized in the pericellular matrix). As with the minor collagen types present in cartilage, the precise roles of these proteoglycans are not fully known. However, it is likely they assist in matrix assembly by associating with the collagen structure during development and repair. Smaller proteoglycans (i.e., biglycan, fibromodulin, and decorin) occur in lower concentrations and contribute to the organization of the matrix and ligand sequestration (Hildebrand et al. 1994; Iozzo 1999).

These smaller proteoglycans in articular cartilage include the SLRPs, which also are comprised of core proteins with various GAG species attached as side chains (Roughley and Lee 1994). However, one atypical family member that lacks the attached GAG chains also exists in cartilage; proline-arginine-rich end leucine-rich repeat protein (PRELP). The proline-arginine-rich amino terminal end allows for interaction with heparin sulfate and perlecan, functionally forming a link between perlecan and collagen bundles. Meanwhile, the typical type SLRPs can be divided into three classes, two of which are found in articular cartilage.

Decorin and biglycan belong to the Class I SLRPs. Decorin, the most abundant SLRP in cartilage, is localized to the interterritorial matrix, with concentrations of decorin increasing with age (Roughley et al. 1994). The structure of decorin is semicircular with one dermatan or chondroitin sulfate attached. This concave structure supports its proposed function in associating with the collagen triple helix during fibril formation and regulating fibril spacing, as decorin has been observed "decorating" type II collagen fibrils. Interestingly, although decorin knockout mice have reduced tendon and skin tensile properties, resulting in skin fragility, the articular cartilage in adult mice appears normal (Reed and Iozzo 2002). Biglycan is localized to the pericellular matrix, with two dermatan or chondroitin sulfates attached. It is a regulator of bone formation, as biglycan knockout mice experience retarded skeletal growth (Young et al. 2002). Interestingly, both decorin and biglycan bind TGF-β. Fibromodulin, lumican, and prolargin belong to the Class II SLRPs, with both fibromodulin and lumican increasing in concentration with age. All three SLRPs bind to collagens. Fibromodulin has been linked to regulation of collagen fibril diameter (Hedbom and Heinegard 1989; Hedlund et al. 1994). The Class III SLRP epiphycan is found in the growth plate (Johnson et al. 1997).

1.3.5 Additional Molecules Critical for Articular Cartilage Function

In addition to the proteoglycans and collagens, articular cartilage also contains noncollagenous proteins, many of which have critical structure and lubricating functions. For example, SZP has been shown to play an important role in the surface properties of articular cartilage through either a lubricating or protective mechanism (Flannery et al. 1999).

1.3.5.1 Boundary Lubrication by SZP/PRG4

SZP (also known as PRG4) is a glycoprotein secreted by, and a marker of, chondrocytes in the superficial layer of articular cartilage and is homologous to lubricin (Schumacher et al. 1994; Jay et al. 2001b). SZP is a hyaluronan binding protein (Jay 1992; Jay et al. 2001b) and is found within the synovial fluid and bound as a thin layer to macromolecules in the lamina splendens. SZP functions as a boundary lubricant at the articular cartilage surface (Schmid et al. 2002), a stress dissipater in synovial fluid (Jay et al. 2007), and has cytoprotective, antiadhesive effects (Schaefer et al. 2004; Englert et al. 2005; Rhee et al. 2005).

SZP is the full-length protein (1404 amino acids and 12 exons in humans) of the *PRG4* gene at locus l q 25 (Ikegawa et al. 2000). Of the protein products of *PRG4*, only SZP (~345 kDa) and lubricin (~227 kDa) have identified lubricating functions. SZP is a multidomain protein with ~60% vitronectin homology at the globular ends and a large (~940 amino acids), highly glycosylated mucin-like domain in the middle (Figure 1.27).

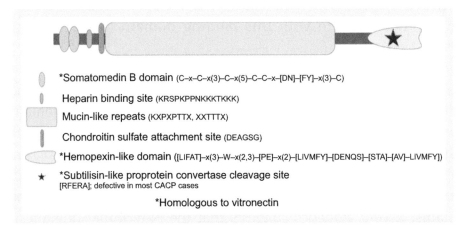

*Somatomedin B domain (C–x–C–x(3)–C–x(5)–C–C–x–[DN]–[FY]–x(3)–C)

Heparin binding site (KRSPKPPNKKKTKKK)

Mucin-like repeats (KXPXPTTX, XXTTTX)

Chondroitin sulfate attachment site (DEAGSG)

*Hemopexin-like domain ([LIFAT]–x(3)–W–x(2,3)–[PE]–x(2)–[LIVMFY]–[DENQS]–[STA]–[AV]–LIVMFY])

★ *Subtilisin-like proprotein convertase cleavage site
[RFERA]; defective in most CACP cases

*Homologous to vitronectin

Figure 1.27 Functional and structural domains of SZP. The mucin domain is approximately 67% of the total length of the protein in humans, with the remainder of the protein in the globular end domains.

SZP contains both O-linked glycosylation and a chondroitin sulfate substitution site, which is likely unoccupied in lubricin (Jay et al. 2001b). In humans, exon 6 encodes a chondroitin sulfate attachment site (DEAGSG) and mucin-like repeats KXPXPTTX (76-78 repeats) and XXTTTX (6-8 repeats). The number of mucin-like repeats is highly species specific and may correspond to body size or joint loading as larger-sized species exhibit an increased number of repeats compared with smaller-sized species (Ikegawa et al. 2000). These oligosaccharides are thought to be responsible for the majority of SZP's lubricating ability, as removal of the (1-3) Gal-GalNAc moieties by endo-*N*-acetyl-D-galactos-aminidase reduces lubricating ability by 77.2% (Jay et al. 2001a).

The C-terminal hemopexin-like domain is critically important for the function of SZP and features a subtilisin-like proprotein covertase cleavage site (RFERA) in exon 10 of human *PRG4*. This domain is cleaved but remains attached to the main protein through disulfide bonds. This domain allows for substrate binding (Jones et al. 2007), and failure to cleave or reduction of these bonds results in a loss of binding and loss of lubricating ability of the molecule (Marcelino et al. 1999; Rhee et al. 2005). The majority of camptodactyly-arthropathy-coxa vara-pericarditis (CACP) cases, the symptoms of which include a lack of functional lubricin, result from mutations in the C-terminal domain that interfere with this binding domain (Marcelino et al. 1999).

The N-terminal domain features two somatomedin B domains and a heparin binding domain. In vitronectin, the somatomedin B domain is able to bind plasminogen activator inhibitor 1 (PAI-1) (Keijer et al. 1991; Kost et al. 1992; Tomasini-Johansson et al. 1998) and inhibit plasmin; thus, SZP may have similar functions. The N-terminal domain undergoes heavy alternative splicing, which can result in the removal of these domains. Recent evidence suggests that the N-terminal domain also acts to bind the extracellular matrix (Zappone et al. 2007; DuRaine et al. 2011), resulting in a potential horseshoe conformation of SZP with each end bound and the mucin domain exposed.

SZP exists at a minimum in both monomeric and disulfide bonded dimeric forms with higher-order multimers likely (Schmidt et al. 2009). Production of recombinant truncated N-terminal proteins has identified at least one dimerization domain within the somatomedin B domain (Jones et al. 2007; Schmidt et al. 2009) of exon 3 (DuRaine et al. 2011). Differences in lubrication between the monomer and dimer may exist *in vivo* and have been demonstrated in artificial systems (Zappone et al. 2007). In addition to its function as a boundary lubricant, SZP inhibits integrative cartilage repair and synovial cell overgrowth. SZP appears to reduce the ability of cells to bind to the articular surface (Schaefer et al. 2004; Englert et al. 2005; Rhee et al. 2005).

1.3.5.2 Molecules for Structural Integrity

Many of the minor proteinaceous components of articular cartilage have been identified through their increased expression during disease progression or through the use of knockout mouse models. These include fibronectin, COMP, tenascin, matrix-GLA (glycine-leucine-alanine) protein, and chondrocalcin (Guilak et al. 2000) (Table 1.3). The functions of these molecules are currently being investigated toward a better understanding of the intricacies associated with cartilage performance. Other matrix constituents in articular cartilage include lipids, phospholipids, glycoproteins, and inorganic crystal compounds (Boskey 1981; Pritzker et al. 1988; Heinegard and Oldberg 1989; Poole et al. 1989).

1.4 ARTICULAR CARTILAGE BIOMECHANICAL PROPERTIES

The primary role of articular cartilage is to provide a low-friction, wear-resistant surface that can withstand large loads over decades of constant use. Section 1.3 described how the biological structure of cartilage is specifically organized for this task. Functionally, the collagen network encapsulating aggrecan provides tensile strength to resist the expansion of the proteoglycans (Stockwell 1990). This results in the collagen achieving a prestrain due to the presence of proteoglycans even in unloaded tissue.

Table 1.3 Other proteins of note in articular cartilage (see also Figure 1.28)

Protein	Function
Cartilage intermediate-layer protein (CILP)	Upregulated in early osteoarthritis and can be causative in an animal disease model. Marker of middle zone in articular cartilage (Lorenzo et al. 1998; Yao et al. 2004).
Cartilage oligomeric matrix protein (COMP)	Matrix aggregation/structural protein; pentameric structure; identified as a potential early osteoarthritis marker. COMP directly binds to collagen, although this requires the presence of zinc (Newton et al. 1994; Petersson et al. 1997; Halasz et al. 2007).
Chondrocalcin	Associated with calcifying cartilage (Poole and Rosenberg 1986).
Matrilins 1 and 3	Matrilins 1 and 3 bind strongly to aggrecan and likely to collagens and COMP (Winterbottom et al. 1992; Hauser et al. 1996; Chen et al. 1999, 2007).
Matrix-GLA (glycine-leucine-alanine) protein	Associated with calcifying cartilage. Knockout mice display increased cartilage calcification (Hale et al. 1988; Luo et al. 1997).
Tenascin	Increased in osteoarthritis as an inverse correlation exists between the presence of tenascin and osteochondral ossification (Pacifici et al. 1993; Veje et al. 2003).

The biochemical and biomechanical characteristics of articular cartilage directly affect how it performs in the joint. Changes in these characteristics can dramatically change the loading profile, thereby beginning a process of degradation that can eventually result in tissue loss.

Within the body, articular cartilage functions to facilitate load support and load transfer while allowing for translation and rotation between bones. The degree of loading in an articulating joint is dependent on its location in the body. The force exerted on the hip has been calculated to be 3.3 times a person's body weight. The knee experiences a load of approximately 3.5 times body weight, the ankle 2.5 times body weight, and the shoulder 1.5 times body weight (Mow et al. 2000). Experimentally, compressive stresses in the hip routinely reach 7-10 MPa and have been measured up to 18 MPa during more stressful activities, such as standing up (Hodge et al. 1989). Within the lower limbs, this loading is cyclical in nature due to the leg gait, with, on average, forces going from a near-zero minimum to maximum loading at a frequency of approximately 1 Hz. It is the contact area of the opposing cartilage surfaces covered by a thin fluid film that transmits these forces, which are then distributed into the rest of the bulk tissue.

The deformation characteristics of articular cartilage play an important role in its mechanical functionality and stem from the combination of interactions between the fluid and solid phases. Articular cartilage is a highly complex material, essentially a fluid-saturated, fiber-reinforced, porous, permeable composite matrix (Mow et al. 1984). The material properties of cartilage can be described as viscoelastic (time or rate dependent), anisotropic (dependent on orientation), and nonlinear (e.g., dependent on magnitude of strain) (Guilak et al. 2000). The time- or rate-dependent behavior of articular cartilage stems from interstitial fluid flow through the solid matrix and is manifested via creep, stress relaxation, and energy dissipation or hysteresis (Hayes and Mockros 1971; Mak 1986; Mow et al. 1989; Setton et al. 1993). Mathematical models have been developed that attempt to describe these properties, which are dependent on the interaction among the different phases in cartilage (solid, fluid, and ionic). Functionally, this viscoelastic behavior plays out as sudden loading during the gait cycle is initially borne by the fluid phase of the cartilage, helping to absorb the energy of impact that would otherwise be felt by the solid phase. This initially raises the contact stress experienced by articular cartilage that is decreased as the tissue deforms upon loading, since the area of contact between surfaces increases.

Loading and deformation of articular cartilage generate a combination of tensile, compressive, and shear stresses within the tissue (Guilak et al. 2000). Healthy cartilage can withstand many decades of rigorous use without deterioration or failure. This section describes the primary mechanical forces acting on articular cartilage.

1.4.1 Compressive Characteristics

Compressive loading is one of the primary types of mechanical stress experienced by articular cartilage. The compressive aggregate modulus, H_A, of cartilage ranges from 0.08 to 2 MPa and varies by depth in the tissue, location on the joint, and species (Athanasiou et al. 1991, 1994, 1995, 1998; Schinag et al. 1997). Compression of articular cartilage is governed primarily by the movement of fluid through the interconnected pore structure of the solid matrix. Hydraulic permeability, a measure of the ease or difficulty of fluid movement through a solid matrix, is related to the pore size, structure, and connectivity (Maroudas and Bullough 1968; Mansour and Mow 1976; Mow et al. 1984). Cartilage has low permeability and resists fluid flow, resulting in high drag forces as the interstitial fluid moves through the solid matrix. Interstitial fluid pressures are very large under compression, which is a significant mechanism for load support in the joint (Maroudas and Bullough 1968; Mansour and Mow 1976; Lai et al. 1981; Mow et al. 1984; Park et al. 2003), and is illustrated in Figure 1.15. The frictional drag associated with interstitial fluid flow through the porous, permeable solid matrix is the dominant dissipative mechanism for cartilage (Setton et al. 1993). However, this functionality might be significantly impaired if the tissue structure is disrupted or otherwise not intact (Figure 1.28).

As fluid redistributes within the tissue, time-dependent changes occur in fluid movement that contribute to the viscoelastic properties of the tissue. As fluid pressure decreases over time, more load is supported by the solid fraction of the matrix, giving rise to creep and stress relaxation behaviors (Mow et al. 1980) (Figure 1.29). The change from support of load from the fluid to the solid fraction is further slowed by both the low permeability of

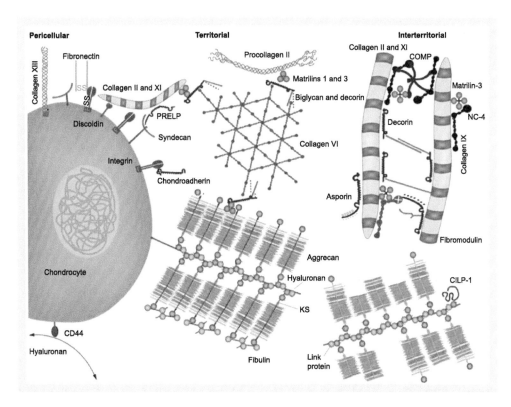

Figure 1.28 The cartilage matrix has a multitude of matrix proteins (described in the text and Table 1.3) with varied localization dependent on proximity to the chondrocytes. (From Heinegard, D., and T. Saxne, *Nat Rev Rheumatol* 7(1): 50-56, 2011. With permission.)

the subchondral bone and the pressurization of the surrounding cartilage, which results in only a small available fluid pressure gradient.

Calculated compressive strains are not uniform throughout the tissue thickness, since the fluid flow is nonhomogeneous (i.e., it changes from location to location). Fluid flow is greatest at the surface of cartilage, resulting in compressive strains as high as 50% due to compaction of the superficial zone (Teeple et al. 2007), with the fluid flow decreasing as a function of increasing tissue depth, resulting in compressive strains of <5% in the middle to deep zones due to the impermeability of the subchondral bone and the bulk of the adjacent cartilage. The mechanical deformation that would occur with compressive loading is restrained

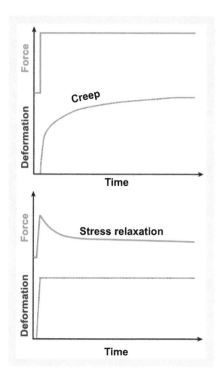

Figure 1.29 Compression testing schematic of different forms of loading and displacement applied to cartilage and the resulting viscoelastic behavior. Creep test is load controlled; a constant load (force) is applied nearly instantaneously (top, green line) and displacement (creep) is measured until plateau (top, red line). The stress relaxation test is displacement controlled: a constant rate of displacement is applied to a specific strain and held (bottom, red line). Loading (force) reaches a peak and then decreases (stress relaxation) until equilibrium loading is reached (bottom, green).

not only by the initial fluid pressurization, but also by the resistance of both the surrounding cartilage and the subchondral bone, which acts to stabilize the cartilage directly under the area of contact. This drives fluid flow to occur from both the areas of cartilage directly under the contact area (assisting with lubrication) and the areas directly adjacent to the loaded region. Volumetric changes occur as fluid is extruded from the tissue under compression.

Upon removal of the compressive load, articular cartilage recovers its initial dimensions. This is possible through the combination of the elasticity of the solid matrix and the imbibition of surrounding fluid due to the hydrostatic tension created by the compaction of the matrix of repeated cycles of use (Linn and Sokoloff 1965). Compression and recovery occur repeatedly at the microscale level during normal joint movement. However, over the course of a day, the bulk cartilage tissue is compressed slightly compared with its initial state. This results in total compressive strains of 15-20% (Armstrong et al. 1979). However, a period of inactivity (e.g., a good night's sleep) will allow the tissue to recover. These compressive strains are always accompanied by corresponding tensile strains generated by the gait cycle.

1.4.2 Tensile Characteristics

Tension can occur when two articular cartilage surfaces slide across one another and pull in a single direction. At the surface of the tissue, tension also occurs when the cartilage is indented or compressed, pulling the surrounding regions toward the point of loading. As cartilage is loaded in tension, the collagen fibrils within the solid matrix align and stretch along the axis of loading; this is described in further detail in Section 5.4.2. The frictional properties of the tissue should help limit the magnitude of tensile strains, but small, repeated periods of tensile loading still occur during normal joint movement.

The tensile properties of articular cartilage are nonlinear due largely to the behavior of collagen fibers in the tissue. For small deformations, collagen fibers realign in the direction of loading. As tension increases, the cross-linked collagen fibers themselves begin to stretch, which results in the tissue exhibiting a higher stiffness at larger strains (Kempson et al. 1968; Woo et al. 1979; Roth and Mow 1980). Cartilage exhibits linear equilibrium stress-strain behavior up to 15% strain (Akizuki et al. 1986).

The tensile Young's modulus is essentially a measure of the solid collagenous matrix and varies by both depth and orientation in the tissue (Roth and Mow 1980). Other contributing physical parameters include collagen fiber density, fiber diameter, amount of cross-linking, and the

57

strength of ionic bonds and frictional interactions between the collagen and proteoglycan networks (Kempson et al. 1973; Schmidt et al. 1990).

The tensile modulus of healthy human cartilage varies from 5 to 25 MPa depending on the location on the joint and depth in the tissue (Kempson et al. 1968; Woo et al. 1976; Akizuki et al. 1986). In general, the superficial zone of cartilage is stiffer in tension than the middle or deep zones (Roth and Mow 1980). Furthermore, the upper regions of cartilage tissue are also stiffer when oriented along split lines (the predominant collagen fiber orientation at the cartilage surface) (Kempson et al. 1973; Woo et al. 1976). Piercing the cartilage surface with a needle dipped in India ink produces a "split" that follows the plane of the collagen fibrils. This technique provides a simple way of visualizing fibril orientation at the cartilage surface (Figure 1.30).

The tensile properties of cartilage are also dependent on interactions between the collagen and proteoglycan networks. Enzymatic extraction of GAGs has been shown to effect a significant increase in collagen fiber alignment, which alters the rate of deformation, or creep, for cartilage samples under tension (Schmidt et al. 1990). While the collagen-proteoglycan interactions appear to affect rate changes in the

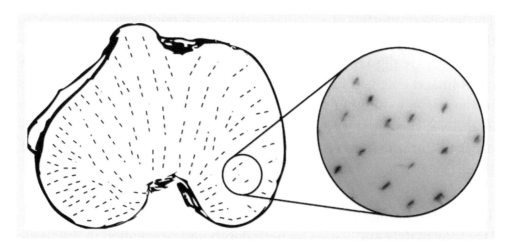

Figure 1.30 Split lines of the distal femur indicate the fibril orientation at the surface of the articular cartilage.

deformation of articular cartilage, the intrinsic stiffness of the solid collagenous matrix is what primarily contributes to the stress-strain behavior and failure properties of cartilage in tension.

1.4.3 Shear Characteristics

Articular cartilage undergoes shear through its depth from normal rotational and translational movements in the joint (Figure 1.31). Shear properties at equilibrium help to characterize the interaction among solid components in cartilage, without having to account for the contribution from fluid flow effects. The equilibrium shear modulus for articular cartilage has been found to vary from 0.05 to 0.25 MPa (Abbot et al. 2003).

Shear testing in articular cartilage is often performed by applying an oscillatory torsional strain over a range of frequencies. This results in the calculation of a dynamic shear modulus (G^*), which indicates the stiffness of the matrix, and a loss angle (δ), which indicates the dissipation

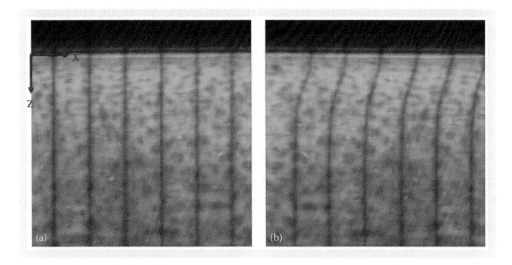

Figure 1.31 Confocal images of human articular cartilage before (a) and during (b) shear. Cartilage was stained with 5-DTAF for visualization and lines were photobleached into the tissue to observe shear deformation. (From Buckley, M. R. et al., *J Biomech* 43(4): 796-800, 2010. With permission.)

of internal friction. A perfectly elastic material would have a loss angle of 0°, whereas a perfectly viscous fluid would have an angle of 90°. The shear behavior of articular cartilage is due to the interaction between collagen fibers and proteoglycan networks. Dynamic shear moduli for human, bovine, and canine samples vary from 0.1 to 4 MPa, with the loss angle being ~10° (Hayes and Mockros 1971; Simon et al. 1990; Zhu et al. 1993; Setton et al. 1995). These values are higher than those for the equilibrium modulus due to the transitory nature of the loading, which is normal for viscoelastic materials.

1.4.4 Friction and Wear Characteristics

Tribology, from Greek *tribo* (τρίβω), meaning "to rub"

Tribology is the science of friction, wear, and lubrication of surfaces moving against each other. Tribological interactions between two surfaces or the environment can result in loss of material from one or both surfaces as wear. Generally, wear can be divided into four main categories: erosion, corrosion, abrasion, and adhesion (also known as friction). In bearing surfaces, wear of surfaces is unwanted, so modification of the surface or the addition of lubrication is used to mitigate wear. Lubricants can reduce frictional and abrasive wear, decreasing the energy necessary for surface movement and increasing the lifespan of the material or, in this case, the articular cartilage.

Articulating joints are complex biomechanical and biochemical systems in which mixed modes of lubrication, including hydrodynamic, elastohydrodynamic, squeeze film lubrication, and boundary lubrication (see Section 5.5) (Lewis and McCutchen 1959; Radin et al. 1970; Mow and Ateshian 1997; Schwarz and Hills 1998), allow for normal activities, such as locomotion (Figure 1.32). In hydrodynamic lubrication, the mechanical load is transmitted via a thin layer of fluid lubricant between two articulating surfaces. The measured friction coefficients may approach 0.001 (Mow and Ateshian 1997). The coefficient of friction

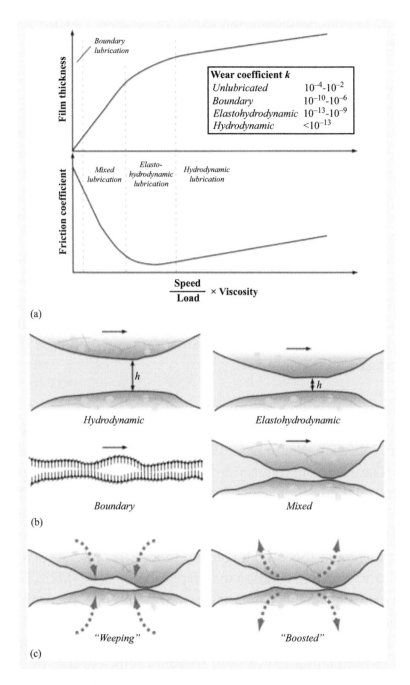

Figure 1.32 Stribeck curve demonstrating changes in friction coefficient and film thickness as a function of speed and load. As the speed-to-load ratio changes, different lubricating regimens and wear coefficients (inset a, b, c) are encountered. (From Neu, C. P. et al., *Tissue Eng Part B Rev* 14(3): 235-247, 2008. With permission.)

for a cartilage-on-cartilage interface is lower than that for any other known bearing.

Several different mechanisms have been proposed to explain the low friction values between articular cartilage surfaces; these include fluid pressurization (McCutchen 1962; Forster and Fisher 1996; Ateshian et al. 1998; Krishnan et al. 2004), elastohydrodynamic lubrication (Dowson and Jin 1986; Suciu et al. 2003), squeeze film lubrication (Hou et al. 1992; Hlavacek 1993), and boundary lubrication (Charnley 1960; Wright and Dowson 1976; Coles et al. 2008). Current findings indicate fluid pressurization is the most influential mechanism for low friction (Ateshian 2009). Experiments focusing on interstitial fluid pressurization show that as pressure decreases 10-fold, the coefficient of friction, which represents the ratio of the tangential frictional force to the compressive force, increases 250-fold. However, normal loading does not allow for interstitial pressures to drop this dramatically, so friction at the cartilage interface remains minimal.

In boundary lubrication, the mechanical load is transmitted directly between two contacting surfaces; one function of SZP/PRG4 is as a boundary lubricant (Radin et al. 1970; Jay 1992; Jay et al. 2001a; Chan et al. 2010). The actions of interacting asperities as the surfaces contact not only increase the friction coefficient, but also increase wear. The measured friction coefficient may approach 0.01 or higher. While hydrodynamic effects in cartilage lubrication are certainly critical to maintaining normal function of the joint, it is likely that in the absence of a boundary lubricant joint degeneration may rapidly propagate (Marcelino et al. 1999). In articular cartilage, boundary lubrication may occur through a "sacrificial layer" mechanism (Schmidt et al. 2005). This type of mechanism is characterized by the removal of the lubricant from contacting surfaces to maintain a low system friction coefficient (i.e., by a "sacrificed" layer), followed by replenishment of the lubricant to the surface. In this mechanism, the lubricating molecule has a strong affinity for the surface attachment by physical adsorption.

1.5 CHAPTER CONCEPTS

- The cartilages of the body include hyaline, elastic, and fibrous; these vary in composition and function.
- Hyaline articular cartilage is a glassy, translucent tissue that is avascular, aneural, and alymphatic.
- The largest joint in the human body is the knee, containing both hyaline articular cartilage and a fibrocartilaginous meniscus.
- Articular cartilage matrix is composed of 70-80% water (per wet weight), 50-75% collagen (per dry weight), and 15-30% proteoglycans (per dry weight).
- The cells of articular cartilage, chondrocytes, reside in lacunae and are responsible for maintaining the extracellular matrix, and, therefore cartilage function.
- Proper function of chondrocytes is dependent on the cytoskeletal organization of actin fibers into a cortical shell for maintenance of their phenotype.
- Chondrocytes, which also require correct mechanical loading to maintain the articular cartilage matrix, employ multiple methods of sensing loading.
- The matrix is divided into superficial, middle, deep, and calcified zones, each with varying biochemical composition, biological function, and biomechanical properties.
- Type II collagen is most abundant in hyaline articular cartilage; type V, VI, IX, and XI collagens are minor components.
- Type II collagen organization and orientation vary by zone. Collagens are responsible for imparting primarily tensile properties.
- Proteoglycans play a central role in resisting compression. The negatively charged keratan and chondroitin sulfates in the aggrecan macromolecule cause the tissue to imbibe and retain water, creating a prestress in the collagen network. Water plays a critical role in resisting applied pressures during compressive loading cycles.

- The synovial fluid reduces friction and plays an important role in the transport of nutrients and metabolic waste.
- PRG4 (SZP), a component of the synovial fluid, is produced by both the synovium and the superficial zone of articular cartilage. It plays a key role as a boundary lubricant.
- The lamina splendens, consisting of collagen fibers oriented along the direction of stress, covers the cartilage surface and serves to resist shear and protect the extracellular matrix.
- The force exerted on the hip and knee joints is more than 3.5 times body weight.
- The compressive aggregate modulus, HA, of cartilage ranges from 0.08 to 2 MPa and varies by depth in the tissue, location on the joint, and species. On average, the aggregate modulus is around 0.8 MPa.
- The tensile modulus of healthy human cartilage varies from 5 to 25 MPa. It is noteworthy that the tensile modulus is about one order of magnitude higher than the compressive modulus.
- The friction coefficient of articular cartilage can be as low as 0.001, lower than any other known bearing surface.

REFERENCES

Abbot, A. E., W. N. Levine et al. (2003). Biomechanics of the articular cartilage and menisci of the adult knee. In *The Adult Knee*, ed. J. J. Callaghan, A. G. Rosenberg, H. E. Rubash, P. T. Simonian, and T. L. Wickiewicz. Philadelphia: Lippincott Williams & Wilkins, pp. 81-103.

Aigner, T., E. Reichenberger et al. (1993). Type X collagen expression in osteoarthritic and rheumatoid articular cartilage. *Virchows Arch B Cell Pathol Incl Mol Pathol* 63(4): 205-211.

Ainsworth, C. (2007). Cilia: Tails of the unexpected. *Nature* 448(7154): 638-641.

Akizuki, S., V. C. Mow et al. (1986). Tensile properties of human knee joint cartilage. I. Influence of ionic conditions, weight bearing, and fibrillation on the tensile modulus. *J Orthop Res* 4(4): 379-392.

Alam, S., D. B. Lovett et al. (2014). Nuclear forces and cell mechanosensing. *Prog Mol Biol Transl Sci* 126: 205-215.

Archer, C. W., J. McDowell et al. (1990). Phenotypic modulation in sub-populations of human articular chondrocytes in vitro. *J Cell Sci* 97(Pt 2): 361-371.

Armstrong, C. G., A. S. Bahrani et al. (1979). In vitro measurement of articular cartilage deformations in the intact human hip joint under load. *J Bone Joint Surg Am* 61(5): 744-755.

Asanbaeva, A., K. Masuda et al. (2008). Cartilage growth and remodeling: Modulation of balance between proteoglycan and collagen network in vitro with beta-aminopropionitrile. *Osteoarthr Cartil* 16(1): 1-11.

Ateshian, G. A. (2009). The role of interstitial fluid pressurization in articular cartilage lubrication. *J Biomech* 42(9): 1163-1176.

Ateshian, G. A., W. M. Lai et al. (1994). An asymptotic solution for the contact of two biphasic cartilage layers. *J Biomech* 27(11): 1347-1360.

Ateshian, G. A., H. Wang et al. (1998). The role of interstitial fluid pressurization and surface porosities on the boundary friction of articular cartilage. *J Tribol* 120: 241-248.

Athanasiou, K. A., A. Agarwal et al. (1994). Comparative study of the intrinsic mechanical properties of the human acetabular and femoral head cartilage. *J Orthop Res* 12(3): 340-349.

Athanasiou, K. A., G. T. Liu et al. (1998). Biomechanical topography of human articular cartilage in the first metatarsophalangeal joint. *Clin Orthop Relat Res* 348: 269-281.

Athanasiou, K. A., G. G. Niederauer et al. (1995). Biomechanical topography of human ankle cartilage. *Ann Biomed Eng* 23(5): 697-704.

Athanasiou, K. A., M. P. Rosenwasser et al. (1991). Interspecies comparisons of in situ intrinsic mechanical properties of distal femoral cartilage. *J Orthop Res* 9(3): 330-340.

Aydelotte, M. B., R. R. Greenhill et al. (1988). Differences between sub-populations of cultured bovine articular chondrocytes. II. Proteoglycan metabolism. *Connect Tissue Res* 18(3): 223-234.

Aydelotte, M. B., and K. E. Kuettner. (1988). Differences between sub-populations of cultured bovine articular chondrocytes. I. Morphology and cartilage matrix production. *Connect Tissue Res* 18(3): 205-222.

Blain, E. J., S. J. Gilbert et al. (2006). Disassembly of the vimentin cytoskeleton disrupts articular cartilage chondrocyte homeostasis. *Matrix Biol* 25(7): 398-408.

Boskey, A. L. (1981). Current concepts of the physiology and biochemistry of calcification. *Clin Orthop Relat Res* (157): 225-257.

Brown, P. D., and P. D. Benya. (1988). Alterations in chondrocyte cytoskeletal architecture during phenotypic modulation by retinoic acid and dihydrocytochalasin B-induced reexpression. *J Cell Biol* 106(1): 171-179.

Buckley, M. R., A. J. Bergou et al. (2010). High-resolution spatial mapping of shear properties in cartilage. *J Biomech* 43(4): 796-800.

Buckwalter, J. A., J. A. Martin et al. (2006). Perspectives on chondrocyte mechanobiology and osteoarthritis. *Biorheology* 43(3-4): 603-609.

Chan, S. M., C. P. Neu et al. (2010). Atomic force microscope investigation of the boundary-lubricant layer in articular cartilage. *Osteoarthr Cartil* 18(7): 956-963.

Charnley, J. (1960). The lubrication of animal joints in relation to surgical reconstruction by arthroplasty. *Ann Rheum Dis* 19: 10-19.

Chen, A. C., M. M. Temple et al. (2002). Induction of advanced glycation end products and alterations of the tensile properties of articular cartilage. *Arthritis Rheum* 46(12): 3212-3217.

Chen, F. H., M. E. Herndon et al. (2007). Interaction of cartilage oligomeric matrix protein/thrombospondin 5 with aggrecan. *J Biol Chem* 282(34): 24591-24598.

Chen, Q., Y. Zhang et al. (1999). Assembly of a novel cartilage matrix protein filamentous network: Molecular basis of differential requirement of von Willebrand factor A domains. *Mol Biol Cell* 10(7): 2149-2162.

Choi, J. B., I. Youn et al. (2007). Zonal changes in the three-dimensional morphology of the chondron under compression: The relationship among cellular, pericellular, and extracellular deformation in articular cartilage. *J Biomech* 40(12): 2596-2603.

Christensen, S. T., S. F. Pedersen et al. (2008). The primary cilium coordinates signaling pathways in cell cycle control and migration during development and tissue repair. *Curr Top Dev Biol* 85: 261-301.

Clark, J. M. (1990). The organisation of collagen fibrils in the superficial zones of articular cartilage. *J Anat* 171: 117-130.

Coles, J. M., J. J. Blum et al. (2008). In situ friction measurement on murine cartilage by atomic force microscopy. *J Biomech* 41(3): 541-548.

Dahl, K. N., A. J. Ribeiro et al. (2008). Nuclear shape, mechanics, and mechanotransduction. *Circ Res* 102(11): 1307-1318.

Daniels, K., and M. Solursh. (1991). Modulation of chondrogenesis by the cytoskeleton and extracellular matrix. *J Cell Sci* 100(Pt 2): 249-254.

Darling, E. M., and K. A. Athanasiou. (2003). Articular cartilage bioreactors and bioprocesses. *Tissue Eng* 9(1): 9-26. [Published erratum appears in *Tissue Eng* 9(3): 565, 2003.]

Darling, E. M., and K. A. Athanasiou. (2005a). Growth factor impact on articular cartilage subpopulations. *Cell Tissue Res* 322(3): 463-473.

Darling, E. M., and K. A. Athanasiou. (2005b). Rapid phenotypic changes in passaged articular chondrocyte subpopulations. *J Orthop Res* 23(2): 425-432.

Darling, E. M., and K. A. Athanasiou. (2005c). Retaining zonal chondrocyte phenotype by means of novel growth environments. *Tissue Eng* 11(3-4): 395-403.

Darling, E. M., J. C. Hu et al. (2004). Zonal and topographical differences in articular chondrocyte gene expression. *J Orthop Res* 22(6): 1182-1187.

Darling, E. M., S. Zauscher et al. (2006). Viscoelastic properties of zonal articular chondrocytes measured by atomic force microscopy. *Osteoarthr Cartil* 14(6): 571-579.

Decker, B., W. McGuckin et al. (1959). Concentration of hyaluronic acid in synovial fluid. *Clin Chem* 5: 465-469.

Deshmukh, K., and M. E. Nimni. (1973). Isolation and characterization of cyanogen bromide peptides from the collagen of bovine articular cartilage. *Biochem J* 133(4): 615-622.

Detamore, M. S., and K. A. Athanasiou. (2003). Structure and function of the temporomandibular joint disc: Implications for tissue engineering. *J Oral Maxillofac Surg* 61(4): 494-506.

Dowson, D., and Z. M. Jin. (1986). Micro-elastohydrodynamic lubrication of synovial joints. *Eng Med* 15(2): 63-65.

Dowthwaite, G. P., J. C. Bishop et al. (2004). The surface of articular cartilage contains a progenitor cell population. *J Cell Sci* 117(Pt 6): 889-897.

Driscoll, T. P., B. D. Cosgrove et al. (2015). Cytoskeletal to nuclear strain transfer regulates YAP signaling in mesenchymal stem cells. *Biophys J* 108(12): 2783-2793.

DuRaine, G. D., S. M. Chan et al. (2011). Effects of TGF-beta1 on alternative splicing of superficial zone protein in articular cartilage cultures. *Osteoarthr Cartil* 19(1): 103-110.

Durr, J., P. Lammi et al. (1996). Identification and immunolocalization of laminin in cartilage. *Exp Cell Res* 222(1): 225-233.

Durrant, L. A., C. W. Archer et al. (1999). Organisation of the chondrocyte cytoskeleton and its response to changing mechanical conditions in organ culture. *J Anat* 194(Pt 3): 343-353.

Eggli, P. S., E. B. Hunziker et al. (1988). Quantitation of structural features characterizing weight- and less-weight-bearing regions in articular cartilage: A stereological analysis of medial femoral condyles in young adult rabbits. *Anat Rec* 222(3): 217-227.

Englert, C., K. B. McGowan et al. (2005). Inhibition of integrative cartilage repair by proteoglycan 4 in synovial fluid. *Arthritis Rheum* 52(4): 1091-1099.

Eyre, D. R., M. A. Weis et al. (2008). Advances in collagen cross-link analysis. *Methods* 45(1): 65-74.

Eyre, D. R., and J. J. Wu. (1995). Collagen structure and cartilage matrix integrity. *J Rheumatol Suppl* 43: 82-85.

Fedorchak, G. R., A. Kaminski et al. (2014). Cellular mechanosensing: Getting to the nucleus of it all. *Prog Biophys Mol Biol* 115(2-3): 76-92.

Fitzgerald, J. B., M. Jin et al. (2008). Shear- and compression-induced chondrocyte transcription requires MAPK activation in cartilage explants. *J Biol Chem* 283(11): 6735-6743.

Flannery, C. R., C. E. Hughes et al. (1999). Articular cartilage superficial zone protein (SZP) is homologous to megakaryocyte stimulating factor precursor and is a multifunctional proteoglycan with potential growth-promoting, cytoprotective, and lubricating properties in cartilage metabolism. *Biochem Biophys Res Commun* 254(3): 535-541.

Fliegauf, M., T. Benzing et al. (2007). When cilia go bad: Cilia defects and ciliopathies. *Nat Rev Mol Cell Biol* 8(11): 880-893.

Forman, J. R., S. Qamar et al. (2005). The remarkable mechanical strength of polycystin-1 supports a direct role in mechanotransduction. *J Mol Biol* 349(4): 861-871.

Forster, H., and J. Fisher. (1996). The influence of loading time and lubricant on the friction of articular cartilage. *Proc Inst Mech Eng H* 210(2): 109-119.

Frost, H. M. (2000). The Utah paradigm of skeletal physiology: An overview of its insights for bone, cartilage and collagenous tissue organs. *J Bone Miner Metab* 18(6): 305-316.

Fry, P., M. L. Harkness et al. (1962). Mechanical properties of tissues of lathyritic animals. *J Physiol* 164: 77-89.

Ghadially, F. N. (1983). *Fine Structure of Synovial Joints: A Text and Atlas of the Ultrastructure of Normal and Pathological Articular Tissues.* London: Butterworths.

Giannoni, P., M. Siegrist et al. (2003). The mechanosensitivity of cartilage oligomeric matrix protein (COMP). *Biorheology* 40(1-3): 101-109.

Glant, T. T., C. Hadhazy et al. (1985). Appearance and persistence of fibronectin in cartilage. Specific interaction of fibronectin with collagen type II. *Histochemistry* 82(2): 149-158.

Glowacki, J., E. Trepman et al. (1983). Cell shape and phenotypic expression in chondrocytes. *Proc Soc Exp Biol Med* 172(1): 93-98.

Grad, S., S. Gogolewski et al. (2006a). Effects of simple and complex motion patterns on gene expression of chondrocytes seeded in 3D scaffolds. *Tissue Eng* 12(11): 3171-3179.

Grad, S., C. R. Lee et al. (2006b). Chondrocyte gene expression under applied surface motion. *Biorheology* 43(3-4): 259-269.

Graham, H. K., D. F. Holmes et al. (2000). Identification of collagen fibril fusion during vertebrate tendon morphogenesis. The process relies on unipolar fibrils and is regulated by collagen-proteoglycan interaction. *J Mol Biol* 295(4): 891-902.

Gray, H., R. Warwick et al. (1980). *Gray's Anatomy.* Philadelphia: Churchill Livingstone.

Guilak, F., L. A. Setton et al. (2000). Structure and function of articular cartilage. In *Principles and Practice of Orthopaedic Sports Medicine*, ed. W. E. Garrett, K. P. Speer, D. T. Kirkendall, and M. D. Kitkowski. Philadelphia: Lippincott Williams & Wilkins, pp. 53-73.

Halasz, K., A. Kassner et al. (2007). COMP acts as a catalyst in collagen fibrillogenesis. *J Biol Chem* 282(43): 31166-31173.

Hale, J. E., J. D. Fraser et al. (1988). The identification of matrix Gla protein in cartilage. *J Biol Chem* 263(12): 5820-5824.

Hardingham, T. E., A. J. Fosang et al. (1994). The structure, function and turnover of aggrecan, the large aggregating proteoglycan from cartilage. *Eur J Clin Chem Clin Biochem* 32(4): 249-257.

Haudenschild, D. R., J. Chen et al. (2011). Vimentin contributes to changes in chondrocyte stiffness in osteoarthritis. *J Orthop Res* 29(1): 20-25.

Hauser, N., M. Paulsson et al. (1996). Interaction of cartilage matrix protein with aggrecan. Increased covalent cross-linking with tissue maturation. *J Biol Chem* 271(50): 32247-32252.

Hayes, A. J., M. Benjamin et al. (1999). Role of actin stress fibres in the development of the intervertebral disc: Cytoskeletal control of extracellular matrix assembly. *Dev Dyn* 215(3): 179-189.

Hayes, W. C., and L. F. Mockros. (1971). Viscoelastic properties of human articular cartilage. *J Appl Physiol* 31(4): 562-568.

Hedbom, E., and D. Heinegard. (1989). Interaction of a 59-kDa connective tissue matrix protein with collagen I and collagen II. *J Biol Chem* 264(12): 6898-6905.

Hedlund, H., S. Mengarelli-Widholm et al. (1994). Fibromodulin distribution and association with collagen. *Matrix Biol* 14(3): 227-232.

Heinegard, D., and A. Oldberg. (1989). Structure and biology of cartilage and bone matrix noncollagenous macromolecules. *FASEB J* 3(9): 2042-2051.

Heinegard, D., and T. Saxne. (2011). The role of the cartilage matrix in osteoarthritis. *Nat Rev Rheumatol* 7(1): 50-56.

Hildebrand, A., M. Romaris et al. (1994). Interaction of the small interstitial proteoglycans biglycan, decorin and fibromodulin with transforming growth factor beta. *Biochem J* 302(Pt 2): 527-534.

Hlavacek, M. (1993). The role of synovial fluid filtration by cartilage in lubrication of synovial joints. II. Squeeze-film lubrication: Homogeneous filtration. *J Biomech* 26(10): 1151-1160.

Hodge, W. A., K. L. Carlson et al. (1989). Contact pressures from an instrumented hip endoprosthesis. *J Bone Joint Surg Am* 71(9): 1378-1386.

Holledge, M. M., S. J. Millward-Sadler et al. (2008). Mechanical regulation of proteoglycan synthesis in normal and osteoarthritic human articular chondrocytes—Roles for alpha5 and alphaVbeta5 integrins. *Biorheology* 45(3-4): 275-288.

Hou, J. S., V. C. Mow et al. (1992). An analysis of the squeeze-film lubrication mechanism for articular cartilage. *J Biomech* 25(3): 247-259.

Huey, D. J., J. C. Hu et al. (2012). Unlike bone, cartilage regeneration remains elusive. *Science* 338(6109): 917-921.

Hughes, L. C., C. W. Archer et al. (2005). The ultrastructure of mouse articular cartilage: Collagen orientation and implications for tissue functionality. A polarised light and scanning electron microscope study and review. *Eur Cell Mater*
9: 68-84.

Hulmes, D. J. (2002). Building collagen molecules, fibrils, and suprafibrillar structures. *J Struct Biol* 137(1-2): 2-10.

Hulmes, D. J., and A. Miller. (1979). Quasi-hexagonal molecular packing in collagen
fibrils. *Nature* 282(5741): 878-880.

Hunziker, E. B., W. Herrmann et al. (1983). Ruthenium hexammine trichloride (RHT)-
mediated interaction between plasmalemmal components and pericellular
matrix proteoglycans is responsible for the preservation of chondrocytic
plasma membranes in situ during cartilage fixation. *J Histochem Cytochem*
31(6): 717-727.

Hunziker, E. B., M. Michel et al. (1997). Ultrastructure of adult human articular cartilage matrix after cryotechnical processing. *Microsc Res Tech* 37(4): 271-284.

Ikegawa, S., M. Sano et al. (2000). Isolation, characterization and mapping of the
mouse and human PRG4 (proteoglycan 4) genes. *Cytogenet Cell Genet* 90
(3-4): 291-297.

Iozzo, R. V. (1999). The biology of the small leucine-rich proteoglycans. Functional
network of interactive proteins. *J Biol Chem* 274(27): 18843-18846.

Jaalouk, D. E., and J. Lammerding. (2009). Mechanotransduction gone awry. *Nat Rev
Mol Cell Biol* 10(1): 63-73.

Jay, G. D. (1992). Characterization of a bovine synovial fluid lubricating factor. I.
Chemical, surface activity and lubricating properties. *Connect Tissue Res*
28(1-2): 71-88.

Jay, G. D., D. A. Harris et al. (2001a). Boundary lubrication by lubricin is mediated by
O-linked beta(1–3)Gal-GalNAc oligosaccharides. *Glycoconj J* 18(10): 807-815.

Jay, G. D., U. Tantravahi et al. (2001b). Homology of lubricin and superficial zone protein (SZP): Products of megakaryocyte stimulating factor (MSF) gene expression by human synovial fibroblasts and articular chondrocytes localized to
chromosome 1q25. *J Orthop Res* 19(4): 677-687.

Jay, G. D., J. R. Torres et al. (2007). The role of lubricin in the mechanical behavior of
synovial fluid. *Proc Natl Acad Sci USA* 104(15): 6194-6199.

Jessop, H. L., S. C. Rawlinson et al. (2002). Mechanical strain and fluid movement
both activate extracellular regulated kinase (ERK) in osteoblast-like cells but
via different signaling pathways. *Bone* 31(1): 186-194.

Johnson, H. J., L. Rosenberg et al. (1997). Characterization of epiphycan, a small
proteoglycan with a leucine-rich repeat core protein. *J Biol Chem* 272(30):
18709-18717.

Johnston, S. A. (1997). Osteoarthritis. Joint anatomy, physiology, and pathobiology.
Vet Clin North Am Small Anim Pract 27(4): 699-723.

Jones, A. R., J. P. Gleghorn et al. (2007). Binding and localization of recombinant lubricin to articular cartilage surfaces. *J Orthop Res* 25(3): 283-292.

Katsumi, A., A. W. Orr et al. (2004). Integrins in mechanotransduction. *J Biol Chem* 279(13): 12001-12004.

Keijer, J., M. Linders et al. (1991). On the target specificity of plasminogen activator inhibitor 1: The role of heparin, vitronectin, and the reactive site. *Blood* 78(5): 1254-1261.

Kempson, G. E., M. A. Freeman et al. (1968). Tensile properties of articular cartilage. *Nature* 220(5172): 1127-1128.

Kempson, G. E., H. Muir et al. (1973). The tensile properties of the cartilage of human femoral condyles related to the content of collagen and glycosaminoglycans. *Biochim Biophys Acta* 297(2): 456-472.

Kiani, C., L. Chen et al. (2002). Structure and function of aggrecan. *Cell Res* 12(1): 19-32.

Knudson, W., and R. F. Loeser. (2002). CD44 and integrin matrix receptors participate in cartilage homeostasis. *Cell Mol Life Sci* 59(1): 36-44.

Koo, S., and T. P. Andriacchi. (2007). A comparison of the influence of global functional loads vs. local contact anatomy on articular cartilage thickness at the knee. *J Biomech* 40(13): 2961-2966.

Kornblatt, J. A., and M. J. Kornblatt. (2002). The effects of osmotic and hydrostatic pressures on macromolecular systems. *Biochim Biophys Acta* 1595(1-2): 30-47.

Kost, C., W. Stuber et al. (1992). Mapping of binding sites for heparin, plasminogen activator inhibitor-1, and plasminogen to vitronectin's heparin-binding region reveals a novel vitronectin-dependent feedback mechanism for the control of plasmin formation. *J Biol Chem* 267(17): 12098-12105.

Kotch, F. W., I. A. Guzei et al. (2008). Stabilization of the collagen triple helix by O-methylation of hydroxyproline residues. *J Am Chem Soc* 130(10): 2952-2953.

Krishnan, R., M. Kopacz et al. (2004). Experimental verification of the role of interstitial fluid pressurization in cartilage lubrication. *J Orthop Res* 22(3): 565-570.

Kumar, P., M. Oka et al. (2001). Role of uppermost superficial surface layer of articular cartilage in the lubrication mechanism of joints. *J Anat* 199(Pt 3): 241-250.

Lai, W. M., V. C. Mow et al. (1981). Effects of nonlinear strain-dependent permeability and rate of compression on the stress behavior of articular cartilage. *J Biomech Eng* 103(2): 61-66.

Lazarides, E. (1980). Intermediate filaments as mechanical integrators of cellular space. *Nature* 283(5744): 249-256.

Leung, M. K., L. I. Fessler et al. (1979). Separate amino and carboxyl procollagen peptidases in chick embryo tendon. *J Biol Chem* 254(1): 224-232.

Lewis, P. R., and C. W. McCutchen. (1959). Experimental evidence for weeping lubrication in mammalian joints. *Nature* 184: 1285.

Li, K. W., A. S. Wang et al. (2003). Microenvironment regulation of extracellular signal-regulated kinase activity in chondrocytes: Effects of culture configuration, interleukin-1, and compressive stress. *Arthritis Rheum* 48(3): 689-699.

Linn, F. C., and L. Sokoloff. (1965). Movement and composition of interstitial fluid of cartilage. *Arthritis Rheum* 8: 481-494.

Little, K., L. H. Pimm et al. (1958). Osteoarthritis of the hip: An electron microscope study. *J Bone Joint Surg Br* 40-B(1): 123-131.

Lorenzo, P., M. T. Bayliss et al. (1998). A novel cartilage protein (CILP) present in the mid-zone of human articular cartilage increases with age. *J Biol Chem* 73(36): 23463-23468.

Luo, G., P. Ducy et al. (1997). Spontaneous calcification of arteries and cartilage in mice lacking matrix GLA protein. *Nature* 386(6620): 78-81.

Mac, C. M. (1951). The movements of bones and joints; the mechanical structure of articulating cartilage. *J Bone Joint Surg Br* 33B(2): 251-257.

Mak, A. F. (1986). The apparent viscoelastic behavior of articular cartilage—The contributions from the intrinsic matrix viscoelasticity and interstitial fluid flows. *J Biomech Eng* 108(2): 123-130.

Makris, E. A., P. Hadidi et al. (2011). The knee meniscus: Structure-function, pathophysiology, current repair techniques, and prospects for regeneration. *Biomaterials* 32(30): 7411-7431.

Makris, E. A., D. J. Responte et al. (2014). Developing functional musculoskeletal tissues through hypoxia and lysyl oxidase-induced collagen cross-linking. *Proc Natl Acad Sci USA* 111(45): E4832-E4841.

Malaviya, P., and R. M. Nerem. (2002). Fluid-induced shear stress stimulates chondrocyte proliferation partially mediated via TGF-beta1. *Tissue Eng* 8(4): 581-590.

Malone, A. M., C. T. Anderson et al. (2007). Primary cilia mediate mechanosensing in bone cells by a calcium-independent mechanism. *Proc Natl Acad Sci USA* 104(33): 13325-13330.

Mankin, H. J., and L. Lippiello. (1969). The turnover of adult rabbit articular cartilage. *J Bone Joint Surg Am* 51(8): 1591-1600.

Mansour, J. M., and V. C. Mow. (1976). The permeability of articular cartilage under compressive strain and at high pressures. *J Bone Joint Surg Am* 58(4): 509-516.

Marcelino, J., J. D. Carpten et al. (1999). CACP, encoding a secreted proteoglycan, is mutated in camptodactyly-arthropathy-coxa vara-pericarditis syndrome. *Nat Genet* 23(3): 319-322.

Maroudas, A. (1975). Glycosaminoglycan turn-over in articular cartilage. *Philos Trans R Soc Lond B Biol Sci* 271(912): 293-313.

Maroudas, A. (1979). Physicochemical properties of articular cartilage. In *Adult Articular Cartilage*, ed. M. Freeman. Tunbridge Wells, UK: Pitman Medical, pp. 215-290.

Maroudas, A., and P. Bullough. (1968). Permeability of articular cartilage. *Nature* 219(5160): 1260-1261.

Maroudas, A., H. Muir et al. (1969). The correlation of fixed negative charge with gly-cosaminoglycan content of human articular cartilage. *Biochim Biophys Acta* 177(3): 492-500.

Maroudas, A. I. (1976). Balance between swelling pressure and collagen tension in normal and degenerate cartilage. *Nature* 260(5554): 808-809.

Marshall, W. F., and S. Nonaka. (2006). Cilia: Tuning in to the cell's antenna. *Curr Biol* 16(15): R604-R614.

Martinac, B. (2004). Mechanosensitive ion channels: Molecules of mechanotrans-duction. *J Cell Sci* 117(Pt 12): 2449-2460.

Mason, R. M. (1981). Recent advances in the biochemistry of hyaluronic acid in car-tilage. *Prog Clin Biol Res* 54: 87-112.

Mayan, M. D., R. Gago-Fuentes et al. (2015). Articular chondrocyte network medi-ated by gap junctions: Role in metabolic cartilage homeostasis. *Ann Rheum Dis* 74(1): 275-284.

McCutchen, C. W. (1962). The frictional properties of animal joints. *Wear* 5(1): 1-17.

McDevitt, C. A., J. Marcelino et al. (1991). Interaction of intact type VI collagen with hyaluronan. *FEBS Lett* 294(3): 167-170.

McGlashan, S. R., M. M. Knight et al. (2010). Mechanical loading modulates chondro-cyte primary cilia incidence and length. *Cell Biol Int* 34(5): 441-446.

Meachim, G., and S. R. Sheffield. (1969). Surface ultrastructure of mature adult human articular cartilage. *J Bone Joint Surg Br* 51(3): 529-539.

Millward-Sadler, S. J., M. O. Wright et al. (2000). Mechanotransduction via integrins and interleukin-4 results in altered aggrecan and matrix metalloproteinase 3 gene expression in normal, but not osteoarthritic, human articular chondro-cytes. *Arthritis Rheum* 43(9): 2091-2099.

Mizuno, S. (2005). A novel method for assessing effects of hydrostatic fluid pressure on intracellular calcium: A study with bovine articular chondrocytes. *Am J Physiol Cell Physiol* 288(2): C329-337.

Mow, V. C., and G. A. Ateshian. (1997). Lubrication and wear of diarthrodial joints. In *Basic Orthopaedic Biomechanics*, ed. V. C. Mow and W. C. Hayes. Philadelphia: Lippincott-Raven, pp. 275-315.

Mow, V. C., N. Bachrach et al. (1994). Stress, strain, pressure, and flow fields in articular cartilage. In *Cell Mechanics and Cellular Engineering*, ed. V. C. Mow, F. Guilak, R. Tran-Son-Tay, and R. Hochmuth. New York: Springer Verlag, pp. 345-379.

Mow, V. C., E. L. Flatow et al. (2000). Biomechanics. *Orthopaedic Basic Science: Biology and Biomechanics of the Musculoskeletal System*, ed. J. A. Buckwalter, T. A. Einhorn, and S. R. Simon. Rosemont, IL: American Academy of Orthopaedic Surgeons, pp. 140-142.

Mow, V. C., M. C. Gibbs et al. (1989). Biphasic indentation of articular cartilage. II. A numerical algorithm and an experimental study. *J Biomech* 22(8-9): 853-861.

Mow, V. C., M. H. Holmes et al. (1984). Fluid transport and mechanical properties of articular cartilage: A review. *J Biomech* 17(5): 377-394.

Mow, V. C., S. C. Kuei et al. (1980). Biphasic creep and stress relaxation of articular cartilage in compression? Theory and experiments. *J Biomech Eng* 102(1): 73-84.

Muir, H., P. Bullough et al. (1970). The distribution of collagen in human articular cartilage with some of its physiological implications. *J Bone Joint Surg Br* 52(3): 554-563.

Neu, C. P., A. Khalafi et al. (2007). Mechanotransduction of bovine articular cartilage superficial zone protein by transforming growth factor beta signaling. *Arthritis Rheum* 56(11): 3706-3714.

Neu, C. P., K. Komvopoulos et al. (2008). The interface of functional biotribology and regenerative medicine in synovial joints. *Tissue Eng Part B Rev* 14(3): 235-247.

Newton, G., S. Weremowicz et al. (1994). Characterization of human and mouse cartilage oligomeric matrix protein. *Genomics* 24(3): 435-439.

Ng, L., A. J. Grodzinsky et al. (2003). Individual cartilage aggrecan macromolecules and their constituent glycosaminoglycans visualized via atomic force microscopy. *J Struct Biol* 143(3): 242-257.

O'Hara, B. P., J. P. Urban et al. (1990). Influence of cyclic loading on the nutrition of articular cartilage. *Ann Rheum Dis* 49(7): 536-539.

Orazizadeh, M., H. S. Lee et al. (2008). CD47 associates with alpha 5 integrin and regulates responses of human articular chondrocytes to mechanical stimulation in an in vitro model. *Arthritis Res Ther* 10(1): R4.

Pacifici, M., M. Iwamoto et al. (1993). Tenascin is associated with articular cartilage development. *Dev Dyn* 198(2): 123-134.

Papachristou, D. J., P. Pirttiniemi et al. (2005). JNK/ERK-AP-1/Runx2 induction "paves the way" to cartilage load-ignited chondroblastic differentiation. *Histochem Cell Biol* 124(3-4): 215-223.

Park, S., R. Krishnan et al. (2003). Cartilage interstitial fluid load support in unconfined compression. *J Biomech* 36(12): 1785-1796.

Pavalko, F. M., S. M. Norvell et al. (2003). A model for mechanotransduction in bone cells: The load-bearing mechanosomes. *J Cell Biochem* 88(1): 104-112.

Petersson, I. F., L. Sandqvist et al. (1997). Cartilage markers in synovial fluid in symptomatic knee osteoarthritis. *Ann Rheum Dis* 56(1): 64-67.

Plaas, A. H., S. Wong-Palms et al. (1997). Chemical and immunological assay of the nonreducing terminal residues of chondroitin sulfate from human aggrecan. *J Biol Chem* 272(33): 20603-20610.

Pollard, T. D., and G. G. Borisy. (2003). Cellular motility driven by assembly and disassembly of actin filaments. *Cell* 112(4): 453-465.

Poole, A. R., Y. Matsui et al. (1989). Cartilage macromolecules and the calcification of cartilage matrix. *Anat Rec* 224(2): 167-179.

Poole, A. R., I. Pidoux et al. (1982). An immunoelectron microscope study of the organization of proteoglycan monomer, link protein, and collagen in the matrix of articular cartilage. *J Cell Biol* 93(3): 921-937.

Poole, A. R., G. Rizkalla et al. (1993). Osteoarthritis in the human knee: A dynamic process of cartilage matrix degradation, synthesis and reorganization. *Agents Actions Suppl* 39: 3-13.

Poole, A. R., and L. C. Rosenberg. (1986). Chondrocalcin and the calcification of cartilage. A review. *Clin Orthop Relat Res* 208: 114-118.

Poole, C. A., S. Ayad et al. (1988a). Chondrons from articular cartilage. I. Immunolocalization of type VI collagen in the pericellular capsule of isolated canine tibial chondrons. *J Cell Sci* 90(Pt 4): 635-643.

Poole, C. A., M. H. Flint et al. (1987). Chondrons in cartilage: Ultrastructural analysis of the pericellular microenvironment in adult human articular cartilages. *J Orthop Res* 5(4): 509-522.

Poole, C. A., M. H. Flint et al. (1988b). Chondrons extracted from canine tibial cartilage: Preliminary report on their isolation and structure. *J Orthop Res* 6(3): 408-419.

Pritzker, K. P., P. T. Cheng et al. (1988). Calcium pyrophosphate crystal deposition in hyaline cartilage. Ultrastructural analysis and implications for pathogenesis. *J Rheumatol* 15(5): 828-835.

Radin, E. L., and R. M. Rose. (1986). Role of subchondral bone in the initiation and progression of cartilage damage. *Clin Orthop Relat Res* 213: 34-40.

Radin, E. L., D. A. Swann et al. (1970). Separation of a hyaluronate-free lubricating fraction from synovial fluid. *Nature* 228(5269): 377-378.

Ralphs, J. R., R. N. Tyers et al. (1992). Development of functionally distinct fibrocartilages at two sites in the quadriceps tendon of the rat: The suprapatella and the attachment to the patella. *Anat Embryol* 185(2): 181-187.

Redler, I., V. C. Mow et al. (1975). The ultrastructure and biomechanical significance of the tidemark of articular cartilage. *Clin Orthop Relat Res* 112: 357-362.

Reed, C. C., and R. V. Iozzo. (2002). The role of decorin in collagen fibrillogenesis and skin homeostasis. *Glycoconj J* 19(4-5): 249-255.

Rhee, D. K., J. Marcelino et al. (2005). The secreted glycoprotein lubricin protects cartilage surfaces and inhibits synovial cell overgrowth. *J Clin Invest* 115(3): 622-631.

Rieppo, J., M. M. Hyttinen et al. (2009). Changes in spatial collagen content and collagen network architecture in porcine articular cartilage during growth and maturation. *Osteoarthr Cartil* 17(4): 448-455.

Ropes, M. W., G. A. Bennett et al. (1939). The origin and nature of normal synovial fluid. *J Clin Invest* 18(3): 351-372.

Roth, V., and V. C. Mow. (1980). The intrinsic tensile behavior of the matrix of bovine articular cartilage and its variation with age. *J Bone Joint Surg Am* 62(7): 1102-1117.

Roughley, P. J., and E. R. Lee. (1994). Cartilage proteoglycans: Structure and potential functions. *Microsc Res Tech* 28(5): 385-397.

Roughley, P. J., L. I. Melching et al. (1994). Changes in the expression of decorin and biglycan in human articular cartilage with age and regulation by TGF-beta. *Matrix Biol* 14(1): 51-59.

Ryan, J. A., E. A. Eisner et al. (2009). Mechanical compression of articular cartilage induces chondrocyte proliferation and inhibits proteoglycan synthesis by activation of the ERK pathway: Implications for tissue engineering and regenerative medicine. *J Tissue Eng Regen Med* 3(2): 107-116.

Schaefer, D. B., D. Wendt et al. (2004). Lubricin reduces cartilage—Cartilage integration. *Biorheology* 41(3-4): 503-508.

Schinagl, R. M., D. Gurskis et al. (1997). Depth-dependent confined compression modulus of full-thickness bovine articular cartilage. *J Orthop Res* 15(4): 499-506.

Schmid, T., G. Homandberg et al. (2002). Superficial zone protein (SZP) binds to macromolecules in the lamina splendens of articular cartilage. Presented at 48th Annual Meeting of the Orthopaedic Research Society, Dallas, TX.

Schmidt, M. B., V. C. Mow et al. (1990). Effects of proteoglycan extraction on the tensile behavior of articular cartilage. *J Orthop Res* 8(3): 353-363.

Schmidt, T. A., A. H. Plaas et al. (2009). Disulfide-bonded multimers of proteoglycan 4 (PRG4) are present in normal synovial fluids. *Biochim Biophys Acta* 1790(5): 375-384.

Schmidt, T. A., B. L. Schumacher et al. (2005). PRG4 contributes to a "sacrificial layer" mechanism of boundary lubrication of aricular cartilage. Presented at 51st Annual Meeting of the Orthopaedic Research Society, Washington, DC.

Schumacher, B. L., J. A. Block et al. (1994). A novel proteoglycan synthesized and secreted by chondrocytes of the superficial zone of articular cartilage. *Arch Biochem Biophys* 311(1): 144-152.

Schwartz, M. A. (2010). Integrins and extracellular matrix in mechanotransduction. *Cold Spring Harb Perspect Biol* 2(12): a005066.

Schwarz, I. M., and B. A. Hills. (1998). Surface-active phospholipid as the lubricating component of lubricin. *Br J Rheumatol* 37(1): 21-26.

Sekiya, I., K. Tsuji et al. (2000). SOX9 enhances aggrecan gene promoter/enhancer activity and is up-regulated by retinoic acid in a cartilage-derived cell line, TC6. *J Biol Chem* 275(15): 10738-10744.

Setton, L. A., V. C. Mow et al. (1995). Mechanical behavior of articular cartilage in shear is altered by transection of the anterior cruciate ligament. *J Orthop Res* 13(4): 473-482.

Setton, L. A., W. Zhu et al. (1993). The biphasic poroviscoelastic behavior of articular cartilage: Role of the surface zone in governing the compressive behavior. *J Biomech* 26(4-5): 581-592.

Shepherd, D. E., and B. B. Seedhom. (1999). Thickness of human articular cartilage in joints of the lower limb. *Ann Rheum Dis* 58(1): 27-34.

Siczkowski, M., and F. M. Watt. (1990). Subpopulations of chondrocytes from different zones of pig articular cartilage. Isolation, growth and proteoglycan synthesis in culture. *J Cell Sci* 97(Pt 2): 349-360.

Simon, W. H., A. Mak et al. (1990). The effect of shear fatigue on bovine articular cartilage. *J Orthop Res* 8(1): 86-93.

Singh, I. (2006). *Textbook of Human Histology with Colour Atlas*. New Delhi: Jaypee Brothers Medical Publishers.

Singla, V., and J. F. Reiter. (2006). The primary cilium as the cell's antenna: Signaling at a sensory organelle. *Science* 313(5787): 629-633.

Soltz, M. A., and G. A. Ateshian. (1998). Experimental verification and theoretical prediction of cartilage interstitial fluid pressurization at an impermeable contact interface in confined compression. *J Biomech* 31(10): 927-934.

Stockwell, R. A. (1971). The interrelationship of cell density and cartilage thickness in mammalian articular cartilage. *J Anat* 109(3): 411-421.

Stockwell, R. A. (1990). Cartilage failure in osteoarthritis: Relevance of normal structure and function. A review. *Clin Anat* 4(3): 161-191.

Sucheston, M. E., and M. S. Cannon. (1969). Variations in the appearance of human elastic cartilage. *Ohio J Sci* 69(6): 366-371.

Suciu, A. N., T. Iwatsubo et al. (2003). Theoretical investigation of an artificial joint with micro-pocket-covered component and biphasic cartilage on the opposite articulating surface. *J Biomech Eng* 125(4): 425-433.

Szafranski, J. D., A. J. Grodzinsky et al. (2004). Chondrocyte mechanotransduction: Effects of compression on deformation of intracellular organelles and relevance to cellular biosynthesis. *Osteoarthr Cartil* 12(12): 937-946.

Teeple, E., B. C. Fleming et al. (2007). Frictional properties of Hartley guinea pig knees with and without proteolytic disruption of the articular surfaces. *Osteoarthr Cartil* 15(3): 309-315.

Tomasini-Johansson, B. R., J. Milbrink et al. (1998). Vitronectin expression in rheumatoid arthritic synovia—Inhibition of plasmin generation by vitronectin produced in vitro. *Br J Rheumatol* 37(6): 620-629.

Tompson, S. W., B. Merriman et al. (2009). A recessive skeletal dysplasia, SEMD aggrecan type, results from a missense mutation affecting the C-type lectin domain of aggrecan. *Am J Hum Genet* 84(1): 72-79.

Trippel, S. B., M. G. Ehrlich et al. (1980). Characterization of chondrocytes from bovine articular cartilage. I. Metabolic and morphological experimental studies. *J Bone Joint Surg Am* 62(5): 816-820.

Tschumperlin, D. J., G. Dai et al. (2004). Mechanotransduction through growth-factor shedding into the extracellular space. *Nature* 429(6987): 83-86.

Van der Heiden, K., B. C. Groenendijk et al. (2006). Monocilia on chicken embryonic endocardium in low shear stress areas. *Dev Dyn* 235(1): 19-28.

van der Rest, M., and R. Garrone. (1991). Collagen family of proteins. *FASEB J* 5(13): 2814-2823.

Veje, K., J. L. Hyllested-Winge et al. (2003). Topographic and zonal distribution of tenascin in human articular cartilage from femoral heads: Normal versus mild and severe osteoarthritis. *Osteoarthr Cartil* 11(3): 217-227.

Veland, I. R., A. Awan et al. (2009). Primary cilia and signaling pathways in mammalian development, health and disease. *Nephron Physiol* 111(3): 39-53.

Venn, M., and A. Maroudas. (1977). Chemical composition and swelling of normal and osteoarthrotic femoral head cartilage. I. Chemical composition. *Ann Rheum Dis* 36(2): 121-129.

Vertel, B. M., A. Velasco et al. (1989). Precursors of chondroitin sulfate proteoglycan are segregated within a subcompartment of the chondrocyte endoplasmic reticulum. *J Cell Biol* 109(4 Pt 1): 1827-1836.

Vinall, R. L., and A. H. Reddi. (2001). The effect of BMP on the expression of cytoskeletal proteins and its potential relevance. *J Bone Joint Surg Am* 83(Suppl 1, Pt 1): S63-S69.

Wang, N., J. P. Butler et al. (1993). Mechanotransduction across the cell surface and through the cytoskeleton. *Science* 260(5111): 1124-1127.

Wang, N., J. D. Tytell et al. (2009). Mechanotransduction at a distance: Mechanically coupling the extracellular matrix with the nucleus. *Nat Rev Mol Cell Biol* 10(1): 75-82.

Watanabe, H., Y. Yamada et al. (1998). Roles of aggrecan, a large chondroitin sulfate proteoglycan, in cartilage structure and function. *J Biochem* 124(4): 687-693.

Williamson, A. K., A. C. Chen et al. (2003a). Tensile mechanical properties of bovine articular cartilage: Variations with growth and relationships to collagen network components. *J Orthop Res* 21(5): 872-880.

Williamson, A. K., K. Masuda et al. (2003b). Growth of immature articular cartilage in vitro: Correlated variation in tensile biomechanical and collagen network properties. *Tissue Eng* 9(4): 625-634.

Winterbottom, N., M. M. Tondravi et al. (1992). Cartilage matrix protein is a component of the collagen fibril of cartilage. *Dev Dyn* 193(3): 266-276.

Woo, S. L., W. H. Akeson et al. (1976). Measurements of nonhomogeneous, directional mechanical properties of articular cartilage in tension. *J Biomech* 9(12): 785-791.

Woo, S. L., P. Lubock et al. (1979). Large deformation nonhomogeneous and directional properties of articular cartilage in uniaxial tension. *J Biomech* 12(6): 437-446.

Woods, A., G. Wang et al. (2005). RhoA/ROCK signaling regulates Sox9 expression and actin organization during chondrogenesis. *J Biol Chem* 280(12): 11626-11634.

Wotton, S. F., V. C. Duance et al. (1988). Type IX collagen: A possible function in articular cartilage. *FEBS Lett* 234(1): 79-82.

Wright, V., and D. Dowson. (1976). Lubrication and cartilage. *J Anat* 121(Pt 1): 107-118.

Wu, J. P., T. B. Kirk et al. (2008). Study of the collagen structure in the superficial zone and physiological state of articular cartilage using a 3D confocal imaging technique. *J Orthop Surg* 3: 29.

Wu, Q., Y. Zhang et al. (2001). Indian hedgehog is an essential component of mechanotransduction complex to stimulate chondrocyte proliferation. *J Biol Chem* 276(38): 35290-35296.

Wu, W., R. C. Billinghurst et al. (2002). Sites of collagenase cleavage and denaturation of type II collagen in aging and osteoarthritic articular cartilage and their relationship to the distribution of matrix metalloproteinase 1 and matrix metalloproteinase 13. *Arthritis Rheum* 46(8): 2087-2094.

Yao, Z., H. Nakamura et al. (2004). Characterisation of cartilage intermediate layer protein (CILP)-induced arthropathy in mice. *Ann Rheum Dis* 63(3): 252-258.

Yoder, B. K. (2007). Role of primary cilia in the pathogenesis of polycystic kidney disease. *J Am Soc Nephrol* 18(5): 1381-1388.

Youn, I., J. B. Choi et al. (2006). Zonal variations in the three-dimensional morphology of the chondron measured in situ using confocal microscopy. *Osteoarthr Cartil* 14(9): 889-897.

Young, M. F., Y. Bi et al. (2002). Biglycan knockout mice: New models for musculoskeletal diseases. *Glycoconj J* 19(4-5): 257-262.

Young, S. R., R. Gerard-O'Riley et al. (2009). Focal adhesion kinase is important for fluid shear stress-induced mechanotransduction in osteoblasts. *J Bone Miner Res* 24(3): 411-424.

Zanetti, M., A. Ratcliffe et al. (1985). Two subpopulations of differentiated chondrocytes identified with a monoclonal antibody to keratan sulfate. *J Cell Biol* 101(1): 53-59.

Zappone, B., M. Ruths et al. (2007). Adsorption, lubrication, and wear of lubricin on model surfaces: Polymer brush-like behavior of a glycoprotein. *Biophys J* 92(5): 1693-1708.

Zhu, W., V. C. Mow et al. (1993). Viscoelastic shear properties of articular cartilage and the effects of glycosidase treatments. *J Orthop Res* 11(6): 771-781.

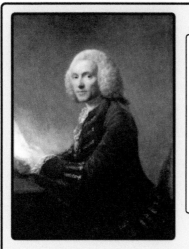

"Articulating cartilage is an elastic substance uniformly compact, of a white colour, and somewhat diaphanous, having a smooth polished surface covered with a membrane; harder and more brittle than a ligament, softer and more pliable than a bone." Hunter is most famous for his quote, "If we consult the standard chirurgical writers from Hippocrates down to the present age, we shall find, that an ulcerated cartilage is universally allowed to be a very troublesome disease; that it admits of a cure with more difficulty than carious bone; and that, when destroyed, it is not recovered."
William Hunter (1718-1783), Scottish physician and anatomist

"My more limited examinations of the human foetus have led me also to the conclusions that during the most early periods the cartilage of the epiphyseal extremities of bones does not contain any blood-vessels, and that notwithstanding their absence, the cells of this cartilage are developed, and its growth carried on; and that at the same time the cells of the epiphyseal and the articular cartilage are formed and developed without the presence of vessels. Into the substance of healthy (adult) articular cartilages I have never been able to trace blood-vessels, and my researches induce me to believe that they do not possess any."
Joseph Toynbee (1815-1866), English otologist

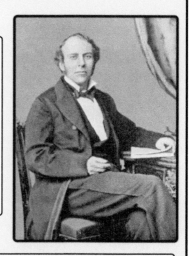

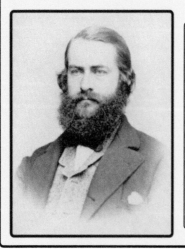

"[Cartilage is] thickest in those [joints] which are most moveable and subject to attrition." "We find all the conditions of a nutritive fluid due to the articular cartilage in the synovia, and it is particularly rich in albumen, the main element of nutrition of the cartilage. From several experiments I find the articular cartilages are quite capable of imbibing the synovial fluid…. [T]he wear of the articular cartilages must be more considerable than is generally supposed, although we really perceive but the slightest degree of diminution after a lapse of many years…. That such a repair is constantly going on is also rendered probable by the condition of the more superficial stratum of the articular cartilage."
Joseph Leidy (1823-1891), American paleontologist

Articular Cartilage Development

2

- Cartilage formation during embryogenesis
- Growth and maturation
- Signaling pathways during growth and maintenance

Classically, developmental biology has focused on articular cartilage from initial limb bud formation and chondrogenesis *in utero* until formation of an initial anlage of cartilage tissue shortly before birth. Following description of embryonic cartilage development, we discuss the overall growth, maturation, and life of articular cartilage through skeletal maturity and aging.

In Section 2.1, we begin our discussion of cartilage formation from embryonic limb bud development to the formation of the synovial joint. While the time for cartilage development varies by species, the steps of limb bud formation are similar. For example, in the mouse limb bud formation begins around day 9, with birth between days 17 and 21. In humans, limb bud initiation begins at week 4.5, and the limbs form during weeks 7-9 of fetal development, with birth at approximately week 40. While development occurs on the order of days to months, as contrasted to potentially decades for cartilage's maturation and serviceable life, the developmental period is extremely biologically complex.

We discuss in Section 2.2 how postnatal cartilage matures and changes with age to both skeletal maturity and beyond (Figure 2.1). Changes during this time are more gradual and less complex than those seen during development and represent adaptations to external forces due to daily activities. However, these changes may presage the events that lead to potential degradation (discussed in Chapter 3).

Changes during development, growth, maturation, and aging are mediated by multiple factors and signaling pathways. In Section 2.3, we discuss the exogenous morphogens and growth factors that feed into the signaling pathways and transcription factors during the life of cartilage (Figure 2.2). In Chapter 3, we discuss how misregulation of these pathways results in disease and degeneration.

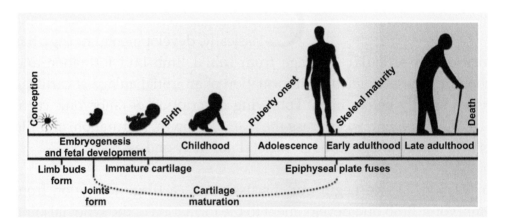

Figure 2.1 Development, growth, maturation, and aging of cartilage, in relation to human development and life (not to scale). Cartilage formation progresses from development in embryogenesis to formation of an initial immature cartilage. Tissue growth and maturation during infancy, childhood, and adolescence are marked by structural and biochemical changes until skeletal maturity in early adulthood. During early to middle adulthood (20s to mid-40s), cartilage properties are relatively stable, exhibiting only subtle changes. In late adulthood (50s onward), chondrocyte and cartilage properties may begin to decline with disease progression.

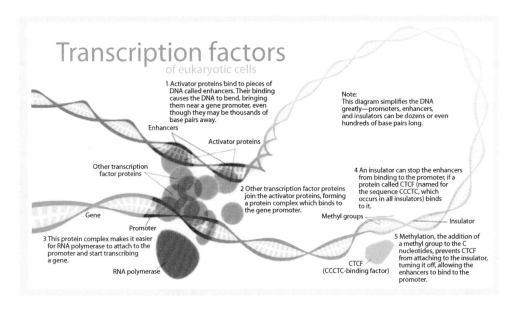

Figure 2.2 Schematic giving a general view of transcription factor function. Table 2.2 lists common transcription factors relevant in limb and cartilage. (From Creative Commons Attribution 3.0 Unported image by Kelvin Song.)

Morphogenesis and Morphogens: Morphogenesis is the developmental process of pattern formation and body plan establishment that culminates in the adult form of the whole human body, including component tissues and organs, such as articular cartilage and joints. Morphogens are extracellularly secreted proteins governing morphogenesis during development. They comprise four evolutionarily conserved protein families: bone morphogenetic proteins (BMPs), fibroblast growth factors (FGFs), hedgehog proteins (HHs), and wingless and int-related proteins (Wnts). These morphogen families exhibit redundant and reiterative signaling with distinct spatial and temporal expression during initiation of morphogenesis, including pattern formation, body plan establishment, bilateral symmetry, and attendant cytodifferentiation.

Bone Morphogenetic Proteins: Bone grafts have been used for more than a century by orthopedic surgeons to aid recalcitrant bone healing. Marshall Urist made the key discovery in 1965 (Urist 1965) that demineralized, lyophilized segments of rabbit bone induced new bone at sites of intramuscular implantation. Thus, the signals for bone formation are resident in the bone matrix. The signals inducing bone morphogenesis, the BMPs, were isolated from demineralized bone matrix by extraction in guanidine, heparin affinity chromatography, and preparative electrophoresis (Reddi 1998a,b). The activity of BMPs was bioassayed by reconstitution with insoluble collagenous bone matrix and implantation in rats (Reddi and Huggins 1972). The resultant stages of bone morphogenesis recapitulate embryonic endochondral bone formation, including chemotaxis, mitosis, and differentiation initially of cartilage that is transient, followed by lasting bone differentiation from stem or progenitor cells. Thus, BMPs direct and induce cartilage and bone morphogenesis *in vivo*.

The human genome encodes for 20 BMPs. BMPs are dimeric proteins that are critically dependent on a single intermolecular disulfide bond for their activity in bone and cartilage morphogenesis. The BMP family consists of four distinct subfamilies:

- BMP2 and 4
- BMP3 and 3B; also known as growth/differentiation factor 10 (GDF10)
- BMP5-8
- GDF5-7; also known as cartilage-derived morphogenetic proteins (CDMPs) 1-3, respectively

It is noteworthy that BMP1 is not a member of the BMP family, but rather is a procollagen C-proteinase involved in the proteolytic processing of soluble procollagen, resulting in self-assembly of insoluble collagen fibers in the extracellular matrix (Reddi 1996).

Fibroblast Growth Factors: FGFs were originally identified and isolated as mitogens for fibroblasts and mesenchymal cells; hence, they were named *fibroblast growth factors*. In the initial stages of investigations, two isoforms were identified: acidic and basic FGFs, also known as FGF1 and FGF2, respectively. There are, at present, 28 isoforms of FGFs implicated in a variety of diverse functions, including morphogenesis of the limb buds in chick and mouse embryos. FGF2 has been demonstrated to be functional in articular cartilage regeneration (Itoh and Ornitz 2011).

Hedgehog Proteins: The hedgehog proteins are signaling molecules initially identified in classic genetic screens in fruit flies, *Drosophila melanogaster* (Nusslein-Volhard and Wieschaus 1980). Homologous genes were subsequently isolated in mice and humans and named *sonic hedgehog* (Shh), *Indian hedgehog* (Ihh), and *desert hedgehog* (Dhh). Members of the hedgehog family bind to their cognate receptors patched (PTC) and also bind transmembrane protein smoothened (Smo) (Figure 2.3). Activation of the hedgehog signaling pathway results in functional activation of the Gli family of transcription factors. The sonic and Indian hedgehog proteins have been implicated in prehypertrophic chondrocytes in the epiphyseal growth plate, and, therefore, in chondrogenesis and longitudinal growth of mammals (Beachy et al. 2010).

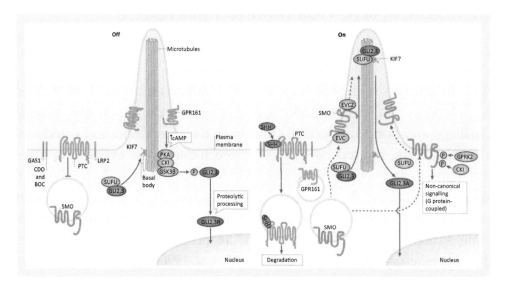

Figure 2.3 Hedgehog-patched (HH-PTC) signaling pathway interaction with the primary cilium. In the off state (left), PTC acts to inhibit smoothened (Smo) activity and is localized near and within the primary cilium. In the on state (right), with the addition of Shh, Smo is activated by phosphorylation and enters the primary cilium while PTC exits. This activation of Smo is also thought to activate the non-canonical signaling pathway. (Adapted from Briscoe, J., and P. P. Therond, *Nat Rev Mol Cell Biol* 14(7): 416-429, 2013. With permission.)

Wingless and int-Related Proteins: Originally, the wingless genes were identified in *Drosophila* wing development pathways. Nusse et al. (1984) first described the int family of genes in virus-induced mammary tumors. The int genes were homologous to *Drosophila* wingless genes, and the nomenclature Wnts derives from the fusion of Wingless and ints. There are about 20 Wnt genes in mammals. Wnts signal via the Frizzled family of cell surface receptors. In the absence of the Wnt ligand, the enzyme glycogen synthase kinase 3 (GSK3) phosphorylates β-catenin and targets it for degradation by proteosomes. However, when Wnt activates the cognate cell surface Frizzled receptors, the GSK3 activity is blocked, rendering the β-catenin stable and resulting in translocation into the nucleus to activate the transcription factor lymphoid enhancer factor (LEF)/T-cell transcription factor (TCF). Wnts have been implicated in articular cartilage homeostasis and function (Nusse 2005).

2.1 CELLULAR BEHAVIOR DURING EMBRYOGENESIS

2.1.1 Limb Precursor Cell Origin

As in all animals with bilateral symmetry, human embryos develop three germ layers, endoderm, mesoderm, and ectoderm, during embryogenesis. Cartilage and bone are derived from both the mesoderm and ectoderm. The mesoderm, interposed between the ectoderm and endoderm, gives rise to articular cartilage of the long bones. From the mesoderm, the axial skeleton forms from the somites. The somites give rise to muscle, skin, and cartilage, and this process is initiated by its splitting into myotome, dermatome, syndetome, and sclerotome. The lateral plate mesoderm generates the appendicular skeleton (limbs) (Olson et al. 1996), specifically the bony and cartilaginous components of the limb, while cells from the myotome eventually form the muscular components. The craniofacial cartilages arise from the ectoderm in response to cells migrating from the neural crest.

During development of the limbs, the limb precursor cells migrate from the originating germ-layer structures following a chemotactic trail to their eventual location, where they undergo mesenchyme cell-to-cell adhesion

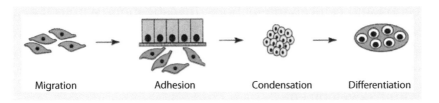

Figure 2.4 The initiating steps in limb development are dependent on cell migration, adhesion, condensation (mitosis and aggregation), and differentiation. (From Hall, B. K., and T. Miyake, *Bioessays* 22(2): 138-147, 2000. With permission.)

mediated by the actions of integrins and cadherins. This migration is driven by chemotaxis, the act of cells moving toward, or away from, a concentration gradient of a specific molecule. The signals that induce chemotaxis are the chemokines, small 8-10 kDa proteins that direct cell movement. This migration is dependent on control of the cytoskeleton and interactions with cell adhesion receptors and the extracellular matrix substrate.

Once these precursor cells have migrated to their destination, they undergo mesenchymal condensation (Hall and Miyake 1992, 2000). Adhesion is a prerequisite for condensation; aggregation and mitosis increase cell density. Condensation leads to differentiation, which produces the correct cell types that lead to cartilage formation (Figure 2.4).

2.1.1.1 Cell Adhesion Molecules

Cell adhesion mechanisms were initially proposed based on a series of experiments performed in the 1950s and 1960s by Aaron Moscona that examined the reaggregation of cells from disassociated embryos (Moscona and Moscona 1952; Moscona 1968). This led to the *differential adhesion hypothesis* by Malcom Steinberg to explain the sorting of mixtures consisting of different cell types (Steinberg and Roth 1964). Sorting was based on differences in the surface tension of various cells, modeled as viscoelastic fluids (Steinberg and Takeichi 1994). This hypothesis would be further elaborated upon with the identification of specific cell adhesion molecules. In cartilage development, the main molecules active in cell adhesion are the cadherins and integrins. Areas of mesenchymal condensation initiate further differentiation, which is dependent on cell aggregation and cell-cell interactions. Investigations with cell aggregation inhibitors, such as carboxymethyl cellulose, can block differentiation of prechondrogenic cells into chondrocytes (Tacchetti et al. 1992). Table 2.1 lists the most common adhesion molecules in cartilage and during limb development.

Table 2.1 Cell adhesion molecules in cartilage and limb development

Family/name	Ligand/extracellular substrate	Binding site
Cadherins		
N-cadherin (a.k.a. neural cadherin, NCAD, or cadherin 2 [CDH2])	Cadherin (homophilic binding)	EC1 domain
Cadherin 11	Cadherin (homophilic binding)	EC1 domain
Integrins		
$\alpha_1\beta_1$	Collagen, laminin	DGEA
$\alpha_2\beta_1$	Collagen, laminin	DGEA
$\alpha_3\beta_1$	Collagen, laminin, fibronectin	
$\alpha_4\beta_1$	Fibronectin (type III connecting domain)	EILDV
$\alpha_5\beta_1$	Fibronectin (RGD [Arg-Gly-Asp]-containing domain)	RGD
$\alpha_{10}\beta_1$	Collagen	RGD
$\alpha_V\beta_3$	Denatured collagen, vitronectin, fibrinogen, fibulin, osteopontin	RGD
$\alpha_V\beta_5$	Vitronectin	RGD
Other molecules		
CD44	Hyaluronan, collagen, matrix metalloproteinases (MMPs), osteopontin	HA binding domain
N-CAM (neural cell adhesion molecule)	N-CAM (homophilic binding)	Ig domain
Syndecan	Tenascin, fibronectin (heparin binding domain)	Chondroitin sulfate, heparin sulfate

2.1.1.1.1 Cadherins

Cadherin (calcium-dependent adhesion) molecules are transmembrane proteins first identified by Masatoshi Takeichi as a specific cell adhesion factor (Takeichi 1977). Extracellularly, cadherins preferentially bind to other cadherins of the same type; for example, N-cadherin (neural cadherin, first identified in neural cells) prefers to complex with other N-cadherins. Intracellularly, cadherins are regulated through association with catenins and the actin cytoskeleton (Figure 2.5), and this association plays a role in signal transduction (Miller and Moon 1996). Studies using N-cadherin-perturbing antibodies have shown that N-cadherin plays a critical role in condensation, though work using organ culture of N-cadherin-deficient limb buds demonstrated that mesenchymal condensation and chondrogenesis were not affected (Luo et al. 2005). In adult cartilage where cell-to-cell contacts are minimal, cadherins are sparse (Widelitz et al. 1993; Oberlender and Tuan 1994a,b).

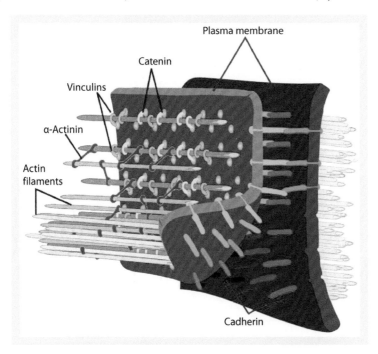

Figure 2.5 Schematic of cadherin-based adherens cell-cell junction and associated proteins. Cadherins ultimately link to the actin cytoskeleton via a series of structural proteins. (Modified from image by Mariana Ruiz, public domain.)

2.1.1.1.2 Integrins

Integrins are heterodimeric transmembrane proteins that interact with both the extracellular matrix and the intracellular actin cytoskeleton through focal adhesions and play a key role in transducing extracellular signals into the cytoskeleton. While integrins were proposed and named by Hynes in the 1980s (Tamkun et al. 1986; Hynes 1987), Pytela et al. (1985) were the first to purify and sequence an integrin while looking for a cell surface receptor for fibronectin. Integrin substrates (listed in Table 2.1) are numerous, reflecting the broad array of tissues involved; however, a common element to these substrates is the presence of an Arg-Gly-Asp (RGD) peptide that interacts with the integrin binding region (Figure 2.6).

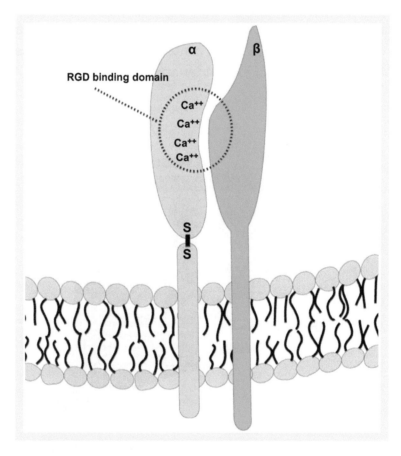

Figure 2.6 Schematic of integrins as heterodimeric transmembrane proteins with calcium-dependent binding domain.

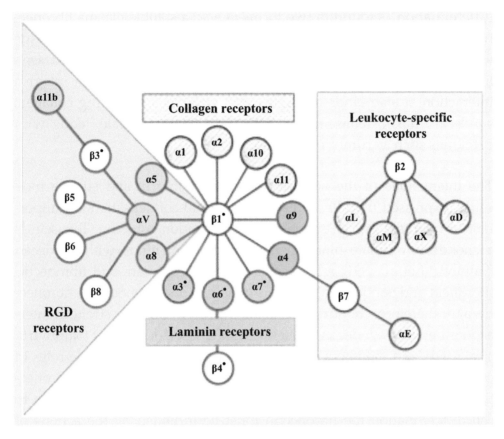

Figure 2.7 Schematic representation of mammalian integrin receptor αβ subunit combinations and their extracellular matrix interactions. (From Hynes, R. O., *Cell* 110(6): 673-687, 2002. With permission.)

Common extracellular matrix binding substrates include fibronectin, vitronectin, laminin, and the collagens (Figure 2.7). Interactions between cadherins and integrins have also been described (Wang et al. 2009).

2.1.1.1.3 Integrin-Extracellular Matrix Interactions

Fibronectin was discovered simultaneously by multiple researchers in the early 1970s (Hakomori 1973; Hynes 1973; Ruoslahti et al. 1973; Vaheri and Ruoslahti 1974; Yamada et al. 1978) and was given a multitude of names. These early papers described a disulfide-bonded glycoprotein dimer with ~250 kDa subunits that was expressed by normal, but not tumor, cells. Fibronectin, involved in cell adhesion, migration, and differentiation, is found in two forms *in vivo*: a soluble plasma fibronectin of 200-250 kDa and a 550 kDa insoluble tissue fibronectin. The tissue form is found in relatively high abundance in the cartilage extracellular matrix. While fibronectin contains an RGD sequence for integrin interaction, it also binds multiple other molecules, including collagen, syndecan, fibrin, tenascin, heparin, and heparan sulfate, along with cytokines such as tumor necrosis factor α (TNF-α).

The interactions of the nascent extracellular matrix and surface molecules expressed by cells in the mesenchymal condensation are important in maintaining cell shape and condensation cohesion. Tenascin is a chondroitin sulfate binding glycoprotein that binds with syndecan (Salmivirta et al. 1991), a heparin sulfate proteoglycan, and fibronectin (Bernfield and Sanderson 1990); this interaction helps modulate fibronectin and, therefore, chondrogenesis. Interestingly, binding strength interactions between syndecan and tenascin are tissue dependent (Salmivirta et al. 1991), and members of the syndecan family have multiple roles in condensation organization and eventual differentiation. While fibronectin helps to maintain condensation (Leonard et al. 1991), to progress to cell differentiation the fibronectin must be inhibited by the actions of tenascin (Pacifici et al. 1993). Mouse knockouts of tenascin develop normal condensations, indicating that other compensatory genes may play a role (Saga et al. 1992). As these factors help to shape the condensate edges, noggin (a BMP antagonist) is expressed and then binds to BMPs to curtail cell proliferation, halting condensation growth (Capdevila and Johnson 1998; McMahon et al. 1998).

While similar to fibronectin in action and containing the integrin RGD interacting sequence, vitronectin is a 75 kDa cell adhesion glycoprotein with an N-terminal somatomedin B domain (Keijer et al. 1991; Kost et al. 1992; Tomasini-Johansson et al. 1998) and central and C-terminal hemopexin homology (Jenne and Stanley 1985). Vitronectin has a critical role in coagulation and inhibition of cell damage during complement activation and has been linked to regulation of cell migration and adhesion during cancer metastasis. *In vitro*, chondrocytes bind readily to vitronectin or fibronectin-coated surfaces.

Chondronectin is a glycoprotein with modes of action similar to those of fibronectin. Chondronectin mediates attachment of chondrocytes to type II collagen but requires interactions with proteoglycan monomers to achieve attachment; it is also found interacting with type II collagen in the vitreous of the eye (Hewitt et al. 1982a,b; Burton-Wurster et al. 1988).

Laminins were initially identified as noncollagenous, large molecular polypeptide chains (220 and 440 kDa) of the basement membrane of a transplantable mouse tumor (Timpl et al. 1979). Laminins are heterotrimeric extracellular glycoproteins consisting of α, β, and γ chains that can self-bind to form lattice structures, while also having domains to bind collagen, integrins, and proteoglycans. In chondrocytes, laminin 1 (LN-1) binds to β_1 integrin, specifically integrin $\alpha_6\beta_1$ (Durr et al. 1996). Laminins are present in most tissues and help to resist tensile forces in the basal laminae through the production of their lattice structural network.

2.1.1.1.4 Other Cell Adhesion Molecules in Limb Development

The differentiation of cells in mesenchymal condensation is mediated by epithelial-mesenchymal interactions, initiated by transforming growth factor β (TGF-β) (Chiquet-Ehrismann et al. 1989; Vaahtokari et al. 1991). TGF-β participates in condensation by regulating fibronectin (Leonard et al. 1991), which in turn regulates neural cell adhesion molecule (N-CAM) (Chimal-Monroy and Diaz de Leon 1999), which is required for maintenance of condensation along with N-cadherin (Oberlender and Tuan 1994a,b; Tavella et al. 1994; Woodward and Tuan 1999). N-CAM is not required for initiating condensation (Chimal-Monroy and Diaz de Leon 1999) but instead in its maintenance. Activin, a member of the TGF-β superfamily, also increases expression of N-CAM (Jiang et al. 1993) and furthers chondrogenesis. The presence of syndecan results in inactivated N-CAM, thus, setting the boundaries for condensation (Widelitz et al. 1993).

2.1.1.2 Initiation of Limb

Initiation of the forelimbs and hindlimbs is controlled by expression of different T-box (Tbx) DNA binding domain-containing transcription factors. Based on initial overexpression models, Tbx4 and 5 were thought to regulate forelimb and hindlimb discrimination, as the expression of *tbx* genes 5 and 4 differs, respectively, between forelimbs and hindlimbs. However, these have been reclassed as limb initiators, not as determiners of forelimb or hindlimb (Minguillon et al. 2005). Instead, induction of morphology specific to the hindlimb has been supported as a role for Pitx1 (DeLaurier et al. 2006). Interestingly, although the molecular components and steps of limb bud initiation are similar between eutherian (placental) and marsupial mammals, the forelimb initiation and subsequent development occur at a much earlier developmental stage, enabling *ex utero* migration of the joey to the pouch (Keyte and Smith 2010). A rough timeline of limb and cartilage formation is depicted in Figure 2.8.

Interactions between the encapsulating ectodermal cells and the limb bud mesenchymal cells result in the formation of the limb, arising from the limb field, as the ectodermal cells secrete FGFs (FGF7 and 10) (Martin 1998; Yonei-Tamura et al. 1999) to produce the limb organizing structure known as the apical ectodermal ridge (AER), which determines the proximal-distal axis.

The limb bud expresses the transcription factors homeobox protein aristaless-like 4 (Alx4) in the anterior region and homeobox protein b8 (Hoxb8) in the posterior region (Figure 2.10). The zone of polarizing activity (ZPA), which determines the anterior-posterior axis of the developing limb, arises where Hoxb8's expression intersects the AER (Charite et al. 1994). The ZPA is marked by the expression of Shh, BMP2, BMP4, and FGF4. FGF4 and BMP2 regulate the proliferation of the underlying mesenchyme with counteracting roles; FGF4 stimulates proliferation, while BMP2 inhibits proliferation and initiates chondrogenesis (Niswander and Martin 1993a,b; Niswander et al. 1994). The AER produces a feedback loop of FGF8 (initiated by Wnt3a and interacting with

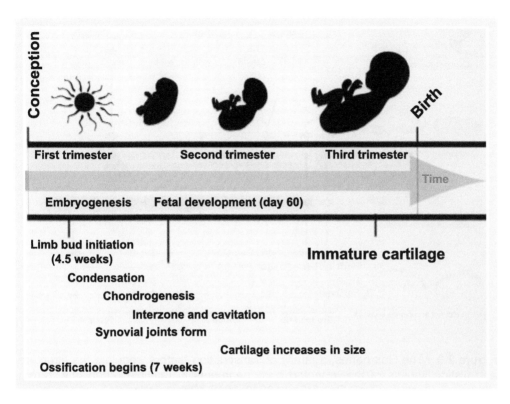

Figure 2.8 As described in the text, changes in the developing embryo and cartilage occur rapidly during the first 9 weeks following conception, when the limb buds and synovial joints form.

FGF10) and FGF4 (which regulates Shh) (Moon and Capecchi 2000). Shh signaling helps maintain FGF10 secretion, which induces proliferation in the mesoderm; it also upregulates the BMP antagonist Gremlin in the mesenchyme, inhibiting BMP and maintaining proliferation (Zuniga et al. 1999). Maintenance of the FGF10 expression is also under control by two different Wnt family members (Wnt2b and Wnt8c). Experimental work in chick limb buds has demonstrated that the function of the AER can be duplicated by the implantation of an FGF4 bead at the site where the AER was removed (Niswander et al. 1994). This is sufficient to upregulate Msx1 expression, which is then maintained by FGF2 and BMP4 (Tickle 2002, 2003). DLX5 (distal-less homeobox) transcription factor is also transiently expressed with implantation of FGF2-soaked beads, and chick limb studies indicate DLX5 may be needed to maintain the AER (Ferrari et al. 1999). The DLX family has been implicated in the regulation

97

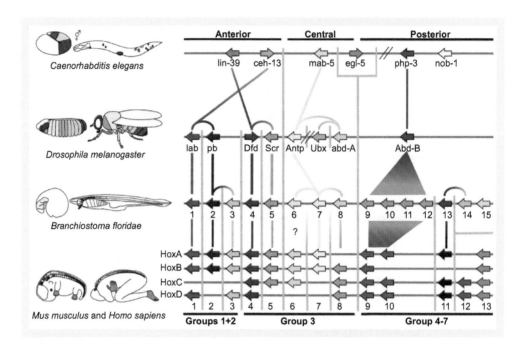

Figure 2.9 The Hox genes, a family of transcription factors, regulate the structure and distinctiveness of the repeated body segments in multiple organisms. (From Hueber, S. D. et al., *PLoS One* 5(5): e10820, 2010. With permission.)

of craniofacial cartilages in zebrafish models (Ellies et al. 1997). DLX5 is expressed in hypertrophic chondrocytes and areas of chondrocytes initiating differentiation, and appears to be under the control of BMP7 (Holleville et al. 2003). It should be noted that while a somewhat linear process is described above, the precise hierarchical relationship and cross-regulation of these factors by Hox genes are still unclear.

Other relevant transcription factors during cartilage development include Pax1 and scleraxis (Table 2.2), which activate cartilage-specific genes (Cserjesi et al. 1995; Sosic et al. 1997). Members of the Sox protein family, specifically Sox9, Sox5, and Sox6, are also expressed in prechondrogenic cells, with Sox9 being necessary for the mesenchymal aggregation (Bi et al. 1999). This differentiation of mesenchymal cells into chondroblasts and further into chondrocytes is under the control of BMP2, BMP4 and 7, and TGF-β (Cole et al. 2003; Tickle 2003). A temporal expression profile of various transcription factors is depicted in Figure 2.11.

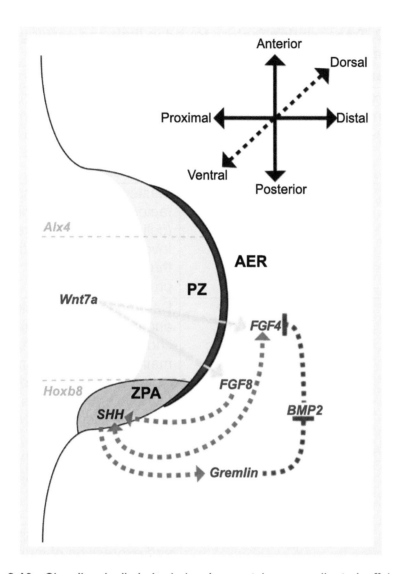

Figure 2.10 Signaling in limb bud development is a coordinated affair among several factors (signaling factors in blue, transcription factors in green). The apical ectodermal ridge (AER) is the limb organizing structure; it provides spatial and temporal cues (growth factors) along the proximal-distal axis to shape the developing limb. The progress zone (PZ), which drives limb bud lengthening, is adjacent to the AER. The ZPA determines the anterior-posterior axis. The transcription factors Hoxb8 and Alx4 determine the initial anterior-posterior axis.

Table 2.2 Transcription factors found in limb and cartilage development and maintenance

Gene family	Members	Function
Sox: Sex-determining region Y (SRY)-box		Main cartilage transcription factors that contain an HMG (High-Mobility Group) box domain that binds the sequence AACAAT.
	Sox9	Master cartilage transcription factor; required for Col2a1 (collagen type II) expression. Involved in condensation through chondrocyte prehypertrophy.
	L-Sox5 (L = long)	Dependent on BMP signaling and expression of multiple chondrocyte extracellular matrix proteins. Has multiple isoforms with the L isoform found in chondrocytes. Activates Col2a1 and AGC1 (collagen type II and aggrecan). Involved in chondrocyte differentiation through chondrocyte prehypertrophy.
	Sox6	Dependent on BMP signaling and expression of multiple chondrocyte extracellular matrix proteins; interacts with other Sox members. Involved in chondrocyte differentiation through chondrocyte prehypertrophy.

(Continued)

Table 2.2 (Continued) Transcription factors found in limb and cartilage development and maintenance

Gene family	Members	Function
Hox (HoxA, HoxD) (homeobox) (Figure 2.9)		Main transcription factors that determine body patterning through spatial and temporal regulation (Figure 2.9). Homeobox genes are found in clusters designated A, B, C, and D that correspond to body regions.
	Hoxa2	Determines condensation boundary; regulated by BMPs.
	Hoxa11, Hoxd11	Controls cell morphogenesis and differentiation; necessary for proper forelimb formation.
	Hoxd12	Regulates Shh.
	Hoxa13, Hoxd13	Involved in adhesion during condensation, and differentiation; necessary for proper forelimb and hindlimb formation.
Tbx: T-box protein		Differentially expressed between hindlimbs and forelimbs. Initiates limb bud formation by activating Wnt and FGF.
	Tbx4	Expressed in hindlimb buds but not forelimbs.
	Tbx5	Expressed in forelimb buds but not hindlimbs.
DLX: Distal-less homeobox		Linked to a hox cluster; homolog of *Distal-less* in *Drosophila*.

(Continued)

Table 2.2 (Continued) Transcription factors found in limb and cartilage development and maintenance

Gene family	Members	Function
	DLX5	Interacts with Msx1 and Msx2. Regulated by BMPs involved in osteoblast differentiation.
Pitx: Paired-like homeodomain		Family of transcription factors involved in organ development and left and right asymmetry.
	Pitx1	Required for development of hindlimb buds; initiates the hindlimb buds; upstream of Tbx4.
	Pitx2	Regulates expression of lysyl hydroxylase, which is necessary for collagen stabilization (Section 1.3.3).
PAX: Paired-box transcription factor		Controls pattern formation, and early axial and limb skeletal development.
	Pax1	Expressed in anterior proximal domain of limb bud; inhibited by BMPs.
	Pax9	Downstream of Gli3 and Shh; interacts with Msx1. Involved in skeletal morphogenesis; expressed in the AER.
PRX: Paired-box homeodomain		Necessary for limb development; some redundancy between Prx1 and Prx2.
	Prx1	Expressed in mesenchyme of the developing limb.

(Continued)

Table 2.2 (Continued) Transcription factors found in limb and cartilage development and maintenance

Gene family	Members	Function
	Prx2	Expressed in mesenchyme of the developing limb.
MSX: msh (muscle segment homeobox in *Drosophila*) homeobox homolog		Initiates epithelial-mesenchyme interaction, involved in limb patterning, and expressed in the AER. Redundancy between Msx1 and Msx2.
	Msx1, Msx2	Distal limb mesenchyme in the AER; helps to specify dorsal and ventral boundaries.
Other important transcription factors		
Runx2: (Cbfa1, Osf2)-runt-domain transcription factor		Chondroblast differentiation, osteoblast differentiation, and skeletal morphogenesis. Part of a larger DNA binding complex.
Scleraxis		A basic helix-loop-helix transcription factor; involved in mesoderm formation and mesenchymal progenitors for tendon; interacts with Sox9.
Fra2: FOS-like antigen		Leucine zipper containing transcription factor; forms AP1 complex; helps chondrocyte differentiation from proliferative to hypertrophic.
Lef1 (Tcf): Lymphoid enhancer binding factor		Wnt3a modulated in the AER; needed for limb bud development.

(Continued)

Table 2.2 (Continued) Transcription factors found in limb and cartilage development and maintenance

Gene family	Members	Function
Gli: Isolated initially in glioblastoma		C2H2 zinc-finger transcription factors that regulate Shh signaling; some redundancy between Gli1, Gli2, and Gli3. All are found in the AER.
	Gli2	Downstream of Shh and also regulates Shh expression, and Shh target genes.
	Gli3	Modulates Shh signaling; Shh activates Gli3 in the posterior region of the ZPA, and induces expression of Gli1 (also required for limb development).
SP(XKLF): Initially isolated using a Sephacryl and phosphocellulose column		Zinc-finger transcription factors that bind to GT and CACCC box sequences.
	Epiprofin (Epfn/Sp6)	Modulates Wnt signaling in the AER.
	Osterix (Sp7)	Required for osteoblast differentiation; downstream of Runx2.
Alx4: Aristaless-like homeobox		Interacts with Gli3, Lef1, and Shh in the AER mesenchyme. Helps to regulate anterior and posterior patterning in the developing limb.
Chicken winged-helix-loop/ forkhead transcription factor 1 (cFKH-1)	Related to mammalian MFH (mesenchyme forkhead) family	Like MFH-1, cFKH-1 regulates proliferation of cells in mesenchymal condensation. This is mediated by regulation of Smads in the TGF-β pathway.

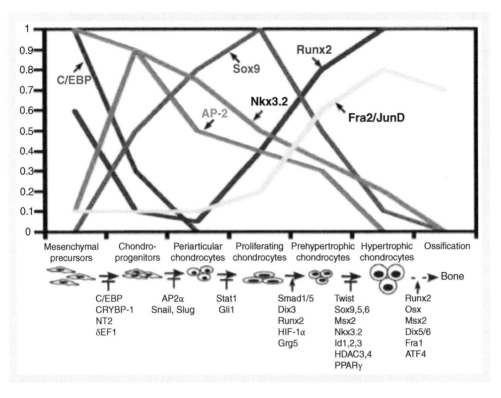

Figure 2.11 Temporal expression of selected transcription factors during bone formation. The y-axis represents arbitrary expression units. Descriptions for these transcription factors can be found in Table 2.2. (From Goldring, M. B. et al., *J Cell Biochem* 97(1): 33-44, 2006. With permission.)

The axial skeleton forms from mesenchymal cells derived from the paraxial mesoderm segmentation into somites (Christ and Wilting 1992). Examples of axial skeleton cartilages include rib, intervertebral disc, and facet joint cartilages. The craniofacial cartilage and bone are derived from neural crest cells of ectodermal origin (Noden 1983). The temporomandibular joint cartilages (i.e., disc, condyle, and fossa), along with auricular and nasal cartilages, are examples of craniofacial cartilages. The sequential development of cartilage described below appears to be similar in cartilages originating from the neural crest and from the lateral plate mesoderm (e.g., cartilage of the hip, knee, and ankle).

2.1.2 Chondrocyte Differentiation and Joint Development

The development of the skeletal elements and the synovial joints begins with the developing limb, through which cell migration, proliferation, and apoptosis are precisely coordinated in three dimensions (Pacifici et al. 2006). This development is orchestrated by the correct temporal and spatial expression (and overlap) of multiple secreted signals, including the FGFs, HHs, Wnts, and TGF family members, including BMPs and GDFs (Martin 1998; Hartmann and Tabin 2001; Tickle 2002; Settle et al. 2003; Rountree et al. 2004).

Within the developing limb, two distinct lineages of chondrocytes will form, those destined to form the growth plate and those which will form the articular cartilage at the ends of the bones. In articular cartilage, the chondrocytes proliferate and produce type II collagen and other matrix proteins and begin to form cartilaginous tissue within the anlage; this will persist as cartilage throughout life. However, in the growth plate the chondrocytes will ultimately undergo hypertrophy and be replaced with bone.

It is the growth plate cartilage that determines the longitudinal growth of long bones. The chondrocytes of the growth plate have characteristic stages of differentiation and proliferation by region (as diagrammed in Figure 2.12). During postnatal growth, the action of proliferating and differentiating chondrocytes increases the bone length through interstitial growth. Shortly before birth, a secondary ossification center will form at the epiphysis of the cartilage anlage, forming the epiphyseal plate. This will be replaced with bone as the organism ages, until skeletal maturation, usually in the mid-20s in humans. Endochondral ossification of the epiphyseal plate (growth plate) may resemble the stages of matrix destruction associated with osteoarthritis (Dreier 2010), as discussed in Section 3.1.3. Many of the experiments determining signaling pathways in chondrocyte differentiation and development derive from studies in mouse mutations, as disruption of genetic components commonly presents as easily

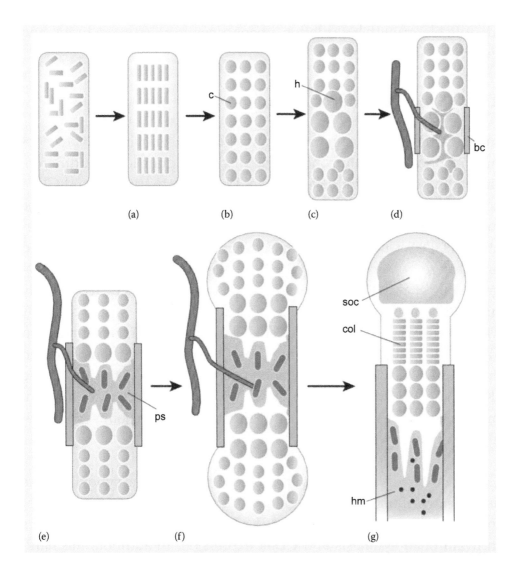

Figure 2.12 Development of the growth plate and the stages of endochondral bone formation proceed from mesenchymal cell condensation (a) to chondrocyte (indicated by the letter c) differentiation (b) and hypertrophy (letter h) (c). The bone collar (bc) forms from osteoblasts; this is mineralized and vascularized and will become cortical bone (d). This indicates initiation of the primary ossification center. The primary spongiosa (ps) (e) forms from osteoblasts following vascularization (f). This will become the trabecular bone, and the bone continues to lengthen at the ends due to columnar chondrocyte proliferation (col) as the secondary ossification center (soc) forms (g). As the bone matures, hematopoietic marrow (hm) fills the central region. (From Kronenberg, H. M., *Nature* 423(6937): 332-336, 2003. With permission from Nature Publishing Group.)

107

identifiable growth retardation phenotypes (e.g., stunted limbs and dwarfism) (Kronenberg 2003).

2.1.2.1 Synovial Joint Formation

In the cartilage anlage, in presumptive areas of synovial joint development, a prominent interzone can be discerned prior to overt differentiation. In fields of joint development, Wnt5, Wnt14 (Wnt9a), and GDF5 cooperate to induce joint formation. Wnt14 is critical in determining the location of the joint in the developing skeleton; this requires the cooperation of GDF5. Under these signals, the interzone cells become flattened and change from expressing type II collagen to expressing type I collagen (Craig et al. 1987). Induction of the interzone cells is not completely understood and may have species variations (Francis-West et al. 1999). The interzone cells appear to selectively express Wnt14 (Hartmann and Tabin 2001) and act as a signaling center through expression of noggin and chordin for control of cavitation and production of the joint space (Koyama et al. 2007; Seemann et al. 2009). Noggin is critical for joint morphogenesis, as mice lacking noggin fail to produce joints (Brunet et al. 1998; Tylzanowski et al. 2006).

Cavitation begins as a multistep process that forms the synovial space as the extracellular matrix degrades or changes through the death of interzone cells, differential growth (Kavanagh et al. 2002), and increases in hyaluronan synthesis and CD44 expression. In addition, mechanical forces play an important role in cavitation (Dowthwaite et al. 1998). Repression of chondrogenic signals by the interzone likely promotes differentiation of the other tissues of the joint into tendon and ligament, which also form from mesenchymal condensations and are produced in concert with the developing joint cartilage (Figure 2.13) (Pacifici et al. 2006). In the knee, the interzone will also form the fibrocartilaginous meniscus (Merida-Velasco et al. 1997). Following cavitation and interzone formation, the cells undergo differentiation via transcriptional activation of Hoxd11-13 (Goff and Tabin 1997). The molecular events

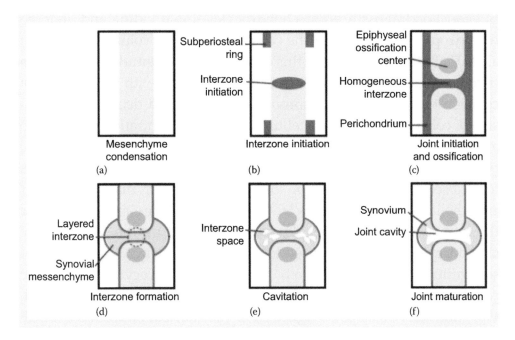

Figure 2.13 Interzone and cavitation in joint formation, progressing from mesenchyme condensation (a), initiation of the interzone and joint formation (b), to ossification of the epiphyseal centers (c). As the interzone forms, it differentiates into a layered structure, and the synovial mesenchyme appears (d). This interzone space then forms cavities through selective apoptosis that will form the joint cavity (e). The initial blueprint for the joint is established (f); however, the joint will continue to mature until skeletal maturity is reached.

described earlier correspond to the point of chondrogenesis and perichondrium formation.

2.1.3 Tissue Hypertrophy and Ossification

Developmentally, cartilage serves as a template for bone morphogenesis. Osteogenesis can occur via intramembranous ossification, which is the direct conversion of mesenchymal tissue into bone, or via endochondral ossification, which is through the calcification of cartilage tissue (Horton 1990). For example, endochondral ossification occurs in cartilages of the somites to form the vertebrae by stopping just short of the facet joint. Similarly, the articulating cartilages of the limbs are preserved as ossification progresses through cartilages of the lateral plate.

In endochondral ossification, chondrocytes stop dividing and undergo hypertrophy, during which the cells increase their volume (Farnum et al. 2002). In the growth plate, this contributes to longitudinal expansion (Kronenberg 2003). The cartilage matrix is altered with the addition of collagen type X, increased fibronectin content, and decreased expression of collagen type II. Intracellular calcium concentration also rises to aid in the production of exocytotic vesicles, which will release alkaline phosphatases, metalloproteinases (MMPs), and calcium phosphates for subsequent mineralization of the extracellular matrix. Vascular endothelial growth factor (VEGF), which mediates angiogenesis or the formation of blood vessels, is also secreted by the hypertrophic chondrocytes (Descalzi Cancedda et al. 1995; Gilbert 2003). Blood vessels infiltrate the cartilage, the hypertrophic chondrocytes die, and the cells that surrounded the cartilage become osteoblasts (Thompson et al. 1989) (the last two steps of Figure 2.14). Vascularization from the VEGF secreted by hypertrophic chondrocytes lays the groundwork for invasion by osteoblasts and osteoclasts (Gerber et al. 1999; Carlevaro et al. 2000). Hypertrophic chondrocytes die through apoptosis, and the cartilage matrix serves as a template for bone formation by osteoblasts. The hypertrophic chondrocyte can be thought of as the regulator of matrix calcification, vascularization, and future ossification.

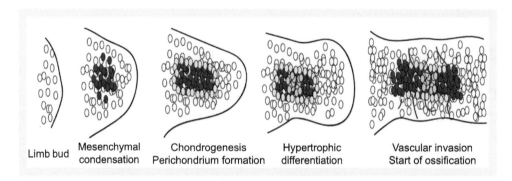

| Limb bud | Mesenchymal condensation | Chondrogenesis Perichondrium formation | Hypertrophic differentiation | Vascular invasion Start of ossification |

Figure 2.14 Mesenchymal condensation and chondrogenesis in the formation of the cartilage anlage. From left to right, cells first condense (red) and differentiate into chondrocytes. Boundaries are defined as the perichondrium forms (in yellow). Certain chondrocytes undergo hypertrophy (green cells) to eventually mineralize, resulting in bone formation through endochondral ossification.

It has been shown that hypertrophy follows chondrocytes switching from aerobic to anaerobic respiration. Evidence for this is provided by examining creatine kinase, an enzyme that catalyzes the formation of ATP in tissues under oxygen stress. Creatine kinase activity is related to both chondrocyte maturation and hypertrophy, and the activity of this enzyme increases to prepare for a hypoxic state (Shapiro et al. 1992). Growth factors that have been shown to affect hypertrophy include the BMPs and TGF-β. BMP2, 4, 6, and 7 have all been implicated in chondrocyte hypertrophy. Of these, BMP6 and 7 are expressed in hypertrophic chondrocytes (Gitelman et al. 1994; Houston et al. 1994), and the exogenous addition of BMP2 and 4 results in increases in chondrocyte hypertrophy (De Luca et al. 2001; Shum et al. 2003). BMP-induced bone formation can occur without cartilage formation, leading to their use for bone repair and tissue engineering (Sasano et al. 1993; Reddi 1998b). Regulation of hypertrophy by BMP also seems to involve GDF5, as overexpression of GDF5 results in enhanced chondrocyte maturation and hypertrophy (Coleman and Tuan 2003a,b).

Developmental principles of endochondral ossification can be applied to tissue engineering of articular cartilage to inhibit chondrocyte hypertrophy. Tissue-engineered cartilages formed from differentiated chondrocytes have seldom been reported as undergoing calcification, except for select cases where chondrocytes from the calcified zone were used (Kandel et al. 1997). However, expansion of the field into stem cells would require a fine control of cell differentiation, and knowledge of how cartilage calcifies might aid in the development of methods to inhibit unwanted calcification in tissue-engineered articular cartilage.

Exogenous methods to control hypertrophy and type X collagen deposition include the reduction of calcium concentrations (Reginato et al. 1993). TGF-β1/Smad3 signals inhibit hypertrophy (Yang et al. 2001), as does FGF2, which has been shown to reduce hypertrophy when added to the culture medium (Mancilla et al. 1998). As Rac1 and Cdc42 overexpression has been shown to accelerate hypertrophy, the pharmacological inhibition of p38 signaling, which blocks the effects of Rac1 and Cdc42 overexpression, also reduces hypertrophy (Wang and Beier 2005). It has also been shown that blocking the $\alpha_1\beta_1$ integrin prevents factor 13A (FXIIIA), a transglutaminase, from inducing chondrocyte hypertrophy (Johnson et al. 2008). BMP7 is another candidate whose inhibition lowers the expression of type X collagen (Haaijman et al. 1997). Parathyroid hormone-related protein has also been shown to have inhibitory effects on type X collagen expression (O'Keefe et al. 1997). Lastly, overexpression of Smad6 in chondrocytes results in delayed hypertrophy to the point of abolishing BMP2's expected effect of inducing hypertrophy (Horiki et al. 2004). Thyroxine has been shown to prevent Meckel's cartilage from undergoing hypertrophy hand (Kavumpurath and Hall 1990). Particularly interesting is the observation that type X collagen was upregulated by stretch-induced matrix deformation (Wu and Chen 2000), hinting that mechanical stimulation may also play a role in hypertrophy.

2.2 ARTICULAR CARTILAGE GROWTH AND MATURATION

2.2.1 Postnatal through Childhood, Adolescence, and Skeletal Maturity

Cartilage from skeletally immature, mature, and older humans displays several prominent differences. Adult articular cartilage is avascular, but immature cartilage may contain vascular channels during development, potentially functioning to provide nutrition for the developing tissue. Remodeling and thickness changes occur during maturation, and the articular cartilage responds to mechanical forces generated as the organism grows. From the cartilage anlage to cartilage in the skeletally mature adult, the cartilage thins toward the cartilage surface as hypertrophy and ossification convert cartilage to bone. Because of this, immature cartilage also appears thicker than mature cartilage, and cartilage continues to decrease in thickness as a person ages (Meachim 1971; Armstrong and Gardner 1977; Meachim et al. 1977). Cartilage must also grow in size to accompany the size increases in the skeleton until epiphyseal closure and subsequent skeletal maturity in young adulthood.

2.2.2 Matrix Changes with Maturation and Aging

Aside from gross morphological changes, postnatal changes occur in the biochemical content and matrix arrangement in cartilage (Figure 2.15). Collagen cross-linking has been observed to increase with age (Eyre et al. 1988), as discussed in Section 1.3.3. The collagen fiber arrangement changes with maturation from child to adolescence, starting from a more randomly organized mesh in the deep zone, to that of a perpendicular alignment with respect to the tidemark (Wei et al. 1998). Collagen density also increases with maturation of cartilage (van Turnhout et al. 2010). Increased nonenzymatic glycosylation of collagen occurs with age, making cartilage stiffer (Bank et al. 1998). Older cartilage displays greater birefringence, indicative of a greater degree of collagen alignment, compared with younger tissues (Hyttinen et al. 2001). Lastly, collagen type XI fragments are only seen in young cartilage (less

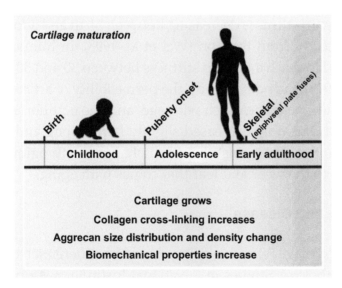

Figure 2.15 Changes in cartilage with maturation from infant to skeletally mature young adult. Maturation of extracellular matrix continues past skeletal maturity, albeit at a slower rate throughout the life of the individual.

than 19 years of age), a possible indication that collagen turnover slows down significantly beyond this point (Vaughan-Thomas et al. 2008).

Significant changes are seen with the proteoglycan content of cartilage with age. As the tissue matures and ages, proteoglycan content decreases with concomitant reductions in the protein core size, resulting in molecular weight decreases in aggrecan (Axelsson and Bjelle 1979). The chondroitin sulfate content decreases (Triphaus et al. 1980), and link protein fragments with time (Wells et al. 2003). Together, this reduces the amount of aggrecan in the tissue. In contrast, the concentration of keratan sulfate increases rapidly up to maturation and continues to do so throughout life, although this concentration increase postmaturation is mostly due to the decrease in aggrecan molecular weight (Bjelle 1975; Bayliss and Ali 1978). Hyaluronan content also increases with maturation from fetal to adult cartilage and in areas of higher cartilage loading (Thonar et al. 1978).

In rats, no changes in biomechanical properties were detected with aging (Athanasiou et al. 2000). In a rabbit knee model, changes in cartilage stiffness (instantaneous and 50-second creep moduli) were seen with maturation, with stiffness decreasing between birth and adolescence but remaining steady from then on (Wei et al. 1998). In humans, cartilage was observed to reach a peak in stiffness between 30 and 50 years of age (Ding et al. 1998). In another study, the permeability of articular cartilage was not found to change much with age, and the equilibrium modulus value of the tissue only decreased slightly (Armstrong and Mow 1982). It is important to distinguish between changes with aging *per se* and changes due to the wear and tear that comes with aging.

2.2.3 Aging and Disease

Changes in cartilage related to aging should be differentiated from those related to pathology. Studies in a National Institute of Aging rat model, which permits the analysis of changes solely due to aging, independent of disease, demonstrated that outside of maturational changes, cartilage functional biomechanical properties do not degrade with advancing age

(Athanasiou et al. 2000). Whether functional deficits in humans are solely due to aging or to other factors remains an open question. It has been hypothesized that changes in cartilage characterized as "normal aging" may be due to a failure of homeostasis (exacerbated by age), which begins the initiation of degradation (Lotz and Carames 2011). Interestingly, recent work suggests that it may be the presence of still living but senescent cells that contributes to the phenotypes seen with aging (Baker et al. 2011).

2.2.4 Cellular Changes

2.2.4.1 Aging Cells

Articular cartilage is somewhat unique from other tissues in that following skeletal maturity (and outside of disease states), chondrocyte proliferation is almost nonexistent. This results in cells that, for humans, can exist for several decades without replacement. Naturally, articular cartilage undergoes a decrease in cellularity, as cells die through attrition. In humans, the decline in cellularity in articular cartilage is most prevalent from prenatal to just past skeletal maturity, with minimal decline in cellularity in healthy individuals into near the ninth decade (Stockwell 1967; Lothe et al. 1979). Particularly problematic is the lack of a sufficient healing response displayed by these cells, a response that further diminishes with age.

In addition to fewer chondrocytes, age also brings about lowered metabolic activity, increased apoptosis, and reduced response to growth factors (Martin et al. 1997; Adams and Horton 1998; Barbero et al. 2004). These characteristics not only hinder natural cartilage healing, but also make it difficult to use older chondrocytes in tissue engineering. Older or osteoarthritic chondrocytes display a reduced production of anabolic factors, such as BMPs, due to increased promoter methylation, resulting in decreased expression of insulin-like growth factor 1 (IGF-1) and matrix genes (Loeser et al. 2009). Older cells also have reduced sensitivity to IGF-1, producing less matrix (Rousseau et al. 1998; Okuda et al. 2001; Yin et al. 2009). This may be mediated through the PI-3K (phosphoinositide 3-kinase) pathway, since older equine chondrocytes display resistance to Akt phosphorylation but not to extracellular signal-regulated kinase (ERK) phosphorylation following addition of IGF-1 (Boehm et al. 2007). This decrease in sensitivity to IGF-1 for PI-3K activation could be recovered by the addition of antioxidants, indicating a role in aging for oxidative stress inhibition of signaling. Mechanistically, oxidative stress results in phosphorylation of inhibitory residues on insulin receptor substrate 1 (IRS-1), an upstream component of the PI-3K pathway, resulting in inhibited phosphorylation of Akt (Yin et al. 2009), as described in the next section.

Autophagy is a lysosomal-mediated mechanism for digesting internal cellular components and for maintaining homeostasis between synthesis and degradation (Figure 2.16). Autophagy is a necessary part of normal tissue

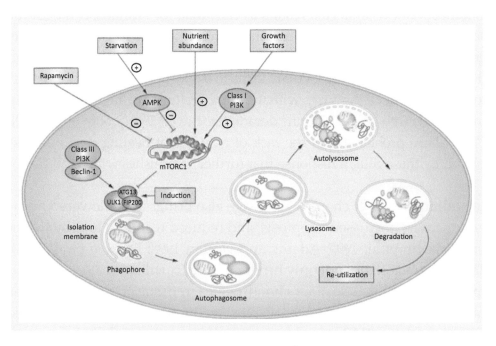

Figure 2.16 Regulation of autophagy is controlled through mammalian target of rapamycin (mTOR) complex 1 (mTORC1). Activation of mTOR causes complex formation resulting in inhibition of autophagy. Inhibiting mTOR initiates the cascade of reactions leading to autophagy. This begins with production of the phagophore and closure into the autophagosome, which fuses with the lysosome, resulting in degradation and reutilization of the enclosed materials. (From Lotz, M. K., and B. Carames, *Nat Rev Rheumatol* 7(10): 579-587, 2011. With permission.)

development and growth. In chondrocytes, autophagy is a primary mechanism for removing damaged organelles, and it prevents protein aggregation within the cell by removing stress-induced, misfolded proteins. Decreased autophagy is noted in older and diseased chondrocytes, which can result in increased oxidative stress from damaged mitochondrial-produced reactive oxygen species or nonapoptotic programmed cell death (also referred to as type II cell death) (Lotz and Carames 2011).

In many ways, these cellular changes in aging cells are distinct from changes during osteoarthritis. As discussed in Chapter 3, osteoarthritis is marked by cellular proliferation, increased protease expression, cell activation, differentiation toward a hypertrophic phenotype, and the presence of inflammatory mediators (Lotz and Carames 2011).

2.3 SIGNALING PATHWAYS DURING DEVELOPMENT AND MAINTENANCE OF ARTICULAR CARTILAGE

While the morphogens inducing the development of articular cartilage have been discussed earlier, the signaling pathways are discussed here. The interplay of these signaling factors, cell-to-cell signaling, mechanical stimuli, and oxygen tension produce a complex web of signals. These signals provide the cues needed to generate the complex geometry and multiple tissue types of the synovial joint. Mouse transgenic models have been crucial in elucidating many of these mechanisms in cartilage development. However, formation of articular cartilage does not happen in isolation; the adjacent tissues, biomechanics, and biological signals all contribute to the formation of the joint (Pacifici et al. 2000, 2006). The cell responds to these signals via transcription factor activation, gene expression, and protein synthesis.

2.3.1 Signaling Factors

2.3.1.1 Morphogens and Growth Factors

BMPs are pleiotropic regulators of the cartilage and bone differentiation cascade, regulating chemotaxis of progenitor cells, mitosis of mesenchymal stem cells, and differentiation of cartilage and bone (Reddi 1998b). BMPs regulate almost every aspect of chondrocytes, including proliferation, differentiation, and maintenance. BMPs induce new bone and cartilage formation *in vitro* and *in vivo* (Pecina et al. 2002). BMP7, also known as human osteogenic protein 1 (OP-1), plays an important role in cartilage homeostasis and repair (Luyten et al. 1992; Flechtenmacher et al. 1996; Chubinskaya et al. 2000; Hidaka et al. 2003). Multiple studies have shown that BMP7 and TGF-β1 can synergistically increase cell survival and matrix synthesis in normal and osteoarthritic human articular chondrocytes (Yaeger et al. 1997; O'Connor et al. 2000; Loeser et al. 2003). TGF-β1 has been identified as one of the strongest pro-cartilage growth factors for maintenance of cartilage and chondrocyte phenotype and appears to be crucial in mediating responses to mechanical loading and in regulating lubrication (Neu et al. 2007; DuRaine et al. 2009, 2011). This superfamily is discussed in more detail in Section 2.3.2.

Other factors, such as FGF2, IGF-1, and platelet-derived growth factor (PDGF), are anabolic for chondrocytes and have been described to have functional roles in cartilage development (Cuevas et al. 1988; Luyten et al. 1988; Fujimoto et al. 1999; O'Connor et al. 2000; Fortier et al. 2002; Mierisch et al. 2002; Wang et al. 2003; Gaissmaier et al. 2005). As noted in Section 2.1.1.2, BMP and FGF have counteracting purposes in the growth plate (Yoon et al. 2006).

Wnts are a family of palmitoylated extracellular signaling proteins that have pleiotropic effects on cell differentiation, embryonic development, and cellular patterning and migration (Klaus and Birchmeier 2008). While Wnt7a blocks chondrogenesis, others, such as Wnt9a, are required for cartilage formation (Stott et al. 1999; Fischer et al. 2002; Hartmann 2002; Daumer et al. 2004; Hwang et al. 2005; Yano et al. 2005; Jin et al. 2006; Spater et al. 2006). Wnts signal through both a canonical and noncanonical pathway, with the actions of the canonical pathway being dominant during chondrogenesis (Figure 2.17). Generically, the

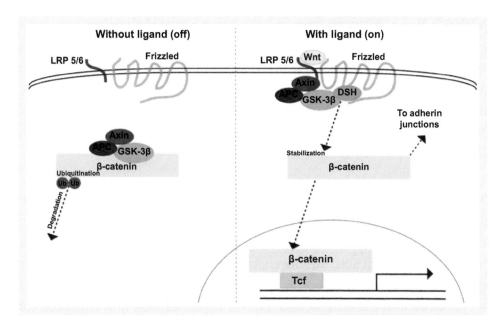

Figure 2.17 Canonical Wnt signaling pathway. Addition of Wnt increases stability of β-catenin, leading to translocation of β-catenin to the nucleus and to adheren junctions.

canonical pathway is activated by the binding of Wnt to a Frizzled cell surface receptor, which activates the intracellular Dishevelled (Dsh) protein and blocks GSK-3β activity, increasing β-catenin stability, leading to nuclear localization and transcription (Klaus and Birchmeier 2008).

2.3.1.2 Mechanical Stimuli

Articular cartilage experiences multiple types of mechanical stimuli, even in embryonic development. The developing muscles of the fetus help to contribute movement and nascent mechanobiological signals to the developing articular cartilage (Bastow et al. 2005). Mechanobiology is important for morphogenesis to form the developing synovial joint. For example, fetus immobilization studies have incisively demonstrated the need for movement in the development of synovial joints, and, therefore, articular cartilage (Dowthwaite et al. 2003). A thorough review of the role of biomechanics in articular cartilage development is provided by Responte et al. (2012).

Evidence has also come forward that in postnatal developing articular cartilage, before skeletal maturity, the thickness and biochemical composition of articular cartilage is directly related to the mechanical loading applied (Brama et al. 2000). Mechanical loading may act to inhibit hypertrophic differentiation to maintain the necessary cartilage thicknesses for function in the loaded areas (Koo and Andriacchi 2007).

During maintenance of cartilage, mechanical stimuli are required. These mechanical stimuli include hydrostatic pressure, compression, tension, and shear. Although the upstream effectors differ with mechanical forces, these factors activate downstream signaling pathways that overlap and cooperate with those activated by other exogenous factors, such as cytokines and growth factors. For example, tension and compression activate various mitogen-activated protein kinase (MAPK) and growth factor pathways (e.g., TGF signaling pathway), as does shear (see Section 2.3.2). Hydrostatic pressure regulates calcium ion channels, which activates MAPK. So while mechanical stimuli are separate from biological or biochemical stimuli, the signaling pathways activated are often the same. The mechanisms of action and the downstream effects are detailed in Sections 1.4 and 4.5.

2.3.1.3 Oxygen Tension

Chondrocytes in mature cartilage exist in a relatively low-oxygen environment. Multiple studies have demonstrated that low oxygen tension promotes and maintains chondrogenesis and cartilage formation (Robins et al. 2005; Schipani 2005; Provot et al. 2007). The initial steps in bone healing with formation of the cartilaginous callous are thought to be, in part, driven by low oxygen tension at the site of the fracture. Failure to sufficiently vascularize this callous can result in the formation of a nonunion at the fracture site (Fassbender et al. 2011) and eventual pseudoarthrosis, neocartilage formation driven by improper fracture fixation (Loboa et al. 2001).

Mechanistically, low oxygen tension is sensed by stabilization of hypoxia-inducible factor 1α (HIF-1α) by impairing its degradative hydroxylation. HIF-1α is a transcription factor that drives gene expression of pro-vascularization signals, such as VEGF, in hypertrophic cartilage and pro-chondrogenic expression in articular cartilage (Robins et al. 2005; Schipani 2005). This is required for neovascularization in the hypertrophic to ossification step. Mouse mutants with impaired HIF-1α or associated components have extremely short limbs; however, condensation progresses normally, although overall chondrogenesis is slowed and joint development is impaired (Provot et al. 2007).

2.3.2 Signaling Cascades

2.3.2.1 Morphogen Signaling

Of the signaling cascades involved in cartilage formation, actions of members of the TGF-β superfamily in initiating key events are crucial, along with their cartilage-specific downstream targets.

2.3.2.2 BMP/TGF-β Superfamily

Several groups of cytokines belong to the TGF-β superfamily, including TGFs, activins, BMPs, and GDFs, comprising a total of 29 ligands (Table 2.3). In mammals, these ligands are complimented by five type II receptors and seven type I receptors (Derynck and Zhang 2003). Of these cytokines, TGF-β1 is the founding member (Shi and Massague 2003) and has been characterized with regard to proliferation, differentiation, motility, and apoptosis, depending on cell type and origin. The BMP subfamily contains over 20 members. TGF-β is part of a large family of extracellular ligands highly conserved within the animal kingdom that control cell growth, differentiation, motility, and apoptosis. Three isoforms are known for mammals, all of which bind to the same receptors. Of these isoforms, TGF-β1 is the best characterized, beginning with its ability to reversibly allow anchorage-dependent, nonneoplastic fibroblast cells to form colonies under anchorage-independent

Table 2.3 TGF-β superfamily of ligands

Ligand	Alternative names	Subgroup
TGF-β/activin		
TGF-β1		TGF-βs
TGF-β2		
TGF-β3		
Activin A	Activin β_A-β_A subunits	Activins
Activin B	β_B-β_B	
Activin AB	β_A-β_B	
Inhibin A	Inhibin α-activin β_A subunits	Inhibins
Inhibin B	α-β_B	
Nodal	Ndr	Nodal
Lefty1	Lefty A/EBAF	Lefty
Lefty2	Lefty B	
BMP/GDF		
BMP2	BMP2A	BMP2/4
BMP4	BMP2B	
BMP5		BMP5/6/7
BMP6	Vgr1/DVR6	
BMP7	OP1	
BMP8A	OP2	
BMP8B	OP3/PC8	
GDF1		GDF1
GDF3	Vgr2	
GDF5	CDMP1	GDF5/6/7
GDF6	CDMP2/BMP13	
GDF7	BMP12	
BMP9	GDF2	BMP9/10
BMP10		
BMP3	Osteogenin	BMP3
BMP3b	GDF10/Sumitomo-BIP	

(Continued)

Table 2.3 (Continued) TGF-β superfamily of ligands

Ligand	Alternative names	Subgroup
GDF9		GDF9
GDF9b	BMP15	
GDF15	MIC1/PLAB/PTGFB/PDF	
GFD8	Myostatin	GDF8
GDF11	BMP11	
MIS (Mullerian inhibitory substance)	MIF/AMH	MIS

Source: Adapted from de Caestecker, M., *Cytokine Growth Factor Rev* 15(1): 1-11, 2004.

conditions in soft agar (de Larco and Todaro 1978; Roberts et al. 1983). This transformation to anchorage-independent, mitogenic activity led to the TGF moniker *transforming growth factor.* TGF-β2 and TGF-β3 have been shown to act similarly in some cell culture conditions, although the results are highly context specific.

2.3.2.3 Receptors and Smads

TGF-β and BMP signaling is based on the interactions of four different kinds of molecules. Signaling pathways in the TGF-β superfamily are composed of different, albeit similar, components for both the BMP and TGF-β ligand groups (Table 2.4), such as cell surface receptors (and secondary binding receptors such as decorin) and internal signaling molecules called Smad, which were originally identified as homologs of Mad in *Drosophila* and Sma in *Caenorhabditis elegans* (Sekelsky et al. 1995; Savage et al. 1996). Once activated, these ligands bind to type II transmembrane receptors, which then recruit and phosphorylate type I receptors, both of which exist as homodimers. The serine/threonine kinase activity of the type I receptor is then able to phosphorylate the carboxy-terminus of the receptor-activated Smads (R-Smad). For BMPs and GDFs, two type I receptors (BMPRIA and BMPRIB), which exist as heterodimers, complex with the type II receptor (BMPRII), which

Table 2.4 Known receptors TGF-β superfamily ligands

Receptors	Alternative names	Ligands
Type I receptors		
Alk 1 (activin receptor-like kinase 1) group		
Alk1	TSR1/SKR3/ACVRL1	TGF-β, activin A
Alk2	TSK7L/ActRIA/SKR1	TGF-β, activin A, MIS, BMP6/7
Alk 3 group		
Alk3	BMPRI/BMPRIA/ BRK1/Tfr11/ACVRLK3	BMP2/4, BMP6/7
Alk6	BMPRIB/BRK2	BMP2/4, GDF5/6, GDF9b, MIS, BMP6/7
Alk 5 group		
Alk4	ActRIB/ACVR1BSKR2	Activin A, GDF1 and Nodal (with EGF-CFC), GDF11
Alk5	TGF-β RI/SKR4	TGF-β
Alk7		Nodal
Type II receptors		
TGF-β RII		TGF-β
BMP RII	BRK3/T-Alk	Inhibin A (with TGFRIII), BMP2/4, BMP6/7, GDF5/6, GDF9b
Act RII (activin type II receptor)	ACVR2	Activin A, inhibin A/B, GDF1 and Nodal (with EGF-CFC), BMP2, BMP6/7, GDF5, GDF9b, GDF8/11
Act RIIB	ACVR2B	Activin A, inhibin A/B, Nodal, BMP2, BMP6/7, GDF5, GDF8/11
MIS RII (MIS type II receptor)	AMHR2	MIS

Source: Adapted from de Caestecker, M., *Cytokine Growth Factor Rev* 15(1): 1-11, 2004.

exists as a homodimer. These recruit and phosphorylate Smad1, 5, and 8, which interact with the common Smad (Smad4) with both TGF-β and BMP pathways (Figure 2.18). For TGF-β, the key players are the TGFRI and TGFRII receptors, which interact with Smad2 or 3 and then Smad4 (Derynck and Zhang 2003; Shi and Massague 2003; Miyazono et al. 2005). Recent evidence also indicates that cartilage oligomeric matrix protein (COMP) plays a role in binding to and presenting TGF-β to these receptors, resulting in enhanced signaling (Haudenschild et al. 2011).

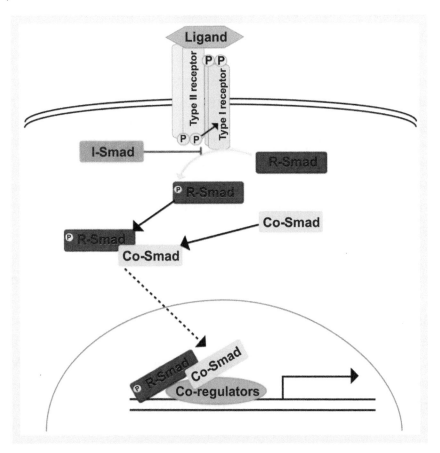

Figure 2.18 Canonical TGF-β superfamily signaling pathway, including TGF and BMP pathways. Ligand binding to the type II receptor and complexing and phosphorylation of the type I receptor drive receptor (R)-Smad phosphorylation. Inhibitory (I)-Smads can block this phosphorylation of R-Smads. Once phosphorylated, R-Smads then bind to the common (Co)-Smad and locate to the nucleus where interactions with coregulators drive gene transcription.

Generally for this pathway, once activated, two R-Smads bind to Smad4 in a heterotrimer and translocate to the nucleus to activate target genes in concert with other transcription factors, although translocation in the absence of Smad4 has been observed (Sirard et al. 2000). Inhibitory Smads, Smad6 and 7, act to inhibit Smad2 and 3 by competing for binding to the type I receptor through an MH2 domain conserved across Smads. However, they lack the MH1 domain and are unable to be phosphorylated and interact with Smad4 (Shi and Massague 2003). Although the R-Smads and Smad4 exist in most cell types, expression of inhibitory Smads is induced by TGF-β or BMP stimulation in an inhibition feedback mechanism.

While the type I receptor activating R-Smads is described as the canonical pathway for TGF-β or BMP (Figure 2.18), Smad-independent (or modifying) pathways exist. Protein interaction with the type II receptor has been described (Massague 2000), and TGF-β can activate various MAPK pathways, ERK, JNK (c-Jun N-terminal kinase), and p38 (Nakamura et al. 1999), which then modulate the actions of Smads, though the mechanism of actions for these pathways is not as well understood (Shi and Massague 2003).

2.3.2.4 MAPK and Rho GTPase Signaling in Articular Cartilage

The assortment of morphogens and growth factors acting on articular cartilage also overlaps with other well-defined signaling pathways, such as the MAPK pathways, PI-3K, and the Rho GTPases. Many of these pathway components and regulatory mechanisms were first described in cancer cells, as they often have strong effects on proliferation and migration. Genetic analysis of these pathways in mouse models has unfortunately been somewhat limited, as knockouts are commonly embryonic lethal. However, although the majority of the work on elucidating the structure of these pathways has been accomplished in more amenable systems, the results can be applied to cartilage.

MAPK pathways have been identified as signaling pathways in all eukaryotic cells (Figure 2.19). They are involved in signal transduction in response to various external cell stimuli and can lead to proliferation, differentiation, migration, and multiple other cellular responses (Krishna and Narang 2008). Five distinct MAPK groups have been described in mammals: ERK1 and 2 (1/2), p38, JNK, ERK3 and 4 (3/4), and ERK5. Of these five pathways, three have been extensively described in the literature: ERK, p38, and JNK. These MAPK groups are distinguished by the amino acid (X) situated between the threonine-X-tyrosine (TXY) phosphorylation site.

Generally, the MAPK pathways are composed of three sequential signaling molecules/kinases, the MAPK, the MAPK kinase (MAPKK),

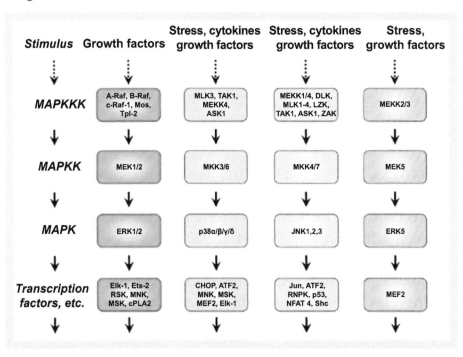

Figure 2.19 Simplified schematic and overview of the mammalian ERK1/2, p38, JNK, and ERK5 MAPK cascades. These represent the five major pathways. While the generic pattern of activation and signaling of the pathways have commonality, the final substrate acted upon (often transcription factors) allows for a wide range of responses. See the text for particular pathway component descriptions. (From Roberts, P. J., and C. J. Der, *Oncogene* 26(22): 3291-3310, 2007. With permission.)

and the MAPK kinase kinase (MAPKKK or MAP3K). These commonly tie G protein-coupled receptors (GPCRs) into the pathway. The MAPKs respond to stress cytokines, either pro-inflammatory or mitogenic, to activate through a cascade of phosphorylation events and eventual transcriptional activity (Pouyssegur et al. 2002; Chong et al. 2003; Chadee and Kyriakis 2004). Specifically, the generic pathway consists of a stimulus activating a MAP3K, which activates a MAPKK, which activates a MAPK, which induces a response, commonly modulation of gene expression. However, MAPK phosphorylates multiple substrates other than transcription factors, including cytoskeletal proteins and phospholipases. Each of these steps results in an amplification of the signal induced by the initial stimuli. These kinase pathways function through phosphorylation events of individual signaling members. Significant crosstalk between the pathways has been observed, with some MAPKKs being activated by multiple MAP3Ks (Junttila et al. 2008). The exact role some member proteins play in activation of specific pathways remains unclear, although scaffolding proteins have been identified that modulate the specificity of pathway activation (Kolch 2005; Sacks 2006).

2.3.2.4.1 ERK1/2

Of the MAPKs, ERK1 and 2 (ERK1/2) were the first described in the literature (Boulton and Cobb 1991; Boulton et al. 1991a,b). These have 83% amino acid sequence identity, with a conserved Thr-Glu-Tyr (TEY) phosphorylation activation loop (Yao et al. 2000). Compared with JNK and p38, ERK1/2 responds more favorably to serum, growth factor, or phorbol ester stimulation, as opposed to stress stimuli. However, multiple other stimuli have been identified, including multiple cytokines, osmotic stress, cytoskeletal disruption, and mechanical stimulation. The current model of ERK activation is a kinase cascade initially activated almost always by an extracellular signal from a tyrosine kinase or GPCR that activates the membrane-associated GTPase Ras through interaction with the guanine nucleotide exchange factor SOS (son of sevenless) (Figure 2.20). Changing the Ras-bound GDP to GTP allows Ras to become active and to interact with and activate MAP3K, in this case a Raf family member (A-Raf,

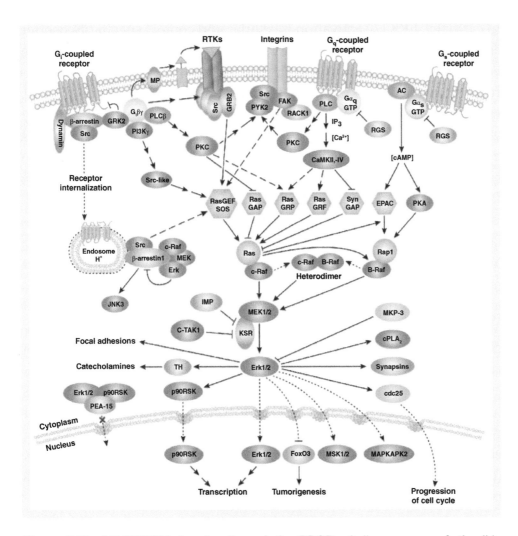

Figure 2.20 MAPK/ERK signaling through the GPCRs. A diverse array of stimuli is able to activate GPCRs. This results in G protein exchanging GDP for GTP, causing the dissociation of the GTP-bound α and β/γ subunits and further downstream signaling. (With permission from Cell Signaling Technologies.)

B-Raf or Raf-1). Activated Raf then phosphorylates and activates MAPKK Mek (Mek1 and 2) and then MAPK ERK (ERK1 and 2). ERK1/2 can then phosphorylate multiple substrates, including other kinases (MSK1/2 and MNK1/2), transcription factors (Elk1 and SAP1), membrane-bound proteins, nuclear proteins, and cytoskeletal proteins. Commonly, pharmacological inhibition of this pathway targets MEK, with two nonrelated compounds widely used, specifically U0126 and PD98059.

129

In cartilage, ERK1/2 activation is cellular and context specific (Schaeffer and Weber 1999). Both stimulatory and inhibitory roles in cartilage have been reported for ERK1/2, likely dependent on the duration, magnitude, and activation kinetics (Nakamura et al. 1999; Hung et al. 2000; Murakami et al. 2000; Yoon et al. 2002; Bobick and Kulyk 2004; Zakany et al. 2005; Ryan et al. 2009; Prasadam et al. 2010). Articular cartilage is a highly mechanoregulated tissue, and the ERK pathway is known to respond to mechanical signals in other cell types (Reusch et al. 1997; Jessop et al. 2002; Hatton et al. 2003; Laboureau et al. 2004; Bastow et al. 2005; Liu et al. 2006; Kook et al. 2009). The ERK1/2 pathway is also regulated by growth factors, such as TGF-β1 and FGF2 (Murakami et al. 2000; Yonekura et al. 1999). In murine primary chondrocytes (Murakami et al. 2000), Sox9 expression is induced by activation of the ERK pathway, and this is required for TGF-β signaling during chondrogenesis (Li et al. 2010). It is noteworthy that during chondrogenesis of chick mesenchymal cells, activation of ERK is decreased, and blocking the upstream signaling component MEK, and, therefore, ERK, enhances chondrogenesis (Oh et al. 2000). Downregulation of cartilage matrix components has also been linked to activation of ERK in primary chondrocytes or cartilage due to FGF2 released following impact (Ryan et al. 2009; Ding et al. 2010). Chondrocyte hypertrophic differentiation also requires ERK (Beier and LuValle 1999; Beier et al. 1999a), indicating the dual role this pathway plays in cartilage tissue.

2.3.2.4.2 p38

The p38 protein has four distinct isoforms, α, β, γ, and δ (50% identity to ERK2 for p38α), with each of these isoforms having different substrate specificity. p38 is denoted by the presence of a conserved Thr-Gly-Tyr (TGY) sequence in the phosphorylation activation loop. p38 was initially identified as being activated by lipopolysaccharide (LPS) (Han et al. 1993, 1994). Common stimuli include environmental stresses, such as UV, oxidative stress, osmotic shock, hypoxia, mechanical loading, and inflammatory cytokines (interleukin 1 [IL-1], TNF-α), but rarely growth factors. Not surprisingly, given these activation stimuli, p38 plays a role in immune and inflammatory reactions, cell differentiation, and apoptosis.

The p38 cascade consists of multiple MAP3Ks (MEKK1-4), MLK2 and 3, DLK, ASK1, Tpl2, and Tak1. The MAPKKs are MEK3 (for isoforms α and β preferentially) and EK6 (all isoforms) and somewhat MEK4, which overlaps with JNK. p38 becomes activated by the phosphorylation of site Thr-180 and Tyr-182 by MAPKK (Raingeaud et al. 1995). Phosphorylated substrates of p38 are numerous and include transcription factors (MEF2, ATF1 and 2, Elk1, NF-kB, p53, and others), cytoskeletal associated proteins (Tau), and phospholipase A2 (Zarubin and Han 2005). Pharmacological inhibition of p38 isoforms α and β can be achieved using SB203580 or SB202190, which both have minimal inhibitory overlap with JNK.

Interestingly, p38 is required for chondrogenesis; GDF5-induced chondrogenic differentiation in ATDC5 cells requires p38 signaling, as does cartilage nodule formation in chick mesenchymal cells (Nakamura et al. 1999; Oh et al. 2000). Chondrocyte hypertrophy also requires p38 signaling (Stanton et al. 2004), with transcription of type X collagen being dependent on p38 activation and MEF2 bindings site in the collagen X promoter (Harada et al. 1997; Beier and LuValle 1999; Beier et al. 1999b). Activation of p38 has also been identified to play a role in cartilage matrix resorption and degradation.

2.3.2.4.3 JNK

JNK (also known as SAPK) was initially identified in cycloheximide-treated rat livers (Kyriakis and Avruch 1990). It is commonly coactivated along with p38. Three JNK genes have been identified, JNK1-3, which share a conserved Thr-Pro-Tyr (TPY) sequence in the phosphorylation activation loop. JNKs are activated by many of the same stimuli as p38, including UV, oxidative stress, heat shock, DNA damage, mechanical shear, inflammatory cytokines (TNF family members, IL-1, Fas and Rank ligand, and others), and protein synthesis inhibitors (such as cycloheximide). Although not strongly activated by growth factors, JNK can be activated by TGF-β (Atfi et al. 1997; Wang et al. 1997).

The JNK pathway components are composed of a variety of MAP3Ks (MEKK1-4, MLK1-3, DLK, Tp12, ASK1 and 2, TAO1 and 2, and TAK1) (Weston and Davis 2002). Downstream, the MAPKKs (MKK4 and 7) phosphorylate the dual Thr and Tyr of the three JNK genes, of which 10 isoforms exist. Activated JNK is able to phosphorylate multiple transcription factors, including ATF2, NF-ATc1, HSF01, Stat3, and c-Jun. Of these transcription factors, c-Jun is the best known, and phosphorylation of Ser63 and 73 leads to increased transcription of c-Jun targets. Pharmacological inhibition of JNK can be accomplished by the use of SP600125 (Bennett et al. 2001). Interestingly, JNK plays a limited role in chondrogenesis. JNK is unresponsive to GDF5 treatment, and the phosphorylation state of JNK does not change during chondrogenesis (Nakamura et al. 1999).

2.3.2.4.4 PI-3K

The PI-3K-Akt pathway is involved in proliferation, differentiation, matrix synthesis, and differentiated cell survival, with downstream kinases of PI-3 consisting of AKT1-3 (Figure 2.21).

Stimuli for PI-3K include activators of tyrosine kinase receptors, such as growth factors like IGF-1. TGF-β also activates AKT phosphorylation, although with different kinetics that indicates an indirect method of activation (Figure 2.22). PI-3K is required for hypertrophic cell differentiation (Ulici et al. 2008, 2010). Activation of PI-3k in adult cartilage enhances synthesis of proteoglycans, type II collagen, and Sox9 (Cheng et al. 2009), and promotes cell survival. While inhibition decreases GAG synthesis and decreases cell survival (Oh and Chun 2003; Li et al. 2009), PI-3K interacts strongly with the Runx2 transcription factor (Fujita et al. 2004). Pharmacological inhibition by LY294002 has been used extensively to elucidate the functions of this pathway.

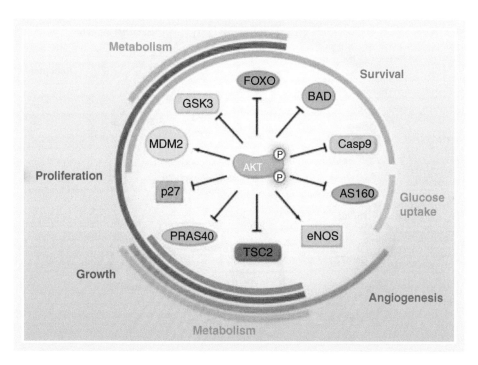

Figure 2.21 Schematic of the multiple and overlapping cellular functions of the Akt signaling pathway. (From Manning, B. D., and L. C. Cantley, *Cell* 129(7): 1261-1274, 2007. With permission.)

2.3.2.4.5 Rho GTPases

Rho family small GTPases are activated by switching from an inactive GDP-bound molecule to an active GTP-bound form. Switching to the active form is controlled by guanine nucleotide exchange factors (GEFs), while switching to the inactive form is regulated by GTPase activating proteins (GAPs). GEFs and GAPs are under the control of a multitude of cell surface receptors, including integrins, serine/threonine and tyrosine kinase receptors, and GPCRs. They link extracellular matrix signaling to changes in the cytoskeleton and cell shape.

For chondrocytes, cell shape is important for maintaining the differentiated phenotype. In articular cartilage, the normal actin organization of the cell is cortical, and the chondrocyte maintains a rounded phenotype.

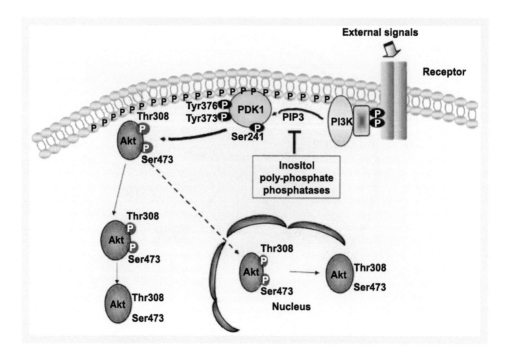

Figure 2.22 PI-3K/AKT pathway. Extracellular signals activate the PI-3K/AKT pathway, resulting in phosphorylation and activation of AKT by PDK1. Once activated, AKT leaves the plasma membrane and translocates to the nucleus (dotted line) or the cytosol, resulting in phosphorylation of other effector proteins and downstream signaling. (From Du, K., and P. N. Tsichlis, *Oncogene* 24(50): 7401-7409, 2005. With permission.)

In chondrocytes, RhoA and its downstream kinases ROCK1/2 have been studied extensively. Activation of RhoA induces actin stress fiber formation, which is associated with the fibroblastic dedifferentiated phenotype. Not surprisingly, inhibition of RhoA supports chondrogenesis and differentiation, while overexpression of RhoA inhibits these actions through modulation of Sox9 (Figure 2.23) (Woods et al. 2005; Woods and Beier 2006; Kumar and Lassar 2009; Haudenschild et al. 2010).

2.3.3 Transcription Factors

When activated by various stimuli and signaling pathways, transcription factors function by locating to the nucleus, binding DNA, and enhancing transcription, and, therefore, translation and protein expression.

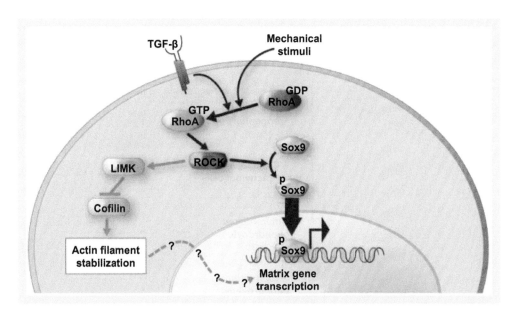

Figure 2.23 Rho GTPase signaling pathway and Sox9 interact. (From Haudenschild, D. R. et al., *Arthritis Rheum* 62(1): 191-200, 2010. With permission.)

Sox5, Sox6, and Sox9 are members of the Sox (sex-determining region Y-box) protein family and the High-Mobility Group (HMG) super family of DNA binding proteins, which are characterized by sequence homology to the HMG domain of the sex-determining region on the Y chromosome. Sox9 is the master regulator of chondrocyte differentiation and is coexpressed with Sox5 (as L-Sox5) and Sox6 (Akiyama et al. 2002; Akiyama 2008).

Regulation of Sox9 expression is under the control of BMP signaling, with BMP2 indicated in direct upregulation of Sox9 (Healy et al. 1999; Zehentner et al. 1999). Sox9 maintains the chondrocyte phenotype and prevents chondrocytes from undergoing terminal differentiation and hypertrophy (Figure 2.24). Loss of Sox9, Sox5, and Sox6 presages differentiation into hypertrophic chondrocytes (Lefebvre et al. 2001; Okubo and Reddi 2003). Sox9 is also directly responsible for regulating the expression of multiple extracellular matrix components that define cartilage, including aggrecan; types II, IX, and XI collagens; and COMP (Zhou et al. 1998; Liu et al. 2000; Sekiya et al. 2000; Panda et

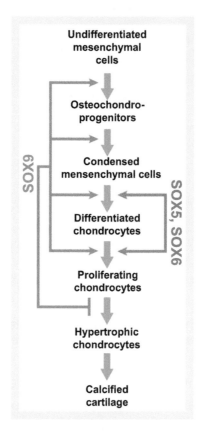

Figure 2.24 The role and actions of Sox9 as the master regulator of the chondrocyte phenotype. Sox9 commits undifferentiated mesenchymal cells to become osteochondro progenitors. During development, Sox9 is critical for mesenchymal condensation to occur. Sox5 and Sox6 also work with Sox9 to regulate chondrocyte differentiation, proliferation, and prevention of hypertrophy. (Modified from Akiyama, H. et al., *Genes Dev* 16(21): 2813-2828, 2002.)

al. 2001; Zhang et al. 2003), although regulation of type II collagen by Sox9 is dependent on the state of differentiation (Aigner et al. 2003; Kypriotou et al. 2003). Also important in chondroblast differentiation is the MAPK-controlled Runx2, which becomes important for cells in entering the hypertrophic stage (Papachristou et al. 2005). These transcription factors function not only during development but also during tissue maintenance and maturation. Changes in their expression and regulation, for a variety of reasons, mediate differences in gene expression as cartilage ages.

2.3.4 Cartilage Homeostasis

Homeostasis, from Greek *hómoios* (ὅμοιος), meaning "similar," and *stasis* (στάσις), meaning "standing still"

Homeostasis is defined as the steady-state maintenance of a tissue. In articular cartilage, this involves the interplay between mechanical and biochemical signals, such as cytokines, as detailed in Figure 2.25 (Reddi 2003). Changes in articular cartilage homeostasis are considered to precede the initiation of osteoarthritis (Moos et al. 1999).

With reference to cytokines, articular cartilage homeostasis has been modeled as the balance between the actions of morphogens and growth factors, such as TGF-β, BMP, and IGF, and the actions of catabolic cytokines, such as interleukins (e.g., IL-1β) and TNF-α. Introduction of excess inflammatory (catabolic) cytokines, such as IL-1β, to the diarthrodial

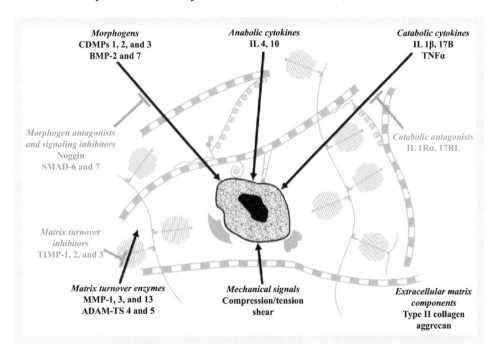

Figure 2.25 Balancing act of anabolic and catabolic factors in cartilage homeostasis, necessary to maintain articular cartilage health. (Courtesy of Dr. Corey Neu. Modified from Reddi, A. H., *Ann Rheum Dis* 62(Suppl 2): ii73-ii78, 2003. With permission.)

joint reduces the production of matrix molecules and leads to changes in matrix constitution that result in reduced mechanical strength and ability to maintain normal articular cartilage function (van den Berg et al. 1999; Tetlow et al. 2001). However, it should be remembered that remodeling and cartilage degradation are necessary parts of normal function, with MMPs, tissue inhibitors of metalloproteinases (TIMPs), and ADAMTS4 and 5 all leading to matrix component degradation. It is the disturbance of this balancing act between anabolic and catabolic processes that leads to disease progression.

The signaling pathways described in Section 2.3.2 play a role not only in development and homeostasis, but also in disease. Increased cytokines, degradative cartilage products (e.g., collagen and fibronectin fragments), and increased growth factor expression due to an improper healing response can combine to disrupt homeostasis and activate multiple pathways. For example, all three MAPK families have been identified to be active during osteoarthritis: phosphorylated ERK is present in normal articular cartilage homeostasis as well as in osteoarthritis. p38 and JNK phosphorylation is increased in osteoarthritic cartilage (Clancy et al. 2001; Rowan 2001; Sondergaard et al. 2010). Fibronectin fragments can activate the $\alpha_5\beta_1$ integrin, resulting in stimulation of all three pathways and upregulation of MMP13 (Forsyth et al. 2002; Yasuda et al. 2003). Likewise, basic FGF (released from the matrix during cartilage injury) also activates all three MAPKs, inducing MMP13 expression (Im et al. 2007). Interestingly, all three pathways are required for this induction of MMP13, with inhibition of any single MAPK resulting in inhibited MMP13 secretion (Im et al. 2007). The association between increases in MAPK activation and increases in degradative enzyme expression, such as MMPs and aggrecanases, is just an example of how disruption in homeostasis results in articular cartilage degeneration (Muddasani et al. 2007; Sondergaard et al. 2010).

It is worth noting that systemic changes to the body can also affect articular cartilage properties. For instance, a study performed on ovariectomized sheep showed decreased articular cartilage material properties if left untreated with estrogen replacement (Turner et al. 1997). This result is relevant to menopausal women. Diabetes, too, can affect cartilage properties adversely (Athanasiou et al. 1999). Anti-inflammatory treatments have also been shown to decrease cartilage material properties (Murray et al. 1998; Ding et al. 2009). While the exact signaling pathways for these changes are yet to be fully elucidated, all these factors resulting in decreased biomechanical properties can make articular cartilage more prone to injuries.

2.4 CHAPTER CONCEPTS

- Morphogenesis is the developmental process of pattern formation that leads to the body plan.
- Morphogenesis is initiated by the combined and coordinated actions of the morphogens BMP, FGF, HHs, and Wnts.
- Limb bud morphogenesis requires sequential processes of migration, adhesion, condensation, proliferation, and differentiation of lateral mesodermal cells.
- A variety of biological signals, such as TGF-β, BMP, VEGF, and Shh, regulate the process of articular cartilage formation. These signals have been employed to study cartilage formation and to recapitulate it for the regeneration of tissues.
- The Hox genes control the formation of the body plan and segments; they have been conserved during evolution.
- Mesenchymal condensation during limb bud formation is driven in part by cell adhesion molecules such as N-CAM, cadherins, and integrins.
- Formation of the skeletal limb elements and synovial joints is initiated by multiple morphogens and signaling factors.
- During hypertrophy, chondrocyte proliferation is arrested and cellular volume increases. Hypertrophy is heralded by production of type X collagen and decreased production of type II collagen.

- Chondrocytes in the growth plate undergo proliferation; hypertrophy and ossification drive the longitudinal growth of the bones.
- The factors and signaling pathways used during development are the same as those in cartilage maintenance. Dysregulation of those pathways leads to disease progression.
- The morphogens of the TGF-β superfamily are potent regulators of cartilage development and maintenance.
- During aging, there are alterations in collagen cross-linking, accompanied by changes in collagen alignment, decreased collagen and proteoglycan content, and decreased matrix turnover.
- As chondrocytes age, their metabolic activity decreases. This may be due to oxidative stress and changes in autophagy.
- It is important to bear in mind that changes in articular cartilage due to aging cannot be easily distinguished from those changes caused by disease progression.
- Signaling cascades in articular cartilage development, maintenance, and aging include the MAPK and the Rho GTPase pathways. The MAPK pathways are composed of three primary kinases: ERK1/2, p38, and JNK.
- The transcriptional regulation by Sox9 plays a key role in development, maintenance, and aging of articular cartilage.
- Homeostasis of articular cartilage involves the interplay between mechanical and biochemical signals in the steady-state maintenance of the tissue. Changes in homeostasis are considered to precede the initiation of osteoarthritis.

References

Adams, C. S., and W. E. Horton Jr. (1998). Chondrocyte apoptosis increases with age in the articular cartilage of adult animals. *Anat Rec* 250(4): 418-425.

Aigner, T., P. M. Gebhard et al. (2003). SOX9 expression does not correlate with type II collagen expression in adult articular chondrocytes. *Matrix Biol* 22(4): 363-372.

Akiyama, H. (2008). Control of chondrogenesis by the transcription factor Sox9. *Mod Rheumatol* 18(3): 213-219.

Akiyama, H., M. C. Chaboissier et al. (2002). The transcription factor Sox9 has essential roles in successive steps of the chondrocyte differentiation pathway and is required for expression of Sox5 and Sox6. *Genes Dev* 16(21): 2813-2828.

Armstrong, C. G., and D. L. Gardner. (1977). Thickness and distribution of human femoral head articular cartilage. Changes with age. *Ann Rheum Dis* 36(5): 407-412.

Armstrong, C. G., and V. C. Mow. (1982). Variations in the intrinsic mechanical properties of human articular cartilage with age, degeneration, and water content. *J Bone Joint Surg Am* 64(1): 88-94.

Atfi, A., S. Djelloul et al. (1997). Evidence for a role of Rho-like GTPases and stress-activated protein kinase/c-Jun N-terminal kinase (SAPK/JNK) in transforming growth factor beta-mediated signaling. *J Biol Chem* 272(3): 1429-1432.

Athanasiou, K. A., J. G. Fleischli et al. (1999). Effects of diabetes mellitus on the biomechanical properties of human ankle cartilage. *Clin Orthop Relat Res* 368: 182-189.

Athanasiou, K. A., C. F. Zhu et al. (2000). Effects of aging and dietary restriction on the structural integrity of rat articular cartilage. *Ann Biomed Eng* 28(2): 143-149.

Axelsson, I., and A. Bjelle. (1979). Proteoglycan structure of bovine articular cartilage. Variation with age and in osteoarthrosis. *Scand J Rheumatol* 8(4): 217-221.

Baker, D. J., T. Wijshake et al. (2011). Clearance of p16(Ink4a)-positive senescent cells delays ageing-associated disorders. *Nature* 479: 232-236.

Bank, R. A., M. T. Bayliss et al. (1998). Ageing and zonal variation in post-translational modification of collagen in normal human articular cartilage. The age-related increase in non-enzymatic glycation affects biomechanical properties of cartilage. *Biochem J* 330(Pt 1): 345-351.

Barbero, A., S. Grogan et al. (2004). Age related changes in human articular chondrocyte yield, proliferation and post-expansion chondrogenic capacity. *Osteoarthr Cartil* 12(6): 476-484.

Bastow, E. R., K. J. Lamb et al. (2005). Selective activation of the MEK-ERK pathway is regulated by mechanical stimuli in forming joints and promotes pericellular matrix formation. *J Biol Chem* 280(12): 11749-11758.

Bayliss, M. T., and S. Y. Ali. (1978). Age-related changes in the composition and struc-ture of human articular-cartilage proteoglycans. *Biochem J* 176(3): 683-693.

Beachy, P. A., S. G. Hymowitz et al. (2010). Interactions between Hedgehog proteins and their binding partners come into view. *Genes Dev* 24(18): 2001-2012.

Beier, F., and P. LuValle. (1999). Serum induction of the collagen X promoter requires the Raf/MEK/ERK and p38 pathways. *Biochem Biophys Res Commun* 262(1): 50-54.

Beier, F., A. C. Taylor et al. (1999a). The Raf-1/MEK/ERK pathway regulates the expres-sion of the p21(Cip1/Waf1) gene in chondrocytes. *J Biol Chem* 274(42): 30273-30279.

Beier, F., A. C. Taylor et al. (1999b). Raf signaling stimulates and represses the human collagen X promoter through distinguishable elements. *J Cell Biochem* 72(4): 549-557.

Bennett, B. L., D. T. Sasaki et al. (2001). SP600125, an anthrapyrazolone inhibitor of Jun N-terminal kinase. *Proc Natl Acad Sci USA* 98(24): 13681-13686.

Bernfield, M., and R. D. Sanderson. (1990). Syndecan, a developmentally regulated cell surface proteoglycan that binds extracellular matrix and growth factors. *Philos Trans R Soc Lond B Biol Sci* 327(1239): 171-186.

Bi, W., J. M. Deng et al. (1999). Sox9 is required for cartilage formation. *Nat Genet* 22(1): 85-89.

Bjelle, A. (1975). Content and composition of glycosaminoglycans in human knee joint cartilage: Variation with site and age in adults. *Connect Tissue Res* 3(2): 141-147.

Bobick, B. E., and W. M. Kulyk. (2004). The MEK-ERK signaling pathway is a negative regulator of cartilage-specific gene expression in embryonic limb mesen-chyme. *J Biol Chem* 279(6): 4588-4595.

Boehm, A. K., M. Seth et al. (2007). Hsp90 mediates insulin-like growth factor 1 and interleukin-1beta signaling in an age-dependent manner in equine articular chondrocytes. *Arthritis Rheum* 56(7): 2335-2343.

Boulton, T. G., and M. H. Cobb. (1991). Identification of multiple extracellular signal-regulated kinases (ERKs) with antipeptide antibodies. *Cell Regul* 2(5): 357-371.

Boulton, T. G., J. S. Gregory et al. (1991a). Purification and properties of extracellular signal-regulated kinase 1, an insulin-stimulated microtubule-associated pro-tein 2 kinase. *Biochemistry* 30(1): 278-286.

Boulton, T. G., S. H. Nye et al. (1991b). ERKs: A family of protein-serine/threonine kinases that are activated and tyrosine phosphorylated in response to insu-lin and NGF. *Cell* 65(4): 663-675.

Brama, P. A., J. M. Tekoppele et al. (2000). Functional adaptation of equine articular cartilage: The formation of regional biochemical characteristics up to age one year. *Equine Vet J* 32(3): 217-221.

Briscoe, J., and P. P. Therond. (2013). The mechanisms of hedgehog signalling and its roles in development and disease. *Nat Rev Mol Cell Biol* 14(7): 416-429.

Brunet, L. J., J. A. McMahon et al. (1998). Noggin, cartilage morphogenesis, and joint formation in the mammalian skeleton. *Science* 280(5368): 1455-1457.

Burton-Wurster, N., V. J. Horn et al. (1988). Immunohistochemical localization of fibronectin and chondronectin in canine articular cartilage. *J Histochem Cytochem* 36(6): 581-588.

Capdevila, J., and R. L. Johnson. (1998). Endogenous and ectopic expression of noggin suggests a conserved mechanism for regulation of BMP function during limb and somite patterning. *Dev Biol* 197(2): 205-217.

Carlevaro, M. F., S. Cermelli et al. (2000). Vascular endothelial growth factor (VEGF) in cartilage neovascularization and chondrocyte differentiation: Auto-paracrine role during endochondral bone formation. *J Cell Sci* 113(Pt 1): 59-69.

Chadee, D. N., and J. M. Kyriakis. (2004). MLK3 is required for mitogen activation of B-Raf, ERK and cell proliferation. *Nat Cell Biol* 6(8): 770-776.

Charite, J., W. de Graaff et al. (1994). Ectopic expression of Hoxb-8 causes duplication of the ZPA in the forelimb and homeotic transformation of axial structures. *Cell* 78(4): 589-601.

Cheng, C. C., Y. Uchiyama et al. (2009). PI3K/AKT regulates aggrecan gene expression by modulating Sox9 expression and activity in nucleus pulposus cells of the intervertebral disc. *J Cell Physiol* 221(3): 668-676.

Chimal-Monroy, J., and L. Diaz de Leon. (1999). Expression of N-cadherin, N-CAM, fibronectin and tenascin is stimulated by TGF-beta1, beta2, beta3 and beta5 during the formation of precartilage condensations. *Int J Dev Biol* 43(1): 59-67.

Chiquet-Ehrismann, R., P. Kalla et al. (1989). Participation of tenascin and transforming growth factor-beta in reciprocal epithelial-mesenchymal interactions of MCF7 cells and fibroblasts. *Cancer Res* 49(15): 4322-4325.

Chong, H., H. G. Vikis et al. (2003). Mechanisms of regulating the Raf kinase family. *Cell Signal* 15(5): 463-469.

Christ, B., and J. Wilting. (1992). From somites to vertebral column. *Ann Anat* 174(1): 23-32.

Chubinskaya, S., C. Merrihew et al. (2000). Human articular chondrocytes express osteogenic protein-1. *J Histochem Cytochem* 48(2): 239-250.

Clancy, R., J. Rediske et al. (2001). Activation of stress-activated protein kinase in osteoarthritic cartilage: Evidence for nitric oxide dependence. *Osteoarthr Cartil* 9(4): 294-299.

Cole, N. J., M. Tanaka et al. (2003). Expression of limb initiation genes and clues to the morphological diversification of threespine stickleback. *Curr Biol* 13(24): R951-952.

Coleman, C. M., and R. S. Tuan. (2003a). Functional role of growth/differentiation factor 5 in chondrogenesis of limb mesenchymal cells. *Mech Dev* 120(7): 823-836.

Coleman, C. M., and R. S. Tuan. (2003b). Growth/differentiation factor 5 enhances chondrocyte maturation. *Dev Dyn* 228(2): 208-216.

Craig, F. M., G. Bentley et al. (1987). The spatial and temporal pattern of collagens I and II and keratan sulphate in the developing chick metatarsophalangeal joint. *Development* 99(3): 383-391.

Cserjesi, P., D. Brown et al. (1995). Scleraxis: A basic helix-loop-helix protein that prefigures skeletal formation during mouse embryogenesis. *Development* 121(4): 1099-1110.

Cuevas, P., J. Burgos et al. (1988). Basic fibroblast growth factor (FGF) promotes cartilage repair in vivo. *Biochem Biophys Res Commun* 156(2): 611-618.

Daumer, K. M., A. C. Tufan et al. (2004). Long-term in vitro analysis of limb cartilage development: Involvement of Wnt signaling. *J Cell Biochem* 93(3): 526-541.

de Caestecker, M. (2004). The transforming growth factor-beta superfamily of receptors. *Cytokine Growth Factor Rev* 15(1): 1-11.

de Larco, J. E., and G. J. Todaro. (1978). Growth factors from murine sarcoma virus-transformed cells. *Proc Natl Acad Sci USA* 75(8): 4001-4005.

DeLaurier, A., R. Schweitzer et al. (2006). Pitx1 determines the morphology of muscle, tendon, and bones of the hindlimb. *Dev Biol* 299(1): 22-34.

De Luca, F., K. M. Barnes et al. (2001). Regulation of growth plate chondrogenesis by bone morphogenetic protein-2. *Endocrinology* 142(1): 430-436.

Derynck, R., and Y. E. Zhang. (2003). Smad-dependent and Smad-independent pathways in TGF-beta family signalling. *Nature* 425(6958): 577-584.

Descalzi Cancedda, F., A. Melchiori et al. (1995). Production of angiogenesis inhibitors and stimulators is modulated by cultured growth plate chondrocytes during in vitro differentiation: Dependence on extracellular matrix assembly. *Eur J Cell Biol* 66(1): 60-68.

Ding, C., F. Cicuttini et al. (2009). Do NSAIDs affect longitudinal changes in knee cartilage volume and knee cartilage defects in older adults? *Am J Med* 122(9): 836-842.

Ding, L., E. Heying et al. (2010). Mechanical impact induces cartilage degradation via mitogen activated protein kinases. *Osteoarthr Cartil* 18(11): 1509-1517.

Ding, M., M. Dalstra et al. (1998). Mechanical properties of the normal human tibial cartilage-bone complex in relation to age. *Clin Biomech (Bristol, Avon)* 13(4-5): 351-358.

Dowthwaite, G. P., J. C. Edwards et al. (1998). An essential role for the interaction between hyaluronan and hyaluronan binding proteins during joint development. *J Histochem Cytochem* 46(5): 641-651.

Dowthwaite, G. P., C. R. Flannery et al. (2003). A mechanism underlying the movement requirement for synovial joint cavitation. *Matrix Biol* 22(4): 311-322.

Dreier, R. (2010). Hypertrophic differentiation of chondrocytes in osteoarthritis: The developmental aspect of degenerative joint disorders. *Arthritis Res Ther* 12(5): 216.

Du, K., and P. N. Tsichlis. (2005). Regulation of the Akt kinase by interacting proteins. *Oncogene* 24(50): 7401-7409.

DuRaine, G., C. P. Neu et al. (2009). Regulation of the friction coefficient of articular cartilage by TGF-beta1 and IL-1beta. *J Orthop Res* 27(2): 249-256.

DuRaine, G. D., S. M. Chan et al. (2011). Effects of TGF-beta1 on alternative splicing of superficial zone protein in articular cartilage cultures. *Osteoarthr Cartil* 19(1): 103-110.

Durr, J., P. Lammi et al. (1996). Identification and immunolocalization of laminin in cartilage. *Exp Cell Res* 222(1): 225-233.

Ellies, D. L., R. M. Langille et al. (1997). Specific craniofacial cartilage dysmorphogenesis coincides with a loss of dlx gene expression in retinoic acid-treated zebrafish embryos. *Mech Dev* 61(1-2): 23-36.

Eyre, D. R., I. R. Dickson et al. (1988). Collagen cross-linking in human bone and articular cartilage. Age-related changes in the content of mature hydroxypyridinium residues. *Biochem J* 252(2): 495-500.

Farnum, C. E., R. Lee et al. (2002). Volume increase in growth plate chondrocytes during hypertrophy: The contribution of organic osmolytes. *Bone* 30(4): 574-581.

Fassbender, M., C. Strobel et al. (2011). Local inhibition of angiogenesis results in an atrophic non-union in a rat osteotomy model. *Eur Cell Mater* 22: 1-11.

Ferrari, D., A. Harrington et al. (1999). Dlx-5 in limb initiation in the chick embryo. *Dev Dyn* 216(1): 10-15.

Fischer, L., G. Boland et al. (2002). Wnt signaling during BMP-2 stimulation of mesenchymal chondrogenesis. *J Cell Biochem* 84(4): 816-831.

Flechtenmacher, J., K. Huch et al. (1996). Recombinant human osteogenic protein 1 is a potent stimulator of the synthesis of cartilage proteoglycans and collagens by human articular chondrocytes. *Arthritis Rheum* 39(11): 1896-1904.

Forsyth, C. B., J. Pulai et al. (2002). Fibronectin fragments and blocking antibodies to alpha2beta1 and alpha5beta1 integrins stimulate mitogen-activated protein kinase signaling and increase collagenase 3 (matrix metalloproteinase 13) production by human articular chondrocytes. *Arthritis Rheum* 46(9): 2368-2376.

Fortier, L. A., H. O. Mohammed et al. (2002). Insulin-like growth factor-I enhances cell-based repair of articular cartilage. *J Bone Joint Surg Br* 84(2): 276-288.

Francis-West, P. H., J. Parish et al. (1999). BMP/GDF-signalling interactions during synovial joint development. *Cell Tissue Res* 296(1): 111-119.

Fujimoto, E., M. Ochi et al. (1999). Beneficial effect of basic fibroblast growth factor on the repair of full-thickness defects in rabbit articular cartilage. *Arch Orthop Trauma Surg* 119(3-4): 139-145.

Fujita, T., R. Fukuyama et al. (2004). Dexamethasone inhibits insulin-induced chondrogenesis of ATDC5 cells by preventing PI3K-Akt signaling and DNA binding of Runx2. *J Cell Biochem* 93(2): 374-383.

Gaissmaier, C., J. Fritz et al. (2005). Effect of human platelet supernatant on proliferation and matrix synthesis of human articular chondrocytes in monolayer and three-dimensional alginate cultures. *Biomaterials* 26(14): 1953-1960.

Gerber, H. P., T. H. Vu et al. (1999). VEGF couples hypertrophic cartilage remodeling, ossification and angiogenesis during endochondral bone formation. *Nat Med* 5(6): 623-628.

Gilbert, S. F. (2003). *Developmental Biology*. Sunderland, MA: Sinauer Associates.

Gitelman, S. E., M. S. Kobrin et al. (1994). Recombinant Vgr-1/BMP-6-expressing tumors induce fibrosis and endochondral bone formation in vivo. *J Cell Biol* 126(6): 1595-1609.

Goff, D. J., and C. J. Tabin. (1997). Analysis of Hoxd-13 and Hoxd-11 misexpression in chick limb buds reveals that Hox genes affect both bone condensation and growth. *Development* 124(3): 627-636.

Goldring, M. B., K. Tsuchimochi et al. (2006). The control of chondrogenesis. *J Cell Biochem* 97(1): 33-44.

Haaijman, A., R. N. D'Souza et al. (1997). OP-1 (BMP-7) affects mRNA expression of type I, II, X collagen, and matrix Gla protein in ossifying long bones in vitro. *J Bone Miner Res* 12(11): 1815-1823.

Hakomori, S. (1973). Glycolipids of tumor cell membrane. *Adv Cancer Res* 18: 265-315.

Hall, B. K., and T. Miyake. (1992). The membranous skeleton: The role of cell condensations in vertebrate skeletogenesis. *Anat Embryol (Berl)* 186(2): 107-124.

Hall, B. K., and T. Miyake. (2000). All for one and one for all: Condensations and the initiation of skeletal development. *Bioessays* 22(2): 138-147.

Han, J., J. D. Lee et al. (1993). Endotoxin induces rapid protein tyrosine phosphorylation in 70Z/3 cells expressing CD14. *J Biol Chem* 268(33): 25009-25014.

Han, J., J. D. Lee et al. (1994). A MAP kinase targeted by endotoxin and hyperosmolarity in mammalian cells. *Science* 265(5173): 808-811.

Harada, S., T. K. Sampath et al. (1997). Osteogenic protein-1 up-regulation of the collagen X promoter activity is mediated by a MEF-2-like sequence and requires an adjacent AP-1 sequence. *Mol Endocrinol* 11(12): 1832-1845.

Hartmann, C. (2002). Wnt-signaling and skeletogenesis. *J Musculoskelet Neuronal Interact* 2(3): 274-276.

Hartmann, C., and C. J. Tabin. (2001). Wnt-14 plays a pivotal role in inducing syno-vial joint formation in the developing appendicular skeleton. *Cell* 104(3): 341-351.

Hatton, J. P., M. Pooran et al. (2003). A short pulse of mechanical force induces gene expression and growth in MC3T3-E1 osteoblasts via an ERK 1/2 pathway. *J Bone Miner Res* 18(1): 58-66.

Haudenschild, D. R., J. Chen et al. (2010). Rho kinase-dependent activation of SOX9 in chondrocytes. *Arthritis Rheum* 62(1): 191-200.

Haudenschild, D. R., E. Hong et al. (2011). Enhanced activity of TGF-beta1 bound to cartilage oligomeric matrix protein. *J Biol Chem* 286(50): 43250-43258.

Healy, C., D. Uwanogho et al. (1999). Regulation and role of Sox9 in cartilage forma-tion. *Dev Dyn* 215(1): 69-78.

Hewitt, A. T., H. H. Varner et al. (1982a). The isolation and partial characterization of chondronectin, an attachment factor for chondrocytes. *J Biol Chem* 257(5): 2330-2334.

Hewitt, A. T., H. H. Varner et al. (1982b). The role of chondronectin and cartilage proteoglycan in the attachment of chondrocytes to collagen. *Prog Clin Biol Res* 110(Pt B): 25-33.

Hidaka, C., L. R. Goodrich et al. (2003). Acceleration of cartilage repair by genetically modified chondrocytes over expressing bone morphogenetic protein-7. *J Orthop Res* 21(4): 573-583.

Holleville, N., A. Quilhac et al. (2003). BMP signals regulate Dlx5 during early avian skull development. *Dev Biol* 257(1): 177-189.

Horiki, M., T. Imamura et al. (2004). Smad6/Smurf1 overexpression in cartilage delays chondrocyte hypertrophy and causes dwarfism with osteopenia. *J Cell Biol* 165(3): 433-445.

Horton, W. A. (1990). The biology of bone growth. *Growth Genet Horm* 6(2): 1-3.

Houston, B., B. H. Thorp et al. (1994). Molecular cloning and expression of bone mor-phogenetic protein-7 in the chick epiphyseal growth plate. *J Mol Endocrinol* 13(3): 289-301.

Hueber, S. D., G. F. Weiller et al. (2010). Improving Hox protein classification across the major model organisms. *PLoS One* 5(5): e10820.

Hung, C. T., D. R. Henshaw et al. (2000). Mitogen-activated protein kinase signaling in bovine articular chondrocytes in response to fluid flow does not require calcium mobilization. *J Biomech* 33(1): 73-80.

Hwang, S. G., S. S. Yu et al. (2005). Wnt-3a regulates chondrocyte differentiation via c-Jun/AP-1 pathway. *FEBS Lett* 579(21): 4837-4842.

Hynes, R. O. (1973). Alteration of cell-surface proteins by viral transformation and by proteolysis. *Proc Natl Acad Sci USA* 70(11): 3170-3174.

Hynes, R. O. (1987). Integrins: A family of cell surface receptors. *Cell* 48(4): 549-554.

Hynes, R. O. (2002). Integrins: Bidirectional, allosteric signaling machines. *Cell* 110(6): 673-687.

Hyttinen, M. M., J. P. Arokoski et al. (2001). Age matters: Collagen birefringence of superficial articular cartilage is increased in young guinea-pigs but decreased in older animals after identical physiological type of joint loading. *Osteoarthr Cartil* 9(8): 694-701.

Im, H. J., P. Muddasani et al. (2007). Basic fibroblast growth factor stimulates matrix metalloproteinase-13 via the molecular cross-talk between the mitogen-activated protein kinases and protein kinase Cdelta pathways in human adult articular chondrocytes. *J Biol Chem* 282(15): 11110-11121.

Itoh, N., and D. M. Ornitz. (2011). Fibroblast growth factors: From molecular evolution to roles in development, metabolism and disease. *J Biochem* 149(2): 121-130.

Jenne, D., and K. K. Stanley. (1985). Molecular cloning of S-protein, a link between complement, coagulation and cell-substrate adhesion. *EMBO J* 4(12): 3153-3157.

Jessop, H. L., S. C. Rawlinson et al. (2002). Mechanical strain and fluid movement both activate extracellular regulated kinase (ERK) in osteoblast-like cells but via different signaling pathways. *Bone* 31(1): 186-194.

Jiang, T. X., J. R. Yi et al. (1993). Activin enhances chondrogenesis of limb bud cells: Stimulation of precartilaginous mesenchymal condensations and expression of NCAM. *Dev Biol* 155(2): 545-557.

Jin, E. J., S. Y. Lee et al. (2006). BMP-2-enhanced chondrogenesis involves p38 MAPK-mediated down-regulation of Wnt-7a pathway. *Mol Cells* 22(3): 353-359.

Johnson, K. A., D. M. Rose et al. (2008). Factor XIIIA mobilizes transglutaminase 2 to induce chondrocyte hypertrophic differentiation. *J Cell Sci* 121(Pt 13): 2256-2264.

Junttila, M. R., S. P. Li et al. (2008). Phosphatase-mediated crosstalk between MAPK signaling pathways in the regulation of cell survival. *FASEB J* 22(4): 954-965.

Kandel, R. A., J. Boyle et al. (1997). In vitro formation of mineralized cartilagenous tissue by articular chondrocytes. *In Vitro Cell Dev Biol Anim* 33(3): 174-181.

Kavanagh, E., M. Abiri et al. (2002). Division and death of cells in developing synovial joints and long bones. *Cell Biol Int* 26(8): 679-688.

Kavumpurath, S., and B. K. Hall. (1990). Lack of either chondrocyte hypertrophy or osteogenesis in Meckel's cartilage of the embryonic chick exposed to epithelia and to thyroxine in vitro. *J Craniofac Genet Dev Biol* 10(3): 263-275.

Keijer, J., M. Linders et al. (1991). On the target specificity of plasminogen activator inhibitor 1: The role of heparin, vitronectin, and the reactive site. *Blood* 78(5): 1254-1261.

Keyte, A. L., and K. K. Smith. (2010). Developmental origins of precocial forelimbs in marsupial neonates. *Development* 137(24): 4283-4294.

Klaus, A., and W. Birchmeier. (2008). Wnt signalling and its impact on development and cancer. *Nat Rev Cancer* 8(5): 387-398.

Kolch, W. (2005). Coordinating ERK/MAPK signalling through scaffolds and inhibitors. *Nat Rev Mol Cell Biol* 6(11): 827-837.

Koo, S., and T. P. Andriacchi. (2007). A comparison of the influence of global functional loads vs. local contact anatomy on articular cartilage thickness at the knee. *J Biomech* 40(13): 2961-2966.

Kook, S. H., J. M. Hwang et al. (2009). Mechanical force induces type I collagen expression in human periodontal ligament fibroblasts through activation of ERK/JNK and AP-1. *J Cell Biochem* 106(6): 1060-1067.

Kost, C., W. Stuber et al. (1992). Mapping of binding sites for heparin, plasminogen activator inhibitor-1, and plasminogen to vitronectin's heparin-binding region reveals a novel vitronectin-dependent feedback mechanism for the control of plasmin formation. *J Biol Chem* 267(17): 12098-12105.

Koyama, E., T. Ochiai et al. (2007). Synovial joint formation during mouse limb skeletogenesis: Roles of Indian hedgehog signaling. *Ann NY Acad Sci* 1116: 100-112.

Krishna, M., and H. Narang. (2008). The complexity of mitogen-activated protein kinases (MAPKs) made simple. *Cell Mol Life Sci* 65(22): 3525-3544.

Kronenberg, H. M. (2003). Developmental regulation of the growth plate. *Nature* 423(6937): 332-336.

Kumar, D., and A. B. Lassar. (2009). The transcriptional activity of Sox9 in chondrocytes is regulated by RhoA signaling and actin polymerization. *Mol Cell Biol* 29(15): 4262-4273.

Kypriotou, M., M. Fossard-Demoor et al. (2003). SOX9 exerts a bifunctional effect on type II collagen gene (COL2A1) expression in chondrocytes depending on the differentiation state. *DNA Cell Biol* 22(2): 119-129.

Kyriakis, J. M., and J. Avruch. (1990). Insulin, epidermal growth factor and fibroblast growth factor elicit distinct patterns of protein tyrosine phosphorylation in BC3H1 cells. *Biochim Biophys Acta* 1054(1): 73-82.

Laboureau, J., L. Dubertret et al. (2004). ERK activation by mechanical strain is regulated by the small G proteins rac-1 and rhoA. *Exp Dermatol* 13(2): 70-77.

Lefebvre, V., R. R. Behringer et al. (2001). L-Sox5, Sox6 and Sox9 control essential steps of the chondrocyte differentiation pathway. *Osteoarthr Cartil* 9(Suppl A): S69-S75.

Leonard, C. M., H. M. Fuld et al. (1991). Role of transforming growth factor-beta in chondrogenic pattern formation in the embryonic limb: Stimulation of mesenchymal condensation and fibronectin gene expression by exogeneous TGF-beta and evidence for endogenous TGF-beta-like activity. *Dev Biol* 145(1): 99-109.

Li, J., Z. Zhao et al. (2010). MEK/ERK and p38 MAPK regulate chondrogenesis of rat bone marrow mesenchymal stem cells through delicate interaction with TGF-beta1/Smads pathway. *Cell Prolif* 43(4): 333-343.

Li, X., M. Ellman et al. (2009). Prostaglandin E2 and its cognate EP receptors control human adult articular cartilage homeostasis and are linked to the pathophysiology of osteoarthritis. *Arthritis Rheum* 60(2): 513-523.

Liu, J., L. Zou et al. (2006). ERK, as an early responder of mechanical signals, mediates in several mechanotransduction pathways in osteoblast-like cells. *Biochem Biophys Res Commun* 348(3): 1167-1173.

Liu, Y., H. Li et al. (2000). Identification of an enhancer sequence within the first intron required for cartilage-specific transcription of the alpha2(XI) collagen gene. *J Biol Chem* 275(17): 12712-12718.

Loboa, E. G., G. S. Beaupre et al. (2001). Mechanobiology of initial pseudarthrosis formation with oblique fractures. *J Orthop Res* 19(6): 1067-1072.

Loeser, R. F., H. J. Im et al. (2009). Methylation of the OP-1 promoter: Potential role in the age-related decline in OP-1 expression in cartilage. *Osteoarthr Cartil* 17(4): 513-517.

Loeser, R. F., C. A. Pacione et al. (2003). The combination of insulin-like growth factor 1 and osteogenic protein 1 promotes increased survival of and matrix synthesis by normal and osteoarthritic human articular chondrocytes. *Arthritis Rheum* 48(8): 2188-2196.

Lothe, K., M. A. Spycher et al. (1979). Human articular cartilage in relation to age, a morphometric study. *Exp Cell Biol* 47(1): 22-28.

Lotz, M. K., and B. Carames. (2011). Autophagy and cartilage homeostasis mechanisms in joint health, aging and OA. *Nat Rev Rheumatol* 7(10): 579-587.

Luo, Y., I. Kostetskii et al. (2005). N-cadherin is not essential for limb mesenchymal chondrogenesis. *Dev Dyn* 232(2): 336-344.

Luyten, F. P., N. S. Cunningham et al. (1992). Advances in osteogenin and related bone morphogenetic proteins in bone induction and repair. *Acta Orthop Belg* 58(Suppl 1): 263-267.

Luyten, F. P., V. C. Hascall et al. (1988). Insulin-like growth factors maintain steady-state metabolism of proteoglycans in bovine articular cartilage explants. *Arch Biochem Biophys* 267(2): 416-425.

Mancilla, E. E., F. De Luca et al. (1998). Effects of fibroblast growth factor-2 on longitudinal bone growth. *Endocrinology* 139(6): 2900-2904.

Manning, B. D., and L. C. Cantley. (2007). AKT/PKB signaling: Navigating downstream. *Cell* 129(7): 1261-1274.

Martin, G. R. (1998). The roles of FGFs in the early development of vertebrate limbs. *Genes Dev* 12(11): 1571-1586.

Martin, J. A., S. M. Ellerbroek et al. (1997). Age-related decline in chondrocyte response to insulin-like growth factor-I: The role of growth factor binding proteins. *J Orthop Res* 15(4): 491-498.

Massague, J. (2000). How cells read TGF-beta signals. *Nat Rev Mol Cell Biol* 1(3): 169-178.

McMahon, J. A., S. Takada et al. (1998). Noggin-mediated antagonism of BMP signaling is required for growth and patterning of the neural tube and somite. *Genes Dev* 12(10): 1438-1452.

Meachim, G. (1971). Effect of age on the thickness of adult articular cartilage at the shoulder joint. *Ann Rheum Dis* 30(1): 43-46.

Meachim, G., G. Bentley et al. (1977). Effect of age on thickness of adult patellar articular cartilage. *Ann Rheum Dis* 36(6): 563-568.

Merida-Velasco, J. A., I. Sanchez-Montesinos et al. (1997). Development of the human knee joint. *Anat Rec* 248(2): 269-278.

Mierisch, C. M., P. C. Anderson et al. (2002). Treatment with insulin-like growth factor-1 increases chondrogenesis by periosteum in vitro. *Connect Tissue Res* 43(4): 559-568.

Miller, J. R., and R. T. Moon. (1996). Signal transduction through beta-catenin and specification of cell fate during embryogenesis. *Genes Dev* 10(20): 2527-2539.

Minguillon, C., J. Del Buono et al. (2005). Tbx5 and Tbx4 are not sufficient to determine limb-specific morphologies but have common roles in initiating limb outgrowth. *Dev Cell* 8(1): 75-84.

Miyazono, K., S. Maeda et al. (2005). BMP receptor signaling: Transcriptional targets, regulation of signals, and signaling cross-talk. *Cytokine Growth Factor Rev* 16(3): 251-263.

Moon, A. M., and M. R. Capecchi. (2000). Fgf8 is required for outgrowth and patterning of the limbs. *Nat Genet* 26(4): 455-459.

Moos, V., S. Fickert et al. (1999). Immunohistological analysis of cytokine expression in human osteoarthritic and healthy cartilage. *J Rheumatol* 26(4): 870-879.

Moscona, A., and H. Moscona. (1952). The dissociation and aggregation of cells from organ rudiments of the early chick embryo. *J Anat* 86(3): 287-301.

Moscona, A. A. (1968). Cell aggregation: Properties of specific cell-ligands and their role in the formation of multicellular systems. *Dev Biol* 18(3): 250-277.

Muddasani, P., J. C. Norman et al. (2007). Basic fibroblast growth factor activates the MAPK and NFkappaB pathways that converge on Elk-1 to control production of matrix metalloproteinase-13 by human adult articular chondrocytes. *J Biol Chem* 282(43): 31409-31421.

Murakami, S., M. Kan et al. (2000). Up-regulation of the chondrogenic Sox9 gene by fibroblast growth factors is mediated by the mitogen-activated protein kinase pathway. *Proc Natl Acad Sci USA* 97(3): 1113-1118.

Murray, R. C., R. M. DeBowes et al. (1998). The effects of intra-articular methylprednisolone and exercise on the mechanical properties of articular cartilage in the horse. *Osteoarthr Cartil* 6(2): 106-114.

Nakamura, K., T. Shirai et al. (1999). p38 mitogen-activated protein kinase functionally contributes to chondrogenesis induced by growth/differentiation factor-5 in ATDC5 cells. *Exp Cell Res* 250(2): 351-363.

Neu, C. P., A. Khalafi et al. (2007). Mechanotransduction of bovine articular cartilage superficial zone protein by transforming growth factor beta signaling. *Arthritis Rheum* 56(11): 3706-3714.

Niswander, L., and G. R. Martin. (1993a). FGF-4 and BMP-2 have opposite effects on limb growth. *Nature* 361(6407): 68-71.

Niswander, L., and G. R. Martin. (1993b). Mixed signals from the AER: FGF-4 and Bmp-2 have opposite effects on limb growth. *Prog Clin Biol Res* 383B: 625-633.

Niswander, L., C. Tickle et al. (1994). Function of FGF-4 in limb development. *Mol Reprod Dev* 39(1): 83-88; discussion 88-89.

Noden, D. M. (1983). The role of the neural crest in patterning of avian cranial skeletal, connective, and muscle tissues. *Dev Biol* 96(1): 144-165.

Nusse, R. (2005). Wnt signaling in disease and in development. *Cell Res* 15(1): 28-32.

Nusse, R., A. van Ooyen et al. (1984). Mode of proviral activation of a putative mammary oncogene (int-1) on mouse chromosome 15. *Nature* 307(5947): 131-136.

Nusslein-Volhard, C., and E. Wieschaus. (1980). Mutations affecting segment number and polarity in *Drosophila*. *Nature* 287(5785): 795-801.

Oberlender, S. A., and R. S. Tuan. (1994a). Expression and functional involvement of N-cadherin in embryonic limb chondrogenesis. *Development* 120(1): 177-187.

Oberlender, S. A., and R. S. Tuan. (1994b). Spatiotemporal profile of N-cadherin expression in the developing limb mesenchyme. *Cell Adhes Commun* 2(6): 521-537.

O'Connor, W. J., T. Botti et al. (2000). The use of growth factors in cartilage repair. *Orthop Clin North Am* 31(3): 399-410.

Oh, C. D., S. H. Chang et al. (2000). Opposing role of mitogen-activated protein kinase subtypes, erk-1/2 and p38, in the regulation of chondrogenesis of mesenchymes. *J Biol Chem* 275(8): 5613-5619.

Oh, C. D., and J. S. Chun. (2003). Signaling mechanisms leading to the regulation of differentiation and apoptosis of articular chondrocytes by insulin-like growth factor-1. *J Biol Chem* 278(38): 36563-36571.

O'Keefe, R. J., L. S. Loveys et al. (1997). Differential regulation of type-II and type-X collagen synthesis by parathyroid hormone-related protein in chick growth-plate chondrocytes. *J Orthop Res* 15(2): 162-174.

Okubo, Y., and A. H. Reddi. (2003). Thyroxine downregulates Sox9 and promotes chondrocyte hypertrophy. *Biochem Biophys Res Commun* 306(1): 186-190.

Okuda, S., A. Myoui et al. (2001). Mechanisms of age-related decline in insulin-like growth factor-I dependent proteoglycan synthesis in rat intervertebral disc cells. *Spine (Phila Pa 1976)* 26(22): 2421-2426.

Olson, E. N., D. Brown et al. (1996). A new subclass of helix-loop-helix transcription factors expressed in paraxial mesoderm and chondrogenic cell lineages. *Ann NY Acad Sci* 785: 108-118.

Pacifici, M., M. Iwamoto et al. (1993). Tenascin is associated with articular cartilage development. *Dev Dyn* 198(2): 123-134.

Pacifici, M., E. Koyama et al. (2000). Development of articular cartilage: What do we know about it and how may it occur? *Connect Tissue Res* 41(3): 175-184.

Pacifici, M., E. Koyama et al. (2006). Cellular and molecular mechanisms of synovial joint and articular cartilage formation. *Ann NY Acad Sci* 1068: 74-86.

Panda, D. K., D. Miao et al. (2001). The transcription factor SOX9 regulates cell cycle and differentiation genes in chondrocytic CFK2 cells. *J Biol Chem* 276(44): 41229-41236.

Papachristou, D. J., P. Pirttiniemi et al. (2005). JNK/ERK-AP-1/Runx2 induction "paves the way" to cartilage load-ignited chondroblastic differentiation. *Histochem Cell Biol* 124(3-4): 215-223.

Pecina, M., M. Jelic et al. (2002). Articular cartilage repair: The role of bone morphogenetic proteins. *Int Orthop* 26(3): 131-136.

Pouyssegur, J., V. Volmat et al. (2002). Fidelity and spatio-temporal control in MAP kinase (ERKs) signalling. *Biochem Pharmacol* 64(5-6): 755-763.

Prasadam, I., S. van Gennip et al. (2010). ERK-1/2 and p38 in the regulation of hypertrophic changes of normal articular cartilage chondrocytes induced by osteoarthritic subchondral osteoblasts. *Arthritis Rheum* 62(5): 1349-1360.

Provot, S., D. Zinyk et al. (2007). Hif-1alpha regulates differentiation of limb bud mesenchyme and joint development. *J Cell Biol* 177(3): 451-464.

Pytela, R., M. D. Pierschbacher et al. (1985). Identification and isolation of a 140 kd cell surface glycoprotein with properties expected of a fibronectin receptor. *Cell* 40(1): 191-198.

Raingeaud, J., S. Gupta et al. (1995). Pro-inflammatory cytokines and environmental stress cause p38 mitogen-activated protein kinase activation by dual phosphorylation on tyrosine and threonine. *J Biol Chem* 270(13): 7420-7426.

Reddi, A. H. (1996). BMP-1: Resurrection as procollagen C-proteinase. *Science* 271(5248): 463.

Reddi, A. H. (1998a). Initiation of fracture repair by bone morphogenetic proteins. *Clin Orthop Relat Res* 355(Suppl): S66-S72.

Reddi, A. H. (1998b). Role of morphogenetic proteins in skeletal tissue engineering and regeneration. *Nat Biotechnol* 16(3): 247-252.

Reddi, A. H. (2003). Cartilage morphogenetic proteins: Role in joint development, homoeostasis, and regeneration. *Ann Rheum Dis* 62(Suppl 2): ii73-ii78.

Reddi, A. H., and C. Huggins. (1972). Biochemical sequences in the transformation of normal fibroblasts in adolescent rats. *Proc Natl Acad Sci USA* 69(6): 1601-1605.

Reginato, A. M., R. S. Tuan et al. (1993). Effects of calcium deficiency on chondrocyte hypertrophy and type X collagen expression in chick embryonic sternum. *Dev Dyn* 198(4): 284-295.

Responte, D. J., J. K. Lee et al. (2012). Biomechanics-driven chondrogenesis: From embryo to adult. *FASEB J* 26(9): 3614-3624.

Reusch, H. P., G. Chan et al. (1997). Activation of JNK/SAPK and ERK by mechanical strain in vascular smooth muscle cells depends on extracellular matrix composition. *Biochem Biophys Res Commun* 237(2): 239-244.

Roberts, A. B., M. A. Anzano et al. (1983). Purification and properties of a type beta transforming growth factor from bovine kidney. *Biochemistry* 22(25): 5692-5698.

Roberts, P. J., and C. J. Der. (2007). Targeting the Raf-MEK-ERK mitogen-activated protein kinase cascade for the treatment of cancer. *Oncogene* 26(22): 3291-3310.

Robins, J. C., N. Akeno et al. (2005). Hypoxia induces chondrocyte-specific gene expression in mesenchymal cells in association with transcriptional activation of Sox9. *Bone* 37(3): 313-322.

Rountree, R. B., M. Schoor et al. (2004). BMP receptor signaling is required for postnatal maintenance of articular cartilage. *PLoS Biol* 2(11): e355.

Rousseau, N., P. Brazeau et al. (1998). Effect of aging on growth hormone-induced insulin-like growth factor-I secretion from cultured rat chondrocytes. *Growth Horm IGF Res* 8(5): 403-409.

Rowan, A. D. (2001). Cartilage catabolism in arthritis: Factors that influence homeostasis. *Expert Rev Mol Med* 2001: 1-20.

Ruoslahti, E., A. Vaheri et al. (1973). Fibroblast surface antigen: A new serum protein. *Biochim Biophys Acta* 322(2): 352-358.

Ryan, J. A., E. A. Eisner et al. (2009). Mechanical compression of articular cartilage induces chondrocyte proliferation and inhibits proteoglycan synthesis by activation of the ERK pathway: Implications for tissue engineering and regenerative medicine. *J Tissue Eng Regen Med* 3(2): 107-116.

Sacks, D. B. (2006). The role of scaffold proteins in MEK/ERK signalling. *Biochem Soc Trans* 34(Pt 5): 833-836.

Saga, Y., T. Yagi et al. (1992). Mice develop normally without tenascin. *Genes Dev* 6(10): 1821-1831.

Salmivirta, M., K. Elenius et al. (1991). Syndecan from embryonic tooth mesenchyme binds tenascin. *J Biol Chem* 266(12): 7733-7739.

Sasano, Y., E. Ohtani et al. (1993). BMPs induce direct bone formation in ectopic sites independent of the endochondral ossification in vivo. *Anat Rec* 236(2): 373-380.

Savage, C., P. Das et al. (1996). *Caenorhabditis elegans* genes sma-2, sma-3, and sma-4 define a conserved family of transforming growth factor beta pathway components. *Proc Natl Acad Sci USA* 93(2): 790-794.

Schaeffer, H. J., and M. J. Weber. (1999). Mitogen-activated protein kinases: Specific messages from ubiquitous messengers. *Mol Cell Biol* 19(4): 2435-2444.

Schipani, E. (2005). Hypoxia and HIF-1 alpha in chondrogenesis. *Semin Cell Dev Biol* 16(4-5): 539-546.

Seemann, P., A. Brehm et al. (2009). Mutations in GDF5 reveal a key residue mediating BMP inhibition by NOGGIN. *PLoS Genet* 5(11): e1000747.

Sekelsky, J. J., S. J. Newfeld et al. (1995). Genetic characterization and cloning of mothers against dpp, a gene required for decapentaplegic function in *Drosophila melanogaster. Genetics* 139(3): 1347-1358.

Sekiya, I., K. Tsuji et al. (2000). SOX9 enhances aggrecan gene promoter/enhancer activity and is up-regulated by retinoic acid in a cartilage-derived cell line, TC6. *J Biol Chem* 275(15): 10738–10744.

Settle, S. H., Jr., R. B. Rountree et al. (2003). Multiple joint and skeletal patterning defects caused by single and double mutations in the mouse Gdf6 and Gdf5 genes. *Dev Biol* 254(1): 116-130.

Shapiro, I. M., K. Debolt et al. (1992). Developmental regulation of creatine kinase activity in cells of the epiphyseal growth cartilage. *J Bone Miner Res* 7(5): 493-500.

Shi, Y., and J. Massague. (2003). Mechanisms of TGF-beta signaling from cell membrane to the nucleus. *Cell* 113(6): 685-700.

Shum, L., X. Wang et al. (2003). BMP4 promotes chondrocyte proliferation and hypertrophy in the endochondral cranial base. *Int J Dev Biol* 47(6): 423-431.

Sirard, C., S. Kim et al. (2000). Targeted disruption in murine cells reveals variable requirement for Smad4 in transforming growth factor beta-related signaling. *J Biol Chem* 275(3): 2063-2070.

Sondergaard, B. C., N. Schultz et al. (2010). MAPKs are essential upstream signaling pathways in proteolytic cartilage degradation—Divergence in pathways leading to aggrecanase and MMP-mediated articular cartilage degradation. *Osteoarthr Cartil* 18(3): 279-288.

Sosic, D., B. Brand-Saberi et al. (1997). Regulation of paraxis expression and somite formation by ectoderm- and neural tube-derived signals. *Dev Biol* 185(2): 229-243.

Spater, D., T. P. Hill et al. (2006). Wnt9a signaling is required for joint integrity and regulation of Ihh during chondrogenesis. *Development* 133(15): 3039-3049.

Stanton, L. A., S. Sabari et al. (2004). p38 MAP kinase signalling is required for hypertrophic chondrocyte differentiation. *Biochem J* 378(Pt 1): 53-62.

Steinberg, M. S., and S. A. Roth. (1964). Phases in cell aggregation and tissue reconstruction an approach to the kinetics of cell aggregation. *J Exp Zool* 157: 327-338.

Steinberg, M. S., and M. Takeichi. (1994). Experimental specification of cell sorting, tissue spreading, and specific spatial patterning by quantitative differences in cadherin expression. *Proc Natl Acad Sci USA* 91(1): 206-209.

Stockwell, R. A. (1967). The cell density of human articular and costal cartilage. *J Anat* 101(Pt 4): 753-763.

Stott, N. S., T. X. Jiang et al. (1999). Successive formative stages of precartilaginous mesenchymal condensations in vitro: Modulation of cell adhesion by Wnt-7A and BMP-2. *J Cell Physiol* 180(3): 314-324.

Tacchetti, C., S. Tavella et al. (1992). Cell condensation in chondrogenic differentiation. *Exp Cell Res* 200(1): 26-33.

Takeichi, M. (1977). Functional correlation between cell adhesive properties and some cell surface proteins. *J Cell Biol* 75(2 Pt 1): 464-474.

Tamkun, J. W., D. W. DeSimone et al. (1986). Structure of integrin, a glycoprotein involved in the transmembrane linkage between fibronectin and actin. *Cell* 46(2): 271-282.

Tavella, S., P. Raffo et al. (1994). N-CAM and N-cadherin expression during in vitro chondrogenesis. *Exp Cell Res* 215(2): 354-362.

Tetlow, L. C., D. J. Adlam et al. (2001). Matrix metalloproteinase and proinflammatory cytokine production by chondrocytes of human osteoarthritic cartilage: Associations with degenerative changes. *Arthritis Rheum* 44(3): 585-594.

Thompson, T. J., P. D. Owens et al. (1989). Intramembranous osteogenesis and angiogenesis in the chick embryo. *J Anat* 166: 55-65.

Thonar, E. J., M. B. Sweet et al. (1978). Hyaluronate in articular cartilage: Age-related changes. *Calcif Tissue Res* 26(1): 19-21.

Tickle, C. (2002). Molecular basis of vertebrate limb patterning. *Am J Med Genet* 112(3): 250-255.

Tickle, C. (2003). Patterning systems—From one end of the limb to the other. *Dev Cell* 4(4): 449-458.

Timpl, R., H. Rohde et al. (1979). Laminin—A glycoprotein from basement membranes. *J Biol Chem* 254(19): 9933-9937.

Tomasini-Johansson, B. R., J. Milbrink et al. (1998). Vitronectin expression in rheumatoid arthritic synovia—Inhibition of plasmin generation by vitronectin produced in vitro. *Br J Rheumatol* 37(6): 620-629.

Triphaus, G. F., A. Schmidt et al. (1980). Age-related changes in the incorporation of [35S]sulfate into two proteoglycan populations from human cartilage. *Hoppe Seylers Z Physiol Chem* 361(12): 1773-1779.

Turner, A. S., K. A. Athanasiou et al. (1997). Biochemical effects of estrogen on articular cartilage in ovariectomized sheep. *Osteoarthr Cartil* 5(1): 63-69.

Tylzanowski, P., L. Mebis et al. (2006). The Noggin null mouse phenotype is strain dependent and haploinsufficiency leads to skeletal defects. *Dev Dyn* 235(6): 1599-1607.

Ulici, V., K. D. Hoenselaar et al. (2008). The PI3K pathway regulates endochondral bone growth through control of hypertrophic chondrocyte differentiation. *BMC Dev Biol* 8: 40.

Ulici, V., C. G. James et al. (2010). Regulation of gene expression by PI3K in mouse growth plate chondrocytes. *PLoS One* 5(1): e8866.

Urist, M. R. (1965). Bone: Formation by autoinduction. *Science* 150(3698): 893-899.

Vaahtokari, A., S. Vainio et al. (1991). Associations between transforming growth factor beta 1 RNA expression and epithelial-mesenchymal interactions during tooth morphogenesis. *Development* 113(3): 985-994.

Vaheri, A., and E. Ruoslahti. (1974). Disappearance of a major cell-type specific surface glycoprotein antigen (SF) after transformation of fibroblasts by Rous sarcoma virus. *Int J Cancer* 13(5): 579-586.

van den Berg, W. B., L. A. Joosten et al. (1999). Role of tumour necrosis factor alpha in experimental arthritis: Separate activity of interleukin 1beta in chronicity and cartilage destruction. *Ann Rheum Dis* 58(Suppl 1): I40-I48.

van Turnhout, M. C., H. Schipper et al. (2010). Postnatal development of depth-dependent collagen density in ovine articular cartilage. *BMC Dev Biol* 10: 108.

Vaughan-Thomas, A., J. Dudhia et al. (2008). Modification of the composition of articular cartilage collagen fibrils with increasing age. *Connect Tissue Res* 49(5): 374-382.

Wang, G., and F. Beier. (2005). Rac1/Cdc42 and RhoA GTPases antagonistically regulate chondrocyte proliferation, hypertrophy, and apoptosis. *J Bone Miner Res* 20(6): 1022-1031.

Wang, J., D. Elewaut et al. (2003). Insulin-like growth factor 1-induced interleukin-1 receptor II overrides the activity of interleukin-1 and controls the homeostasis of the extracellular matrix of cartilage. *Arthritis Rheum* 48(5): 1281-1291.

Wang, N., J. D. Tytell et al. (2009). Mechanotransduction at a distance: Mechanically coupling the extracellular matrix with the nucleus. *Nat Rev Mol Cell Biol* 10(1): 75-82.

Wang, W., G. Zhou et al. (1997). Activation of the hematopoietic progenitor kinase-1 (HPK1)-dependent, stress-activated c-Jun N-terminal kinase (JNK) pathway by transforming growth factor beta (TGF-beta)-activated kinase (TAK1), a kinase mediator of TGF beta signal transduction. *J Biol Chem* 272(36): 22771-22775.

Wei, X., T. Rasanen et al. (1998). Maturation-related compressive properties of rabbit knee articular cartilage and volume fraction of subchondral tissue. *Osteoarthr Cartil* 6(6): 400-409.

Wells, T., C. Davidson et al. (2003). Age-related changes in the composition, the molecular stoichiometry and the stability of proteoglycan aggregates extracted from human articular cartilage. *Biochem J* 370(Pt 1): 69-79.

Weston, C. R., and R. J. Davis. (2002). The JNK signal transduction pathway. *Curr Opin Genet Dev* 12(1): 14-21.

Widelitz, R. B., T. X. Jiang et al. (1993). Adhesion molecules in skeletogenesis. II. Neural cell adhesion molecules mediate precartilaginous mesenchymal condensations and enhance chondrogenesis. *J Cell Physiol* 156(2): 399-411.

Woods, A., and F. Beier. (2006). RhoA/ROCK signaling regulates chondrogenesis in a context-dependent manner. *J Biol Chem* 281(19): 13134-13140.

Woods, A., G. Wang et al. (2005). RhoA/ROCK signaling regulates Sox9 expression and actin organization during chondrogenesis. *J Biol Chem* 280(12): 11626-11634.

Woodward, W. A., and R. S. Tuan. (1999). N-Cadherin expression and signaling in limb mesenchymal chondrogenesis: Stimulation by poly-L-lysine. *Dev Genet* 24(1-2): 178-187.

Wu, Q. Q., and Q. Chen. (2000). Mechanoregulation of chondrocyte proliferation, maturation, and hypertrophy: Ion-channel dependent transduction of matrix deformation signals. *Exp Cell Res* 256(2): 383-391.

Yaeger, P. C., T. L. Masi et al. (1997). Synergistic action of transforming growth factor-beta and insulin-like growth factor-I induces expression of type II collagen and aggrecan genes in adult human articular chondrocytes. *Exp Cell Res* 237(2): 318-325.

Yamada, K. M., K. Olden et al. (1978). Transformation-sensitive cell surface protein: Isolation, characterization, and role in cellular morphology and adhesion. *Ann NY Acad Sci* 312: 256-277.

Yang, X., L. Chen et al. (2001). TGF-beta/Smad3 signals repress chondrocyte hypertrophic differentiation and are required for maintaining articular cartilage. *J Cell Biol* 153(1): 35-46.

Yano, F., F. Kugimiya et al. (2005). The canonical Wnt signaling pathway promotes chondrocyte differentiation in a Sox9-dependent manner. *Biochem Biophys Res Commun* 333(4): 1300-1308.

Yao, Z., Y. Dolginov et al. (2000). Detection of partially phosphorylated forms of ERK by monoclonal antibodies reveals spatial regulation of ERK activity by phosphatases. *FEBS Lett* 468(1): 37-42.

Yasuda, T., M. Shimizu et al. (2003). Matrix metalloproteinase production by COOH-terminal heparin-binding fibronectin fragment in rheumatoid synovial cells. *Lab Invest* 83(2): 153-162.

Yin, W., J. I. Park et al. (2009). Oxidative stress inhibits insulin-like growth factor-I induction of chondrocyte proteoglycan synthesis through differential regulation of phosphatidylinositol 3-kinase-Akt and MEK-ERK MAPK signaling pathways. *J Biol Chem* 284(46): 31972-31981.

Yonei-Tamura, S., T. Endo et al. (1999). FGF7 and FGF10 directly induce the apical ectodermal ridge in chick embryos. *Dev Biol* 211(1): 133-143.

Yonekura, A., M. Osaki et al. (1999). Transforming growth factor-beta stimulates articular chondrocyte cell growth through p44/42 MAP kinase (ERK) activation. *Endocr J* 46(4): 545-53.

Yoon, B. S., R. Pogue et al. (2006). BMPs regulate multiple aspects of growth-plate chondrogenesis through opposing actions on FGF pathways. *Development* 133(23): 4667-4678.

Yoon, Y. M., S. J. Kim et al. (2002). Maintenance of differentiated phenotype of articular chondrocytes by protein kinase C and extracellular signal-regulated protein kinase. *J Biol Chem* 277(10): 8412-8420.

Zakany, R., Z. Szijgyarto et al. (2005). Hydrogen peroxide inhibits formation of cartilage in chicken micromass cultures and decreases the activity of calcineurin: Implication of ERK1/2 and Sox9 pathways. *Exp Cell Res* 305(1): 190-199.

Zarubin, T., and J. Han. (2005). Activation and signaling of the p38 MAP kinase pathway. *Cell Res* 15(1): 11-18.

Zehentner, B. K., C. Dony et al. (1999). The transcription factor Sox9 is involved in BMP-2 signaling. *J Bone Miner Res* 14(10): 1734-1741.

Zhang, P., S. A. Jimenez et al. (2003). Regulation of human COL9A1 gene expression. Activation of the proximal promoter region by SOX9. *J Biol Chem* 278(1): 117-123.

Zhou, G., V. Lefebvre et al. (1998). Three High Mobility Group-like sequences within a 48-base pair enhancer of the Col2a1 gene are required for cartilage-specific expression in vivo. *J Biol Chem* 273(24): 14989-14997.

Zuniga, A., A. P. Haramis et al. (1999). Signal relay by BMP antagonism controls the SHH/FGF4 feedback loop in vertebrate limb buds. *Nature* 401(6753): 598-602.

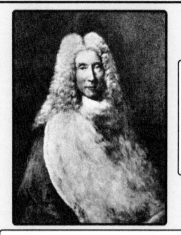

"[Orthopedics]…of two Greek words, viz. orthos, which signifies straight, free from deformity, and pais, a child. Out of these two words I have compounded that of orthopaedia, to express in one term the design I propose, which is to teach the different methods of preventing and correction of deformities of children." (Orthopédie 1741) Nicolas Andry de Bois-Regard (1658-1742), French physician and writer

"It would indeed be as reasonable to attempt to cure a fever patient by kicking him out of bed, as to benefit joint disease by a wriggling at the articulation." Healing requires "…enforced, uninterrupted and prolonged rest." While later work would show that minimal passive motion had the best results, this work was extremely successful for the time and led to the innovation of multiple orthopedic splints that bear his name (e.g., Thomas splint, Thomas collar). However, due to his abrasive personality, many of these innovations would not be well-recognized until championed by his nephew Sir Robert Jones during WWI, more than 25 years after Thomas' death. Hugh Owen Thomas (1834-1891), Welsh surgeon considered the father of orthopedic surgery in Britain

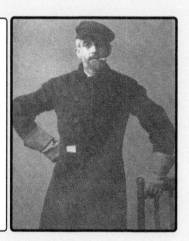

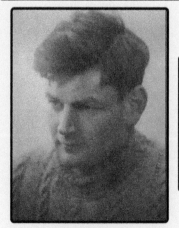

He is best known for development of the Pridie drilling cartilage repair technique. This procedure consists of surgical debridement of the defect with subsequent drilling of small holes into the subchondral bone plate allowing a clot and cells to fill the cartilage defect and form a fibrocartilage repair. This was later modified into the widely used microfracture technique for cartilage defect filling. Kenneth Hampden Pridie (1906-1963), eminent English orthopedic surgeon and athlete

Articular Cartilage Pathology and Therapies

3

- Arthritis
- Cartilage injuries
- Current and emerging therapies
- Motivation for tissue engineering

3.1 ARTHRITIS

Arthritis, from Greek (ἀρθρίτις), from arthron (ἄρθρον), meaning "joint/limb," and suffix -itis, denoting inflammation

Arthritis, defined as joint inflammation, is often painful and can have multiple causes. Of the diseases that affect articular cartilage, a distinction can be made between genetic and metabolic diseases and those caused by injury, wear and tear, and immune-mediated processes. For the period 2007-2009, the Centers for Disease Control and Prevention (CDC) National Health Interview Survey reported that 22% of adults (50 million individuals) in the United States had been doctor-diagnosed with some form of arthritis. Currently, more than 100 different types of arthritis have been documented and are listed in the appendix of this chapter, compiled from the Arthritis Foundation (arthritis.org) and based on prior work (Montgomery and Poske 1968). Although the focus of this book is on articular cartilage, and by extension damage to articular cartilage by disease, arthritis is a whole organ (the joint) disease with a broad spectrum of disorders in multiple tissues. This section primarily focuses on the changes in articular cartilage associated with the initiation and progression of the most common arthritis, osteoarthritis.

3.1.1 Osteoarthritis and Rheumatoid Arthritis

3.1.1.1 Osteoarthritis

Osteoarthritis is the most common type of arthritis and is a significant problem, as it poses great costs both financially and to the patient's quality of life. Osteoarthritis is marked by destruction of cartilage (Hadler 1985; Hamerman 1988; Aluisio et al. 1998) that affects mostly the aged population. Colloquially, it is seen as a "wearing out" or slow degeneration of the tissue. Osteoarthritis inevitably leads to progressive damage to articular cartilage (Figure 3.1). With the aging population, the incidence of osteoarthritis has increased from an estimated 21 million in 1995 to nearly 27 million a decade later (Lawrence et al. 2008). Broken down by age, surveys show that in the United States more than one-fifth of the population over 45 and almost one-half over 65 develop osteoarthritis (Hart et al. 1999), with the prevalence higher in women

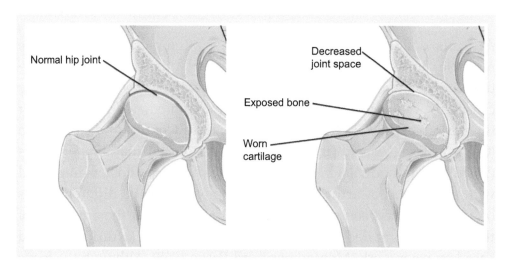

Figure 3.1 Illustration detailing osteoarthritic changes in the hip. (Image used with a Creative Commons Attribution License Unported 3.0. From http://cnx.org /contents/14fb4ad7-39a1-4eee-ab6e-3ef2482e3e22@6.27.)

than men. Osteoarthritis has even been linked to a decrease in lifespan (Nuesch et al. 2011).

Damage to articular cartilage by osteoarthritis represents a common event during aging and has widespread clinical and quality of life implications. During the progression of osteoarthritis, cartilage typically decreases in collagen and proteoglycan content and increases in water content (Setton et al. 1999), with subsequent changes in biomechanical characteristics. As illustrated in Figure 3.2, fibrillation and fissures may develop that extend to the subchondral bone (Aluisio et al. 1998). Broadly, osteoarthritis can be further divided into subtypes, including generalized versus joint-specific, secondary (in response to joint injury) versus primary (multiple interactions), painful versus nonpainful (quality of life factors), and biomechanically malaligned versus nonmalaligned. Treatment needs to focus on these specific subtypes by first identifying and distinguishing among subtypes.

The incidence and severity of osteoarthritis increases with age, and the clinical standard of treatment for advanced stages is joint arthroplasty.

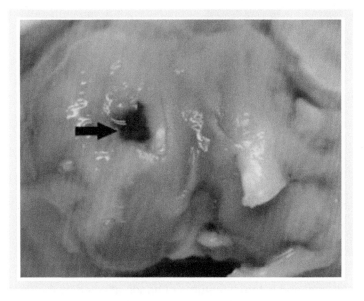

Figure 3.2 Osteoarthritis of a rabbit (leporine) patellofemoral groove, displaying a defect (arrow) penetrating into the subchondral bone.

165

Treatment during early stage osteoarthritis is mostly control of pain symptoms. Effective long-term treatment of osteoarthritis will most likely arise from not only an understanding of the etiology of the disease, but also a deeper understanding of the nature of articular cartilage biology. Finally, efforts to tissue engineer replacement biological materials can be combined with adjunctive therapies to manage the inflammatory environment.

3.1.1.2 Rheumatoid Arthritis

Approximately 1% of the population suffers from rheumatoid arthritis. Although rheumatoid arthritis results in joint destruction, it differs from the injury or aging etiology of osteoarthritis, as the cause is immune-mediated (Figure 3.3). This results in systemic chronic inflammation (synovitis). Unfortunately, the initiating antigens in susceptible patients have not yet been identified definitively. Females are more than

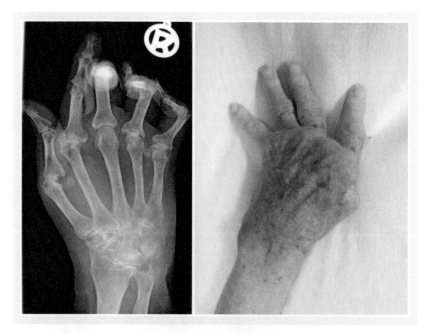

Figure 3.3 Internal and external features of hands affected by rheumatoid arthritis. (Courtesy of Creative Commons Attribution-ShareAlike 3.0 Unported [CC BY-SA 3.0] License, attributed to Bernd Brägelmann [left] and James Heilman [right].)

twice as susceptible as men to rheumatoid arthritis, and this has been hypothesized to be due to differences in estrogen effects on T-cell function (Ahmed et al. 1999; Pernis 2007).

Onset of rheumatoid arthritis is most common in the fourth decade of life, though individuals of any age can be afflicted. Juvenile rheumatoid arthritis, afflicting individuals before 18 years of age, affects 294,000 children (Sacks et al. 2007) in the United States alone. Symptoms mirror those of other types of arthritis, including pain, swelling, loss of joint function, and joint contracture.

Although rheumatoid arthritis primarily targets the joints, as a systemic autoimmune disease, multiple organs can be affected. While the cause of rheumatoid arthritis is known to be immune-mediated, the initiating event for the immune reaction is still unclear. However, environmental factors such as infection, chemical or antigen exposure, along with genetic factors, have all been implicated in initiating rheumatoid arthritis (Firestein 2003; Oliver and Silman 2006). Current treatments have seen success recently by blocking inflammatory mediators, such as tumor necrosis factor α (TNF-α). This can be accomplished pharmacologically or using recombinant antibodies. However, these treatments are associated with a host of side effects (Toussirot and Wendling 2004, 2007), such as increased risks for infection and certain types of cancer.

3.1.2 Etiology and Epidemiology

The main factors that lead to osteoarthritis can be classified into three categories: genetic, abnormal biomechanics and injury, and aging. These categories, considered the triad of primary osteoarthritis factors, are used to further subdivide osteoarthritis into subtypes and phenotypes. Of course, these factors are not observed in isolation, as they have complex interactions. They are also induced or exacerbated by secondary factors, such as metabolic disorders, biochemical and biomechanical changes, and inflammation. Of the main factors, injury and genetics have been the most amenable to much of the basic research in this field.

It is still unclear if aging may be considered a contributor to both genetics and injury or a separate entity. Clearly, incidence of osteoarthritis is correlated to advancing age, but is the contribution of age the result of wear and tear that merely accumulates over time? See Section 2.2.3 for further discussion of aging and disease. As discussed in Chapters 1 and 2, changes in matrix composition due to increased accumulations of advanced glycation endproducts (AGEs) result in increases in matrix brittleness, but does this predispose cartilage to injuries, and, therefore, osteoarthritis? It should be noted that not only the accumulation of wear and tear, but also the absence of function results in degeneration and arthritis (Buckwalter 1995). This makes sense within the context of mechanobiology, where it is known that the effects of overuse are tantamount to disuse insofar as cartilage degeneration is concerned.

Studies employing animal models have generated much of the information we have on the biology of osteoarthritis (see Chapter 6 for a description of various animal models used) (van den Berg 2001; Brandt 2002; Pritzker 2011). Tissues in the diarthrodial joints of animal models have analogous anatomical structures in humans, and all are involved in degenerative joint disease. However, in animals the rate of osteoarthritis progression is often much faster, with induced osteoarthritis in rodents occurring in weeks to months in some cases. Models of osteoarthritis in animals are almost exclusively based on *induced* osteoarthritis, as, for example, by surgical transection of the anterior cruciate ligament (ACL), although naturally occurring osteoarthritis models do exist. For example, in the small animal realm, rabbits have been identified as progressing to natural osteoarthritis (Arzi et al. 2011) (Figures 3.2 and 3.4). Many of the changes identified in osteoarthritic joints described in the following sections, especially early changes, are from animal models.

The factors that initiate the often inexorable descent to osteoarthritis, including the tissues from which the disease originates, are still unclear. Evidence linking osteoarthritis to changes in articular cartilage, secretion by the surrounding synovium of catabolic factors, and defects in

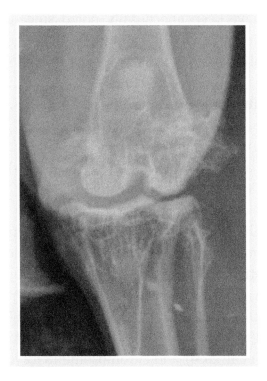

Figure 3.4 Radiographic evidence of naturally occurring osteoarthritis in the rabbit knee with advancing age. Dorsal-ventral view of a 6-year-old rabbit with Grade 3 osteoarthritis. (Courtesy of Dr. Boaz Arzi.)

the underlying bone (or combinations of all these issues) suggest that osteoarthritis may have multifactorial causes.

3.1.2.1 Genetic and Metabolic Defects

Increasingly strong evidence demonstrates that genetics is central to the incidence of idiopathic osteoarthritis. However, the genetic factors that lead to idiopathic osteoarthritis in seemingly phenotypically "normal" individuals are likely complex, with subtle differences in the expression of one gene when combined with others, resulting in increased osteoarthritis incidences (Sandell 2012). Recent patterns have been identified that may be useful in predicting later stage osteoarthritis due to genetic issues. Genetic factors likely involve multiple genes affecting osteoarthritis susceptibility and progression. Incidences of osteoarthritis within families have been anecdotally noted since early times, leading to the hypothesis that subtle changes in many genes occurring in the right combinations can result in osteoarthritis. Only within the last 50 years have the implications of familial osteoarthritis been linked to genetics. Studies in families, in siblings, and in twins, along with modern genome-wide scans for osteoarthritis-associated genes, have identified strong genetic associations in osteoarthritis incidence (Kellgren 1963; Kellgren et al. 1963; Bijkerk et al. 1999; Holderbaum et al. 1999; Ingvarsson et al. 2000; Valdes and Spector 2011).

From these population studies, differences in genetic linkages influencing the anatomical location of osteoarthritis development have also been noted. Potential linkage sites (Lee et al. 2006; Loughlin 2006) have been identified on chromosomes 1, 7, 9, 13, and 19 for hand osteoarthritis (Demissie et al. 2002; Hunter et al. 2004; Livshits et al. 2007); chromosomes 2, 4, 11 (11q), and 19 for hip osteoarthritis (Chapman et al. 1999; Loughlin et al. 1999; Forster et al. 2004); and chromosome 13 for knee osteoarthritis (in the LRCH1 gene at 13q14) (Spector et al. 2006; Snelling et al. 2007).

Not surprisingly, many of the candidate genes identified are those of the articular cartilage extracellular matrix. Candidate genes identified through familial studies are matrix genes such as *COL2A1*, *COL1A1*, cartilage oligomeric matrix protein (*COMP*), aggrecan (*ACAN*), matrilin 3 (*MATN3*), and asporin (*ASPN*) (Bleasel et al. 1999; Meulenbelt et al. 1999; Mustafa et al. 2000; Stefansson et al. 2003; Kizawa et al. 2005). However, more distantly associated genes involved in the development and maintenance of the joint have also been implicated (Sandell 2012).

Some notable examples of genetic defects that lead to osteoarthritis are described here: Alkaptonuria is an autosomal recessive genetic disorder resulting in abnormal phenylalanine and tyrosine metabolism, wherein the tyrosine metabolic byproduct is not cleared (homogentisic acid, or alkapton) and builds up in cartilage (ochronosis), heart valves, and the kidneys. Ochronosis leads to articular cartilage degeneration. The defect lies in the homogentisate 1,2-dioxygenase enzyme produced by the *HGD* gene on chromosome 3. This enzyme participates in tyrosine metabolism by converting homogentistic acid into 4-maleylacetoacetate (Figure 3.5).

Marfan syndrome is a dominant genetic disorder in the connective tissue extracellular matrix component fibrillin 1 gene (*FBN1*) on chromosome 15, which is a TGF-β binding protein. The phenotype can range from mild to severe. Patients with Marfan syndrome tend to have above-average height, long fingers and limbs, hyperflexible joints, and earlier onset osteoarthritis. Other skeletal abnormalities may exist of the spine, sternum, and palate. Life-threatening defects may be present in the aorta and heart valve, and secondary problems may exist with the eyes and lungs. How reduced TGF-β binding and sequestration in the matrix due to reduced FBN1 leads to the disease is still unclear, although mutations in the *TGFBR2* (a TGF-β receptor) gene lead to Loeys-Dietz syndrome, which has similar clinical features (Singh et al. 2006; Stheneur et al. 2008; Arslan-Kirchner et al. 2011).

Stickler syndrome is a rare autosomal dominant disease linked to collagen types II and XI, specifically the procollagen genes *COL2A1* and

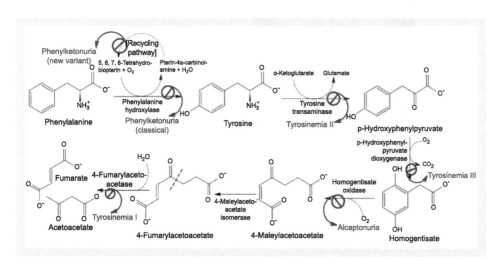

Figure 3.5 Metabolic pathway and corresponding deficiencies leading to alkaptonuria. (Image used with a Creative Commons 3.0 License LCheM.)

COL11A1 or *COL11A2* (Francomano et al. 1987; Knowlton et al. 1989; Sirko-Osadsa et al. 1998; Faber et al. 2000). In addition to early onset of osteoarthritis, pathologies of the eye also occur, including retinal detachment and vitreous degeneration in *COL2A1* linkages (~50-75% of affected families). Facial, palate, and other joint and skeletal abnormalities may also be present.

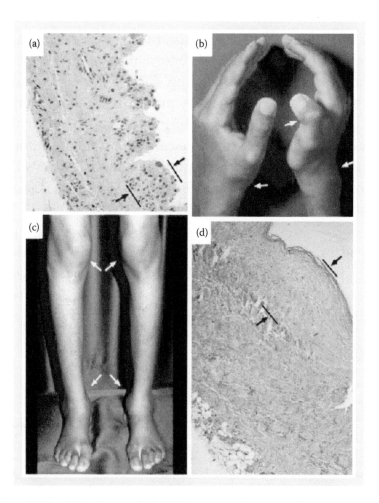

Figure 3.6 Clinical features of CACP patients lacking functional *PRG4* gene products. These features include (a) hyperplasia of synoviocytes without inflammation (arrowheads), (b) flexion deformity of the fingers and swelling of the wrists (arrows), (c) swelling of the knee and ankle joints (arrows), and (d) hyperplasia of the intimal cells of the pericardium (arrows). (From Marcelino, J. et al., *Nat Genet* 23(3): 319-322, 1999. With permission.)

Camptodactyly-arthropathy-coxa vara-pericarditis (CACP) is an auto-somal recessive disease characterized by hyperplasia of synovium without evidence of inflammation, where ineffective lubrication leads to precocious arthropathy (Figure 3.6) (Marcelino et al. 1999). A muta-tion in *PRG4* located in human chromosome locus l q 25 and encoding superficial zone protein (SZP) has been linked to CACP syndrome. It has also been reported that *PRG4* is differently expressed in the synovium of rheumatoid arthritis and osteoarthritis, implying a possible role in the pathogenesis of these diseases (Justen et al. 2000). Mice lacking a functional *PRG4* gene demonstrated disappearance of the superficial zone, synovial hyperplasia, and precocious failure of joint function (Rhee et al. 2005). However, the joint initially develops normally.

3.1.2.2 Crystal Pathologies

Many crystal pathologies have strong genetic associations, such as mutations in the procollagen type II gene (Reginato et al. 1994) or familial chondrocalcinosis (Marcos et al. 1981; Fernandez Dapica and Gomez-Reino 1986). Commonly, dietary issues (e.g., alcohol consump-tion in gout) are coassociated, such as hypophosphatasia-induced cal-cium pyrophosphate (CPP) disease or the association between gout and diabetes mellitus. Chemically, crystals are commonly derived from two sources, calcium and uric acid, although an unknown source of silicon dioxide crystals has also been reported in synovial fluid (Oliviero et al. 2008). Crystals cause joint problems due to their deposition within the joint and associated tissues, inducing not only mechanical dam-age through third-body wear but also inflammation. The presence of crystals within the joint space has been linked to cartilage lesions, induced by mechanical damage, as detected in cadaveric samples of the ankle (Muehleman et al. 2008). Interestingly, of the crystals identified, approximately one-third were CPP, while the remaining two-thirds were monosodium urate (MSU). The crystals also induce biochemical changes in both the chondrocyte and synoviocytes and activate inflam-matory processes (McCarty 1970, 1999; Halverson and Derfus 2001; Landis and Haskard 2001; Akahoshi et al. 2007). Inflammation due to

173

crystal arthropathies is mediated through neutrophil infiltration and macrophage recruitment (Akahoshi et al. 2007).

3.1.2.2.1 Monosodium Urate (Gout)

Gout is a buildup of uric acid crystals in the blood and synovial fluid, leading to inflammatory arthritis. This increase in uric acid levels in the blood can be due to a lack of uric acid excretion by the kidneys or increased dietary intake of foods high in purine, a uric acid precursor. Excessive alcohol consumption is also commonly associated with increased uric acid concentrations (Saker et al. 1967; Liberopoulos et al. 2004; Fam 2005; Zhang et al. 2006; Choi and Curhan 2007), although the role of alcohol in gout progression is increasingly being questioned (Hennigan and Terkeltaub 2007). Gout has been described since ancient times by both the Babylonians and Egyptians, with Hippocrates providing one of the classical descriptions in the fifth century BC, relating it to dietary intake of alcohol and certain foods. The most common joint affected is the first metatarsophalangeal joint (big toe). Other disorders associated with increased uric acid concentration include tophus formation (large MSU crystals) and renal calculi (Figure 3.7).

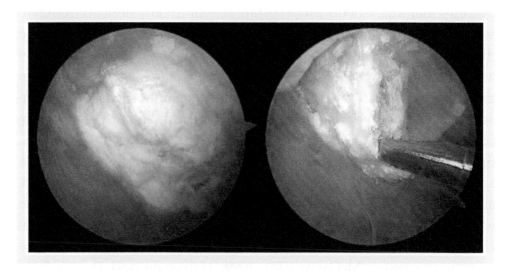

Figure 3.7 Arthroscopic image of tophus removal in the knee. (Public domain image.)

3.1.2.2.2 Calcium-Based Crystals

Radiologically seen as calcification of the cartilage, there is some doubt regarding calcium crystals' coassociation with osteoarthritis. Calcium-based crystals include CPP, also known as CPP dehydrate (CPPD), and basic calcium phosphate hydroxy-apatite (BCP). These crystals are a common cofinding, with their increased presence corresponding to worse osteoarthritis radiological scoring (Derfus et al. 2002). Chondrocyte vesicle digests can form calcium crystals of apatite or pyrophosphate from ATP, the pyrophosphate being formed via action of triphosphate pyrophosphohydrolase. Calcium crystal formation is more common in older women (>60 years), and risk factors include magnesium or phosphate deficiency, increased blood or synovial fluid levels of calcium or pyrophosphate, gout, and thyroid diseases. In osteoarthritic patients with BCP, soft-tissue calcium deposits (calcinosis), inflammatory arthritis, periarthritis (inflammation of tissues surrounding the joint), and cartilage destruction are all noted. However, radiographic determination of chondrocalcinosis does not correlate with increased risk of cartilage loss (Zhang et al. 2006). CPP may be generated by osteoarthritis degeneration of cartilage. It may also be a self-amplifying process during the early stages of osteoarthritis; through initiating trauma, abnormal loading, and cartilage damage, the formation of CPP crystals is initiated, which leads to additional CPP crystal deposition (Mankin 1971; Rosenthal 2006). However, the role of calcium crystals in initiating osteoarthritis (Halverson 1996; Rosenthal 2006) is unclear. Both calcium crystals promote inflammatory reactions, and their deposition within and upon the cartilage may increase expression of matrix degradative enzymes, such as collagenase and metalloproteinases (Cheung et al. 1996; McCarthy et al. 1998; Brogley et al. 1999; Molloy et al. 2008).

3.1.2.3 Biomechanics, Loading, and Injury

Osteoarthritis is an interaction of biomechanical factors and biological factors, with both having complex feedback loops that result in the initiation and progression of pathology. Changes in the biomechanics, and, therefore, the loads to which the cartilage has adapted, can cause a wide range of changes in the biochemical response and matrix composition. The knee joint has been the focus of much of the literature dealing with biomechanics due to its anatomical and mechanical complexity, ease of access, and high rate of osteoarthritis incidence.

3.1.2.3.1 Abnormal Biomechanics and Altered Loading of Articular Cartilage

Clinically, early signs of abnormal loading and biomechanics with a link to osteoarthritis have been determined using gait analysis of the external knee adduction moment (movement of the knee toward the body midline during normal gait) (Goh et al. 1993; Sharma et al. 1998; Hurwitz et al. 2002; Foroughi et al. 2009, 2010; Vanwanseele et al. 2010; Robbins et al. 2011). In the knee, osteoarthritis preferentially targets the medial condyle, as this location experiences the highest loads during walking; 60-80% of the total knee compressive load is applied to the medial compartment (Andriacchi 1994). Changes in medial loading can be measured indirectly from changes in the peak knee adduction moment (Birmingham et al. 2007); this is predictive of disease progression of osteoarthritis in the medial compartment (Miyazaki et al. 2002). Larger knee adduction moments are seen during osteoarthritis of the medial compartment, and these larger moments induce larger stresses on this compartment (Sharma et al. 1998) (Figure 3.8). Radiologically, osteoarthritic patients with larger knee adduction moments have more narrowing of the medial joint space (Andriacchi 1994; Miyazaki et al. 2002).

Abnormal increases in joint loading push articular cartilage from repair and maintenance to degeneration. Abnormal loading can be due to either overloading or underloading. Further refinement of these conditions would include the frequency and type of load, as these factors are known to alter the response by chondrocytes and effectively upset the delicate homeostasis of the joint. Interestingly, the changes seen with load are more easily identified in underloaded (or unloaded) conditions, where

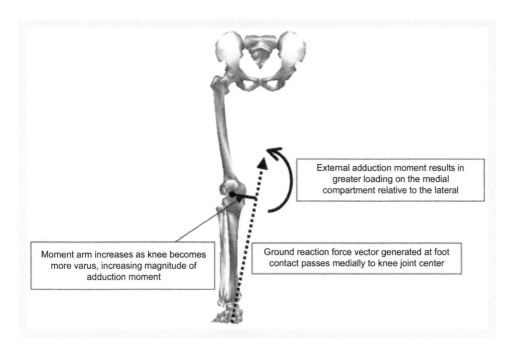

Figure 3.8 Diagram of knee adduction moment and the change in forces acting on the medial compartment. (From Hinman, R. S., and K. L. Bennell, *Curr Opin Rheumatol* 21(2): 164-170, 2009. With permission.)

grossly the articular cartilage may appear normal early on. However, even early on histological and mechanical testing can detect changes in matrix composition. Given the rapid nature of proteoglycan metabolism and turnover compared with collagen (discussed in Chapter 1), the short-term changes seen are those of proteoglycan loss (Slowman and Brandt 1986), which manifests biomechanically as reduced tissue compressive properties and thickness (Hudelmaier et al. 2006). Depending on how loading is reapplied, this situation may only be temporary, and the cartilage may be able to recover.

More common is the case of overloading, which is also thought to be the mechanism behind malalignment and degeneration. Specifically, by causing malalignment or instability of the joint (e.g., by ACL transection), areas of the cartilage not normally exposed or adapted to loads of a specific magnitude are overloaded via stress concentrations (Koo and Andriacchi 2007). For instance, the altered biomechanical environment resulting from ACL transection has long been used as a model to induce osteoarthritis. Contributive to the degeneration is the increased knee abduction moment post-ACL transection (Butler et al. 2009), which alters the biomechanical environment of the chondrocytes. Biologically, extracellular matrix maintenance by the chondrocytes is dependent on both the frequency and magnitude of loading, with increased chondrocyte matrix synthesis noted at frequencies of loading analogous to normal walking (~1 Hz) (Kock et al. 2009). Abnormal shear has also been linked with chondrocyte death and secretion of pro-inflammatory factors (Smith et al. 1995; Healy et al. 2005). With the changes in loading, the chondrocyte behavior is altered, resulting in degenerative changes in the articular cartilage.

Acceleration of osteoarthritis can also be neurogenic in nature. In a transected cruciate ligament model of the dog, osteoarthritis typically develops in 4 years, but this can be shortened to 8 weeks when accompanied by nerve transection (O'Connor et al. 1992). This loss of nerve function results in altered ability to control the musculature and, therefore, mechanics of the joint. Proprioceptive impairment has been detected in human patients with osteoarthritis, although its contribution to pathogenesis is unclear (Sharma and Pai 1997). It has been postulated that the resultant alteration in biomechanics with loss of muscle control is partially responsible for osteoarthritis development due to the muscles' role in energy absorption (Palmieri-Smith and Thomas 2009). As a result, weakness of the quadriceps has been associated with knee osteoarthritis and may be a risk factor in disease progression (Slemenda et al. 1997; Brandt et al. 1999). The altered loading leads not only to possible lesions (Pond and Nuki 1973; Johnson and Poole 1990) but also to different compressive loads or loading rates applied to chondrocytes that may lead to catabolism (Guilak et al. 1994; Ragan et al. 2000; Kisiday et al. 2009), potentially mimicking a disuse situation. At-home exercise regimens to strengthen the quadriceps therefore remain a common knee osteoarthritis method of care. However, this may place abnormal loading onto the cartilage of osteoarthritic patients with malalignments or joint laxity (Sharma 2003; Sharma et al. 2003).

Obesity is a special risk factor as it covers lifestyle, genetics, and biomechanics. Obesity has been strongly linked to osteoarthritis, especially in the knee (Felson et al. 1988; Davis et al. 1990; Hart et al. 1999; Al-Arfaj 2002; Browning and Kram 2007). In obesity, changes in the adduction moment with increasing weight result in abnormal and excessive loading. Obesity in some cases has a strong genetic cause. For example, systemic metabolic effects due to genetic conditions can result in an increased incidence of osteoarthritis. However, leptin-deficient mice (high body weight and body fat percentage) do not have increases in the incidence of osteoarthritis (Griffin et al. 2009). Interestingly, obesity and articular cartilage degradation in non-weight-bearing joints (e.g., hand) are also linked (Carman et al. 1994), indicating that a component of this degeneration is not necessarily biomechanically driven. Current thought is the increased osteoarthritis incidence is linked to the increased presence of inflammatory processes. While injury may alter the biomechanics of the joint through various mechanisms (described below) injuries also alter other facets of joint biology.

3.1.2.3.2 Role of the Meniscus in Osteoarthritis

The meniscus functions to transmit loads in the knee by increasing the surface area of contact and conformity of the surfaces between the tibial plateau and femoral condyles (Figure 3.9). While originally thought to function as a "shock absorber," this model has come under criticism (Andrews et al. 2011). Meniscus injuries have been linked to osteoarthritis, and meniscectomy has been linked to both increased prevalence and severity of articular cartilage injuries due to altered biomechanics (Mills et al. 2008). As modeled by finite element analysis with partial meniscectomy, maximum contact stress increased approximately 50-100% in the adjacent articular cartilage as the contact area between the articular cartilage and remaining meniscus decreased. A complete meniscectomy increased maximum contact stress by more than 270% (Pena et al. 2005).

An established experimental method to induce osteoarthritis via meniscectomy has shown that the patellar cartilage is adversely affected

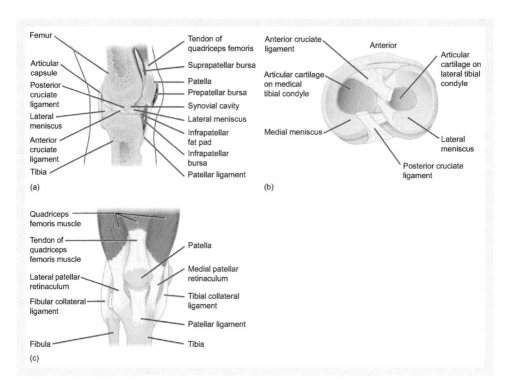

Figure 3.9 Illustration of the human knee joint. (a) Sagittal section through the right knee joint with anatomy labeled. (b) Superior view of the right tibia in the knee joint, showing the menisci and cruciate ligaments, covering the tibial condyles. (c) Anterior view of the right knee with musculature and ligaments labeled. (Image used with a Creative Commons Attribution License Unported 3.0. From http://cnx.org /contents/14fb4ad7-39a1-4eee-ab6e-3ef2482e3e22@6.27.)

within 3 months in an ovine model (Appleyard et al. 1999). A murine, destabilized medial meniscus model shows progression to osteoarthritis in 12-16 weeks following transection of the medial meniscal horn. Clinical studies of patients with meniscectomy have shown that, after 21 years, mild radiographic changes were found in 71% of the knees, while more advanced changes were seen in 48% (Roos et al. 1998).

3.1.2.3.3 Injury Leading to Osteoarthritis

In the clinical setting, osteoarthritis is categorized as primary or secondary. Primary osteoarthritis is idiopathic with unidentified causes, whereas secondary osteoarthritis arises from identifiable causes or conditions. A majority of secondary osteoarthritis cases is attributable to traumatic joint injury that may have occurred years previously and is termed posttraumatic osteoarthritis (Roos et al. 1995; Buckwalter and Mankin 1998; Buckwalter 2002; Lohmander et al. 2004). Trauma was first linked to osteoarthritis by Hunter in 1743 (Hunter 1743). Athletes with a history of joint injury have a higher incidence of osteoarthritis than non-athletes (Kern et al. 1988). ACL injury causes immediate changes in bio-mechanics (Georgoulis et al. 2003; Andriacchi and Dyrby 2005; Li et al. 2006), which may lead to osteoarthritis (Andriacchi et al. 2004, 2006). For instance, the quadriceps and surrounding muscles of the knee are pre-vented from full activation in injured knees, and this muscle inhibition has been observed in patients with ACL and other joint injuries (Hurley et al. 1994; Palmieri et al. 2004; McVey et al. 2005; Sedory et al. 2007).

Mechanical injuries, such as those that happen during motor vehicle collisions, falls, and sports injuries, have been implicated in the devel-opment of posttraumatic osteoarthritis, though the precise pathophysi-ology is not yet fully elucidated (Figure 3.10) (Chrisman et al. 1981; Borrelli and Ricci 2004; Olson and Guilak 2006). Other factors that may play a role in whether initial trauma progresses to osteoarthritis include genetic variability, patient factors (e.g., physical therapy compliance), smoking, socioeconomic status, and the degree of injury. Also, treat-ment factors must be considered following injury, for example, to the meniscus or the ACL. How the tissue (meniscus or ligament) is sur-gically treated will affect the biomechanical environment of the joint. Similarly, the rehabilitation regimen employed and the time of return to strenuous activity are also expected to influence the progress to osteoarthritis.

Identification of comorbidities or susceptibilities to the initial injury, especially in meniscal tears, may help to predict the clinical progres-sion. The progression of osteoarthritis following injury, however, can be broken down into a series of steps, which may allow earlier interven-tion. These steps include the trigger event, acute phase, chronic phase, and biomechanical derangement. These likely encompass the cascade of

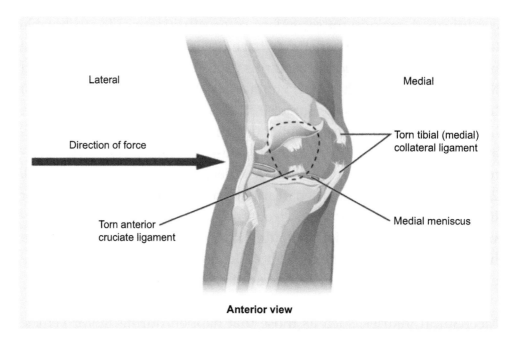

Figure 3.10 Illustration of damage to the knee joint leading to tearing of the ligaments. (Image used with a Creative Commons Attribution License Unported 3.0. From http://cnx.org/contents/14fb4ad7-39a1-4eee-ab6e-3ef2482e3e22@6.27.)

both degradative factors, including matrix metalloproteinases (MMPs) and aggrecanases, and changes in joint biomechanics following injury. Biomechanical factors may also contribute to the initiation and progression of posttraumatic osteoarthritis. For instance, articular surface integrity is destroyed during the early stages of joint degeneration (Guilak et al. 2004), and as a result, the frictional properties of the tissue are altered. However, the mechanisms underlying the biochemical decline in matrix quality and biomechanical changes are not clear (Wilson et al. 2008).

The need for early detection of degradative biochemical and biomechanical changes in cartilage is important, as these changes in the matrix lead to a "death spiral" of increasing matrix degradation and poorer biomechanical properties (Andriacchi et al. 2009). Fissure propagation is affected by cartilage thickness and the ratio between the compliance of the cartilage and its underlying bone (Kuo and Keer 1993). Modeling has shown that higher stresses are found in the thicker of two contacting biphasic layers of articular cartilage (Wu et al. 1996). Considering that osteoarthritis reduces both cartilage stiffness and thickness, these models provide evidence that the disease results in a degenerative cycle. A three-phase (collagen, matrix, and synovial fluid), transversely isotropic, unconfined half-space model of articular cartilage has also been developed for studying surface fissures (Kafka 2002). Interestingly, it was shown that collagen is in tension for the first 10 to 20 seconds of a rapidly applied compressive load, switching to compression thereafter if the load is held constant. The tensile stresses generated within this model were within the range of reported tensile strength of collagen fibers, showing that failure of collagen could lead to surface fissuring. This was not the case for slowly applied loads. In another study (Wilson et al. 2006), mediators of collagen damage due to mechanical injury were investigated in a fibril-reinforced poroviscoelastic model of articular cartilage. Using differential immunohistochemistry, wherein distinct antibodies were used to separate staining of enzymatically cleaved collagen from other damaged collagen, it was shown that shear and maximum strain in the collagen fibers corresponded to area staining for mechanically damaged collagen. These results implicate collagen as having a key role in keeping the surface intact when subjected to injurious mechanical loading.

Wear in the joint during osteoarthritis likely also plays a role in the destruction of articular cartilage. It should be noted that it is still unclear whether osteoarthritis initiation is due to wear or some unknown etiology. Wear in the superficial zone during osteoarthritis results in loss of SZP-producing cells; SZP is further initially downregulated by the presence of various catabolic cytokines and during the early stages of osteoarthritis induced by abnormal loading (Young et al. 2006; Jones and Flannery 2007). In conclusion, both biochemical and biomechanical factors play critical roles in initiating early changes in osteoarthritis (Figure 3.11).

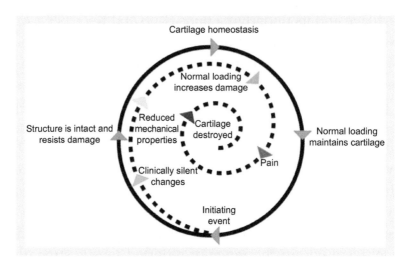

Figure 3.11 While the initiating event and early changes may be clinically silent, as the cartilage matrix degrades, and the biomechanical properties are reduced, normal loading increases matrix damage, leading to an increasing feedback loop of cartilage damage, pain, and destruction.

3.1.2.4 Epidemiology

While osteoarthritis is the most common arthritic disease, other arthritides, or types of arthritis, including rheumatic conditions, are also commonly diagnosed. The estimated numbers of people diagnosed with the most common arthritides and other common rheumatic conditions in the United States are as follows: for osteoarthritis, 27 million as of 2005; for gout, 3 million as of 2005 (Lawrence et al. 2008); and for rheumatoid arthritis, 1.5 million as of 2007 (Myasoedova et al. 2010). Per the CDC, by the year 2030, an estimated 67 million adults will have doctor-diagnosed arthritis, an increase from the 52.5 million adults identified in 2010-2012 (Figure 3.12).

However, the actual incidence of osteoarthritis in the population is probably higher than reported, since generally only symptomatic patients seek treatment. Over the age of 45, the radiographic incidence of osteoarthritis is 27.8% in the knees and 27.0% in the hips (Lawrence et al. 2008). During their lifetimes, 50% of the population is likely to develop symptomatic knee osteoarthritis, rising to 66% if they are obese

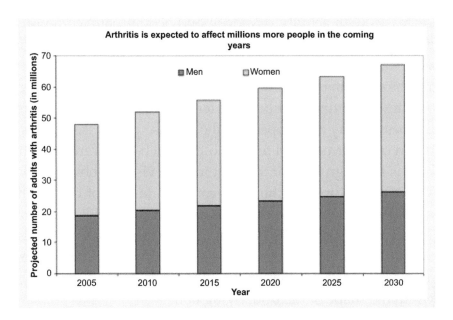

Figure 3.12 The incidence of doctor-diagnosed arthritis is expected to reach 67 million adults by the year 2030. (Public domain image, Centers for Disease Control and Prevention.)

(Murphy et al. 2008). However, it is estimated that by age 65 the true incidence of radiographically detectable osteoarthritis is closer to 80% of the population (Lawrence et al. 2008). These reported values for osteoarthritis incidence are probably lower than those of the actual population, as these tend to be from a self-selecting population, for example, those seeking treatment based on clinical symptoms of pain. It is important to note, though, that the pain may not be from osteoarthritis in the joint (Lawrence et al. 2008). Tissues involved can be any of the tissues within or surrounding the joint, including articular cartilage, meniscus, periosteum, subchondral bone, synovium, tendon, ligament, muscles, or undefined nerve compression.

Clinically, pain is often an initial symptom of osteoarthritis, leading to medical diagnosis. The initial onset can take years to decades to reach a clinically observable level. Symptomatic osteoarthritis manifests itself as frequent pain in a joint, made worse with activity and subsiding with rest. This may initially be a mild and diffuse pain or stiffness

185

that decreases with activity or a deep and aching pain, common after activity or at the end of the day. In later stages, difficulty in performing tasks, loss of function, or problems with rising from a seated position may be evident. Limitation of motion due to joint surface deformity (osteophytes), crepitus, fluid buildup (effusion), flexion contractures, or muscle spasms may also appear as the disease progresses. Joints may be swollen or deformed and tender to the touch. In severe osteoarthritis, obvious malalignment of the joint may be visually obvious. Hands, knees, spine, and hips are the most common targets of osteoarthritis. Diagnosis is by clinical examination and history with radiographic imaging for confirmation. To confirm a diagnosis of osteoarthritis, the clinician will look for changes such as osteophytes, joint space narrowing, voids or deformities in the subchondral bone (sclerosis), and changes in the shape of the underlying bone.

3.1.3 Changes in the Matrix

Osteoarthritis affects all components of the joint. Starting with the capsule, thickening and frequent adherence of the capsule to the underlying bone are seen, with increased vascularization and hemorrhage (Brandt et al. 1991). Amyloid formation is often observed with advanced stages of the disease (Sorensen and Christensen 1973; Egan et al. 1982).

Destruction of the cartilage surface in osteoarthritis occurs in phases. Depending on the joint location, articular cartilage can visually change from a pearly white color to yellow or brownish. Generally, decreased biomechanical properties are also observed, though there can be regions where new, healthy-looking cartilage has formed in small, pebbled patterns. During the early development of osteoarthritis, no visual, functional, or mechanical alterations appear detectable. However, changes may be detectable through imaging modalities such as magnetic resonance imaging (MRI) (Figure 3.13) (Javaid et al. 2010; Wang et al. 2010; Guermazi et al. 2012). Fibrillation, surface erosion, and fissures are the first noticeable signs of the disease by gross observation. From this point on, altered histological staining will show continued decreases in

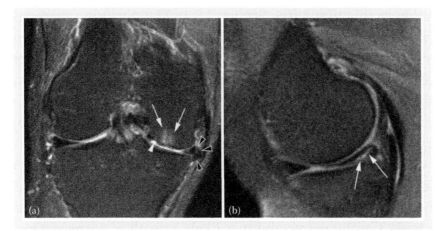

Figure 3.13 During the early development of osteoarthritis, degenerative changes may be clinically and radiographically silent but visible by MRI. Anterior (coronal fat-suppressed proton density-weighted) image (a) of a knee with indications of early stage osteoarthritis, such as medial full-thickness defect (white arrowhead), subchondral lesion (white arrow), and meniscal and medial collateral bulging (black arrowhead). Sagittal (proton density-weighted) image (b) of a knee with a tear of the medial meniscus horn (white arrow), but without observed cartilage or subchondral changes. (From Guermazi, A. et al., *BMJ* 345: e5339, 2012. With permission.)

proteoglycan content. The tidemark begins to appear irregular, punctuated with blood vessels. A second stage of the disease shows greater surface wear and irregularity. Vertical and sometimes horizontal fissures can now be seen in the cartilage. Proteoglycans start to leach out from the fissures, and the lack of proteoglycan staining will spread to the rest of the tissue. These patterns of increased tissue fragmentation and decreased staining continue until the cartilage loses its ability to withstand load, and, therefore, is worn away to expose the subchondral bone. During these cartilage changes, bone and synovium remodeling occurs, setting the stage for further degeneration.

When considering this cascade of events, it is not surprising to note that osteoarthritic cartilage possesses lower biomechanical properties. Gradual proteoglycan loss is the first observable indication. However, osteoarthritic cartilage also increases in water content, an observation that appears counterintuitive, as it is the proteoglycans that drive hydration in this tissue (see Section 1.3.4). The declining proteoglycan content should result in lower Donnan osmotic pressure and attendant water loss. Instead, the observed increase in hydration that accompanies proteoglycan loss is postulated to be due to the loosening of the proteoglycan structure, which allows for macromolecular uncurling and more interstitial space for water to occupy. This theory is supported by the observations that the fraction of aggregating proteoglycans decreases with osteoarthritis and that the proteoglycans are increasingly more extractable with disease progression. Being unable to aggregate, the proteoglycans are thus unable to pack as densely, supporting the uncurling hypothesis. Greater extractability is likely a result of decreased molecular weight or, as has been shown, damaged link proteins that no longer facilitate the formation of aggrecan macromolecules (Mort et al. 1983; Nguyen et al. 1993). In addition, the catabolic cytokines released during osteoarthritis can loosen the collagen network too, to result in more space for water to occupy. Tensile strength, attributed to the collagen in cartilage, has been shown to decrease with osteoarthritis.

Changes in the underlying bone matrix are also seen with osteoarthritis progression. Once the subchondral bone has become exposed, the eburnated bone is no longer protected from loading by the cushioning effects of the overlying cartilage. In response to this load, the subchondral bone remodels by becoming thicker and is replaced by trabecular bone (Kusakabe 1977; Oettmeier and Abendroth 1989). The bone may be entirely exposed as cartilage is denuded during the disease's progression (Figure 3.14). Loss of cartilage can result in areas of bone necrosis and bone cysts, as synovial fluid penetrates into the more permeable bone through the Haversian canals (Landells 1953). Radiological identification of subchondral cysts is a diagnostic for osteoarthritis, although they may spontaneously resolve.

Along with thickening, new bone formation is observed. Osteophytes form as bony outgrowths, usually located along the periphery of degenerating cartilage. While osteophyte formation is used as a clinically relevant finding of osteoarthritis, its initiation process and the cellular source are still debated in the literature. Osteophytes are strongly

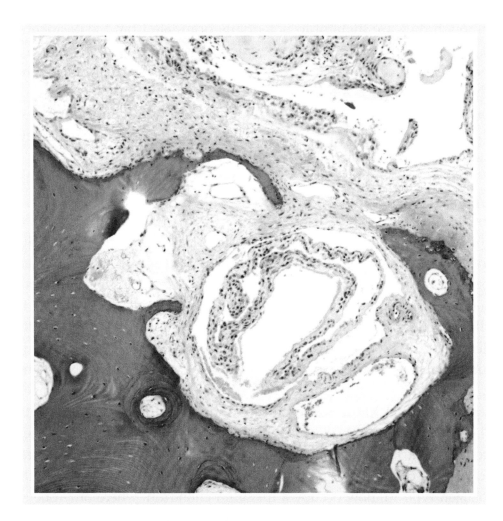

Figure 3.14 Synovial infiltration into an exposed subchondral bone lesion from naturally occurring osteoarthritis in the rabbit knee. (Courtesy of Dr. Boaz Arzi.)

associated with malalignment (Nagaosa et al. 2002; Felson et al. 2005; van der Esch et al. 2005), an identified cause for cartilage lesions that can lead to further degeneration. Although multiple causes can induce osteophyte formation, including osteoarthritis, osteomyelitis (infection of the bone), and diabetic neuropathy (nerve damage due to diabetes), the mechanism of formation is still undetermined. An improper healing response and changes in the balance of catabolic and anabolic factors have been proposed as likely candidates (Felson and Neogi 2004). The source of cells that initiate osteophyte formation is still undetermined,

189

although they are thought to potentially originate from the peripheral cartilage (Peng et al. 2000). These bone spurs often result in reduced mobility, pain, and, in the spine, numbness due to nerve impingement. The remodeling and formation of osteophytes alter the contours of the joint. Symptomatic osteophytes may require surgical removal. Further studies on osteophyte initiation and growth are needed to develop new therapeutic approaches.

3.1.4 Cellular Changes

The cellular changes in osteoarthritis can be classified in terms of proliferation, catabolism, and cell death. With changes occurring in the interterritorial and territorial matrices, the chondrocyte-containing chondrons may become swollen and distended, signaling the cells to proliferate to fill up the additional space. Interleukin 1 (IL-1) upregulation then initiates the destruction of the fibrillar collagen environment, which results in additional chondron distortion, and proliferation continues. TNF-α and IL-1β can induce aggrecanase and decrease matrix integrity. Collagen types II, IX, and XI are rendered more soluble by the catabolic activity. The breakup of the collagen network results in TGF-β being released from the matrix, and greater collagen type VI production and sequestration by the cells ensue. Finally, many cells, encapsulated by a sheath of collagen type VI, now occupy a distorted chondron, where only one or two cells used to reside in healthy cartilage (Figure 3.15) (Poole 1997).

How, then, does inflammation wreak such havoc on this tissue? As the disease progresses, the thickening and increasingly hypervascular synovium secretes MMPs and aggrecanases. The cleavage of aggrecan and the subsequent degradation of compressive properties are mediated by these aggrecanases. Aggrecanases belong to the A Disintegrin and Metalloproteinase with Thrombospondin motifs (ADAMTS) family, which includes ADAMTS4 and 5 (aggrecanase 1 and 2, respectively). IL-1 and TNF-α modulate the expression of ADAMTS4 to induce catabolism (Tortorella et al. 2001). However, ADAMTS5 is constitutively expressed (McCulloch et al. 2009); it must be remembered, though, given

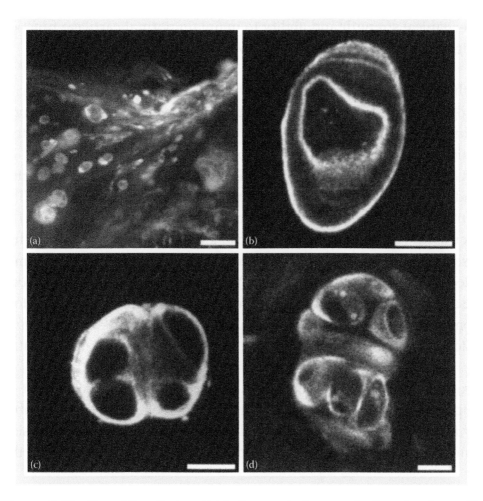

Figure 3.15 Type VI collagen distribution and changes in the chondron with osteoarthritis. Overview of osteoarthritic tissue indicating pericellular distribution of type VI collagen (a) (scale bar 100 μm). Subsequent changes with progressing osteoarthritis (b-d), including increase in size of the chondron (b), division of the chondrocyte (c), and formation of a clonal cluster of chondrocytes occupying a single chondron (d) (scale bar 10 μm). (From Poole, C. A., *J Anat* 191(Pt 1): 1-13, 1997. With permission.)

the shorter half-life of aggrecan, that both aggrecanases have natural functions in tissue remodeling in healthy tissue, versus their function in the disease state.

Introduction of inflammatory (catabolic) cytokines, such as IL-1β, IL-6, and TNF-α, to the joint reduces the production of matrix molecules and leads to changes in matrix constitution. This results in reduced mechanical strength and ability to maintain normal cartilage function (Figure 3.16) (van den Berg et al. 1999; Tetlow et al. 2001).

Other molecular factors that appear to serve as players in osteoarthritis progression include F-spondin, a neuronal extracellular matrix glycoprotein. Approximately a sevenfold increase for this species is seen in osteoarthritic cartilage, and its presence primes TGF-β1 and prostaglandin E2 (PGE2) release (Attur et al. 2009). PGE2 is a pro-inflammatory mediator, and its release is also accompanied by collagen degradation and MMP13 activation when cartilage explants are stimulated with F-spondin. The increased synthesis of COMP by chondrocytes and synoviocytes has also been associated with osteoarthritis, as its production can be stimulated by TGF-β1 (Recklies et al. 1998). This increase in TGF-β1 in the diseased joint is a product of an improper healing response, trying to restore homeostasis (see Section 2.3.4). Upregulation of anabolic factors results in osteophyte formation, which is detrimental to the function of the joint.

Progression of osteoarthritis, as described earlier, is due in part to improper repair responses and increased catabolic signaling. The ability to detect early osteoarthritis and to monitor the disease progression using biomarkers is necessary to determine drug efficacy. Given the

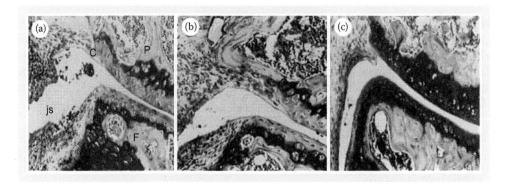

Figure 3.16 Surgically induced osteoarthritis at day 28 in the mouse knee. Loss of proteoglycans (darker areas) from the cartilage surface is seen from controls (a) and TNF-α knockout mice (b), while in panel c, mice lacking IL-1β (knockout) display resistance against loss of proteoglycans. (From van den Berg, W. B. et al., *Ann Rheum Dis* 58(Suppl 1): I40-I48, 1999. With permission.)

slow progress of osteoarthritis, proper utilization of biomarker detection can also shorten the experimental time needed to see if a drug is efficacious. Changes may be detected in months, instead of the years that would be required to observe definitive osteoarthritic changes. Toward this end, there is interest in using serologically detected COMP fragmentation as an alternative detection method for cartilage matrix degradation because COMP fragmentation has been noted in the synovial fluid and blood of arthritic patients (Saxne and Heinegard 1992; Lohmander et al. 1994; Petersson et al. 1997). This and other biomarkers (Table 3.1) can be useful as earlier detection methods than radiographic

Table 3.1 Biological markers of arthritis

Macromolecule	Function	Marker
Aggrecan	*Structural matrix component*	Core protein fragments
Aggrecan	*Structural matrix component*	Keratan sulphate
Aggrecan	*Structural matrix component*	Chondroitin sulphate
Hyaluronan	*Structural matrix component*	Hyaluronan oligosaccharides
Type III collagen	*Structural matrix component*	Type III collagen N-propeptide (PIIINP)
Type II collagen	*Structural matrix component*	Type II collagen C-terminal cross-linking telopeptide
Type II collagen	*Structural matrix component*	Type II collagen C-propeptide
Cartilage oligomeric matrix protein (COMP)	*Structural matrix component*	COMP fragment
MMP1	*Catabolic enzyme*	Collagenase (MMP1)
MMP3	*Catabolic enzyme*	Stromelysin (MMP3)
MMP13	*Catabolic enzyme*	Collagenase (MMP13)
Tissue inhibitors of metalloproteinases (TIMP)	*Inhibitor of MMPs*	Tissue inhibitors of metalloproteinases (TIMP)

measures and also as markers during clinical trials of disease-modifying osteoarthritis drugs (DMOADs).

In addition, chondrocyte death can be observed much earlier than matrix degradation, resulting in the release of secondary necrosis factors that diffuse to initiate apoptosis in neighboring cells. In this case, the dense matrix becomes a space that the chondrocytes cannot escape from, and the chondron a place where phagocytes cannot reach to clear cellular debris to interrupt the cycle of inflammation and necrosis (Polzer et al. 2007).

3.1.5 Costs of Arthritis

The CDC (2007) reports that the costs of arthritis and other rheumatic diseases have increased from $86 billion in 1997 to $128 billion by 2003, with cost increases expected to rise with an aging population. The most common of these arthritic conditions, osteoarthritis, causes significant pain and suffering to individual patients, and the economic burden of this disease for society is great (Yelin 1998). For example, in the United States alone osteoarthritis-related costs exceed $65 billion per year in terms of both medical costs and lost wages (Jackson et al. 2001). Conservatively, it is estimated that one in eight American adults over the age of 25 have clinically manifested osteoarthritis (Lawrence et al. 1998, 2008), making it one of the leading causes of disability in the United States (Borrelli and Ricci 2004).

Increased costs associated with osteoarthritis and rheumatoid arthritis are high, as it has been demonstrated that several other comorbid conditions exist, such as anemia, osteoporosis, and bacterial infection (Gabriel and Michaud 2009). Analyses show that when compared with patients without osteoarthritis and rheumatoid arthritis, significantly more costs are incurred by osteoarthritis and rheumatoid arthritis patients in other health care areas, such as respiratory, cardiovascular, gastrointestinal, neurological, and psychiatric conditions, and also for general medical care. Increased therapeutic procedures, physician services, use of prescription medication, and so forth, are also more prevalent in sufferers of osteoarthritis and rheumatoid arthritis (Gabriel et al. 1997).

Another significant source of costs is loss of productivity. As reported by the CDC (2007), indirect costs (loss of earnings) associated with arthritis and other rheumatic diseases also increased from 1997 to 2003, from $35.1 billion to $47 billion. Indirect costs associated with articular cartilage injuries, that have not yet developed to osteoarthritis, can be four times as much as treatment of the defect itself (Upmeier et al. 2007), and a similar scenario can be expected for osteoarthritis. In addition to costs associated with treating the articular surface, other medical comorbidities observed with osteoarthritis and rheumatoid arthritis contribute significantly to the costs of disease management (Gabriel and Michaud 2009).

3.2 CARTILAGE INJURIES

3.2.1 Osteochondral and Chondral Defects and Microfractures

Injurious impact or repeated loading, joint malalignment, and foreign bodies in the joint can all lead to cartilage injuries. Cartilage injuries are classified as osteochondral defects, chondral defects, and cartilage microfractures (not to be confused with the surgical procedure). Despite its avascular nature, articular cartilage bleeds from an osteochondral defect because the injury extends through the cartilage into the vascularized subchondral bone. Chondral defects are also visible to the naked eye, oftentimes through India ink staining, in contrast to cartilage microfractures. For each type, the changes in tissue appearance, composition, and biomechanical properties will be presented below, along with a description of the resultant cellular responses. The information presented earlier on articular cartilage physiology and aging directly affects the outcomes for cartilage injuries, which often lead eventually to osteoarthritis. For instance, a lack of vasculature and the hyaline nature of articular cartilage result in few cells available to mount an adequate healing response. A degenerative process thus follows, exacerbated by age, as stresses from daily use continue to be applied onto the already weakened tissue, with morphological and cellular changes.

The Outerbridge classification (Figure 3.17) has been used to grade the severity of cartilage lesions, with Grade 0 representing normal cartilage (Outerbridge 1961). Softening or swelling of the cartilage without visible defects is classified as Grade I. Grade II, which is the most frequently

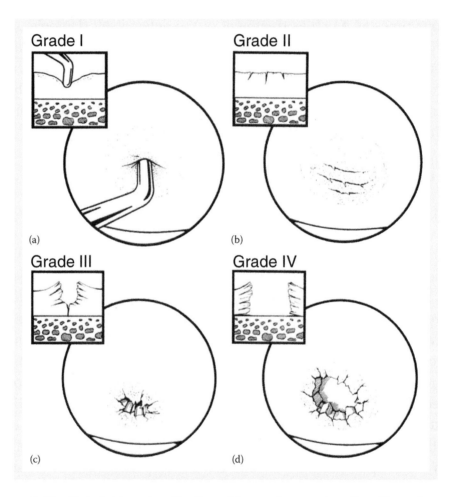

Figure 3.17 Outerbridge classification of increasing grades of cartilage damage. (a) Grade I. Softening of the articular cartilage, but no obvious damage. (b) Grade II. Minor fibrillation or partial-thickness damage is less than 1.5 cm in diameter. (c) Grade III. Fibrillation or partial-thickness lesion larger than 1.5 cm in diameter. (d) Grade IV. Full-thickness lesion extending to the bone. (From Mandelbaum, B. R. et al., *Am J Sports Med* 26(6): 853–861, 1998. With permission.)

observed clinically (Widuchowski et al. 2007), denotes that a defect contains fissures that do not extend to the subchondral bone (i.e., a chondral defect) and that the defect's diameter is less than 1.5 cm. When fissuring extends to the level of the subchondral bone, in an area with a diameter more than 1.5 cm, the lesion is classified as Grade III. Lastly, an articular cartilage injury that results in exposure of the subchondral bone is classified as Grade IV. A similar scale modified from the Outerbridge scale (Beguin et al. 1982) has been shown to correlate well with a scale termed the Histological/Histochemical Grading System (Mankin et al. 1971) when the severity of the lesions was Grade III or below (Acebes et al. 2009). A scale specifically for arthroscopic grading of cartilage has also been developed (Noyes and Stabler 1989). Arthroscopic application of the Outerbridge classification has shown that orthopedic surgeons can use this scale to accurately grade chondral lesions regardless of their level of experience (Cameron et al. 2003). Other grading scales have also been developed for osteoarthritis, including the Osteoarthritis Research Society International (OARSI) Osteoarthritis Cartilage Histopathology Assessment System (OOCHAS) (Custers et al. 2007).

While the Outerbridge score was originally designed to describe a cartilage injury, the International Cartilage Repair Society (ICRS) has developed the ICRS Cartilage Injury Evaluation Package (www.carti lage.org), which includes both injury classification and repair assessment (Figure 3.18), along with other assessments of cartilage. The ICRS classification score is based on lesion depth and size and also considers anatomical location. As with the Outerbridge scoring system, the ICRS classification uses a score of Grade 0 through Grade 4, to describe "normal" to "severely abnormal" cartilage, respectively. A score of Grade 1 (nearly normal) describes the presence of minor or superficial damage to the cartilage or areas where the cartilage is softer. Grade 2 (abnormal) denotes the presence of lesions that penetrate less than 50% of the depth of the tissue. Grade 3 (severely abnormal) is characterized by lesions that penetrate more than 50% of the depth or into the calcified tissue. Finally, Grade 4 (also termed severely abnormal) is descriptive of full-thickness lesions into the subchondral bone.

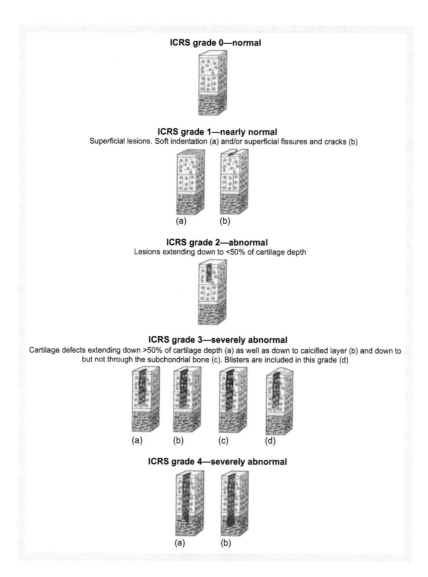

Figure 3.18 Diagram of the ICRS injury classification for scoring chondral and osteochondral lesions based on lesion depth. This classification also considers location and area of defect coverage using a mapping system that is included in the evaluation package. The full ICRS Cartilage Injury Evaluation Package, among other evaluations, includes both a Cartilage Repair Assessment and an Articular Cartilage Injury Classification. (From ICRS Cartilage Injury Evaluation Package [www.cartilage .org]. With permission from the International Cartilage Repair Society.)

Articular cartilage microfractures do not result in immediate changes to the matrix that are visible to the naked eye. However, the damage to the collagen network begins to effect superficial proteoglycan loss (Radin et al. 1978). As the network loosens, increased hydration is also observed (Dekel and Weissman 1978). Microfractures can also lead to altered load distribution of the matrix, resulting in stress concentrations that can cause further damage or a greater proportion of forces borne by the bone. These loading alterations, as well as fractures to the calcified layer that can occur, lead to eventual thickening of the subchondral bone (Mankin et al. 1994). In the subchondral bone, microfracture healing results in decreased blood flow. The calcified layer also thickens as the cartilage thins, leading to further changes in load distribution. Since cartilage is aneural, repeated loading of microfractured cartilage can continue without pain, leading to further degeneration (Buckwalter et al. 1994). Though the proteoglycan loss stimulates chondrocyte activity, the metabolic response is typically inadequate, leading to a net loss of proteoglycan, increased wear, and the eventual development of fissures and progression of pathology (Figure 3.19).

Chondral fissures are defects that do not extend to the subchondral bone. These defects are visible to the naked eye, often via India ink staining. Chondral defects can proceed from cartilage microfractures or

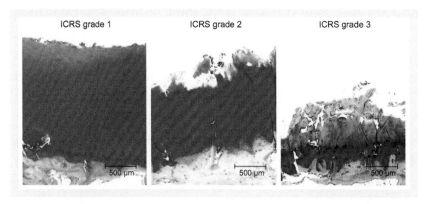

Figure 3.19 Histology of cartilage with osteoarthritis of different ICRS grades, indicating fissuring of the surface, loss of staining associated with glycosaminoglycans, and increasing tissue loss and disorganization. (From Kleemann, R. U. et al., *Osteoarthr Cartil* 13(11): 958-963, 2005. With permission.)

from trauma, improper loading, or foreign bodies. Without blood, the intrinsic metabolic activity after such an injury is insufficient to result in adequate repair, leading to the eventual development of osteochondral fissures (Buckwalter et al. 1994). Osteochondral fissures are lesions that cross the tidemark and penetrate the underlying bone. Osteoarthritis is partially a bone disease, and bone injury, such as microcracks, allows for capillary invasion and bone remodeling (Burr 2004). Though growth factors and progenitor cells are recruited from the bone's vasculature, there is impaired biomechanical functionality of the repair tissue, a mix of fibro- and articular cartilages (Furukawa et al. 1980), resulting in eventual degeneration into osteoarthritis. It is important to recall that with age, both chondrocytes and progenitor cells decrease in number and metabolic activity, thus contributing to the cartilage healing problem.

3.2.2 Causes of Cartilage Injuries

Cartilage injuries can result from impact and repeated loading, and these can occur under a wide range of loads, timescales, and frequencies. Determining thresholds that can correlate to certain elicited cellular responses is important in understanding cartilage injuries and degeneration. Because of the viscoelastic nature of articular cartilage, load rate affects tissue stiffness, and, thus, failure. The rates of applied stress, strain, and load must be considered. For example, using a confined compression loading protocol, the dynamic modulus has been shown to increase from 225 to 850 MPa as the load rate was increased from 25 to 1000 MPa/s (Milentijevic and Torzilli 2005).

As reviewed elsewhere (Komistek et al. 2005), peak forces during normal physiological loading of knee articular cartilage range from 1.9 to 7.2 times body weight. For a 70 kg person, this would correspond to ~1400-4900 N (Natoli and Athanasiou 2008). Taking the medial tibial plateau to have an area of 1670 mm² (Wluka et al. 2005), this corresponds to a maximum stress of ~3 MPa. During normal activities, like running, time to peak force is on the order of 30 ms, leading to a stress rate of

100 MPa/s. One can expect that impact injuries occur on a timescale an order of magnitude smaller, resulting in stress rates of 1,000 MPa/s. Based on data such as these, Aspden et al. (2002) put forth a definition for injurious impact loading as time to peak load on the order of milli-seconds, plus one of the following: (1) stress rate greater than 1,000 MPa/s, (2) strain rate greater than 500 per second, or (3) loading rates in excess of 100 kN/s.

Articular cartilage subjected to loads that do not satisfy Aspden's three criteria for impact can nonetheless result in damage via repeated application. The thresholds of forces and timescales required to pro-duce injuries are important in determining the type of injury sustained and for modeling impact and injurious compression experimentally. Mathematical models of impact and injurious compression have been performed (Armstrong et al. 1984; Anderson et al. 1990; Ateshian et al. 1994; Atkinson et al. 1998; Dunbar et al. 2001), as well as studies of impact done on explants (Jeffrey et al. 1995, 1997; Farquhar et al. 1996; Torzilli et al. 1999; D'Lima et al. 2001; Milentijevic and Torzilli 2005; Scott and Athanasiou 2006; Blumberg et al. 2008; Natoli and Athanasiou 2008; Natoli et al. 2008) and *in vivo* (Thompson and Bassett 1970; Simon et al. 1972; Dekel and Weissman 1978; Mitchell and Shepard 1980; Donohue et al. 1983; Haut et al. 1995; Ewers et al. 2002a,b) based on this and other classifications. The difference between impact and injurious compres-sion is that the latter occurs over a longer time span (Bonassar et al. 2001; Morel and Quinn 2004). However, the strain rate used in injurious compression is important. Studies with very slow strain rates (0.01 per second) and up to 50% strain have resulted in no measurable effect on chondrocytes, while the same strain applied at 0.1-1.0 per second had significant decreases in cell viability and biosynthetic response (Kurz et al. 2001). Under similar loading conditions of 40% strain at 0.1 per second, this decrease in biosynthetic activity has been linked to both increased cell death adjacent to the loaded surface and an increased proliferative response due to enhanced ERK1/2 signaling (Ryan et al. 2009), likely from released basic fibroblast growth factor (bFGF) bound in the matrix (Vincent et al. 2002). This biological response in injurious

201

compression likely parallels that during impact. Using a drop tower device to apply impact on cartilage (Scott and Athanasiou 2006), it was noted that even at levels where no morphological changes were observable immediately, significant cell death and decreases in cartilage stiffness were found 4 weeks after impact, compared with unimpacted controls (Figure 3.20) (Natoli et al. 2008). These data show that "clinically silent" impacts can nonetheless result in articular injuries.

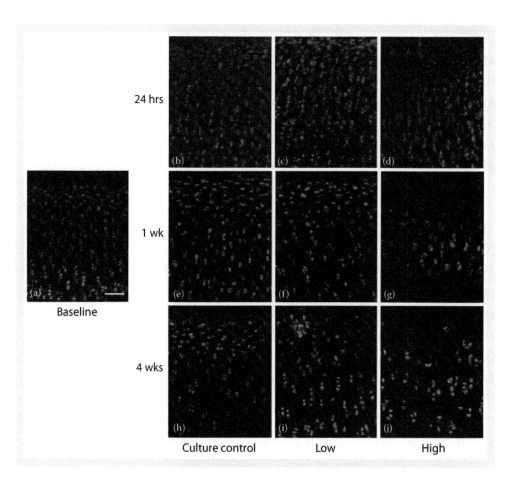

Figure 3.20 Viability staining of impacted cartilage (b-j), using nonimpacted, noncultured cartilage as baseline (a) (green/live and red/dead). Compared with nonimpacted control (b, e, h), increasing impact energy, going from low impact (c, f, i) to high impact (d, g, j), resulted in cell death spreading to deeper zones of the cartilage explant. Cell death also increased with culture time (24 hours to 4 weeks) in all groups. (From Natoli, R. M. et al., *Ann Biomed Eng* 36(5): 780-792, 2008. With permission.)

The superficial zone contains collagen fibers that are oriented parallel to the cartilage surface, aligned in the direction of shear (Meachim and Sheffield 1969). One important function of this higher-collagen- and lower-proteoglycan-density zone is to resist shear stress, and the superficial zone has been shown to be stiffer in tension than the other zones (Roth and Mow 1980). In addition, cartilage is weaker in tension in the direction perpendicular to shear (Kempson et al. 1973; Woo et al. 1976), and this weakness makes it susceptible to torsional injuries. Classifications of torsional injuries with respect to the forces, time frame, and frequencies necessary to generate cartilage microfractures and chondral or osteochondral defects are not as well studied as impact and injurious compression loading. These types of loading are, however, likely to play a role in cases of joint malalignment, as the altered biomechanics can result in repeated nonphysiological focal stresses or torques.

Surgical procedures or injuries to other connective tissues can be a cause of joint malalignment or improper cartilage loading. Also, foreign bodies, such as crystals, can result in damage to the articulating surface. MSU and CPPD (Webb 1978), characteristic in gout and synovitis (Kozin and McCarty 1976; Mandel and Mandel 1976), are strongly associated with cartilage lesions, higher levels of SZP, and collagen X (Muehleman et al. 2008), and are suspected to be linked to arthritis (Rizzoli et al. 1980). Associated lesions appear to be biomechanically induced, and crystals have been observed in joints both before and after the onset of osteoarthritis (Muehleman et al. 2008). Plastics or other debris can also contribute to third-body wear in a joint (Shields et al. 2009).

3.2.3 Cellular Responses to Injury

Cellular responses to osteochondral defects are complex due to the involvement of cells from the articular cartilage but also from elsewhere (e.g., synovium and subchondral bone or vasculature). For cartilage microfractures and chondral defects, the dense matrix keeps other cell types out of the repair response. Radiolabeling and other techniques have shown chondrocyte proliferation and matrix synthesis occurring for about 2 weeks postinjury (DePalma et al. 1966; Cheung et al. 1978). However, before the defect is filled, this anabolic activity ceases and the matrix is left unprepared for the continued rigors of daily use, leading to eventual degeneration as described previously (Fuller and Ghadially 1972; Shapiro et al. 1993).

With osteochondral defects, the repair process extends greatly beyond 2 weeks. The subchondral vasculature delivers progenitor cells that are much more motile and more active than chondrocytes, dominating the healing process. Blood from the bone forms a fibrin clot, which contains platelets that secrete factors to recruit mesenchymal stem cells (MSCs) from the bone. In the 2 weeks following injury, MSCs proliferate and differentiate. Repair continues beyond 2 weeks as differentiated cells produce type II collagen and type I collagen. By 6-8 weeks, the defect is filled (Hjertquist and Lemperg 1971; Cheung et al. 1980; Furukawa et al. 1980). From here on, matrix production slowly shifts from type II collagen to type I collagen such that by the end of 1 year, the repair tissue consists of both hyaline cartilage and fibrocartilage (Hjertquist and Lemperg 1971; Cheung et al. 1978; Shapiro et al. 1993). Since the fibrocartilage does not possess sufficient biomechanical properties for sustained function, continued matrix degeneration via fibrillation (Ghadially et al. 1977), proteoglycan loss (Squires et al. 2003), chondrocyte death and proliferation, and development of deep fissures are observed beyond the first year (Furukawa et al. 1980; Shapiro et al. 1993). Repair responses from both chondrocytes and other cells are also seen with immature cartilage where calcification has yet to be completed and where vasculature still exists close to the articulating surface. However, it has been shown that cartilage defects do not heal even in immature animals (DePalma et al. 1966; Fuller and Ghadially 1972), although surprisingly, superficial defects have been shown to heal in fetal lamb models (Namba et al. 1998). Whereas it has been proposed that "noncritical" defects (less than 3-9 mm in diameter, depending on the animal model) can heal (U.S. Food and Drug Administration [FDA] 2005), the repair tissue is again mechanically inferior fibrocartilage, which eventually degenerates, leading to osteoarthritis.

204

Whereas abundant evidence exists to indicate that osteochondral injuries lead eventually to osteoarthritis, it may not be as obvious that chondral defects and microfractures similarly lead to osteoarthritis. As pointed out earlier, though, when cartilage is subjected to impact, degenerative changes can occur even when no noticeable signs of damage can be observed immediately postimpact (Natoli et al. 2008). Investigations have been performed to see if agents such as P188 (Phillips and Haut 2004; Baars et al. 2006; Natoli and Athanasiou 2008), IGF-I (Natoli and Athanasiou 2008), and doxycycline (Blumberg et al. 2008) can halt or reverse the degenerative process postimpact. For example, P188 was shown to reduce cell death by 75% in the week following impact, while IGF-I decreased glycosaminoglycan loss from the tissue by 49%. However, neither treatment, or their combination, was able to reverse the detrimental change in cartilage stiffness following impact (Natoli and Athanasiou 2008). As the biochemical and biomechanical pathways that lead to osteoarthritis continue to be uncovered, no established methods currently exist in stopping these degenerative changes, leading to significant costs both financially and to the quality of life of osteoarthritic patients.

3.2.4 Costs of Articular Cartilage Injuries

In a retrospective cross-sectional study, the follow-up costs for the first 5 years following arthroscopy and treatment for 1708 Germans between 1997 and 2001 were quantified. The treatments included mostly debridement or cartilage shaving, with abrasion arthroplasty, chondroplasty or laser chondroplasty, and microfracture or subchondral drilling performed at roughly the same frequency. Autologous chondrocyte implantation (ACI), osteochondral allografts, and autografts were also observed, although much less frequently. Not included in the study were cases that were Grade 4 according to the Outerbridge classification system, fully osteoarthritic, or consisting of bacterial infections or tumors. Cumulative costs associated with loss of productivity were found to be almost four times the direct costs, with those who had prior operative history on the knee spending roughly double (Upmeier et al. 2007).

Another source of traumatic injuries posing significant costs is combat trauma. Based on queries to the Department of Defense Medical Metrics (M2) database for hospital admissions and billing data between October 2001 and January 2005 for injuries sustained in Iraq and Afghanistan, estimates of the cost of combat-related joint injuries approach $2 billion (Masini et al. 2009). Without a sufficient healing response, cartilage lesions eventually degenerate to osteoarthritis, which has much greater associated costs—in this case in excess of $65 billion (Jackson et al. 2001).

3.3 CURRENT AND EMERGING THERAPIES FOR ARTICULAR CARTILAGE REPAIR AND ARTHRITIS

In this section, current therapies that involve biological products for articular cartilage repair are described. It is important to note that treatment may include targeting cartilage, bone, synovium, or muscle, as it is unclear at this time whether any one component is the primary cause for injuries that progress to osteoarthritis (Samuels et al. 2008). The efficacy for many of these treatments has been assessed using both clinical trials and meta-analyses.

Comparing clinical trials or studies that contain different numbers of enrollees should take sample size into account because larger sample sizes yield greater statistical power, and even minute differences can be found to be significant. Thus, a therapy that marginally improves articular cartilage repair outcomes can be found to have an effect when a large number of patients are enrolled in the study, even if the actual benefits of such effects are miniscule. Effect size estimates such as Cohen's d and effect size correlation (also termed effect size r) have thus been used as statistical tools for assessing the magnitude of an effect independent of sample size. Using Cohen's d, an effect size of 0.0 indicates that outputs from the treated and untreated groups overlap completely; an effect size of 0.2 is considered small, 0.5 is considered medium, and 0.8 is considered large. Effect sizes for many existing therapies, both nonsurgical and surgical, have been calculated, and newly developed methods should also benefit from this analysis.

As the last treatment option, total joint replacement or arthroplasty will only be briefly mentioned here (Figure 3.21). Improvements in the design of arthroplasty implants have significantly lengthened their usable lifespan, though failure can still occur due to a variety of reasons. Aside from the wear of the articular surface and the failure of the implant itself, failure can result from the mechanical differences between the implant and the surrounding bone. As the stiffer implant is capable of bearing more load, shielding of the surrounding bone occurs, and osteolysis, instability, and implant loosening can occur. The difference in stiffness between the artificial and natural materials can also result in peri-prosthetic fracture. Children and adolescents are not good candidates for these procedures, due to both their developing skeletons

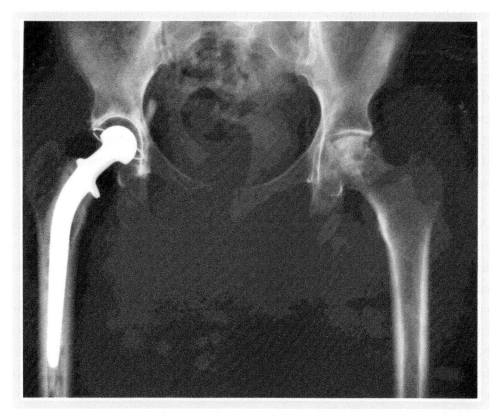

Figure 3.21 Anteroposterior x-ray image of pelvis showing a total hip joint replacement. The prosthesis is composed of a metal stem implanted in the right femur and a plastic cup implanted in the acetabulum. (Public domain image, National Institutes of Health.)

and the fact that their age requires a longer-term solution. In addition, arthroplasty is not the best solution for cases where focal lesions are concerned, as often caused by sports injuries. Thus, here we will discuss nonarthroplasty therapies, divided into nonsurgical and surgical techniques. Surgical transplantation of allogeneic or xenogeneic materials is discussed in Section 3.3.2 with cartilage immunology, as the outcome of these transplants relies heavily on whether the implant is accepted by the body.

3.3.1 Nonsurgical Treatments

Treatment options for osteoarthritis and cartilage damage depend on both the level of progression and the nature of the injury (discussed in Section 3.2). For idiopathic osteoarthritis and secondary osteoarthritis (which may be difficult to distinguish from the former), early symptoms such as diffuse pain are treated with nonsteroidal anti-inflammatory drugs (NSAIDs) (e.g., acetaminophen) to reduce pain and inflammation. Lifestyle changes, including weight loss and exercise, along with gait modification, are recommended to reduce the progression of the disease. When nonsurgical treatments do not help the patient, more aggressive treatments are initiated.

Articular cartilage injuries can be caused by a variety of reasons, as reviewed earlier. Since sports or improper loading are implicated, activity modification, weight and body fat loss, physical therapy, and the use of a cane to lessen the load applied on the problematic joint are all nonsurgical and nonpharmacological methods to address discomfort. For instance, weight reduction in combination with strength exercises has been shown to significantly reduce knee pain in overweight and obese individuals (Christensen et al. 2007; Jenkinson et al. 2009). The reduction of body fat, independent of weight loss, has also been shown to be beneficial (Christensen et al. 2005; Teichtahl et al. 2008). Heating and ice applied to the knee show moderate to large effect sizes (0.69 to 1.03) for pain reduction and improvements in function (Brosseau et al. 2003; Zhang et al. 2010).

208

In addition to modalities with a scientific basis, there seem to exist a plethora of other approaches whose scientific origin, as well as efficacy, is dubious at best, if not charlatanic. For example, it has long been believed by many that items such as copper bracelets can alleviate joint pain caused by arthritis. It has already been determined that the placebo effect is at work in this case (Walker and Keats 1976). The efficacy of similar devices, such as magnetic bracelets (Richmond 2008), is still undergoing investigation, although these, too, appear to function through a placebo effect (Richmond et al. 2009).

The popularity of copper and magnetic bracelets stems from several desirable characteristics, namely, the ease of use, noninvasiveness, the presence of few or no side effects, and the perception that these items are more "natural" than other therapies. Over-the-counter dietary supplements, such as glucosamine and chondroitin, share many of these desirable characteristics. These are of particular interest due to their wide availability and popularity. These products have been recommended by both OARSI in 2007 (Brosseau et al. 2002) and the European League Against Rheumatism (EULAR) in 2003 (Jordan et al. 2003), while being the subject of conflicting results and heated debates. Questions have been raised about study results with regard to design, sample sizes, publication bias, and the choices of controls, all complicated by the overwhelming variety of formulations and derivatives available on the market. The Glucosamine/Chondroitin Arthritis Intervention Trial (GAIT) (NIH 2008), funded by the National Institutes of Health (NIH) and published in 2008, showed that these supplements did not significantly reduce pain compared with a placebo, though this study has itself received similar criticism, as listed above. A recent review of glucosamine in the management of osteoarthritis found that glucosamine sulfate had an effect size greater than or equal to those of common analgesics, basing its recommendation on this and the low incidence of adverse effects (Henrotin et al. 2012). However, the effects of glucosamine appear to be location dependent. Based on its analyses, OARSI recommends glucosamine in management of the knee but not the hip (Zhang et al. 2010), and the same recommendation is given by EULAR (Jordan et al. 2003; Zhang et al. 2005). One recent review of the literature, however, has indicated that there is very little scientific basis for glucosamine supplements in alleviating arthritis (Henrotin et al. 2012).

Other pharmacological interventions include aspirin, ibuprofen, and a variety of cyclooxygenase 2 (COX2) inhibitors, as well as dietary supplements. Not surprisingly, opioids and other COX2 inhibitors have moderate effect sizes on pain reduction, but lower effect sizes for improving joint function; over-the-counter pain relievers have low effect sizes for pain reduction (Zhang et al. 2010). Viscosupplementation (e.g., hyaluronan) via injections (Figure 3.22) and corticosteroids have also been used to relieve joint pain; it should be noted, though, that some steroidal injections have been shown to soften the remaining cartilage (Murray et al. 1998). Overall, these nonsurgical treatments have shown varying degrees of effectiveness for relieving pain and restoring function but are not effective for articular cartilage healing.

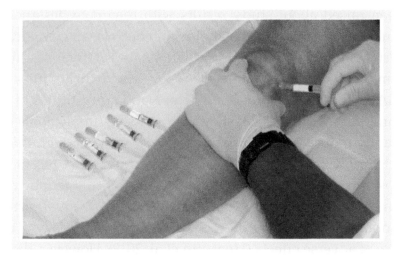

Figure 3.22 Viscosupplementation via injection of sodium hyaluronate into the knee of a patient. (Image used under Creative Commons by 3.0 Ported License. Photo by Dr. Harry Gouvas.)

3.3.2 Surgical Treatments for Articular Cartilage Repair

For smaller focal defects, several treatment options are available that reduce pain and extend the useful life of the joint, prior to total joint replacement (Magnussen et al. 2008). The most common treatments used are microfracture (Steadman et al. 2003), mosaicplasty (Hangody and Fules 2003), ACI (Brittberg et al. 1994), and allogeneic transplants (Gross et al. 1975, 1983). The use of autologous MSCs (from bone marrow, adipose, or synovial tissues) has also been explored for cartilage repair (Caplan et al. 1997; Erickson et al. 2002; Lee et al. 2007, 2010). The choice of the technique and approach is based on the size of the defect to be filled and the health of the surrounding tissue. In each of these techniques, the initial defect will be debrided of torn and loosely attached cartilage. Commonly, an arthroscopic debridement or lavage will be used to remove loose flaps of cartilage or debris, although this is mostly palliative. This technique can be used on small defects and can reduce pain, inflammation, and mechanical impingement.

Though it may be ideal to not have to compromise the joint by introducing foreign matter, surgical methods also provide ways to alleviate pain and restore function. As discussed previously, choice of surgical procedure depends on indication, anatomical location, and accompanying conditions. In the knee, when articular cartilage lesions are less than 2 cm^2 and not accompanied by other conditions, such as inflammatory arthritis, lesions are treated with marrow stimulation techniques, including subchondral drilling and microfracture. A second line of treatments include osteochondral autografts and ACI. For lesions greater than 2 cm^2, debridement and marrow stimulation are also the initial surgical options. Secondary measures include ACI and allografts, since at this point it becomes difficult to source autologous tissue.

3.3.2.1 Debridement

Arthroscopic abrasion arthroplasty is a procedure where the cartilage defect is smoothed and reshaped. This treatment is often combined with others, such as marrow stimulation, for a variety of indications. Burrs, diseased tissue, delaminated cartilage, and flaps can be removed to improve the gliding motion and provide temporary relief. Osteochondral defects can also be treated by removing the dead bone or sclerotic lesions to stimulate fibrocartilage production. This fibrocartilage repair tissue has been reported to last up to 6 years (Johnson 1986). Reports have shown that for chondromalacia patellae, 75% of the patients were satisfied with the procedure when followed up (Federico and Reider 1997). Even for athletes, the procedure has shown quick success, with resumption of sports activities on an average of 10.8 weeks following the procedure (Levy et al. 1996). Cartilage debridement has been applied to various joints, including the knee (Jackson et al. 1997; Chiu and Chen 2007), elbow (Vingerhoeds et al. 2004; Wada et al. 2005), ankle (Gould and Flick 1985), and shoulder (Cuff et al. 2008), oftentimes in combination with other procedures. However, arthroscopic debridement has been demonstrated to be no better than placebo procedure for osteoarthritis of the knee (Moseley et al. 2002).

3.3.2.2 Marrow Stimulation Techniques

Multiple methods have been developed to bring bone marrow to the damaged articular surface. These serve as primary treatments for chondral and osteochondral lesions, both small and large. The overall treatment outcome is a mixture of hyaline and fibrous repair tissues. Microfracture techniques have their origin in Pridie drilling (Pridie 1959), where multiple transcortical holes are drilled after surface debridement, stimulating the marrow for a healing response. To avoid the heat generated by Pridie drilling and to allow for greater instrumentation access, Pridie drilling has now been supplanted by microfracture.

Microfracture is the simplest, quickest, and least expensive treatment option, with arthroscopic operating time being as little as 30-90 minutes. This technique has been widely employed for isolated chondral defects of the knee (Bae et al. 2006; Mithoefer et al. 2006), shoulder (Siebold et al. 2003), and ankle (Becher and Thermann 2005). Microfracture involves having the surgeon cause small fractures into the bone of a full-thickness defect connecting into the underlying bone marrow to allow bleeding and clot formation in the defect (Mithoefer et al. 2006). This also allows for stem cells and other factors in the bone marrow to migrate into the defect. The damaged cartilage is first removed down to the calcified zone to expose healthy adjacent tissue. The calcified cartilage is then removed, and an arthroscopic awl perforates the subchondral plate to a depth of approximately 4 mm, with holes spaced 3-4 mm apart. Blood fills the defect, resulting in a fibrin clot that initiates a healing response. This clot, over a period of 8-12 weeks, will be replaced with fibrocartilage, which, although filling the defect and providing improved outcomes, is less mechanically robust than hyaline cartilage. Thus, fibrocartilage only serves as a temporary treatment.

To improve upon this, microfracture has been used in combination with coverings, such as a periosteal flap (Siebold et al. 2003) or other natural (e.g., chitosan [Hoemann et al. 2005] and collagen [Breinan et al. 2000; Dorotka et al. 2005]) and synthetic (e.g., poly-glycolic acid [PGA] mixed with hyaluronan [Erggelet et al. 2009]) materials. Other improvements to the technique include the addition of a BMP4 carrier, which showed more rapid repair (Zhang et al. 2008). BMP7 has been shown to increase the volume of the repair tissue generated (Kuo et al. 2006). A systematic review of 28 studies describing 3122 patients has shown that the procedure is effective within the first 24 months in improving knee function (Mithoefer et al. 2009). Subsequently, the effectiveness wears off, especially for patients 40 years old and older (Kreuz et al. 2006; Mithoefer et al. 2009), as the fibrocartilage formed eventually degenerates, resulting in recurred loss of function. Many of the new therapies under development consist of new scaffolds and materials intended to augment marrow stimulation. These will be discussed in the context of FDA regulations and clinical trials in upcoming chapters.

3.3.2.3 Autologous Implants

Though limited in source, autologous implants enjoy several advantages as transplant materials, such as not eliciting immune responses and having functionality close to the tissues they are replacing. These may be indicated for defects less than 2 cm² after marrow stimulation has proven to be unsatisfactory. In autologous implantation, low or nonloading areas of the joint are chosen to extract full-thickness punches of articular cartilage to be implanted into the defect region. This is limited in the amount of material that may be harvested to fill the defect. Treatment also requires healthy donor sites to be available and unaccompanied by inflammatory arthritis. Taken from non-load-bearing regions, autologous implants may not be as mechanically suitable for their target defects, but they contain live, autologous cells that have the potential for continued remodeling. Unlike allogeneic tissue, the concern for disease transmission is greatly mitigated in this case. However, the scarcity of source material, donor site morbidity, and differences in shape between the implant and the recipient site limit the use of autologous implants. In allograft procedures, the normal cartilage tissue is procured from donor tissue (deceased), allowing for infill of much larger defects. However, this raises both possible disease transmission and immune issues. Allogeneic and xenogeneic implants are alternatives for the same indications, and these are discussed under Section 6.2, "Immune Response, Immunogenicity, and Transplants." Chondral implants, which do not extend into the subchondral bone, face the significant problem of integration with the adjacent cartilage tissue.

Autologous implants typically fall into two forms, osteochondral plugs and patient-derived cells. Osteochondral plugs are harvested from non-weight-bearing regions and have shown efficacy for as long as 10 years (Marcacci et al. 1999). To better accommodate the differences in curvature between the donor and recipient surfaces, mosaicplasty (Hangody et al. 1997) has been shown to have better results than Pridie drilling, abrasion arthroplasty, microfracture repair, and ACI (Hangody et al. 1997; Hangody and Fules 2003; Dozin et al. 2005), as evaluated by radiography, MRI, biopsy analysis, and other techniques to generate scores from a variety of systems, including the ICRS scoring system. Good to excellent scores have been demonstrated for resurfacing the femoral condyle (92%), tibia (87%), patella or trochlea (79%), and talus (94%) using mosaicplasty (Szerb et al. 2005).

Attempts have been made to use less tissue to reduce donor site morbidity and increase the amount of usable grafts. For example, 6 mm diameter osteochondral plugs have been placed into 10 mm diameter defects in the sheep model to examine whether the resulting 2 mm band around the plug can be filled with repair tissue (Burks et al. 2006). Tissue ingrowth in this ring was observed, but it consisted of fibrocartilage. Since a 6 mm diameter is below the 7 mm "critical defect" size (FDA 2005), a donor site defect of this size or below is expected to recover. However, it has been shown that the repair tissues at the donor sites consist of fibrocartilage (Szerb et al. 2005).

Though osteochondral plugs are taken from non-weight-bearing locations, the material properties of adjacent repair fibrocartilage can nonetheless be inadequate for long-term use. For instance, fibrocartilage repair tissue (and osteoarthritic tissue) has been shown to lack the extent of collagen organization and alignment of healthy articular cartilage (Bi et al. 2005). Even under low loading conditions, shear forces that are an integral aspect of articulation may still prove to be challenging for the relatively unorganized repair tissue. Without proper organization and material properties, the repair tissue from the donor site can degenerate. For this reason, osteochondral autografts are typically employed only after other techniques have been excluded due to their complexity or inadequacy.

In the U.S., the only FDA-approved cell-based articular cartilage repair product is Carticel, developed by Genzyme Corporation and consisting of the implantation of autologous cultured chondrocytes (Seigel and Donlon 1997; Wood et al. 2006). In this procedure, cartilage is first harvested from low-weight-bearing regions of the knee and sent to Genzyme for enzymatic digestion. The released chondrocytes are expanded *in vitro* for several weeks and sent back to the surgeon. Prior to the implantation of these cells, the defect must first be debrided and cleaned. In early versions of the treatment, a membrane obtained from the periosteum was sutured over the defect to protect the cells; at present, a porcine-derived collagenous membrane is used. This flap is stitched over the defect to form a pocket, into which the expanded cells are injected (Brittberg et al. 1994) (Figure 3.23). The tissue that forms from these cells can be hyaline or fibrocartilage, with as few as 15% of the cases reporting hyaline cartilage (Horas et al. 2003; Roberts et al. 2009). Type II collagen that does form is not aligned like native tissue (Kurkijarvi et al. 2007). As a result, the stiffness of the repair tissue has ranged from 62% (Vasara et al. 2005) to 90% (Peterson et al. 2002) of the values of the surrounding cartilage.

ACI has been shown to yield better results for femoral cartilage defects than patella or tibial defects, with the location within each region also affecting clinical outcomes (Erggelet et al. 2008; Niemeyer et al. 2008).

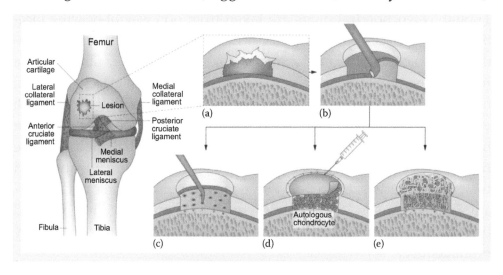

Figure 3.23 Schematic comparison of various cartilage repair techniques for an osteochondral lesion (a), including debridement (b), microfracture (c), ACI (d), and matrix-induced ACI (MACI) (e). Each procedure begins with the debridement of the lesion, including the calcified layer. For ACI, a periosteal flap or collagen type I or III membrane is anchored with horizontal sutures into the cartilage to cover the defect. The lesion is then filled with expanded autologous chondrocytes (12-48 million cells, depending on defect size). For MACI, the autologous chondrocytes are preseeded into a three-dimensional matrix, commonly collagen (I or III) or hyaluronic acid, and implanted into the lesion with fibrin glue. (From Makris, E. A. et al., *Nat Rev Rheumatol* 11(1): 21-34, 2015. With permission.)

It has been shown that 4 years after ACI, 75% of patients were mostly satisfied with the surgical outcome (McNickle et al. 2009). When comparing this technique to microfracture, conflicting findings exist. Better clinical results have been seen for ACI than microfracture, although both show satisfactory outcomes at medium-term follow-ups (Kon et al. 2009). Procedures using autologous chondrocytes have been improved with products such as Carticel II, which uses a fleece carrier, and Arthro Kinetics' CaReS-1S, which consists of a collagen gel carrier. Both of these scaffolds are intended to sequester the delivered chondrocytes, similar to scaffolds used to augment marrow stimulation techniques. Both of these products are available in Europe but not in the United States.

However, for advanced joint damage the gold standard still remains partial or complete joint replacement with synthetic prostheses. This has limitations as reported by the American Academy of Orthopaedic Surgeons (AAOS). These prostheses generally have a lifespan of approximately 10-20 years prior to revision, depending on the type of implant and multiple patient factors. Complications include wear debris particles, stress shielding, and catastrophic material failure, requiring revision surgery.

3.3.2.4 Adjunctive Treatments

Concomitant treatments, such as different rehabilitation regimens (Hambly et al. 2006; Reinold et al. 2006), and patient age (Giannoni et al. 2005) and surgical history (Mithofer et al. 2005) are all factors that influence treatment outcomes. For instance, clinical studies involving joint repair have long established that immobilization inhibits long-term healing in articular cartilage (Kim et al. 1995; Athanasiou et al. 1998; Alfredson and Lorentzon 1999; Lee et al. 2003). Motion is needed to induce movement of fluid and nutrients throughout the joint spaces, as well as to provide mechanical cues that can stimulate the chondrocytic phenotype. However, for emerging therapies, such as engineered articular cartilage, the strenuous mechanical environment of the joint can prove to be too challenging for newly formed tissues, resulting in rapid failure of such implants. Thus, continuous passive motion (CPM) is an adjunctive therapy that is commonly used for the first 2 weeks after surgery to improve the therapeutic outcomes of surgical treatments (Figure 3.24). CPM facilitates the transport of fluid, nutrients, and solutes within the joint, thereby stimulating chondrocyte metabolism (Lee et al. 2003). CPM alone may be insufficient since it does not allow any significant loading of the tissue (Athanasiou et al. 1998). Active motion, including incremental strength and weight-bearing exercises, may be necessary to stimulate repair processes during rehabilitation. As in many *in vitro* experiments, chondrocytes respond favorably when suitable mechanical forces are present.

As discussed previously, treating the cartilage alone may be insufficient to address lesions completely, since other problems may underlie the lesions' formation. The same can be said of therapies using either mosaicplasty or ACI. Joint malalignment can result in lesions, and postoperative joint alignment can affect ACI outcomes (Peterson et al. 2000). In cases of malalignment, excessive contact pressures in the defect area may be reduced back to physiological levels by osteotomy. Osteotomy may be performed independently of articular cartilage treatments to correct alignment, with the target of preventing future damage to the

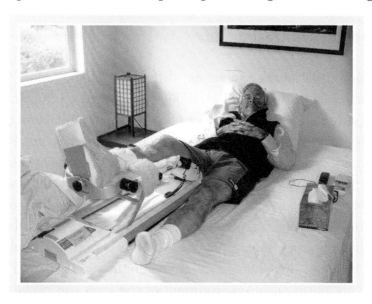

Figure 3.24 CPM device in use by a patient. (Image by Peter Stevens and used under Creative Commons 2.0 License.)

articular surface. Methods include anteromedial transfer of the tibial tubercle to decrease the contact forces on the lateral facet of the patella (Fulkerson et al. 1990); this has been shown to lower contact pressures in the lateral trochlea in a cadaver model (Beck et al. 2005). This, in combination with other surgical techniques such as ACI, can be beneficial to patients with multiple knee disorders (Farr 2007). Currently, the combined consideration of alignment and autologous osteochondral grafting is associated with traumatic reconstruction case studies, and, thus, they are difficult to compare (Rose et al. 2005). Nonetheless, in order to prevent relapse, future cartilage resurfacing methods may consider the accompaniment of additional orthopedic adjustments.

3.3.3 Other Treatments and Emerging Techniques

An alternative to tissue engineering articular cartilage outside the body is to implant a scaffold *in vivo*, with or without cells, and allow regeneration to occur with minimal additional manipulation. Regeneration of hyaline cartilage within the body is complicated by the demanding mechanical environment present in active joints. However, the complex mixture of biochemical and biomechanical cues present in the body may accelerate tissue growth in a way that is difficult to reproduce *in vitro*. Loading is applied naturally by the normal physiological environment, which may be seen as the ideal cartilage bioreactor. Chapter 4 will further describe the factors related to *in vitro* tissue engineering and how these factors commonly seek to replicate the *in vivo* environment.

The *in vivo* growth of cartilage depends on many different factors that cannot be modeled well *in vitro*. For example, many cytokines and bioactive molecules cannot be easily included in a laboratory experiment because of cost and availability. Using serum in the culture media is intended to replicate these conditions, but results can be dramatically different under the dynamic conditions of the body, where the implanted construct communicates with the host. Even in an isolated tissue such as cartilage, chemical and mechanical signals can impact the development of the tissue, whether in an empty defect or in an implanted construct.

Investigations into *in vivo* cartilage engineering have focused on repairing defect sites with transplanted cartilage or cells, synthetic materials, and cell-seeded cross-linkable scaffolds. The first, which was discussed earlier in this chapter, includes autologous and allogeneic cartilage or cell implantation, in which cells or minced tissue are inserted into a defect site and then kept in place with a covering, such as a periosteal flap (Brittberg et al. 1994). The second approach is primarily a stop-gap measure that would provide a mechanically functional insert but does not allow regeneration of the tissue (Falez and Sciarretta 2005; Maiotti et al. 2005; McNickle et al. 2008). The third repair technique includes several different types of synthesized polymers that can transition from a fluid to a stiff gel using either light or heat as initiators (Elisseeff et al. 1999, 2000). These techniques, where the bulk of the tissue formation occurs *in vivo*, all have advantages and disadvantages, although none of the approaches have resulted in long-term, functional repair of articular cartilage comparable to healthy tissue.

ACI has been modified in various ways in animal studies. Instead of a cell slurry, expanded chondrocytes have been condensed into spheroids first and then implanted into severe combined immunodeficiency (SCID) mice (Schubert et al. 2009). Attempts have also been made by embedding cells in an alginate-gelatin hydrogel with subsequent implantation in sheep. Hyaline-like repair tissue formed in both cases, although better histological scores resulted when chondrocytes were included (Schagemann et al. 2009). Attempts have also been made at replacing the periosteum flap with other materials, such as collagen sheets with embedded cells (Mitani et al. 2009; Steinwachs 2009), showing that symptomatic hypertrophy, disturbed fusion, delamination, and graft failure observed with periosteum use can be subsequently reduced (Niemeyer et al. 2008).

A possible approach to *in vivo* articular cartilage replacement is to insert synthetic constructs, which would fill a defect and provide mechanical support and a low-friction surface. These acellular constructs would be nonresorbable and could likely find a niche as a stop-gap measure for patients wanting to delay full arthroscopy procedures (McNickle et al. 2008). Synthetic replacements represent an attractive option due to their ease of handling and modification. Synthetic replacements can provide structural support for limited periods of time, but eventually more drastic procedures will be necessary as the conditions in the joint continue to degrade.

Several cell-scaffold combinations have been examined for resurfacing articular cartilage. BioSeed-C, a fibrin and polymer-based scaffold (poly-lactic-co-glycolic acid [PGLA]/polydioxanone) has been able to mitigate pain and improve knee-related quality of life measures after 0.5, 1, and 4 years (Figure 3.25) (Kreuz et al. 2009; Erggelet et al. 2010). A type I or III collagen mesh with chondrocyte implantation has shown good or excellent outcomes 2 years postoperation in 82% of patients that

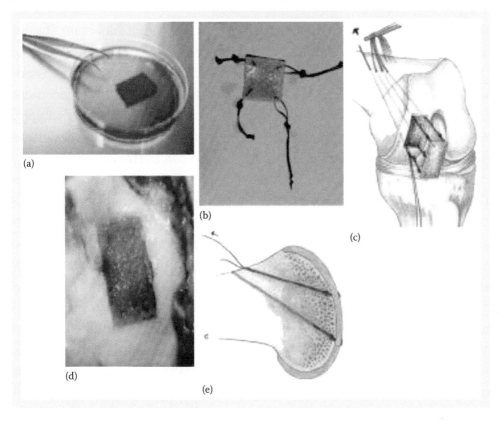

Figure 3.25 BioSeed-C scaffold is seeded with autologous chondrocytes (a) and anchored transosseously through the back of the femur using a combination of Vicryl sutures (b) and k-wires (c). This results in an initial smooth filling of the defect (d, e). (From Erggelet, C. et al., *Arch Orthop Trauma Surg* 130(8): 957-964, 2010. With permission.)

underwent the procedure, although 75% of the defects showed fibrous tissue formation rather than hyaline (Anders et al. 2008). Hyaff-11, by Fidia Advanced Biopolymers, is an esterified hyaluronic acid scaffold that could be implanted using an arthroscopic technique to yield formation of hyaline-like cartilage tissue (Ferruzzi et al. 2008). Outcomes for these products and procedures can depend on the patient population. For instance, young, highly active patients had better outcomes than their less active counterparts after treatment with Hyalograft C (Marcacci et al. 2005a,b). Tables of products currently in clinical trials are provided in Section 6.4.

3.4 MOTIVATION FOR TISSUE ENGINEERING

Based on more than 25,000 arthroscopies surveyed, it has been shown that osteochondral and chondral lesions are the most common types of cartilage damage, accounting for 67% of the observations, while osteoarthritis accounts for 29% (Widuchowski et al. 2007). While replacement cartilage for osteoarthritis will address a significant clinical problem, tissue engineering may be used to repair articular cartilage focal defects before such lesions manifest themselves into osteoarthritis.

The dense, hyaline matrix greatly hinders cell movement and, as discussed earlier, is a barrier to even chondrocytes themselves, precluding a complete healing response as the sequestered chondrocytes are prevented from populating the wound edge. This same dense matrix also serves as a barrier to integration, discussed in Chapter 6. For the time being, it is important to note that unless compromised, the dense tissue locks cells and matrix in and keeps cells out. Articular cartilage has long been considered immunoprivileged due to this dense matrix and because of its avascular and alymphatic nature. This gave hope that xenogeneic cartilage materials might be readily available as replacement tissue sources. However, new research indicates that with introduction of xenogeneic materials into the joint, the immunoprivileged hypothesis may not hold true (Pei et al. 2010), especially for materials of tissue-engineered origin.

As presented earlier, the cartilage's inability to mount a sufficient healing response eventually results in degenerative changes, and the observed proportion of lesions to osteoarthritis is expected to change in the near future due to the large cohort of baby boomers, with concomitant rises in management and treatment costs. Aside from osteoarthritis being linked to the aging population, it is more important to note that these lesions frequently occur in youth, a population whose needs for long-term solutions are much greater than those of older patients.

A need for tissue engineering rises from the prevalence of joint injuries in adolescents. "Little Leaguer's elbow," osteochondrosis, and osteochondritis dissecans are joint diseases that occur mainly in children, due to the increased vulnerability to stress in the growing skeleton (Figure 3.26). One out of three school-aged children will sustain an injury severe enough to require medical treatment. Emergency room

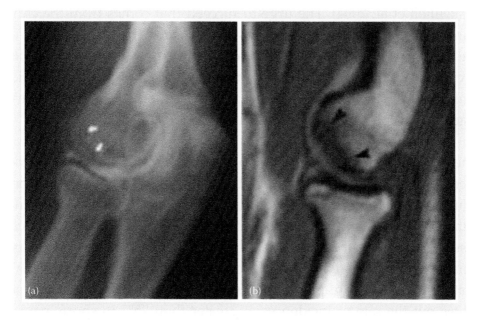

Figure 3.26 Arthrographic x-ray (a) and MRI (b) showing osteochondritis dissecans of the capitellum in a 14-year-old female athlete with elbow pain. White arrows (a) point to a 10 mm lucency in the subchondral bone. Black arrow heads indicate a fibrous repair tissue on a T1-weighted spin-echo MRI in the same location. (Modified from Frostick, S. P. et al., *Br J Sports Med* 33(5): 301-311, 1999. With permission.)

visits are the highest among children and young adults. ACL treatments, as well, are seen in higher frequencies (and are rising) in these two groups (Shea et al. 2003; Utukuri et al. 2006). With the estimated 30 million children who participate in organized sports activities, the yearly costs for injuries within this group have been projected to be $1.8 billion (Adirim and Cheng 2003). Kids may play on multiple teams with overlapping schedules, and it is not uncommon to see the absence of well-defined standards defining when training becomes excessive. Little League began to implement a pilot pitch-count program only in 2005 (Berler 2009), though its initially set standards were quickly relaxed. While elbow injuries (e.g., Figure 3.26) and shoulder injuries are common in baseball, a global survey of adolescent knee injuries put the incidence rate at greater than 25% in sports participants (Louw et al. 2008), particularly in basketball (Jones et al. 2000; Hewett et al. 2005). In terms of articular cartilage defects, young patients with knee injuries show 75% superficial (grade I-II) and 25% deep (grade III-IV) lesions (Eskelinen et al. 2004). The urge to succeed that comes from the child, parents, and coaches has gone to such a degree that overuse injuries are common. It is difficult for some parents to realize that their children's hard work in sports can result in catastrophic cartilage injuries. Unfortunately, no consistently successful solutions exist for the cartilage repair problem in children and adolescents.

The formation of repair fibrocartilage serves only as a temporary biomechanical fix, so a long-term solution for youth afflicted with joint injuries would be ideal. Even in cases where articular cartilage is not damaged in the primary traumatic event, the malalignment that can result (Hunter et al. 2005) has been shown to predict cartilage loss (Sharma et al. 2008). A survey of global adolescent knee injuries shows that females are more prone to these injuries than males. Recent estimates put the rate of incidences at greater than 25% in sports participants (Louw et al. 2008). Basketball has been linked to the highest rates of knee injury, as the frequent jumping associated with this activity results in applied loads that are several times body weight (Jones et al. 2000; Hewett et al. 2005). Indeed, knee and hip cartilage shows greater incidences of lesions than other anatomical regions. A survey of all cartilage lesions across all ages shows that the patellar articular surface and the medial femoral condyle were the most frequently damaged, accounting for 36% and 34%, respectively, of the cases surveyed (Widuchowski et al. 2007). These joints are also the ones that enable mobility and have great impact on quality of life. Arthroscopic evaluation in young Finnish males showed that 73.5% of the lesions were patellar, 12.0% in the medial condyle of the femur, and 8.0% in the femoral groove. Roughly 75% of the patients had superficial (grade I-II) and 25% deep (grade III-IV) lesions (Eskelinen et al. 2004). This is particularly alarming as data from 1995 to 1997 indicate that roughly 20% of the knee injuries in adolescents require surgery (Gomez et al. 1996; Hickey et al. 1997; Powell and Barber-Foss 1999). Unfortunately, current therapies are not sufficient in effecting long-term relief and activity resumption. Follow-up studies of 5, 10, or even more years have consistently shown a need for improvement in the outcomes of arthroplasty, along with osteochondral and autologous cell transplantation. Effective solutions are clearly needed, whether they be improvements on current therapies, *in vivo* tissue engineering approaches such as chondrocyte transplantation, or controlled manipulation of cells and materials *in vitro* to form implantable neocartilage.

3.5 CHAPTER CONCEPTS

- Arthritis encompasses a multitude of diseases that affect the joint; of these, osteoarthritis is the most common.
- Osteoarthritis affects more than one-fifth of the U.S. population over the age of 45 and almost one-half of those over the age of 65.
- In the United States alone, costs of osteoarthritis are in excess of $65 billion per year (both medical costs and lost wages). Comorbidities are common with osteoarthritis and are also costly to manage.
- Causes of arthritis can be due to both the strong actions of a single gene or the subtle interactions of multiple genes. The genetic basis of osteoarthritis is complex and may be due to multiple genes.
- The progression of osteoarthritis can be due to the interaction of biological and biomechanical factors, such as abnormal or altered loading.
- The formation of calcium salt or uric acid crystals in the joint space can lead to several pathologies and cartilage damage.
- Articular cartilage can be injured by impact, repeated loading, torsional loading, joint malalignment, or foreign bodies in the joint space.
- Injury to the fibrocartilage meniscus or ligaments in the joint can lead to osteoarthritis.
- Pain is the predominant symptom that leads to diagnosis of arthritis.
- Traumatic articular cartilage injuries are seen with automobile accidents and in combat.
- During the progression of arthritis, cartilage and adjacent joint tissues, including subchondral bone, are altered at the tissue and cellular levels.
- Loss of proteoglycans in articular cartilage from osteoarthritis results in reduced biomechanical properties and increased wear. Continued wear of the cartilage leads to destruction of the articular cartilage surface with attendant pain.

- Although articular cartilage injuries may not result in gross morphological changes, chondrocyte death and catabolism have been reported to occur even for these clinically silent injuries.
- Chondral lesions do not heal. Osteochondral lesions are filled with mechanically inferior fibrocartilage that is susceptible to breakdown.
- Treatment options for early stage osteoarthritis are usually palliative and consist of alleviation of symptomatic pain.
- Advanced osteoarthritis may be treated by partial or total joint replacement.
- Current approaches to treat osteochondral lesions include microfracture, ACI, and osteochondral grafts.
- Microfracture is a marrow stimulation treatment for chondral lesions, usually less than 2 cm^2, which results in filling of the defect with a blood clot and eventually a fibrocartilage repair tissue.
- Autologous implants employ an osteochondral graft for filling osteochondral lesions in areas of loaded cartilage. This graft is sourced from healthy areas of the patient's own cartilage.
- ACI fills osteochondral lesions using the patient's own chondrocytes, which have been expanded *in vitro*.
- In addition to in the elderly, cartilage injuries in children and adolescents are increasingly observed, with roughly 20% of knee injuries in adolescents requiring surgery.

We would like to thank Nicholas Paschos, MD, PhD, for his careful review and comments during the preparation of this chapter.

APPENDIX

Types of arthritis

Achilles tendinitis	Metastatic carcinomatous arthritis
Achondroplasia	Mixed connective tissue disease (MCTD)
Acromegalic arthropathy	Mixed cryoglobulinemia
Adhesive capsulitis	Mucopolysaccharidosis
Adult onset Still's disease	Multicentric reticulohistiocytosis
Ankylosing spondylitis	Multiple epiphyseal dysplasia
Anserine bursitis	Mycoplasmal arthritis
Arthritis of ulcerative colitis	Myofascial pain syndrome
Avascular necrosis	Neonatal lupus
Behcet's syndrome	Neuropathic arthropathy
Bicipital tendinitis	Nodular panniculitis
Blount's disease	Ochronosis
Brucellar spondylitis	Olecranon bursitis
Bursitis	Osgood-Schlatter disease
Calcaneal bursitis	Osteoarthritis
Calcium pyrophosphate dihydrate (CPPD)	Osteochondromatosis
Caplan's syndrome	Osteogenesis imperfecta
Carpal tunnel syndrome	Osteomalacia
Chondrocalcinosis	Osteomyelitis
Chondromalacia patellae	Osteonecrosis
Chronic recurrent multifocal osteomyelitis	Osteoporosis
Chronic synovitis	Overlap syndrome
Churg-Strauss syndrome	Pachydermoperiostosis
Churg-Strauss syndrome	Paget's disease of bone
Cogan's syndrome	Palindromic rheumatism
Corticosteroid-induced osteoporosis	Patellofemoral pain syndrome

(Continued)

Types of arthritis (Continued)

Costosternal syndrome	Pellegrini-Stieda syndrome
CREST syndrome	Pigmented villonodular synovitis
Cryoglobulinemia	Piriformis syndrome
Crystal deposition disease	Plantar fasciitis
Degenerative joint disease	Polyarteritis nodos
Dermatomyositis	Polymyalgia rheumatica
Diabetic finger sclerosis	Polymyositis
Diffuse idiopathic skeletal hyperostosis (DISH)	Popliteal cysts
Discitis	Posterior tibial tendinitis
Discoid lupus erythematosus	Pott's disease
Drug-induced lupus	Prepatellar bursitis
Duchenne's muscular dystrophy	Prosthetic joint infection
Dupuytren's contracture	Pseudoxanthoma elasticum
Ehlers-Danlos syndrome	Psoriatic arthritis
Enteropathic arthritis	Raynaud's phenomenon
Epicondylitis	Reactive arthritis/Reiter's syndrome
Erosive inflammatory osteoarthritis	Reflex sympathetic dystrophy syndrome
Exercise-induced compartment syndrome	Relapsing polychondritis
Fabry's disease	Retrocalcaneal bursitis
Familial Mediterranean fever	Rheumatic fever
Farber's lipogranulomatosis	Rheumatoid arthritis
Felty's syndrome	Rheumatoid vasculitis
Fibromyalgia	Rotator cuff tendinitis
Fifth's disease	Sacroiliitis
Flat feet	Salmonella osteomyelitis
Foreign body synovitis	Sarcoidosis
Freiberg's disease	Saturnine gout

(Continued)

Types of arthritis (Continued)

Fungal arthritis	Scheuermann's osteochondritis
Gaucher's disease	Scleroderma
Giant cell arteritis	Septic arthritis
Gonococcal arthritis	Seronegative arthritis
Goodpasture's syndrome	Shigella arthritis
Gout	Shoulder-hand syndrome
Granulomatous arteritis	Sickle cell arthropathy
Hemarthrosis	Sjogren's syndrome
Hemochromatosis	Slipped capital femoral epiphysis
Henoch-Schonlein purpura	Spinal stenosis
Hepatitis B surface antigen disease	Spondylolysis
Hip dysplasia	Staphylococcus arthritis
Hurler syndrome	Stickler syndrome
Hypermobility syndrome	Subacute cutaneous lupus
Hypersensitivity vasculitis	Sweet's syndrome
Hypertrophic osteoarthropathy	Sydenham's chorea
Immune complex disease	Syphilitic arthritis
Impingement syndrome	Systemic lupus erythematosus (SLE)
Jaccoud's arthropathy	Takayasu's arteritis
Juvenile ankylosing spondylitis	Tarsal tunnel syndrome
Juvenile dermatomyositis	Tennis elbow
Juvenile rheumatoid arthritis	Tietse's syndrome
Kawasaki disease	Transient osteoporosis
Kienbock's disease	Traumatic arthritis
Legg-Calve-Perthes disease	Trochanteric bursitis
Lesch-Nyhan syndrome	Tuberculosis arthritis
Linear scleroderma	Undifferentiated connective tissue syndrome (UCTS)
Lipoid dermatoarthritis	Urticarial vasculitis

(Continued)

Types of arthritis (Continued)

Lofgren's syndrome	Viral arthritis
Lyme disease	Wegener's granulomatosis
Malignant synovioma	Whipple's disease
Marfan's syndrome	Wilson's disease
Medial plica syndrome	Yersinial arthritis

Source: Modified from the Arthritis Foundation at Arthritis.org and based on Montgomery, M. M., and R. M. Poske, *Dis Mon* 14(6): 1-48, 1968.

References

Acebes, C., J. A. Roman-Blas et al. (2009). Correlation between arthroscopic and histopathological grading systems of articular cartilage lesions in knee osteoarthritis. *Osteoarthr Cartil* 17(2): 205-212.

Adirim, T. A., and T. L. Cheng. (2003). Overview of injuries in the young athlete. *Sports Med* 33(1): 75-81.

Ahmed, S. A., B. D. Hissong et al. (1999). Gender and risk of autoimmune diseases: Possible role of estrogenic compounds. *Environ Health Perspect* 107(Suppl 5): 681-686.

Akahoshi, T., Y. Murakami et al. (2007). Recent advances in crystal-induced acute inflammation. *Curr Opin Rheumatol* 19(2): 146-150.

Al-Arfaj, A. S. (2002). Radiographic osteoarthritis and obesity. *Saudi Med J* 23(8): 938-942.

Alfredson, H., and R. Lorentzon. (1999). Superior results with continuous passive motion compared to active motion after periosteal transplantation. A retrospective study of human patella cartilage defect treatment. *Knee Surg Sports Traumatol Arthrosc* 7(4): 232-238.

Aluisio, F. V., C. P. Christensen et al. (1998). *Orthopaedics*. Philadelphia: Lippincott Williams & Wilkins.

Anders, S., J. Schaumburger et al. (2008). Matrix-associated autologous chondrocyte transplantation (MACT). Minimally invasive technique in the knee (in German). *Oper Orthop Traumatol* 20(3): 208-219.

Anderson, D. D., T. D. Brown et al. (1990). A dynamic finite element analysis of impulsive loading of the extension-splinted rabbit knee. *J Biomech Eng 1* 12 (2): 119-128.

Andrews, S., N. Shrive et al. (2011). The shocking truth about meniscus. *J Biomech* 44(16): 2737-2740.

Andriacchi, T. P. (1994). Dynamics of knee malalignment. *Orthop Clin North Am* 25(3): 395-403.

Andriacchi, T. P., P. L. Briant et al. (2006). Rotational changes at the knee after ACL injury cause cartilage thinning. *Clin Orthop Relat Res* 442: 39-44.

Andriacchi, T. P., and C. O. Dyrby. (2005). Interactions between kinematics and loading during walking for the normal and ACL deficient knee. *J Biomech* 38(2): 293-298.

Andriacchi, T. P., S. Koo et al. (2009). Gait mechanics influence healthy cartilage morphology and osteoarthritis of the knee. *J Bone Joint Surg Am* 91(Suppl 1): 95-101.

Andriacchi, T. P., A. Mundermann et al. (2004). A framework for the in vivo pathomechanics of osteoarthritis at the knee. *Ann Biomed Eng* 32(3): 447-457.

Appleyard, R. C., P. Ghosh et al. (1999). Biomechanical, histological and immuno-histological studies of patellar cartilage in an ovine model of osteoarthritis induced by lateral meniscectomy. *Osteoarthr Cartil* 7(3): 281-294.

Armstrong, C. G., W. M. Lai et al. (1984). An analysis of the unconfined compression of articular cartilage. *J Biomech Eng* 106(2): 165-173.

Arslan-Kirchner, M., J. T. Epplen et al. (2011). Clinical utility gene card for: Loeys-Dietz syndrome (TGFBR1/2) and related phenotypes. *Eur J Hum Genet* 19(10).

Arzi, B., E. R. Wisner et al. (2011). A proposed model of naturally occurring osteoarthritis in the domestic rabbit. *Lab Anim (NY)* 41(1): 20-25.

Aspden, R. M., J. E. Jeffrey et al. (2002). Impact loading of articular cartilage. *Osteoarthr Cartil* 10(7): 588-589; author reply 590.

Ateshian, G. A., W. M. Lai et al. (1994). An asymptotic solution for the contact of two biphasic cartilage layers. *J Biomech* 27(11): 1347-1360.

Athanasiou, K. A., M. P. Rosenwasser et al. (1998). Biomechanical modeling of repair articular cartilage: Effects of passive motion on osteochondral defects in monkey knee joints. *Tissue Eng* 4(2): 185-195.

Atkinson, T. S., R. C. Haut et al. (1998). An investigation of biphasic failure criteria for impact-induced fissuring of articular cartilage. *J Biomech Eng* 120(4): 536-537.

Attur, M. G., G. D. Palmer et al. (2009). F-spondin, a neuroregulatory protein, is up-regulated in osteoarthritis and regulates cartilage metabolism via TGF-beta activation. *FASEB J* 23(1): 79-89.

Baars, D. C., S. A. Rundell et al. (2006). Treatment with the non-ionic surfactant poloxamer P188 reduces DNA fragmentation in cells from bovine chondral explants exposed to injurious unconfined compression. *Biomech Model Mechanobiol* 5(2-3): 133-139.

Bae, D. K., K. H. Yoon et al. (2006). Cartilage healing after microfracture in osteo-arthritic knees. *Arthroscopy* 22(4): 367-374.

Becher, C., and H. Thermann. (2005). Results of microfracture in the treatment of articular cartilage defects of the talus. *Foot Ankle Int* 26(8): 583-589.

Beck, P. R., A. L. Thomas et al. (2005). Trochlear contact pressures after anteromedialization of the tibial tubercle. *Am J Sports Med* 33(11): 1710-1715.

Beguin, J. A., J. F. Heron et al. (1982). Arthroscopy of the knee. Diagnostic value. 1005 cases (in French). *Nouv Presse Med* 11(49): 3619-3621.

Berler, R. (2009). Arms-control breakdown. *New York Times*, August 7, p. MM20.

Bi, X., G. Li et al. (2005). A novel method for determination of collagen orientation in cartilage by Fourier transform infrared imaging spectroscopy (FT-IRIS). *Osteoarthr Cartil* 13(12): 1050-1058.

Bijkerk, C., J. J. Houwing-Duistermaat et al. (1999). Heritabilities of radiologic osteoarthritis in peripheral joints and of disc degeneration of the spine. *Arthritis Rheum* 42(8): 1729-1735.

Birmingham, T. B., M. A. Hunt et al. (2007). Test-retest reliability of the peak knee adduction moment during walking in patients with medial compartment knee osteoarthritis. *Arthritis Rheum* 57(6): 1012-1017.

Bleasel, J. F., A. R. Poole et al. (1999). Changes in serum cartilage marker levels indicate altered cartilage metabolism in families with the osteoarthritis-related type II collagen gene COL2A1 mutation. *Arthritis Rheum* 42(1): 39-45.

Blumberg, T. J., R. M. Natoli et al. (2008). Effects of doxycycline on articular cartilage GAG release and mechanical properties following impact. *Biotechnol Bioeng* 100(3): 506-515.

Bonassar, L. J., A. J. Grodzinsky et al. (2001). The effect of dynamic compression on the response of articular cartilage to insulin-like growth factor-I. *J Orthop Res* 19(1): 11-17.

Borrelli, J., Jr., and W. M. Ricci. (2004). Acute effects of cartilage impact. *Clin Orthop* 423: 33-39.

Brandt, K. D. (2002). Animal models of osteoarthritis. *Biorheology* 39(1-2): 221-235.

Brandt, K. D., D. K. Heilman et al. (1999). Quadriceps strength in women with radiographically progressive osteoarthritis of the knee and those with stable radiographic changes. *J Rheumatol* 26(11): 2431-2437.

Brandt, K. D., S. L. Myers et al. (1991). Osteoarthritic changes in canine articular cartilage, subchondral bone, and synovium fifty-four months after transection of the anterior cruciate ligament. *Arthritis Rheum* 34(12): 1560-1570.

Breinan, H. A., S. D. Martin et al. (2000). Healing of canine articular cartilage defects treated with microfracture, a type-II collagen matrix, or cultured autologous chondrocytes. *J Orthop Res* 18(5): 781-789.

Brittberg, M., A. Lindahl et al. (1994). Treatment of deep cartilage defects in the knee with autologous chondrocyte transplantation. *N Engl J Med* 331(14): 889-895.

Brogley, M. A., M. Cruz et al. (1999). Basic calcium phosphate crystal induction of collagenase 1 and stromelysin expression is dependent on a p42/44 mitogen-activated protein kinase signal transduction pathway. *J Cell Physiol* 180(2): 215-224.

Brosseau, L., K. A. Yonge et al. (2003). Thermotherapy for treatment of osteoarthritis. *Cochrane Database Syst Rev* (4): CD004522.

Brosseau, L. M., D. L. Parker et al. (2002). Designing intervention effectiveness studies for occupational health and safety: The Minnesota Wood Dust Study. *Am J Ind Med* 41(1): 54-61.

Browning, R. C., and R. Kram. (2007). Effects of obesity on the biomechanics of walking at different speeds. *Med Sci Sports Exerc* 39(9): 1632-1641.

Buckwalter, J. A. (1995). Osteoarthritis and articular cartilage use, disuse, and abuse: Experimental studies. *J Rheumatol Suppl* 43: 13-15.

Buckwalter, J. A. (2002). Articular cartilage injuries. *Clin Orthop Relat Res* 402: 21-37.

Buckwalter, J. A., and H. J. Mankin. (1998). Articular cartilage: Degeneration and osteoarthrosis, repair, regeneration, and transplantation. *Instr Course Lect* 47: 487-504.

Buckwalter, J. A., V. C. Mow et al. (1994). Restoration of injured or degenerated articular cartilage. *J Am Acad Orthop Surg* 2(4): 192-201.

Burks, R. T., P. E. Greis et al. (2006). The use of a single osteochondral autograft plug in the treatment of a large osteochondral lesion in the femoral condyle: An experimental study in sheep. *Am J Sports Med* 34(2): 247-255.

Burr, D. B. (2004). The importance of subchondral bone in the progression of osteoarthritis. *J Rheumatol Suppl* 70: 77-80.

Butler, R. J., K. I. Minick et al. (2009). Gait mechanics after ACL reconstruction: Implications for the early onset of knee osteoarthritis. *Br J Sports Med* 43(5): 366-370.

Cameron, M. L., K. K. Briggs et al. (2003). Reproducibility and reliability of the outerbridge classification for grading chondral lesions of the knee arthroscopically. *Am J Sports Med* 31(1): 83-86.

Caplan, A. I., M. Elyaderani et al. (1997). Principles of cartilage repair and regeneration. *Clin Orthop Relat Res* 342: 254-269.

Carman, W. J., M. Sowers et al. (1994). Obesity as a risk factor for osteoarthritis of the hand and wrist: A prospective study. *Am J Epidemiol* 139(2): 119-129.

Chapman, K., Z. Mustafa et al. (1999). Osteoarthritis-susceptibility locus on chromosome 11q, detected by linkage. *Am J Hum Genet* 65(1): 167-174.

Centers for Disease Control and Prevention (CDC). (2007). National and state medical expenditures and lost earnings attributable to arthritis and other rheumatic conditions—United States, 2003. *Morb Mortal Wkly Rep* 56(1): 4-7.

Cheung, H. S., W. H. Cottrell et al. (1978). In vitro collagen biosynthesis in healing and normal rabbit articular cartilage. *J Bone Joint Surg Am* 60(8): 1076-1081.

Cheung, H. S., K. L. Lynch et al. (1980). In vitro synthesis of tissue-specific type II collagen by healing cartilage. I. Short-term repair of cartilage by mature rabbits. *Arthritis Rheum* 23(2): 211-219.

Cheung, H. S., J. D. Sallis et al. (1996). Specific inhibition of basic calcium phosphate and calcium pyrophosphate crystal-induction of metalloproteinase synthesis by phosphocitrate. *Biochim Biophys Acta* 1315(2): 105-111.

Chiu, F. Y., and C. M. Chen. (2007). Surgical debridement and parenteral antibiotics in infected revision total knee arthroplasty. *Clin Orthop Relat Res* 461: 130-135.

Choi, H. K., and G. Curhan. (2007). Alcohol and gout. *Am J Med* 120(10): e5; author reply e7.

Chrisman, O. D., I. M. Ladenbauer-Bellis et al. (1981). 1981 Nicolas Andry Award. The relationship of mechanical trauma and the early biochemical reactions of osteoarthritic cartilage. *Clin Orthop* 161(161): 275-284.

Christensen, R., A. Astrup et al. (2005). Weight loss: The treatment of choice for knee osteoarthritis? A randomized trial. *Osteoarthr Cartil* 13(1): 20-27.

Christensen, R., E. M. Bartels et al. (2007). Effect of weight reduction in obese patients diagnosed with knee osteoarthritis: A systematic review and meta-analysis. *Ann Rheum Dis* 66(4): 433-439.

Cuff, D. J., N. A. Virani et al. (2008). The treatment of deep shoulder infection and glenohumeral instability with debridement, reverse shoulder arthroplasty and postoperative antibiotics. *J Bone Joint Surg Br* 90(3): 336-342.

Custers, R. J., L. B. Creemers et al. (2007). Reliability, reproducibility and variability of the traditional Histologic/Histochemical Grading System vs the new OARSI Osteoarthritis Cartilage Histopathology Assessment System. *Osteoarthr Cartil* 15(11): 1241-1248.

Davis, M. A., W. H. Ettinger et al. (1990). Obesity and osteoarthritis of the knee: Evidence from the National Health and Nutrition Examination Survey (NHANES I). *Semin Arthritis Rheum* 20(3 Suppl 1): 34-41.

Dekel, S., and S. L. Weissman. (1978). Joint changes after overuse and peak overloading of rabbit knees in vivo. *Acta Orthop Scand* 49(6): 519-528.

Demissie, S., L. A. Cupples et al. (2002). Genome scan for quantity of hand osteoarthritis: The Framingham Study. *Arthritis Rheum* 46(4): 946-952.

DePalma, A. F., C. D. McKeever et al. (1966). Process of repair of articular cartilage demonstrated by histology and autoradiography with tritiated thymidine. *Clin Orthop Relat Res* 48: 229-242.

Derfus, B. A., J. B. Kurian et al. (2002). The high prevalence of pathologic calcium crystals in pre-operative knees. *J Rheumatol* 29(3): 570-574.

D'Lima, D. D., S. Hashimoto et al. (2001). Human chondrocyte apoptosis in response to mechanical injury. *Osteoarthr Cartil* 9(8): 712-719.

Donohue, J. M., D. Buss et al. (1983). The effects of indirect blunt trauma on adult canine articular cartilage. *J Bone Joint Surg Am* 65(7): 948-957.

Dorotka, R., U. Windberger et al. (2005). Repair of articular cartilage defects treated by microfracture and a three-dimensional collagen matrix. *Biomaterials* 26(17): 3617-3629.

Dozin, B., M. Malpeli et al. (2005). Comparative evaluation of autologous chondrocyte implantation and mosaicplasty: A multicentered randomized clinical trial. *Clin J Sport Med* 15(4): 220-226.

Dunbar, W. L., Jr., K. Un et al. (2001). An evaluation of three-dimensional diarthrodial joint contact using penetration data and the finite element method. *J Biomech Eng* 123(4): 333-340.

Egan, M. S., D. L. Goldenberg et al. (1982). The association of amyloid deposits and osteoarthritis. *Arthritis Rheum* 25(2): 204-208.

Elisseeff, J., K. Anseth et al. (1999). Transdermal photopolymerization for minimally invasive implantation. *Proc Natl Acad Sci USA* 96(6): 3104-3107.

Elisseeff, J., W. McIntosh et al. (2000). Photoencapsulation of chondrocytes in poly(ethylene oxide)-based semi-interpenetrating networks. *J Biomed Mater Res* 51(2): 164-171.

Erggelet, C., M. Endres et al. (2009). Formation of cartilage repair tissue in articular cartilage defects pretreated with microfracture and covered with cell-free polymer-based implants. *J Orthop Res* 27(10): 1353-1360.

Erggelet, C., J. Holz et al. (2008). Matrix-augmented autologous chondrocyte implantation in the knee—Arthroscopic technique [in German]. *Oper Orthop Traumatol* 20(3): 199-207.

Erggelet, C., P. C. Kreuz et al. (2010). Autologous chondrocyte implantation versus ACI using 3D-bioresorbable graft for the treatment of large full-thickness cartilage lesions of the knee. *Arch Orthop Trauma Surg* 130(8): 957-964.

Erickson, G. R., J. M. Gimble et al. (2002). Chondrogenic potential of adipose tissue-derived stromal cells in vitro and in vivo. *Biochem Biophys Res Commun* 290(2): 763-769.

Eskelinen, A. P., T. Visuri et al. (2004). Primary cartilage lesions of the knee joint in young male adults. Overweight as a predisposing factor. An arthroscopic study. *Scand J Surg* 93(3): 229-233.

Ewers, B. J., V. M. Jayaraman et al. (2002a). Rate of blunt impact loading affects changes in retropatellar cartilage and underlying bone in the rabbit patella. *J Biomech* 35(6): 747-755.

Ewers, B. J., B. T. Weaver et al. (2002b). Chronic changes in rabbit retro-patellar cartilage and subchondral bone after blunt impact loading of the patellofemoral joint. *J Orthop Res* 20(3): 545-550.

Faber, J., A. Winterpacht et al. (2000). Clinical variability of Stickler syndrome with a COL2A1 haploinsufficiency mutation: Implications for genetic counselling. *J Med Genet* 37(4): 318-320.

Falez, F., and F. Sciarretta. (2005). Treatment of osteochondral symptomatic defects of the knee with SaluCartilage. *J Bone Joint Surg Br* 87(Suppl II): 202.

Fam, A. G. (2005). Gout: Excess calories, purines, and alcohol intake and beyond. Response to a urate-lowering diet. *J Rheumatol* 32(5): 773-777.

Farquhar, T., Y. Xia et al. (1996). Swelling and fibronectin accumulation in articular cartilage explants after cyclical impact. *J Orthop Res* 14(3): 417-423.

Farr, J. (2007). Autologous chondrocyte implantation improves patellofemoral cartilage treatment outcomes. *Clin Orthop Relat Res* 463: 187-194.

Federico, D. J., and B. Reider. (1997). Results of isolated patellar debridement for patellofemoral pain in patients with normal patellar alignment. *Am J Sports Med* 25(5): 663-669.

Felson, D. T., J. J. Anderson et al. (1988). Obesity and knee osteoarthritis. The Framingham Study. *Ann Intern Med* 109(1): 18-24.

Felson, D. T., D. R. Gale et al. (2005). Osteophytes and progression of knee osteoarthritis. *Rheumatology (Oxford)* 44(1): 100-104.

Felson, D. T., and T. Neogi. (2004). Osteoarthritis: Is it a disease of cartilage or of bone? *Arthritis Rheum* 50(2): 341-344.

Fernandez Dapica, M. P., and J. J. Gomez-Reino. (1986). Familial chondrocalcinosis in the Spanish population. *J Rheumatol* 13(3): 631-633.

Ferruzzi, A., R. Buda et al. (2008). Autologous chondrocyte implantation in the knee joint: Open compared with arthroscopic technique. Comparison at a minimum follow-up of five years. *J Bone Joint Surg Am* 90(Suppl 4): 90-101.

Firestein, G. S. (2003). Evolving concepts of rheumatoid arthritis. *Nature* 423(6937): 356-361.

Foroughi, N., R. Smith et al. (2009). The association of external knee adduction moment with biomechanical variables in osteoarthritis: A systematic review. *Knee* 16(5): 303-309.

Foroughi, N., R. M. Smith et al. (2010). Dynamic alignment and its association with knee adduction moment in medial knee osteoarthritis. *Knee* 17(3): 210-216.

Forster, T., K. Chapman et al. (2004). Finer linkage mapping of primary osteoarthritis susceptibility loci on chromosomes 4 and 16 in families with affected women. *Arthritis Rheum* 50(1): 98-102.

Francomano, C. A., R. M. Liberfarb et al. (1987). The Stickler syndrome: Evidence for close linkage to the structural gene for type II collagen. *Genomics* 1(4): 293-296.

Frostick, S. P., M. Mohammad et al. (1999). Sport injuries of the elbow. *Br J Sports Med* 33(5): 301-311.

Fulkerson, J. P., G. J. Becker et al. (1990). Anteromedial tibial tubercle transfer without bone graft. *Am J Sports Med* 18(5): 490-496; discussion 496-497.

Fuller, J. A., and F. N. Ghadially. (1972). Ultrastructural observations on surgically produced partial-thickness defects in articular cartilage. *Clin Orthop Relat Res* 86: 193-205.

Furukawa, T., D. R. Eyre et al. (1980). Biochemical studies on repair cartilage resurfacing experimental defects in the rabbit knee. *J Bone Joint Surg Am* 62(1): 79-89.

Gabriel, S. E., C. S. Crowson et al. (1997). Direct medical costs unique to people with arthritis. *J Rheumatol* 24(4): 719-725.

Gabriel, S. E., and K. Michaud. (2009). Epidemiological studies in incidence, prevalence, mortality, and comorbidity of the rheumatic diseases. *Arthritis Res Ther* 11(3): 229.

Georgoulis, A. D., A. Papadonikolakis et al. (2003). Three-dimensional tibiofemoral kinematics of the anterior cruciate ligament-deficient and reconstructed knee during walking. *Am J Sports Med* 31(1): 75-79.

Ghadially, J. A., R. Ghadially et al. (1977). Long-term results of deep defects in articular cartilage. A scanning electron microscope study. *Virchows Arch B Cell Pathol* 25(2): 125-136.

Giannoni, P., A. Pagano et al. (2005). Autologous chondrocyte implantation (ACI) for aged patients: Development of the proper cell expansion conditions for possible therapeutic applications. *Osteoarthr Cartil* 13(7): 589-600.

Goh, J. C., K. Bose et al. (1993). Gait analysis study on patients with varus osteoarthrosis of the knee. *Clin Orthop Relat Res* 294: 223-231.

Gomez, E., J. C. DeLee et al. (1996). Incidence of injury in Texas girls' high school basketball. *Am J Sports Med* 24(5): 684-687.

Gould, N., and A. B. Flick. (1985). Post-fracture, late debridement resection arthroplasty of the ankle. *Foot Ankle* 6(2): 70-82.

Griffin, T. M., J. L. Huebner et al. (2009). Extreme obesity due to impaired leptin signaling in mice does not cause knee osteoarthritis. *Arthritis Rheum* 60(10): 2935-2944.

Gross, A. E., N. H. McKee et al. (1983). Reconstruction of skeletal deficits at the knee. A comprehensive osteochondral transplant program. *Clin Orthop Relat Res* 174: 96-106.

Gross, A. E., E. A. Silverstein et al. (1975). The allotransplantation of partial joints in the treatment of osteoarthritis of the knee. *Clin Orthop Relat Res* 108: 7-14.

Guermazi, A., J. Niu et al. (2012). Prevalence of abnormalities in knees detected by MRI in adults without knee osteoarthritis: Population based observational study (Framingham Osteoarthritis Study). *BMJ* 345: e5339.

Guilak, F., B. Fermor et al. (2004). The role of biomechanics and inflammation in cartilage injury and repair. *Clin Orthop Relat Res* 423: 17-26.

Guilak, F., B. C. Meyer et al. (1994). The effects of matrix compression on proteoglycan metabolism in articular cartilage explants. *Osteoarthr Cartil* 2(2): 91-101.

Hadler, N. M. (1985). Osteoarthritis as a public health problem. *Clin Rheum Dis* 11(2): 175-185.

Halverson, P. B. (1996). Calcium crystal-associated diseases. *Curr Opin Rheumatol* 8(3): 259-261.

Halverson, P. B., and B. A. Derfus. (2001). Calcium crystal-induced inflammation. *Curr Opin Rheumatol* 13(3): 221-224.

Hambly, K., V. Bobic et al. (2006). Autologous chondrocyte implantation postoperative care and rehabilitation: Science and practice. *Am J Sports Med* 34(6): 1020-1038.

Hamerman, D. (1988). Osteoarthritis. *Orthop Rev* 17(4): 353-360.

Hangody, L., and P. Fules. (2003). Autologous osteochondral mosaicplasty for the treatment of full-thickness defects of weight-bearing joints: Ten years of experimental and clinical experience. *J Bone Joint Surg Am* 85-A(Suppl 2): 25-32.

Hangody, L., G. Kish et al. (1997). Arthroscopic autogenous osteochondral mosaicplasty for the treatment of femoral condylar articular defects. A preliminary report. *Knee Surg Sports Traumatol Arthrosc* 5(4): 262-267.

Hart, D. J., D. V. Doyle et al. (1999). Incidence and risk factors for radiographic knee osteoarthritis in middle-aged women: The Chingford Study. *Arthritis Rheum* 42(1): 17-24.

Haut, R. C., T. M. Ide et al. (1995). Mechanical responses of the rabbit patello-femoral joint to blunt impact. *J Biomech Eng* 117(4): 402-408.

Healy, Z. R., N. H. Lee et al. (2005). Divergent responses of chondrocytes and endothelial cells to shear stress: Cross-talk among COX-2, the phase II response, and apoptosis. *Proc Natl Acad Sci USA* 102(39): 14010-14015.

Hennigan, S., and R. Terkeltaub. (2007). Last call for alcohol in gout? *Curr Rheumatol Rep* 9(3): 229-230.

Henrotin, Y., A. Mobasheri et al. (2012). Is there any scientific evidence for the use of glucosamine in the management of human osteoarthritis? *Arthritis Res Ther* 14(1): 201.

Hewett, T. E., G. D. Myer et al. (2005). Biomechanical measures of neuromuscular control and valgus loading of the knee predict anterior cruciate ligament injury risk in female athletes: A prospective study. *Am J Sports Med* 33(4): 492-501.

Hickey, G. J., P. A. Fricker et al. (1997). Injuries of young elite female basketball players over a six-year period. *Clin J Sport Med* 7(4): 252-256.

Hinman, R. S., and K. L. Bennell. (2009). Advances in insoles and shoes for knee osteoarthritis. *Curr Opin Rheumatol* 21(2): 164-170.

Hjertquist, S. O., and R. Lemperg. (1971). Histological, autoradiographic and microchemical studies of spontaneously healing osteochondral articular defects in adult rabbits. *Calcif Tissue Res* 8(1): 54-72.

Hoemann, C. D., M. Hurtig et al. (2005). Chitosan-glycerol phosphate/blood implants improve hyaline cartilage repair in ovine microfracture defects. *J Bone Joint Surg Am* 87(12): 2671-2686.

Holderbaum, D., T. M. Haqqi et al. (1999). Genetics and osteoarthritis: Exposing the iceberg. *Arthritis Rheum* 42(3): 397-405.

Horas, U., D. Pelinkovic et al. (2003). Autologous chondrocyte implantation and osteochondral cylinder transplantation in cartilage repair of the knee joint. A prospective, comparative trial. *J Bone Joint Surg Am* 85-A(2): 185-192.

Hudelmaier, M., C. Glaser et al. (2006). Effects of joint unloading and reloading on human cartilage morphology and function, muscle cross-sectional areas, and bone density—A quantitative case report. *J Musculoskelet Neuronal Interact* 6(3): 284-290.

Hunter, D. J., S. Demissie et al. (2004). A genome scan for joint-specific hand osteoarthritis susceptibility: The Framingham Study. *Arthritis Rheum* 50(8): 2489-2496.

Hunter, D. J., Y. Zhang et al. (2005). Structural factors associated with malalignment in knee osteoarthritis: The Boston osteoarthritis knee study. *J Rheumatol* 32(11): 2192-2199.

Hunter, W. (1743). Of the structure and diseases of articulating cartilages. *Philos Trans R Soc* 43: 514-521.

Hurley, M. V., D. W. Jones et al. (1994). Arthrogenic quadriceps inhibition and rehabilitation of patients with extensive traumatic knee injuries. *Clin Sci (Lond)* 86(3): 305-310.

Hurwitz, D. E., A. B. Ryals et al. (2002). The knee adduction moment during gait in subjects with knee osteoarthritis is more closely correlated with static alignment than radiographic disease severity, toe out angle and pain. *J Orthop Res* 20(1): 101-107.

Ingvarsson, T., S. E. Stefansson et al. (2000). The inheritance of hip osteoarthritis in Iceland. *Arthritis Rheum* 43(12): 2785-2792.

Jackson, D. W., T. M. Simon et al. (2001). Symptomatic articular cartilage degeneration: The impact in the new millennium. *Clin Orthop* 391(Suppl): S14-S25.

Jackson, R. W., J. E. Gilbert et al. (1997). Arthroscopic debridement versus arthroplasty in the osteoarthritic knee. *J Arthroplasty* 12(4): 465-469; discussion 469-470.

Javaid, M. K., J. A. Lynch et al. (2010). Pre-radiographic MRI findings are associated with onset of knee symptoms: The MOST study. *Osteoarthr Cartil* 18(3): 323-328.

Jeffrey, J. E., D. W. Gregory et al. (1995). Matrix damage and chondrocyte viability following a single impact load on articular cartilage. *Arch Biochem Biophys* 322(1): 87-96.

Jeffrey, J. E., L. A. Thomson et al. (1997). Matrix loss and synthesis following a single impact load on articular cartilage in vitro. *Biochim Biophys Acta* 1334(2-3): 223-232.

Jenkinson, C. M., M. Doherty et al. (2009). Effects of dietary intervention and quadriceps strengthening exercises on pain and function in overweight people with knee pain: Randomised controlled trial. *BMJ* 339: b3170.

Johnson, L. L. (1986). Arthroscopic abrasion arthroplasty historical and pathologic perspective: Present status. *Arthroscopy* 2(1): 54-69.

Johnson, R. G., and A. R. Poole. (1990). The early response of articular cartilage to ACL transection in a canine model. *Exp Pathol* 38(1): 37-52.

Jones, A. R., and C. R. Flannery. (2007). Bioregulation of lubricin expression by growth factors and cytokines. *Eur Cell Mater* 13: 40-45; discussion 45.

Jones, D., Q. Louw et al. (2000). Recreational and sporting injury to the adolescent knee and ankle: Prevalence and causes. *Aust J Physiother* 46(3): 179-188.

Jordan, K. M., N. K. Arden et al. (2003). EULAR Recommendations 2003: An evidence based approach to the management of knee osteoarthritis: Report of a Task Force of the Standing Committee for International Clinical Studies Including Therapeutic Trials (ESCISIT). *Ann Rheum Dis* 62(12): 1145-1155.

Justen, H. P., E. Grunewald et al. (2000). Differential gene expression in synovium of rheumatoid arthritis and osteoarthritis. *Mol Cell Biol Res Commun* 3(3): 165-172.

Kafka, V. (2002). Surface fissures in articular cartilage: New concepts, hypotheses and modeling. *Clin Biomech (Bristol, Avon)* 17(1): 73-80.

Kellgren, J. H. (1963). Arthritis in populations. *J Coll Gen Pract* 6(Suppl 3): 2-7.

Kellgren, J. H., J. S. Lawrence et al. (1963). Genetic factors in generalized osteo-arthrosis. *Ann Rheum Dis* 22: 237-255.

Kempson, G. E., H. Muir et al. (1973). The tensile properties of the cartilage of human femoral condyles related to the content of collagen and glycosaminoglycans. *Biochim Biophys Acta* 297(2): 456-472.

Kern, D., M. B. Zlatkin et al. (1988). Occupational and post-traumatic arthritis. *Radiol Clin North Am* 26(6): 1349-1358.

Kim, H. K., R. G. Kerr et al. (1995). Effects of continuous passive motion and immo-bilization on synovitis and cartilage degradation in antigen induced arthritis. *J Rheumatol* 22(9): 1714-1721.

Kisiday, J. D., J. H. Lee et al. (2009). Catabolic responses of chondrocyte-seeded pep-tide hydrogel to dynamic compression. *Ann Biomed Eng* 37(7): 1368-1375.

Kizawa, H., I. Kou et al. (2005). An aspartic acid repeat polymorphism in asporin inhibits chondrogenesis and increases susceptibility to osteoarthritis. *Nat Genet* 37(2): 138-144.

Kleemann, R. U., D. Krocker et al. (2005). Altered cartilage mechanics and histology in knee osteoarthritis: Relation to clinical assessment (ICRS Grade). *Osteoarthr Cartil* 13(11): 958-963.

Knowlton, R. G., E. J. Weaver et al. (1989). Genetic linkage analysis of hereditary arthro-ophthalmopathy (Stickler syndrome) and the type II procollagen gene. *Am J Hum Genet* 45(5): 681-688.

Kock, L. M., R. M. Schulz et al. (2009). RGD-dependent integrins are mechanotrans-ducers in dynamically compressed tissue-engineered cartilage constructs. *J Biomech* 42(13): 2177-2182.

Komistek, R. D., T. R. Kane et al. (2005). Knee mechanics: A review of past and pres-ent techniques to determine in vivo loads. *J Biomech* 38(2): 215-228.

Kon, E., A. Gobbi et al. (2009). Arthroscopic second-generation autologous chondrocyte implantation compared with microfracture for chondral lesions of the knee: Prospective nonrandomized study at 5 years. *Am J Sports Med* 37(1): 33-41.

Koo, S., and T. P. Andriacchi. (2007). A comparison of the influence of global functional loads vs. local contact anatomy on articular cartilage thickness at the knee. *J Biomech* 40(13): 2961-2966.

Kozin, F., and D. J. McCarty. (1976). Protein adsorption to monosodium urate, calcium pyrophosphate dihydrate, and silica crystals: Relationship to the pathogenesis of crystal-induced inflammation. *Arthritis Rheum* 19(Suppl 3): 433-438.

Kreuz, P. C., C. Erggelet et al. (2006). Is microfracture of chondral defects in the knee associated with different results in patients aged 40 years or younger? *Arthroscopy* 22(11): 1180-1186.

Kreuz, P. C., S. Muller et al. (2009). Treatment of focal degenerative cartilage defects with polymer-based autologous chondrocyte grafts: Four-year clinical results. *Arthritis Res Ther* 11(2): R33.

Kuo, A. C., J. J. Rodrigo et al. (2006). Microfracture and bone morphogenetic protein 7 (BMP-7) synergistically stimulate articular cartilage repair. *Osteoarthr Cartil* 14(11): 1126-1135.

Kuo, C. H., and L. M. Keer. (1993). Contact stress and fracture analysis of articular cartilage. *Bimoed Eng Appl Basis Comm* 5: 515-521.

Kurkijarvi, J. E., L. Mattila et al. (2007). Evaluation of cartilage repair in the distal femur after autologous chondrocyte transplantation using T2 relaxation time and dGEMRIC. *Osteoarthr Cartil* 15(4): 372-378.

Kurz, B., M. Jin et al. (2001). Biosynthetic response and mechanical properties of articular cartilage after injurious compression. *J Orthop Res* 19(6): 1140-1146.

Kusakabe, A. (1977). Subchondral cancellous bone in osteoarthrosis and rheumatoid arthritis of the femoral head. A quantitative histological study of trabecular remodelling. *Arch Orthop Unfallchir* 88(2): 185-197.

Landells, J. W. (1953). The bone cysts of osteoarthritis. *J Bone Joint Surg Br* 35-B(4): 643-649.

Landis, R. C., and D. O. Haskard. (2001). Pathogenesis of crystal-induced inflammation. *Curr Rheumatol Rep* 3(1): 36-41.

Lawrence, R. C., D. T. Felson et al. (2008). Estimates of the prevalence of arthritis and other rheumatic conditions in the United States. II. *Arthritis Rheum* 58(1): 26-35.

Lawrence, R. C., C. G. Helmick et al. (1998). Estimates of the prevalence of arthritis and selected musculoskeletal disorders in the United States. *Arthritis Rheum* 41(5): 778-799.

Lee, K. B., J. H. Hui et al. (2007). Injectable mesenchymal stem cell therapy for large cartilage defects—A porcine model. *Stem Cells* 25(11): 2964-2971.

Lee, M. S., T. Ikenoue et al. (2003). Protective effects of intermittent hydrostatic pressure on osteoarthritic chondrocytes activated by bacterial endotoxin in vitro. *J Orthop Res* 21(1): 117-122.

Lee, S. Y., T. Nakagawa et al. (2010). Mesenchymal progenitor cells derived from synovium and infrapatellar fat pad as a source for superficial zone cartilage tissue engineering: Analysis of superficial zone protein/lubricin expression. *Tissue Eng Part A* 16(1): 317-325.

Lee, Y. H., Y. H. Rho et al. (2006). Osteoarthritis susceptibility loci defined by genome scan meta-analysis. *Rheumatol Int* 26(11): 959-963.

Levy, A. S., J. Lohnes et al. (1996). Chondral delamination of the knee in soccer players. *Am J Sports Med* 24(5): 634-639.

Li, G., J. M. Moses et al. (2006). Anterior cruciate ligament deficiency alters the in vivo motion of the tibiofemoral cartilage contact points in both the anteroposterior and mediolateral directions. *J Bone Joint Surg Am* 88(8): 1826-1834.

Liberopoulos, E. N., G. A. Miltiadous et al. (2004). Alcohol intake, serum uric acid concentrations, and risk of gout. *Lancet* 364(9430): 246-247; author reply 247.

Livshits, G., B. S. Kato et al. (2007). Genomewide linkage scan of hand osteoarthritis in female twin pairs showing replication of quantitative trait loci on chromosomes 2 and 19. *Ann Rheum Dis* 66(5): 623-627.

Lohmander, L. S., A. Ostenberg et al. (2004). High prevalence of knee osteoarthritis, pain, and functional limitations in female soccer players twelve years after anterior cruciate ligament injury. *Arthritis Rheum* 50(10): 3145-3152.

Lohmander, L. S., T. Saxne et al. (1994). Release of cartilage oligomeric matrix protein (COMP) into joint fluid after knee injury and in osteoarthritis. *Ann Rheum Dis* 53(1): 8-13.

Loughlin, J. (2006). Osteoarthritis linkage scan: More loci for the geneticists to investigate. *Ann Rheum Dis* 65(10): 1265-1266.

Loughlin, J., Z. Mustafa et al. (1999). Stratification analysis of an osteoarthritis genome screen-suggestive linkage to chromosomes 4, 6, and 16. *Am J Hum Genet* 65(6): 1795-1798.

Louw, Q. A., J. Manilall et al. (2008). Epidemiology of knee injuries among adolescents: A systematic review. *Br J Sports Med* 42(1): 2-10.

Magnussen, R. A., W. R. Dunn et al. (2008). Treatment of focal articular cartilage defects in the knee: A systematic review. *Clin Orthop Relat Res* 466(4): 952-962.

Maiotti, M., C. Massoni et al. (2005). *The Use of Poli-Hydrogel Cylindrical Implants to Treat Deep Chondral Defects of the Knee*. Vancouver, BC: Arthroscopy Association of North America.

Makris, E. A., A. H. Gomoll et al. (2015). Repair and tissue engineering techniques for articular cartilage. *Nat Rev Rheumatol* 11(1): 21-34.

Mandel, N. S., and G. S. Mandel. (1976). Monosodium urate monohydrate, the gout culprit. *J Am Chem Soc* 98(8): 2319-2323.

Mandelbaum, B. R., J. E. Browne et al. (1998). Articular cartilage lesions of the knee. *Am J Sports Med* 26(6): 853-861.

Mankin, H. J. (1971). Biochemical and metabolic aspects of osteoarthritis. *Orthop Clin North Am* 2(1): 19-31.

Mankin, H. J., H. Dorfman et al. (1971). Biochemical and metabolic abnormalities in articular cartilage from osteo-arthritic human hips. II. Correlation of morphology with biochemical and metabolic data. *J Bone Joint Surg Am* 53(3): 523-537.

Mankin, H. J., V. C. Mow et al. (1994). Form and function of articular cartilage. In *Orthopaedic Basic Science*, ed. S. Simon. Rosemont, IL: American Academy of Orthopaedic Surgeons.

Marcacci, M., M. Berruto et al. (2005a). Articular cartilage engineering with Hyalograft C: 3-year clinical results. *Clin Orthop Relat Res* 435: 96-105.

Marcacci, M., E. Kon et al. (1999). Use of autologous grafts for reconstruction of osteochondral defects of the knee. *Orthopedics* 22(6): 595-600.

Marcacci, M., S. Zaffagnini et al. (2005b). Outcomes and results of 2nd generation autologous chondrocyte implantation. Presented at Annual Meeting of the American Orthopaedic Society for Sports Medicine, Keystone, CO.

Marcelino, J., J. D. Carpten et al. (1999). CACP, encoding a secreted proteoglycan, is mutated in camptodactyly-arthropathy-coxa vara-pericarditis syndrome. *Nat Genet* 23(3): 319-322.

Marcos, J. C., M. A. De Benyacar et al. (1981). Idiopathic familial chondrocalcinosis due to apatite crystal deposition. *Am J Med* 71(4): 557-564.

Masini, B. D., S. M. Waterman et al. (2009). Resource utilization and disability outcome assessment of combat casualties from Operation Iraqi Freedom and Operation Enduring Freedom. *J Orthop Trauma* 23(4): 261-266.

McCarthy, G. M. (1999). Crystal-induced inflammation and cartilage degradation. *Curr Rheumatol Rep* 1(2): 101-106.

McCarthy, G. M., H. S. Cheung et al. (1998). Basic calcium phosphate crystal-induced collagenase production: Role of intracellular crystal dissolution. *Osteoarthr Cartil* 6(3): 205-213.

McCarty, D. J. (1970). Crystal-induced inflammation of the joints. *Annu Rev Med* 21: 357-366.

McCulloch, D. R., C. Le Goff et al. (2009). Adamts5, the gene encoding a proteoglycan-degrading metalloprotease, is expressed by specific cell lineages during mouse embryonic development and in adult tissues. *Gene Expr Patterns* 9(5): 314-323.

McNickle, A. G., R. L'Heureux D et al. (2009). Outcomes of autologous chondrocyte implantation in a diverse patient population. *Am J Sports Med* 37(7): 1344-1350.

McNickle, A. G., M. T. Provencher et al. (2008). Overview of existing cartilage repair technology. *Sports Med Arthrosc* 16(4): 196-201.

McVey, E. D., R. M. Palmieri et al. (2005). Arthrogenic muscle inhibition in the leg muscles of subjects exhibiting functional ankle instability. *Foot Ankle Int* 26(12): 1055-1061.

Meachim, G., and S. R. Sheffield. (1969). Surface ultrastructure of mature adult human articular cartilage. *J Bone Joint Surg Br* 51(3): 529-539.

Meulenbelt, I., C. Bijkerk et al. (1999). Haplotype analysis of three polymorphisms of the COL2A1 gene and associations with generalised radiological osteoarthritis. *Ann Hum Genet* 63(Pt 5): 393-400.

Milentijevic, D., and P. A. Torzilli. (2005). Influence of stress rate on water loss, matrix deformation and chondrocyte viability in impacted articular cartilage. *J Biomech* 38(3): 493-502.

Mills, P. M., Y. Wang et al. (2008). Tibio-femoral cartilage defects 3-5 years following arthroscopic partial medial meniscectomy. *Osteoarthr Cartil* 16(12): 1526-1531.

Mitani, G., M. Sato et al. (2009). The properties of bioengineered chondrocyte sheets for cartilage regeneration. *BMC Biotechnol* 9(1): 17.

Mitchell, N., and N. Shepard. (1980). Healing of articular cartilage in intra-articular fractures in rabbits. *J Bone Joint Surg Am* 62(4): 628-634.

Mithoefer, K., T. McAdams et al. (2009). Clinical efficacy of the microfracture technique for articular cartilage repair in the knee: An evidence-based systematic analysis. *Am J Sports Med* 37(10): 2053-2063.

Mithoefer, K., R. J. Williams 3rd et al. (2006). Chondral resurfacing of articular cartilage defects in the knee with the microfracture technique. Surgical technique. *J Bone Joint Surg Am* 88(Suppl 1, Pt 2): 294-304.

Mithofer, K., L. Peterson et al. (2005). Articular cartilage repair in soccer players with autologous chondrocyte transplantation: Functional outcome and return to competition. *Am J Sports Med* 33(11): 1639-1646.

Miyazaki, T., M. Wada et al. (2002). Dynamic load at baseline can predict radiographic disease progression in medial compartment knee osteoarthritis. *Ann Rheum Dis* 61(7): 617-622.

Molloy, E. S., M. P. Morgan et al. (2008). Mechanism of basic calcium phosphate crystal-stimulated matrix metalloproteinase-13 expression by osteoarthritic synovial fibroblasts: Inhibition by prostaglandin E2. *Ann Rheum Dis* 67(12): 1773-1779.

Montgomery, M. M., and R. M. Poske. (1968). Less common types of arthritis. *Dis Mon* 14(6): 1-48.

Morel, V., and T. M. Quinn. (2004). Cartilage injury by ramp compression near the gel diffusion rate. *J Orthop Res* 22(1): 145-151.

Moseley, J. B., K. O'Malley et al. (2002). A controlled trial of arthroscopic surgery for osteoarthritis of the knee. *N Engl J Med* 347(2): 81-88.

Muehleman, C., J. Li et al. (2008). Association between crystals and cartilage degeneration in the ankle. *J Rheumatol* 35(6): 1108-1117.

Murphy, L., T. A. Schwartz et al. (2008). Lifetime risk of symptomatic knee osteoarthritis. *Arthritis Rheum* 59(9): 1207-1213.

Murray, R. C., R. M. DeBowes et al. (1998). The effects of intra-articular methylprednisolone and exercise on the mechanical properties of articular cartilage in the horse. *Osteoarthr Cartil* 6(2): 106-114.

Mustafa, Z., K. Chapman et al. (2000). Linkage analysis of candidate genes as susceptibility loci for osteoarthritis-suggestive linkage of COL9A1 to female hip osteoarthritis. *Rheumatology (Oxford)* 39(3): 299-306.

Myasoedova, E., C. S. Crowson et al. (2010). Is the incidence of rheumatoid arthritis rising? Results from Olmsted County, Minnesota, 1955-2007. *Arthritis Rheum* 62(6): 1576-1582.

Nagaosa, Y., P. Lanyon et al. (2002). Characterisation of size and direction of osteophyte in knee osteoarthritis: A radiographic study. *Ann Rheum Dis* 61(4): 319-324.

Namba, R. S., M. Meuli et al. (1998). Spontaneous repair of superficial defects in articular cartilage in a fetal lamb model. *J Bone Joint Surg Am* 80(1): 4-10.

National Institutes of Health (NIH). (2008). The NIH Glucosamine/Chondroitin Arthritis Intervention Trial (GAIT). *J Pain Palliat Care Pharmacother* 22(1): 39-43.

Natoli, R. M., and K. A. Athanasiou. (2008). P188 reduces cell death and IGF-I reduces GAG release following single-impact loading of articular cartilage. *J Biomech Eng* 130(4): 041012.

Natoli, R. M., C. C. Scott et al. (2008). Temporal effects of impact on articular cartilage cell death, gene expression, matrix biochemistry, and biomechanics. *Ann Biomed Eng* 36(5): 780-792.

Niemeyer, P., J. M. Pestka et al. (2008a). Characteristic complications after autologous chondrocyte implantation for cartilage defects of the knee joint. *Am J Sports Med* 36(11): 2091-2099.

Niemeyer, P., M. Steinwachs et al. (2008b). Autologous chondrocyte implantation for the treatment of retropatellar cartilage defects: Clinical results referred to defect localisation. *Arch Orthop Trauma Surg* 128(11): 1223-1231.

Noyes, F. R., and C. L. Stabler. (1989). A system for grading articular cartilage lesions at arthroscopy. *Am J Sports Med* 17(4): 505-513.

Nuesch, E., P. Dieppe et al. (2011). All cause and disease specific mortality in patients with knee or hip osteoarthritis: Population based cohort study. *BMJ* 342: d1165.

O'Connor, B. L., D. M. Visco et al. (1992). Neurogenic acceleration of osteoarthrosis. The effects of previous neurectomy of the articular nerves on the development of osteoarthrosis after transection of the anterior cruciate ligament in dogs. *J Bone Joint Surg Am* 74(3): 367-376.

Oettmeier, R., and K. Abendroth. (1989). Osteoarthritis and bone: Osteologic types of osteoarthritis of the hip. *Skeletal Radiol* 18(3): 165-174.

Oliver, J. E., and A. J. Silman. (2006). Risk factors for the development of rheumatoid arthritis. *Scand J Rheumatol* 35(3): 169-174.

Oliviero, F., P. Frallonardo et al. (2008). Evidence of silicon dioxide crystals in synovial fluid of patients with osteoarthritis. *J Rheumatol* 35(6): 1092-1095.

Olson, S. A., and F. Guilak (2006). From articular fracture to posttraumatic arthritis: A black box that needs to be opened. *J Orthop Trauma* 20(10): 661-662.

Outerbridge, R. E. (1961). The etiology of chondromalacia patellae. *J Bone Joint Surg Br* 43-B: 752-757.

Palmieri, R. M., C. D. Ingersoll et al. (2004). Arthrogenic muscle response to a simulated ankle joint effusion. *Br J Sports Med* 38(1): 26-30.

Palmieri-Smith, R. M., and A. C. Thomas. (2009). A neuromuscular mechanism of posttraumatic osteoarthritis associated with ACL injury. *Exerc Sport Sci Rev* 37(3): 147-153.

Pei, M., Z. Yan et al. (2010). Failure of xenoimplantation using porcine synovium-derived stem cell-based cartilage tissue constructs for the repair of rabbit osteochondral defects. *J Orthop Res* 28(8): 1064-1070.

Pena, E., B. Calvo et al. (2005). Finite element analysis of the effect of meniscal tears and meniscectomies on human knee biomechanics. *Clin Biomech (Bristol, Avon)* 20(5): 498-507.

Peng, B., S. Hou et al. (2000). Experimental study on mechanism of vertebral osteophyte formation. *Chin J Traumatol* 3(4): 202-205.

Pernis, A. B. (2007). Estrogen and CD4+ T cells. *Curr Opin Rheumatol* 19(5): 414-420.

Peterson, L., M. Brittberg et al. (2002). Autologous chondrocyte transplantation. Biomechanics and long-term durability. *Am J Sports Med* 30(1): 2-12.

Peterson, L., T. Minas et al. (2000). Two- to 9-year outcome after autologous chondrocyte transplantation of the knee. *Clin Orthop Relat Res* 374: 212-234.

Petersson, I. F., L. Sandqvist et al. (1997). Cartilage markers in synovial fluid in symptomatic knee osteoarthritis. *Ann Rheum Dis* 56(1): 64-67.

Phillips, D. M., and R. C. Haut. (2004). The use of a non-ionic surfactant (P188) to save chondrocytes from necrosis following impact loading of chondral explants. *J Orthop Res* 22(5): 1135-1142.

Polzer, K., G. Schett et al. (2007). The lonely death: Chondrocyte apoptosis in TNF-induced arthritis. *Autoimmunity* 40(4): 333-336.

Pond, M. J., and G. Nuki. (1973). Experimentally-induced osteoarthritis in the dog. *Ann Rheum Dis* 32(4): 387-388.

Poole, C. A. (1997). Articular cartilage chondrons: Form, function and failure. *J Anat* 191(Pt 1): 1-13.

Powell, J. W., and K. D. Barber-Foss. (1999). Injury patterns in selected high school sports: A review of the 1995-1997 seasons. *J Athl Train* 34(3): 277-284.

Pridie, K. H. (1959). A method of resurfacing osteoarthritic knee joints. *J Bone Joint Surg Br* 41: 618-619.

Pritzker, K. P. (2011). Osteoarthritis: Joint instability and OA: Do animal models provide insights? *Nat Rev Rheumatol* 7(8): 444-445.

Radin, E. L., M. G. Ehrlich et al. (1978). Effect of repetitive impulsive loading on the knee joints of rabbits. *Clin Orthop* 131(131): 288-293.

Ragan, P. M., V. I. Chin et al. (2000). Chondrocyte extracellular matrix synthesis and turnover are influenced by static compression in a new alginate disk culture system. *Arch Biochem Biophys* 383(2): 256-264.

Recklies, A. D., L. Baillargeon et al. (1998). Regulation of cartilage oligomeric matrix protein synthesis in human synovial cells and articular chondrocytes. *Arthritis Rheum* 41(6): 997-1006.

Reginato, A. J., G. M. Passano et al. (1994). Familial spondyloepiphyseal dysplasia tarda, brachydactyly, and precocious osteoarthritis associated with an arginine 75 → cysteine mutation in the procollagen type II gene in a kindred of Chiloe Islanders. I. Clinical, radiographic, and pathologic findings. *Arthritis Rheum* 37(7): 1078-1086.

Reinold, M. M., K. E. Wilk et al. (2006). Current concepts in the rehabilitation following articular cartilage repair procedures in the knee. *J Orthop Sports Phys Ther* 36(10): 774-794.

Rhee, D. K., J. Marcelino et al. (2005). The secreted glycoprotein lubricin protects cartilage surfaces and inhibits synovial cell overgrowth. *J Clin Invest* 115(3): 622-631.

Richmond, S. J. (2008). Magnet therapy for the relief of pain and inflammation in rheumatoid arthritis (CAMBRA): A randomised placebo-controlled crossover trial. *Trials* 9: 53.

Richmond, S. J., S. R. Brown et al. (2009). Therapeutic effects of magnetic and copper bracelets in osteoarthritis: A randomised placebo-controlled crossover trial. *Complement Ther Med* 17(5-6): 249-256.

Rizzoli, A. J., L. Trujeque et al. (1980). The coexistence of gout and rheumatoid arthritis: Case reports and a review of the literature. *J Rheumatol* 7(3): 316-324.

Robbins, S. M., T. B. Birmingham et al. (2011). Comparative diagnostic accuracy of knee adduction moments in knee osteoarthritis: A case for not normalizing to body size. *J Biomech* 44(5): 968-971.

Roberts, S., J. Menage et al. (2009). Immunohistochemical study of collagen types I and II and procollagen IIA in human cartilage repair tissue following autologous chondrocyte implantation. *Knee* 16(5): 398-404.

Roos, H., T. Adalberth et al. (1995). Osteoarthritis of the knee after injury to the anterior cruciate ligament or meniscus: The influence of time and age. *Osteoarthr Cartil* 3(4): 261-267.

Roos, H., M. Lauren et al. (1998). Knee osteoarthritis after meniscectomy: Prevalence of radiographic changes after twenty-one years, compared with matched controls. *Arthritis Rheum* 41(4): 687-693.

Rose, T., H. Lill et al. (2005). Autologous osteochondral mosaicplasty for treatment of a posttraumatic defect of the lateral tibial plateau: A case report with two-year follow-up. *J Orthop Trauma* 19(3): 217-222.

Rosenthal, A. K. (2006). Calcium crystal deposition and osteoarthritis. *Rheum Dis Clin North Am* 32(2): 401-412, vii.

Roth, V., and V. C. Mow. (1980). The intrinsic tensile behavior of the matrix of bovine articular cartilage and its variation with age. *J Bone Joint Surg Am* 62(7): 1102-1117.

Ryan, J. A., E. A. Eisner et al. (2009). Mechanical compression of articular cartilage induces chondrocyte proliferation and inhibits proteoglycan synthesis by activation of the ERK pathway: Implications for tissue engineering and regenerative medicine. *J Tissue Eng Regen Med* 3(2): 107-116.

Sacks, J. J., C. G. Helmick et al. (2007). Prevalence of and annual ambulatory health care visits for pediatric arthritis and other rheumatologic conditions in the United States in 2001-2004. *Arthritis Rheum* 57(8): 1439-1445.

Saker, B. M., O. B. Tofler et al. (1967). Alcohol consumption and gout. *Med J Aust* 1(24): 1213-1216.

Samuels, J., S. Krasnokutsky et al. (2008). Osteoarthritis: A tale of three tissues. *Bull NYU Hosp Jt Dis* 66(3): 244-250.

Sandell, L. J. (2012). Etiology of osteoarthritis: Genetics and synovial joint development. *Nat Rev Rheumatol* 8(2): 77-89.

Saxne, T., and D. Heinegard. (1992). Cartilage oligomeric matrix protein: A novel marker of cartilage turnover detectable in synovial fluid and blood. *Br J Rheumatol* 31(9): 583-591.

Schagemann, J. C., C. Erggelet et al. (2009). Cell-laden and cell-free biopolymer hydrogel for the treatment of osteochondral defects in a sheep model. *Tissue Eng Part A* 15(1): 75-82.

Schubert, T., S. Anders et al. (2009). Long-term effects of chondrospheres on cartilage lesions in an autologous chondrocyte implantation model as investigated in the SCID mouse model. *Int J Mol Med* 23(4): 455-460.

Scott, C. C., and K. A. Athanasiou. (2006). Design, validation, and utilization of an articular cartilage impact instrument. *Proc Inst Mech Eng H* 220(8): 845-855.

Sedory, E. J., E. D. McVey et al. (2007). Arthrogenic muscle response of the quadriceps and hamstrings with chronic ankle instability. *J Athl Train* 42(3): 355-360.

Seigel, J. P., and J. A. Donlon. (1997). Approval letter—Carticel. Rockville, MD: Department of Health and Human Services, Public Health Service.

Setton, L. A., D. M. Elliott et al. (1999). Altered mechanics of cartilage with osteoar-thritis: Human osteoarthritis and an experimental model of joint degenera-tion. *Osteoarthr Cartil* 7(1): 2-14.

Shapiro, F., S. Koide et al. (1993). Cell origin and differentiation in the repair of full-thickness defects of articular cartilage. *J Bone Joint Surg Am* 75(4): 532-553.

Sharma, L. (2003). Examination of exercise effects on knee osteoarthritis outcomes: Why should the local mechanical environment be considered? *Arthritis Rheum* 49(2): 255-260.

Sharma, L., D. D. Dunlop et al. (2003). Quadriceps strength and osteoarthritis pro-gression in malaligned and lax knees. *Ann Intern Med* 138(8): 613-619.

Sharma, L., F. Eckstein et al. (2008). Relationship of meniscal damage, meniscal extru-sion, malalignment, and joint laxity to subsequent cartilage loss in osteoar-thritic knees. *Arthritis Rheum* 58(6): 1716-1726.

Sharma, L., D. E. Hurwitz et al. (1998). Knee adduction moment, serum hyaluronan level, and disease severity in medial tibiofemoral osteoarthritis. *Arthritis Rheum* 41(7): 1233-1240.

Sharma, L., and Y. C. Pai. (1997). Impaired proprioception and osteoarthritis. *Curr Opin Rheumatol* 9(3): 253-258.

Shea, K. G., P. J. Apel et al. (2003). Anterior cruciate ligament injury in paediatric and adolescent patients: A review of basic science and clinical research. *Sports Med* 33(6): 455-471.

Shields, K. J., J. R. Owen et al. (2009). Biomechanical and biotribological correlation of induced wear on bovine femoral condyles. *J Biomech Eng* 131(6): 061005.

Siebold, R., S. Lichtenberg et al. (2003). Combination of microfracture and periostal-flap for the treatment of focal full thickness articular cartilage lesions of the shoulder: A prospective study. *Knee Surg Sports Traumatol Arthrosc* 11(3): 183-189.

Simon, S. R., E. L. Radin et al. (1972). The response of joints to impact loading. II. In vivo behavior of subchondral bone. *J Biomech* 5(3): 267-272.

Singh, K. K., K. Rommel et al. (2006). TGFBR1 and TGFBR2 mutations in patients with features of Marfan syndrome and Loeys-Dietz syndrome. *Hum Mutat* 27(8): 770-777.

Sirko-Osadsa, D. A., M. A. Murray et al. (1998). Stickler syndrome without eye involve-ment is caused by mutations in COL11A2, the gene encoding the alpha2(XI) chain of type XI collagen. *J Pediatr* 132(2): 368-371.

Slemenda, C., K. D. Brandt et al. (1997). Quadriceps weakness and osteoarthritis of the knee. *Ann Intern Med* 127(2): 97-104.

Slowman, S. D., and K. D. Brandt. (1986). Composition and glycosaminoglycan metab-olism of articular cartilage from habitually loaded and habitually unloaded sites. *Arthritis Rheum* 29(1): 88-94.

Smith, R. L., B. S. Donlon et al. (1995). Effects of fluid-induced shear on articular chondrocyte morphology and metabolism in vitro. *J Orthop Res* 13(6): 824-831.

Snelling, S., J. S. Sinsheimer et al. (2007). Genetic association analysis of LRCH1 as an osteoarthritis susceptibility locus. *Rheumatology (Oxford)* 46(2): 250-252.

Sorensen, K. H., and H. E. Christensen. (1973). Local amyloid formation in the hip joint capsule in osteoarthritis. *Acta Orthop Scand* 44(4): 460-466.

Spector, T. D., R. H. Reneland et al. (2006). Association between a variation in LRCH1 and knee osteoarthritis: A genome-wide single-nucleotide polymorphism association study using DNA pooling. *Arthritis Rheum* 54(2): 524-532.

Squires, G. R., S. Okouneff et al. (2003). The pathobiology of focal lesion development in aging human articular cartilage and molecular matrix changes characteristic of osteoarthritis. *Arthritis Rheum* 48(5): 1261-1270.

Steadman, J. R., K. K. Briggs et al. (2003). Outcomes of microfracture for traumatic chondral defects of the knee: Average 11-year follow-up. *Arthroscopy* 19(5): 477-484.

Stefansson, S. E., H. Jonsson et al. (2003). Genomewide scan for hand osteoarthritis: A novel mutation in matrilin-3. *Am J Hum Genet* 72(6): 1448-1459.

Steinwachs, M. (2009). New technique for cell-seeded collagen matrix-supported autologous chondrocyte transplantation. *Arthroscopy* 25(2): 208-211.

Stheneur, C., G. Collod-Beroud et al. (2008). Identification of 23 TGFBR2 and 6 TGFBR1 gene mutations and genotype-phenotype investigations in 457 patients with Marfan syndrome type I and II, Loeys-Dietz syndrome and related disorders. *Hum Mutat* 29(11): E284-E295.

Szerb, I., L. Hangody et al. (2005). Mosaicplasty: Long-term follow-up. *Bull Hosp Jt Dis* 63(1-2): 54-62.

Teichtahl, A. J., Y. Wang et al. (2008). The longitudinal relationship between body composition and patella cartilage in healthy adults. *Obesity (Silver Spring)* 16(2): 421-427.

Tetlow, L. C., D. J. Adlam et al. (2001). Matrix metalloproteinase and proinflammatory cytokine production by chondrocytes of human osteoarthritic cartilage: Associations with degenerative changes. *Arthritis Rheum* 44(3): 585-594.

Thompson, R. C., Jr., and C. A. Bassett. (1970). Histological observations on experimentally induced degeneration of articular cartilage. *J Bone Joint Surg Am* 52(3): 435-443.

Tortorella, M. D., A. M. Malfait et al. (2001). The role of ADAM-TS4 (aggrecanase-1) and ADAM-TS5 (aggrecanase-2) in a model of cartilage degradation. *Osteoarthr Cartil* 9(6): 539-552.

Torzilli, P. A., R. Grigiene et al. (1999). Effect of impact load on articular cartilage: Cell metabolism and viability, and matrix water content. *J Biomech Eng* 121(5): 433-441.

Toussirot, E., and D. Wendling. (2004). The use of TNF-alpha blocking agents in rheumatoid arthritis: An overview. *Expert Opin Pharmacother* 5(3): 581-594.

Toussirot, E., and D. Wendling. (2007). The use of TNF-alpha blocking agents in rheumatoid arthritis: An update. *Expert Opin Pharmacother* 8(13): 2089-2107.

U.S. Food and Drug Administration (FDA). (2005). Cellular products for joint surface repair—Briefing document. Meeting 38 of the Cellular, Tissue, and Gene Therapies Advisory Committee. Silver Spring, MD: FDA.

Upmeier, H., B. Bruggenjurgen et al. (2007). Follow-up costs up to 5 years after conventional treatments in patients with cartilage lesions of the knee. *Knee Surg Sports Traumatol Arthrosc* 15(3): 249-257.

Utukuri, M. M., H. S. Somayaji et al. (2006). Update on paediatric ACL injuries. *Knee* 13(5): 345-352.

Valdes, A. M., and T. D. Spector. (2011). Genetic epidemiology of hip and knee osteoarthritis. *Nat Rev Rheumatol* 7(1): 23-32.

van den Berg, W. B. (2001). Lessons from animal models of osteoarthritis. *Curr Opin Rheumatol* 13(5): 452-456.

van den Berg, W. B., L. A. Joosten et al. (1999). Role of tumour necrosis factor alpha in experimental arthritis: Separate activity of interleukin 1beta in chronicity and cartilage destruction. *Ann Rheum Dis* 58(Suppl 1): I40-I48.

van der Esch, M., M. Steultjens et al. (2005). Structural joint changes, malalignment, and laxity in osteoarthritis of the knee. *Scand J Rheumatol* 34(4): 298-301.

Vanwanseele, B., F. Eckstein et al. (2010). The relationship between knee adduction moment and cartilage and meniscus morphology in women with osteoarthritis. *Osteoarthr Cartil* 18(7): 894-901.

Vasara, A. I., M. T. Nieminen et al. (2005). Indentation stiffness of repair tissue after autologous chondrocyte transplantation. *Clin Orthop Relat Res* 433: 233-242.

Vincent, T., M. Hermansson et al. (2002). Basic FGF mediates an immediate response of articular cartilage to mechanical injury. *Proc Natl Acad Sci USA* 99(12): 8259-8264.

Vingerhoeds, B., I. Degreef et al. (2004). Debridement arthroplasty for osteoarthritis of the elbow (Outerbridge-Kashiwagi procedure). *Acta Orthop Belg* 70(4): 306-310.

Wada, T., S. Isogai et al. (2005). Debridement arthroplasty for primary osteoarthritis of the elbow. Surgical technique. *J Bone Joint Surg Am* 87(Suppl 1, Pt 1): 95-105.

Walker, W. R., and D. M. Keats. (1976). An investigation of the therapeutic value of the 'copper bracelet'-dermal assimilation of copper in arthritic/rheumatoid conditions. *Agents Actions* 6(4): 454-459.

Wang, Y. X., J. F. Griffith et al. (2010). Non-invasive MRI assessment of the articular cartilage in clinical studies and experimental settings. *World J Radiol* 2(1): 44-54.

Webb, J. (1978). Crystal induced arthritis: Gout and pseudogout. *Aust Fam Physician* 7(8): 959-980.

Widuchowski, W., J. Widuchowski et al. (2007). Articular cartilage defects: Study of 25,124 knee arthroscopies. *Knee* 14(3): 177-182.

Wilson, R., D. Belluoccio et al. (2008). Proteomic characterization of mouse cartilage degradation in vitro. *Arthritis Rheum* 58(10): 3120-3131.

Wilson, W., C. van Burken et al. (2006). Causes of mechanically induced collagen damage in articular cartilage. *J Orthop Res* 24(2): 220-228.

Wluka, A. E., Y. Wang et al. (2005). Tibial plateau size is related to grade of joint space narrowing and osteophytes in healthy women and in women with osteoarthritis. *Ann Rheum Dis* 64(7): 1033-1037.

Woo, S. L., W. H. Akeson et al. (1976). Measurements of nonhomogeneous, directional mechanical properties of articular cartilage in tension. *J Biomech* 9(12): 785-791.

Wood, J. J., M. A. Malek et al. (2006). Autologous cultured chondrocytes: Adverse events reported to the United States Food and Drug Administration. *J Bone Joint Surg Am* 88(3): 503-507.

Wu, J. Z., W. Herzog et al. (1996). Modeling axi-symmetrical joint contact with biphasic cartilage layers—An asymptotic solution. *J Biomech* 29(10): 1263-1281.

Yelin, E. (1998). The economics of osteoarthritis. In *Osteoarthritis*, ed. K. D. Brandt, M. Doherty, and L. S. Lohmander. New York: Oxford University Press, pp. 23-30.

Young, A. A., S. McLennan et al. (2006). Proteoglycan 4 downregulation in a sheep meniscectomy model of early osteoarthritis. *Arthritis Res Ther* 8(2): R41.

Zhang, W., M. Doherty et al. (2005). EULAR evidence based recommendations for the management of hip osteoarthritis: Report of a task force of the EULAR Standing Committee for International Clinical Studies Including Therapeutics (ESCISIT). *Ann Rheum Dis* 64(5): 669-681.

Zhang, W., G. Nuki et al. (2010). OARSI recommendations for the management of hip and knee osteoarthritis. III. Changes in evidence following systematic cumulative update of research published through January 2009. *Osteoarthr Cartil* 18(4): 476-499.

Zhang, X., Z. Zheng et al. (2008). The synergistic effects of microfracture, perforated decalcified cortical bone matrix and adenovirus-bone morphogenetic protein-4 in cartilage defect repair. *Biomaterials* 29(35): 4616-4629.

Zhang, Y., R. Woods et al. (2006). Alcohol consumption as a trigger of recurrent gout attacks. *Am J Med* 119(9): 800 e813-808.

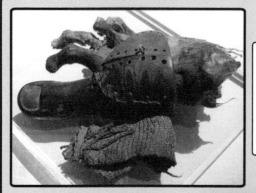

Prosthetic toe dating between 950 and 710 BCE located in the Egyptian Museum (Cairo, Egypt). This prosthesis is one of the oldest known examples and was designed to restore normal locomotion (Finch 2011).

Traditional three-legged Japanese stone lantern. Each of the three legs supports the whole, analogous to the three main pillars of tissue engineering: cells, signals, and scaffolds.

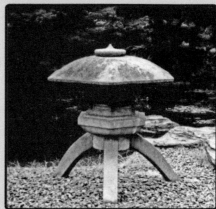

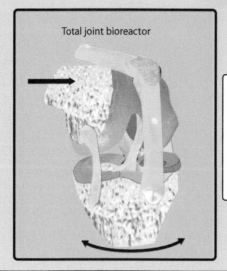

Total joint bioreactor

Total joint bioreactor: in the future such a bioreactor can be employed in tissue engineering toward producing a living total joint assembled from multiple engineered tissues. Such a bioreactor would provide mechanical stimuli along multiple physiologically relevant axes.

Tissue Engineering of Articular Cartilage

- Need for *in vitro* tissue engineering
- Cell source
- Biomaterials and scaffold design
- Bioactive molecules
- Bioreactors and mechanical stimuli
- Convergence of stimuli

In this chapter, we discuss the strategies employed by researchers striving to repair or regenerate articular cartilage through biological means. While methods to repair cartilage using surgery exist (e.g., debridement, microfracture, and mosaicplasty), tissue engineering holds the promise of complete regeneration. Furthermore, engineered constructs can be designed that are mechanically functional from day 1, potentially decreasing recovery time for the patient.

Focus has been placed on the three main pillars of tissue engineering: cell source, scaffold design, and external stimulation through the use of bioactive molecules and mechanical bioreactors (Figure 4.1). Cell sources that are discussed include primary chondrocytes as well as

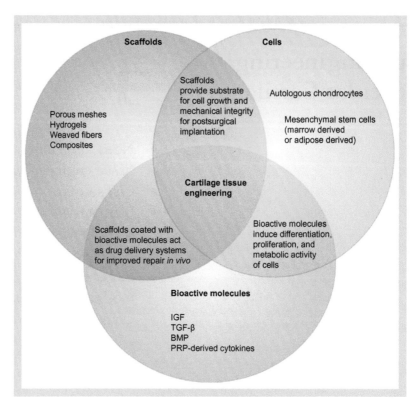

Figure 4.1 Traditional paradigm of tissue engineering consisting of the three components of scaffolds, cells, and bioactive molecules. (From Daher, R. J. et al., *Nat Rev Rheumatol* 5(11): 599–607, 2009. With permission.)

stem and progenitor cells. Natural, synthetic, and hybrid biomaterials have all been used for cartilage engineering, with the latest approaches building upon previous findings to create new and innovative scaffolds suitable for long-term repair. Growth factors and other bioactive molecules are critical components to rapid, complete regeneration of tissues in the body, and those with proven roles in cartilage repair are reviewed here. Finally, a comprehensive discussion of bioreactors and mechanical stimulation is included. Incorporating sufficient mechanical integrity in engineered cartilage (neocartilage) is crucial for its success in the mechanically demanding joint environment. Bioreactors that mimic cartilage's physiological environment are described, along with reported experimental findings using each approach. In all subsections, discussions of specific studies that have taken place in the past couple of decades are used to illustrate the current state of cartilage engineering, as well as future directions in this highly active field of research.

For decades, hyaline articular cartilage has been a primary target for tissue engineering efforts due to the lack of functional regeneration intrinsically within the joint. In addition to focal defects, pathologies such as osteoarthritis can destroy the entire cartilage surface, resulting in loss of function and persistent pain. This chapter highlights both the seminal tissue engineering studies focused on articular cartilage and the latest approaches that incorporate bioreactors, bioactive molecules, and specialized biomaterials.

Tissue engineering, in its classical sense, involves the manipulation of a complex interplay among biomaterials, growth factors, and cell populations (Mikos et al. 2006) to achieve functional improvement or restoration. Articular cartilage has been a high priority for tissue engineers since it does not naturally regenerate after injury. Furthermore, the annual health care costs associated with musculoskeletal diseases and injuries are extremely large (estimated at $874 billion per year), and an effective reparative solution would not only reduce costs but also improve the quality of life for millions (U.S. Bone and Joint Initiative 2014). The average age for patients undergoing arthroscopy who exhibit cartilage defects in the knee is 43, and, combined with the demographical data on adolescent cartilage injuries, as discussed in Chapter 3, the need to create a repair tissue that can last several decades is a major goal (Curl et al. 1997).

The earliest attempts at cartilage regeneration involved transplanting either minced cartilage tissue or dissociated chondrocytes (Chesterman and Smith 1968). Surgical solutions to cartilage defects typically include surface abrasion, microfracture, and debridement, all of which can reduce symptoms. However, the repair tissue formed in response to these procedures is fibrocartilage, which, as discussed elsewhere in this book, has biomechanical properties that are markedly different from those of normal cartilage (Curl et al. 1997). Fibrocartilage does not have the biochemical composition or structural organization to provide proper mechanical function within the joint environment and will degrade over time because of insufficient load-bearing capacity (Hunziker 2002; Smith et al. 2005). Because of this, current research is striving to produce a tissue that is hyaline-like in its biochemical composition and biomechanical properties. The first part of this chapter focuses on *in vitro* tissue engineering approaches. Attempts to tissue engineer within the *in vivo* environment are discussed; germane immunological considerations are presented in Section 6.2.

It is natural to think that the *in vivo* environment probably comprises all conditions necessary to effect successful regeneration. That is, the *in vivo* environment must contain the proper growth factors and mechanical stimuli, delivered in a well-sequenced manner through autocrine and paracrine signaling, to effect proper healing, the major missing component being metabolically active chondrocytes at the defect site. Initial efforts at delivering mechanical stimuli *in vitro* attempted to emulate these signals, the natural thought being that the objective of bioreactors ought to be the creation of signals reminiscent of the native environment, for example, the 1 Hz pace of walking and the low oxygen tension of the joint. Unfortunately, the physiological conditions have not been shown to result in cartilage repair *in vivo*, and the act of mimicking these conditions *in vitro* should be questioned. It may not be that physiological conditions are not required, but just that physiological conditions of a different developmental period may be more beneficial in generating functional cartilage. To investigate this latter case, *in vitro* tissue engineering has been employed to recapitulate developmental conditions.

4.1 The Need for *In Vitro* Tissue Engineering

The primary advantage of *in vitro* tissue engineering is proposed to be immediate functionality. The idea is that a tissue replacement that is mechanically and biologically functional before implantation will have a higher probability for success. This is especially true for mechanically arduous environments, such as articulating joints. Without the requisite mechanical characteristics, a tissue-engineered construct would be quickly destroyed by the high stresses that are part of normal loading of an ambulatory patient. In contrast, a construct that possesses material properties comparable to those of the native tissue would not fracture or degrade. Because of this, many researchers believe articular cartilage engineering should place emphasis on biomimetic construct development *in vitro*. Since the tissue resides in a mechanically demanding environment, the implanted construct needs to be developed to a point that it can withstand or respond to these mechanical loads. Constructs possessing insufficient integrity will collapse in the articular defect, which not only prevents regeneration but also could accelerate degradation of the tissues surrounding it. Also critical in this effort is the issue of integration of the construct with the surrounding tissues, discussed in more detail in Section 6.1.1. Efforts to heal large defects *in vivo* could fail without some means of protecting the structure of newly developed tissues. By growing neocartilage in a laboratory, the culture environment can be carefully controlled with respect to nutrient supply, biological stimuli, and mechanical loading.

For a tissue like articular cartilage, possible treatments often depend on the type of damage to the joint. For example, an osteochondral defect that reaches down into the subchondral bone introduces blood into the defect. This influx of blood and marrow brings a variety of signals and cells to the injury site. However, fibrocartilage will form in the defects if left untreated, filling the site with a disordered mass of fibrous tissue that possesses inferior mechanical functionality. Another type of damage in cartilage is a chondral defect that does not extend through the depth of the tissue to reach vascularity. In this case, some of the chemical and biological factors associated with osteochondral defects are not present. Unfortunately, the mechanical functionality of the articular cartilage is still compromised due to disruption of the tissue's surface. Both osteochondral and chondral defects can be considered focal defects if the damage is localized to a single region.

261

The most difficult type of cartilage injury to treat is a breakdown of the articulating surface caused by diseases, such as osteoarthritis and osteochondritis dissecans. Most tissue engineering approaches create small constructs that can be fit into focal defect sites in the cartilage. However, this would be insufficient for injuries affecting entire joint compartments or larger, since there would be no functional tissue in which to anchor the new constructs. As yet, there are no successful approaches to treating osteoarthritis using tissue engineering. Researchers are continually investigating alternative approaches, such as engineering a replacement tissue or scaffold that can completely resurface the joint (Moutos et al. 2007) (Figure 4.2). Other possibilities include gene therapy or pharmaceuticals, which might have more success in treating systemic degeneration of articular cartilage.

Articular cartilage growth and development are affected by both biomechanical and biological stimuli. On the mechanical side, loading is a required part of the normal joint environment. As seen in previous chapters, while excessive forces can damage cartilage, some stimulation is necessary to promote chondrogenesis (Darling and Athanasiou 2003). Articular cartilage will atrophy in a mechanically static environment (Vanwanseele et al. 2002), so researchers are currently evaluating a variety of loading approaches to prevent this while promoting the regeneration process. An important factor to consider prior to mechanical loading is the choice of scaffold for the engineered construct. The scaffold material not only affects how cells sense mechanical loads but also may provide an environment conducive to cell attachment and matrix synthesis.

In addition to mechanical stimuli, articular cartilage responds dramatically to growth factors that are naturally present in the joint environment or exogenously added. The transforming growth factor β (TGF-β) superfamily includes growth factors that are present in developing bone and articular cartilage, as described in Chapter 2. These molecules play an integral role in the natural development process, and can induce large changes on the growth of musculoskeletal tissues *in vitro*.

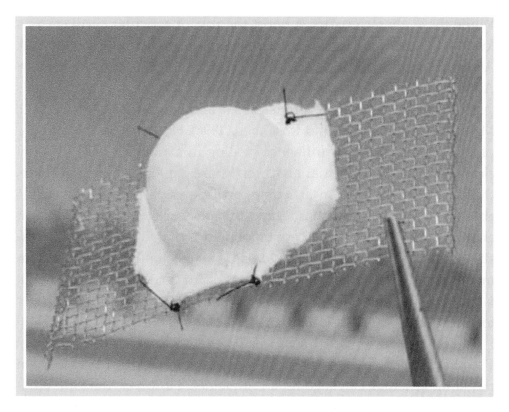

Figure 4.2 Whole joint scaffold using a mold of a sheep femur to shape a fiber-based scaffold. This could then be coated in a cartilage-derived matrix and seeded with cells to form a cap of neocartilage that could be sutured in place. (From Dr. F. Moutos, Duke. With permission.)

This section illustrates the importance of the *in vitro* culture environment on the growth, development, and functionality of native and engineered articular cartilage. Following the paradigm for functional tissue engineering, four main categories are reviewed: cell sources, biomaterials, bioactive molecules, and bioreactors (Guilak 2002).

4.1.1 Characteristics of the *In Vivo* System

Articular cartilage is a specialized tissue, with physiological characteristics that help retain tissue functionality for decades of rigorous use. The composition and structure of articular cartilage, as well as its ambient mechanical microenvironment, are discussed in detail in Chapter 1.

While these characteristics support the role of articular cartilage as a load-bearing surface, they become problematic if the tissue is damaged. Articular cartilage is avascular, alymphatic, and aneural (Revell and Athanasiou 2009). The lack of a blood supply prevents the influx of cells (e.g., stem cells) that can repopulate a site and begin repair (Pridie 1959; Mankin 1982; Hunziker and Rosenberg 1996). How the absence of lymphatics and nerves may influence healing in articular cartilage is not clear. They are all potential areas for future exploration. For instance, the perception of pain in articular cartilage is paradoxical given the absence of nerves in this tissue, and it is unclear from where pain can arise. It is likely that the perception of pain is due to the associated tissues of the joint and subchondral bone. The mechanical microenvironment might be the largest hurdle to successful cartilage repair. While it is necessary for normal tissue homeostasis, it also acts as a major driver to progressive deterioration if damage already exists.

The characteristics of the *in vivo* system present many difficulties when pursuing articular cartilage repair strategies. However, the joint environment may provide some beneficial aspects as well. For instance, it has long been thought that articular cartilage is immunoprivileged, meaning transplanted cells and tissues are less likely to induce a sustained immune response from the body. This is directly related to the avascular and alymphatic nature of articular cartilage. Some amount of immune response is still expected, since almost all procedures will require surgical access to the joint through the capsule or otherwise exposing the synovial space. While the acute inflammation response to surgery or implantation can be severe, it can be limited by the use of arthroscopic or minimally invasive procedures. The immune characteristics of the joint space have allowed for successful outcomes using allograft tissue, for example, osteochondral grafts and anterior cruciate ligament transplants (Barber et al. 2010; Bedi et al. 2010; Bhumiratana et al. 2014). However, it needs to be demonstrated conclusively how xenogeneic tissues fare in a diarthrodial joint environment. A discussion about immunogenicity in response to xenogeneic and allogeneic materials is provided in greater depth in Section 6.2.

In vivo studies of articular cartilage regeneration take one of several forms. Most commonly, cells or engineered constructs are implanted directly into a cartilage defect (Brittberg et al. 1996). These experiments allow for assessment of tissue growth, integration, and longevity in its targeted biological environment. Other approaches have used the *in vivo* environment in a manner similar to that of a bioreactor, implanting engineered constructs subcutaneously (Emans et al. 2010; Responte et al. 2012). This approach exposes the construct to a complex array of biological factors that would otherwise be difficult to apply individually. Since it is difficult to induce vascularization *in vitro*, osteochondral constructs (Figure 4.3) that require vascularization of the engineered bone are often cultured *in vivo* (Emans et al. 2005; Jin et al. 2011; Qu et al. 2011).

Other important differences between the *in vivo* environment and standard cell culture conditions include lower oxygen concentrations (discussed in more detail in Section 4.5.6), lower temperatures, and limited nutrient and waste diffusion. *In vitro* conditions typically use ambient air oxygen tensions (~20%), standard body temperature (37°C), and an excess of culture medium that is changed regularly. Compared with physiological conditions, these *in vitro* conditions are quite different; physiologically, oxygen tension is estimated to be ~7-10% at the surface and ~1% at the subchondral bone (Silver 1975; Malda et al. 2003; Fermor et al. 2007), knee joint temperature is ~35°C (Zaffagnini et al. 1996), and

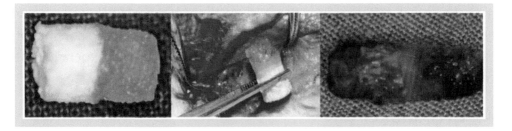

Figure 4.3 *In vivo* culture of polymer (polyvinyl alcohol/gelatin-nano-hydroxyapatite/polyamide 6 [PVA-n-HA/PA6]) osteochondral constructs in an intramuscular pocket for 4 weeks induces vascularization of the construct. Left: Osteochondral PVA-n-HA/PA6 cylinder; left side is n-HA6 and right side is PVA. Implanted in the intramuscular pocket (center) and after 4 weeks (right). (From Qu, D. et al., *J Biomed Mater Res B Appl Biomater* 96(1): 9-15, 2011. With permission.)

diffusion of nutrients from the synovial fluid is restricted (Guilak et al. 2000). The influence of these differences continues to be investigated, and it is not yet clear whether creating a true physiological environment is the best means of growing new articular cartilage.

Major drawbacks to *in vivo* approaches include a limited set of evaluation techniques, as well as the maintenance of well-controlled experiments. The *in vivo* environment contains a multitude of chemical and mechanical signals that are in continuous flux and can be vastly different from one subject to another (Liu et al. 2010; Qu et al. 2011). Growth factors and cytokines circulating in the blood and present in the extracellular matrix can stimulate changes in the implanted cells. Likewise, mechanical loading (see Section 1.2), such as compression, tension, hydrostatic pressure, and shear, can induce changes in the biological response of implanted cells and the structure of implanted constructs (see Section 4.5). Controlling these variables is often difficult and is challenging for studies. The *in vitro* environment allows for precise control of growth factor levels, mechanical stimulation, and other experimental factors (Bobick et al. 2009), but does not replicate the complexity of the physiological system. Because of this, research typically progresses from *in vitro* studies to *in vivo* studies. Ethical and cost considerations also play a role when determining whether a study should be done *in vitro* or *in vivo*. For example, a dose-response study of a novel chemical would require a large number of samples, which can be accomplished in a more cost-effective manner *in vitro* than *in vivo*. While there may not be a direct transfer of findings from *in vitro* to *in vivo*, the benefits of each system help researchers investigate a wide range of experimental conditions important for understanding cartilage regeneration.

4.2 CELL SOURCE

Cells are one of the key components of tissue engineering. Studies have shown that including cells in an engineered construct accelerates regeneration (Tatebe et al. 2005). Furthermore, these implanted cells have been shown to remain in the tissue without being replaced by host cells

(Tatebe et al. 2005). Researchers have several options when choosing a cell source. The cell type most commonly used in early cartilage engineering studies is the autologous chondrocyte. By extracting cells from the patient's own body, any immune response is minimized or totally removed. Furthermore, chondrocytes are already differentiated into the target phenotype and have the capacity to secrete cartilage-specific matrix molecules.

The choice of cell type often depends on the initial condition of the cartilage tissue. In cases of extensive degradation or disease, use of autologous chondrocytes is not an option. One possible alternative is to use allogeneic chondrocytes from donor tissue. This approach is commonly used for general *in vitro* experiments and some *in vivo* studies due to the relatively ready availability of donor tissue. While the cell phenotype is appropriate for the implant environment, problems can arise with respect to tissue availability for humans, as well as possible disease transmission or immune response.

Due to limits on the availability of human tissue, some have suggested that cross-species cell implantations might be an alternative option. Xenogeneic transplants have been reported to be successful in sheep (Homminga et al. 1991), goats (van Susante et al. 1999), and rabbits (Toolan et al. 1998). However, similar difficulties exist with xenogeneic transplants as with allogeneic transplants, namely, immunogenicity concerns. Further complications could arise with cross-species compatibility issues at the cellular and molecular level.

4.2.1 A Need for Alternative Cell Sources

Although articular chondrocytes have been generally used as a cell source, their utility is limited by issues of autologous donor site morbidity and *in vitro* phenotypic stability. Sourcing cells from diseased cartilage is likely not useful. Likewise, tissue engineering typically requires many millions of cells to treat a small region of damage. Articular cartilage is sparsely populated by chondrocytes, which effectively requires *in vitro* expansion of the cells before use. Chondrocytes rapidly dedifferentiate in monolayer, losing chondrocytic gene and protein expressions critical for proper tissue regeneration (Darling and Athanasiou 2005a). Thus, methods to help dedifferentiated chondrocytes regain their lost phenotypes may be useful. Perhaps a better approach may be the identification of alternative cell sources that can mimic the role of chondrocytes

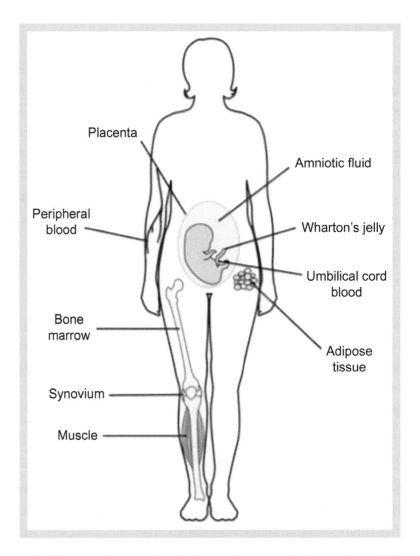

Figure 4.4 Stem cells can be isolated from multiple anatomical locations, encompassing adult and extra-embryonic tissues. The cell sources shown have all been investigated for cartilage regeneration, although mesenchymal sources have been studied much more than other tissues. (From Beane, O. S., and E. M. Darling, *Ann Biomed Eng* 40(10): 2079-2097, 2012. With permission.)

in cartilage while also being able to rapidly regenerate damaged or diseased tissue (Beane and Darling 2012) (Figure 4.4). Possibilities include adult mesenchymal stem cells, embryonic stem cells, and induced pluripotent stem cells.

4.2.2 Chondrogenic Differentiation of Mesenchymal Stem Cells and Progenitor Cell Populations

Progenitor and stem cell populations, in particular mesenchymal stem cells, have been long considered as a promising cell source for cartilage tissue engineering (Hwang and Elisseeff 2009; Beane and Darling 2012). Progenitor cells reside throughout the body and can be differentiated along many different lineages. These populations have been positively identified in synovium, bone marrow, fat, muscle, skin, dental pulp, amniotic fluid, umbilical cord, and neural tissue (Prockop 1997; Jiang et al. 2002; Sekiya et al. 2002; Deng et al. 2007; Kurth et al. 2007; Sanchez-Adams and Athanasiou 2012). For the past two decades, research has focused on inducing stem and progenitor cells to form cartilagenous matrices.

Mesenchymal stem cells from bone marrow and fat tissue are two sources that have been extensively investigated for their promising application to cartilage regeneration (Caplan 1991; Chen and Tuan 2008). Several specific studies will be discussed later in this section.

Mesenchymal stem cells are especially attractive as a cell source for articular cartilage regeneration because they can be taken directly from the patient's own body. Articular cartilage damage and disease render resident chondrocytes unsuitable for tissue engineering approaches. Autologous mesenchymal stem cells may be ideal in these cases since they can be taken from a healthy region of the body. Likewise, as an autologous material, these cells have little to no problems with immunogenicity. Progenitor and stem cells also show a large capacity for proliferation, so only small tissue samples are needed to obtain enough cells to grow the large populations required for tissue engineering. Donor site morbidity and patient pain are dependent on the site of harvest, but

269

for some cell types this is minimal (e.g., skin- and adipose-derived stem cells).

The difficulty with using nonchondrocyte cell sources is successfully inducing chondrocytic expression for short- and long-term applications. This is usually done through chemical means, exposing stem

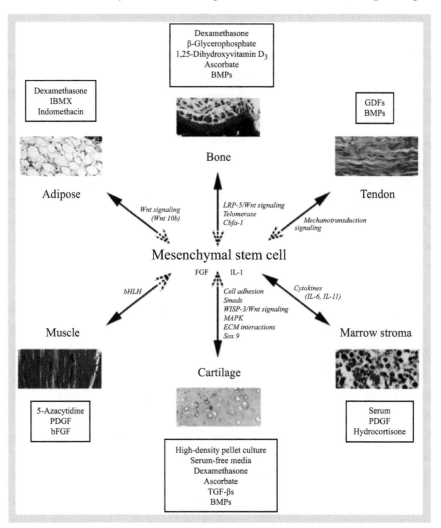

Figure 4.5 Mesenchymal stem cells possess multilineage differentiation potential, with possibilities including bone, cartilage, fat, muscle, tendon, and marrow stroma. Differentiation is induced by stimulating cells with chemical, mechanical, and other environmental factors. (From Tuan, R. S. et al., *Arthritis Res Ther* 5(1): 32-45, 2003. With permission from BioMed Central.)

cells to growth factors and cytokines that upregulate and downregulate multiple genes to achieve a chondrocyte-like state (Tuan et al. 2003). Chondrogenic differentiation can be induced by using combinations of TGF-β, bone morphogenetic proteins (BMPs), and dexamethasone (Caterson et al. 2001; Guilak et al. 2010). Currently, no conclusive evidence exists that these treatments actually change undifferentiated stem cells into fully, and irreversibly, differentiated chondrocytes. Regardless, progress has been made using mesenchymal stem cells for cartilage regeneration. Improvements are continuously made in the composition of differentiation media and customization of growth environments (Figure 4.5). Recently, engineered articular cartilage tissue with physiologically relevant compressive and frictional properties was produced using a pellet culture of human mesenchymal stem cells overlaid onto a demineralized bone support (Bhumiratana et al. 2014). There is reason to believe that autologous mesenchymal stem cells will be one of the primary cell sources for cartilage engineering in the future, though it needs to be conclusively demonstrated that mesenchymal stem cells can produce viable, functional articular chondrocytes.

4.2.3 Chondrogenic Differentiation of Embryonic Stem Cells and Induced Pluripotent Stem Cells

Another possible cell source akin to progenitor populations is embryonic stem cells. While progenitor cells are highly proliferative, extensive expansion in monolayer culture can retard growth rates, shorten telomeres, and reduce multipotency (Bruder et al. 1997; Banfi et al. 2002; Baxter et al. 2004; Parsch et al. 2004; Vacanti et al. 2005). Embryonic stem cells, however, have an unlimited capacity for proliferation, and, hence, are attractive for tissue engineering endeavors that require large cell numbers (Mikos et al. 2006; Koay et al. 2007). These cells are truly pluripotent, showing a capacity to differentiate into any cell type in the body. However, researchers do not currently know the best ways to differentiate embryonic stem cells along every lineage. Some protocols have better efficacy than others, though; for example, by using established differentiation protocols, good results have been obtained for the chondrocytic lineage of human embryonic stem cells (Koay et al. 2007; Hoben et al. 2008; Koay and Athanasiou 2008, 2009; Hwang and Elisseeff 2009). As with all treatments using embryonic stem cells, there are potential problems with teratoma formation, poorly controlled cell proliferation or differentiation, and possible immunogenicity issues since the cells come from an allogeneic source. Ethical concerns have also been raised since an embryo typically has to be destroyed to establish a population of embryonic stem cells.

Induced pluripotent stem cells have risen as an attractive alternative to embryonic stem cells that might assuage ethical and immunogenicity concerns. These cells can be created by transfecting virtually any somatic cell in the body with stem cell-associated genes. Oct-3/4 and Sox2, master transcriptional regulators, are almost always included in this transfection (Takahashi and Yamanaka 2006). Other genes are added to improve induction efficiency and can include Klf4, c-Myc, Nanog, and LIN28 (Yu et al. 2007). Recent work with induced pluripotent stem cells has shown the ability to purify a well-defined cell population with strong chondrogenic potential and usefulness for cartilage tissue engineering, while reducing off-target cell types to minimize risks of teratoma formation (Diekman et al. 2012). The reprogramming of somatic cells provides an autologous, pluripotent cell source capable of differentiating into chondrocytes for cartilage repair. Questions still remain as to the implementation of this technology in the clinical setting and regulatory approval.

4.3 BIOMATERIALS AND SCAFFOLD DESIGN

For tissue engineering, biocompatible scaffolds are often chosen to improve the regeneration of a damaged or diseased tissue. While recent studies have indicated that cartilage constructs can be formed *in vitro* without having to use scaffolds (Hu and Athanasiou 2006a,b; Jubel et al. 2008; Ofek et al. 2008), traditional tissue engineering approaches are based on seeding cells on scaffolds to provide structure to the neocartilage. The architectural structure of the scaffold can affect the mechanical properties of the construct, cell seeding distributions, and diffusional characteristics. Furthermore, the material itself can help or hinder cell attachment, proliferation, and synthesis over the lifetime of the implant.

The scaffold base material and its architecture should fulfill three main requirements: have an interconnected network that allows efficient diffusion of nutrients and wastes; be biocompatible and bioresorbable, with a degradation rate that ideally matches the rate of tissue growth; and allow for cell attachment, proliferation, and differentiation. The last requirement is often fulfilled using bioactive molecules that are either physically tethered to the scaffold or included in the culture medium.

An additional factor for choosing a scaffold is whether it will be used *in vitro* or *in vivo*. If implanted immediately, the scaffold should possess mechanical characteristics that are appropriate for the loading environment. The scaffold should maintain its shape and protect the seeded cells from excessive forces. If bioresorbable, the degradation of the scaffold should correspond with the growth of tissue in the construct, which would gradually take more of the applied load from the scaffold. If chemical initiators are used to cross-link the scaffold either *in vitro* or *in vivo*, then the process should be designed to minimize negative effects on cell viability or metabolism. Some injectable biomaterials are cross-linked in the defect site to achieve sufficient mechanical properties, but this process can involve chemicals that are cytotoxic.

Current research includes injectable cell and polymer solutions (Figure 4.6) that form constructs with robust mechanical properties in the defect site (Bryant and Anseth 2001; Dobratz et al. 2009; Park et al. 2009). Cell-seeded scaffolds cultured *in vitro*, however, may not need the same level of structural integrity, since newly formed tissue should help achieve mechanical characteristics sufficient for the biological environment. These properties would be independent of the degrading scaffold material. This approach simply uses the scaffold as a structure that helps support seeded cells for a period of weeks while new tissue forms. Ideally,

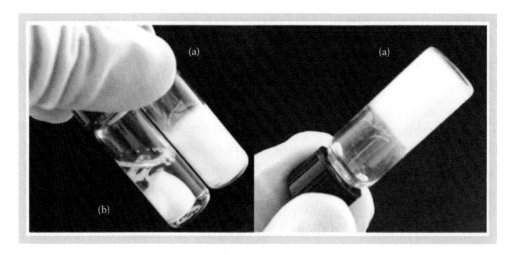

Figure 4.6 Injectable hydrogel in the liquid state (left) undergoes rapid gelation within 1 minute to form a solid gel (right). Stabilization agents can maintain gel volume (a) which may otherwise collapse (b). (From Vo, T. N. et al., *Biomacromolecules* 15(1): 132-142, 2014. With permission.)

once the construct is implanted, the newly formed matrix is capable of functioning in the native loading environment.

In general, biomaterials are classified into three main categories: natural, synthetic, and composite materials. Natural materials are found in living organisms and can be extracted and processed into functional biomaterials. Synthetic materials are created using chemical processes, which allow extensive customization of material properties. However, some processes can also have negative side effects, such as cytotoxicity or immune response activation. Composite scaffolds combine two or more materials into one scaffold to take advantage of special characteristics intrinsic to each substance.

New materials for biological applications are synthesized frequently, but extensive chemical and physical characterization is necessary before a material can be used in the body. The biomaterials summarized in the following paragraphs have been well characterized and shown to be cytocompatible in many tissue engineering studies. Not all have been applied to cartilage tissue engineering, though, and success could be dependent on the cell-surface interactions specific to different cell types.

4.3.1 Natural Scaffolds

Natural materials are often preferred for biological applications because synthetic materials are believed to elicit more immune response. Their structures can vary from hydrogels (a colloidal gel in which water is the dispersion medium) to solid fibers and fragments. Among the natural materials used in articular cartilage engineering are alginate, agarose, chitosan, fibrin glue, type I and II collagens, hyaluronic acid-based materials, and reconstituted tissue matrices. Each material has strengths and weaknesses to its use, and results can vary depending on the application.

Alginate is a polysaccharide extracted from seaweed and can be used to encapsulate cells in a three-dimensional matrix (Figure 4.7). Encapsulation maintains a chondrocyte's rounded morphology, which has been shown to induce redifferentiation of monolayer expanded cells (Murphy and Sambanis 2001a). This approach can also be applied when differentiating stem cells along the chondrocytic lineage. Besides encapsulation, one of the main advantages of alginate is its proven biocompatibility (Hutmacher 2001). For sterile applications, alginate can be purified by filtration, precipitation, or extraction. Alginate is not an ideal material for many tissue engineering applications, however. The material does not degrade rapidly *in vivo*, which can interfere with new tissue growth. The mechanical integrity of alginate scaffolds is insufficient for long-term success of implants (Hutmacher 2001).

Agarose is another polysaccharide derived from seaweed that exhibits temperature-sensitive solubility in water, an attribute convenient for encapsulating cells (Hutmacher 2001) (Figures 4.6 and 4.8). Similar to alginate, agarose provides a biocompatible, three-dimensional environment for culturing chondrocytes. Unfortunately, the degradation properties of agarose are similar to those of alginate and cannot be easily altered to tailor the life of the scaffold. In addition, it is unclear whether agarose is eventually degraded or removed as the cells form matrix. Despite these deficiencies, many *in vitro* studies use agarose as a scaffold material when investigating the effects of mechanical stimuli on

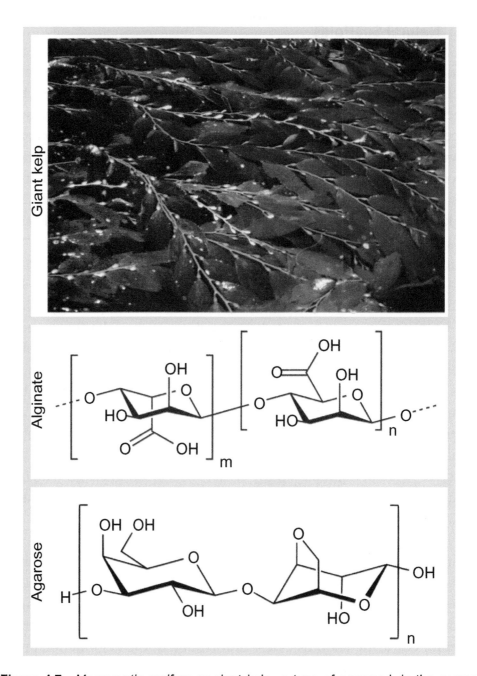

Figure 4.7 *Macrocystis pyrifera* or giant kelp, a type of seaweed, is the source of both algininic acid (alginate) and agarose. (Public domain image, U.S. National Oceanic and Atmospheric Administration.)

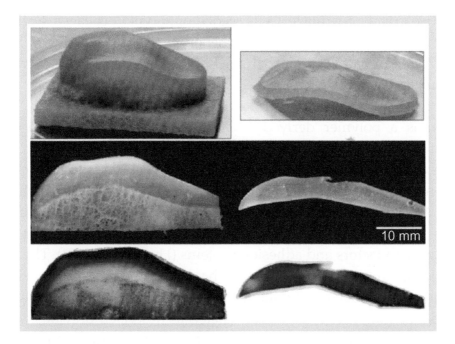

Figure 4.8 Agarose is often used as a scaffold material for articular cartilage tissue engineering in part because it can maintain complex shapes. Shown are osteochondral (left) and agarose-only (right) constructs in the shape of a patella. The bottom row is stained for sulfated glycosaminoglycans, which are a main component of articular cartilage. (From Hung, C. T. et al., *Ann Biomed Eng* 32(1): 35-49, 2004. With permission.)

chondrocytes (Saris et al. 2000; Elder et al. 2001; Hung et al. 2004). Since it is a continuous, hydrogel matrix, applied mechanical forces are transmitted to the embedded chondrocytes, stimulating them to produce extracellular matrix proteins (Mauck et al. 2000).

Another common scaffold material used for cartilage tissue engineering is collagen, specifically type I or II collagen. Collagen is the major component of extracellular matrix in cartilage (see Section 1.3). As with most other natural materials, collagen has to be purified before use to decrease its antigenicity. In studies investigating direct compression, type I collagen scaffolds have facilitated cartilaginous tissue formation (Hunter et al. 2002), as have collagen-glycosaminoglycan composite scaffolds (C. R. Lee et al. 2000; van Susante et al. 2001). However, type I collagen alone can also result in dedifferentiation of chondrocytes (Hutmacher 2001), likely due to the fact that type II collagen, not type I, is the predominant collagen

277

in native articular cartilage. Cells seeded onto type II collagen scaffolds show retention of the chondrocytic phenotype (Nehrer et al. 1997; Chang et al. 2009; Ko et al. 2009). Unfortunately, type II collagen scaffolds can be difficult and expensive to manufacture, due to limited availability.

Chitin is a polymer derived from the exoskeleton of crustaceans (Figure 4.9), although it is also naturally found in many arthropod shells and fungi cell walls. After deacetylation, chitin is termed chitosan and exhibits a high degree of biocompatibility *in vivo* (Hutmacher 2001; Abe et al. 2004; Kuo and Ku 2008). The molecular structure of chitosan is similar to many glycosaminoglycans, allowing it to interact with growth factors and adhesion proteins (Hutmacher 2001). The degradation of chitosan is controlled by the degree of deacetylation within the polymer, which can be altered during processing of the original chitin material. Unlike the natural materials described previously, chitosan scaffolds can degrade rapidly *in vivo* to allow space for the formation of new tissue (Hutmacher 2001). The porosity of the biomaterial can also be controlled during processing, effectively modulating the overall strength and elasticity of the scaffold (Madihally and Matthew 1999). Oftentimes, chitosan is combined with other molecules to create scaffolds that stimulate the secretion of cartilage matrix. In one such study, chondroitin sulfate was cross-linked with chitosan to form

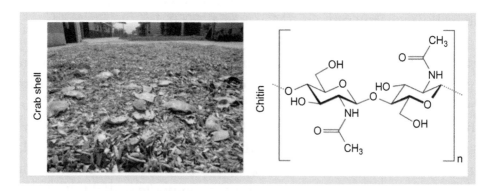

Figure 4.9 Left: Crustacean shells form the starting material for commercial chitin production. Right: Structure of chitin polymer demonstrating two of the *N*-acetylglucosamine units in a β-1,4 linkage. (Crab shell image © Biotech Surindo/ Fraunhofer IGB, Essen Germany. With permission.)

a scaffold that promoted the chondrocytic phenotype (Sechriest et al. 2000). Chitosan and its composites can also influence cell attachment and growth in culture. Endothelial and smooth muscle cells seeded onto a dextran sulfate-chitosan composite, heparin-chitosan composite, or chitosan material alone all showed positive effects in terms of cell attachment and proliferation. However, the glycosaminoglycan-chitosan composite actually inhibited attachment and growth (Chupa et al. 2000). The modification of chitosan scaffolds with glycosaminoglycan can dramatically change the overall characteristics of the scaffold. This flexibility is an attractive attribute that could make chitosan a useful material for articular cartilage engineering.

Silk, a naturally occurring polymer extruded from insects, has been increasingly used in biomedical applications. The material has good biocompatibility, slow degradation rates, and strong mechanical strength, and can be processed into many different forms useful for tissue engineering (Wang et al. 2006). Recent studies investigating silk scaffolds for cartilage engineering have shown good results using either primary chondrocytes or induced stem cells (Makaya et al. 2009; Chao et al. 2010; Y. Wang et al. 2010; Bhardwaj et al. 2011; Chlapanidas et al. 2011; Kawakami et al. 2011). In comparison to collagen-based scaffolds, silk constructs had higher type II collagen and glycosaminoglycan deposition, as well as better chondrocytic gene expressions in constructs seeded with mesenchymal stem cells (Meinel et al. 2004).

Fibrin glue is another naturally derived biomaterial that has been used in tissue regeneration studies (Westreich et al. 2004; Chou et al. 2007; Jung et al. 2010; Scotti et al. 2010; Z. H. Wang et al. 2010). It is made by mixing fibrinogen (Figure 4.10) with thrombin, which acts to solidify the material either in a defect site or in another scaffold material. Fibrin glue is popular because it is completely biodegradable and can be injected before it becomes solid. Unfortunately, the mechanical strength of fibrin glue is low, so its use as a primary scaffold in articular cartilage engineering is limited. Because of this, fibrin is often combined with other materials to enhance its structural integrity. Chondrocytes have been

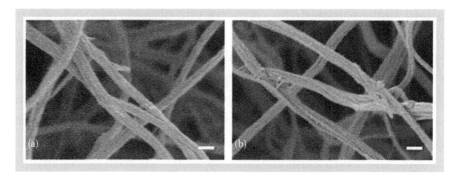

Figure 4.10 Scanning electron micrographs of thrombin-polymerized human fibrinogen at 80,000× (a) and 120,000× (b) magnification. (From Moreno-Arotzena, O. et al., *Materials (Basel)* 8(4): 1636-1651, 2015. Used under Creative Commons BY 4.0 License.)

seeded in pure fibrin glue (Silverman et al. 1999), as well as in mixtures with alginate (Almqvist et al. 2001; Perka et al. 2001) or collagen (Perka et al. 2000). Biochemical results did not show major differences from other scaffold materials. However, genipin cross-linked fibrin scaffolds showed accumulation of type II collagen and aggrecan with a corresponding increase in compressive and shear moduli (Dare et al. 2009).

Hyaluronan (HA) or hyaluronic acid is a polysaccharide that has been used to create biocompatible scaffolds for articular cartilage engineering applications (Yamane et al. 2005; Fan et al. 2010). HA is a nonsulfated glycosaminoglycan that helps in lubrication of the joint and forms the backbone of the proteoglycan macromolecules (see Section 1.3). It can be cross-linked to form a scaffold capable of supporting chondrocytes. Similar to fibrin glue, HA is injectable and performs well as a minimally invasive approach to filling irregularly shaped defects. However, HA has also been investigated for use as a solid, porous scaffold. Scaffolds made of an HA derivative that were implanted *in vivo* showed good histological results for cartilage matrix deposition (Grigolo et al. 2001). Other researchers found that cross-linked HA sponges produced better histological results than benzylated HA, which was, in turn, better than untreated defects (Solchaga et al. 2000). Integration with the host tissue improved in conjunction with histological findings.

A logical hypothesis in the field of tissue engineering is to expect better results when using scaffold materials made from the same molecules as those of the tissue being repaired (Badylak 2007). One method to achieve this is through reconstituted matrices. An early example of demineralized bone matrix scaffold for bone regeneration is the work of Urist (1965). More recent examples include decellularized heart (Figure 4.11) and tracheal tissues (Ott and Matthiesen 2008; Macchiarini et al. 2008). Growth factors and other bioactive molecules resident in harvested tissue are hypothesized to promote the formation of new matrix. Reconstituted matrices use this material to form scaffolds that allow for cell seeding and tissue growth. For example, articular cartilage can be harvested, homogenized, washed, and then frozen and lyophilized to create sponge-like scaffolds that promote chondrogenesis in adult stem cells (Cheng et al. 2008, 2011; Diekman et al. 2010).

Protein mixtures provide another variation on using naturally secreted matrix molecules as scaffold materials. Matrigel, a basement membrane analog, is used extensively in biological experiments (Kleinman et al. 1982). Thus, scaffolds formed from materials naturally present in the body provide an attractive approach toward facilitating the regeneration process.

4.3.2 Synthetic Scaffolds

Synthetic scaffold materials are fabricated commercially or in a research laboratory and, unlike natural polymers, can be customized in terms of their physical and chemical properties. Specific characteristics of a polymer, such as its mechanical strength and degradation profile, can be altered through modification of its chemical composition. This flexibility allows researchers to design scaffolds with known degradation rates, biological activity, or specific mechanical characteristics.

Poly-glycolides, poly-lactides, and their copolymers (Figure 4.12) are commonly used for scaffold materials and other biomedical applications (Athanasiou et al. 1995a,b, 1996, 1997, 1998; Vunjak-Novakovic and Freed 1998). These polymers can be formed into porous scaffolds,

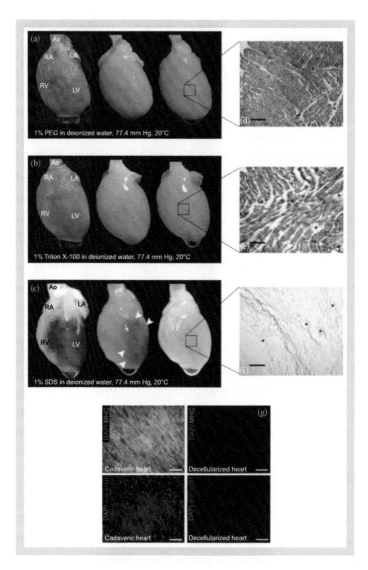

Figure 4.11 Rat hearts become more translucent as they are perfused and decellularized over 12 hours using PEG (a), Triton X-100 (b), or sodium dodecyl sulfate (SDS) (c). Ao, aorta; LA, left atrium; LV, left ventricle; RA, right atrium; RV, right ventricle. Hematoxylin and eosin (H&E) staining of thin sections from LV of rat hearts perfused with PEG (d), Triton X-100 (e), or SDS (f) showing retained nuclei and myofibers except with SDS treatment (scale bars 200 μm). (g) Immunofluorescent staining shows lack of DAPI-positive nuclei (purple), cardiac α-myosin heavy chain (green), or sarcomeric α-actin (red) in SDS decellularized heart (scale bars 50 μm). (From Ott, H. C. et al., *Nat Med* 14(2): 213-221, 2008. With permission.)

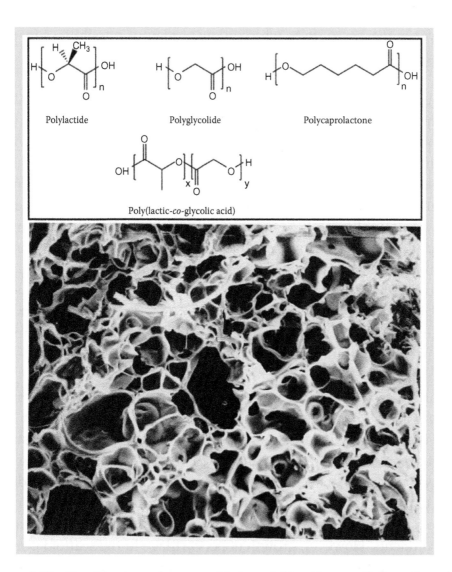

Figure 4.12 Top: Structure of common biodegradable polymers. Bottom: Scanning electron micrograph of microporous PLA-PGA polymer implant showing an average pore size of 150 μm and a porosity of 60% by volume (80× magnification). (Top image from Llorens, E. et al., *Polymers* 5(3): 1115-1157, 2013. Bottom image from Agrawal, C. M. et al., *Tissue Eng* 1(3): 241-252, 1995. With permission.)

nonwoven meshes, or felts, which allow numerous possibilities for scaffold shape and architecture.

Poly-glycolic acid (PGA), perhaps the most commonly used synthetic polymer in articular cartilage engineering, is an alpha polyester that degrades by hydrolytic scission. Total degradation can occur within 4-12 months, which is brief compared with other implanted polyesters (Daniels et al. 1990). Loss of mechanical properties occurs prior to this, sometimes as early as a few weeks. Since the degradation products of PGA are naturally resorbed into the body, it is attractive for many medical applications requiring biocompatibility. PGA can be formed into a porous scaffold by applying a salt-leaching process. The porosity and interconnectivity of the pores can be controlled by adjusting the amount of salt included during fabrication. PGA is often extruded as thin strands (~13 μm in diameter) that can be used for making sutures and threads or weaving three-dimensional structures (Freed et al. 1994a).

For articular cartilage engineering purposes, however, PGA is more commonly used as nonwoven mesh or felt. The porosity in mesh scaffolds is high, allowing good nutrient transfer throughout the construct. Furthermore, the interconnectivity of the pores increases seeding efficiency since cells can infiltrate throughout the scaffold. One major drawback to these mesh scaffolds is their mechanical properties. The initial scaffold structure is too weak to be immediately used in load-bearing environments. However, growth of neocartilage in the scaffold pores is hypothesized to compensate for the mechanical deficiencies of the scaffold itself. Over time, secreted matrix should fill the void space, giving the construct sufficient mechanical integrity to withstand the joint environment. Consistently good extracellular matrix production has been observed using PGA scaffolds, which, along with predictable degradation rates, makes PGA attractive for cartilage engineering experiments (Freed et al. 1993, 1994a, 1998). Past studies have also shown that PGA promotes more proteoglycan synthesis than other materials, such as collagen or poly-glycolide/lactide copolymers (Grande et al. 1997). While the predictable degradation profile of PGA is often seen as a positive trait, it can also cause problems for tissue engineering applications that require scaffold integrity longer than a few weeks. For these applications, other polymers have been investigated.

Another alpha polyester polymer, used extensively in the medical field, is poly-lactic acid (PLA), which, like PGA, has been approved by the Food and Drug Administration (FDA) for implantation in humans. PLA generally degrades more slowly than PGA, with a total degradation time ranging from 12 months to more than 2 years (Middleton and Tipton 2000). As molecular weight loss precedes mass loss, again, the loss of mechanical properties and scaffold integrity occur prior to mass degradation, which could cause an engineered construct to fail prematurely. As with PGA, the degradation products of PLA are resorbable, rendering PLA an attractive and biocompatible material for implantation, though the inability to clear byproducts of bulk degradation may result in adverse effects.

PLA exists in two stereoisometric forms, giving rise to four different types of PLA: poly-D-lactide, poly-L-lactide, poly-D,L-lactide, and poly-meso-lactide (Agrawal et al. 1995; Singhal et al. 1996; Hutmacher et al. 2001). Applications of the PLA isomers range from drug delivery to suture materials. The D- and L-monomers polymerize to form semi-crystalline structures that have been investigated as possible scaffolds for cartilage engineering. PLA scaffolds are primarily made as non-woven meshes due to the previous success of this structure for neocartilage formation. Studies have shown that chondrocytes might not have as great of an affinity for PLA surfaces as PGA surfaces, but over time, total cell numbers on the two materials are similar (Ishaug-Riley et al. 1999). Due to its slower degradation rate, PLA scaffolds allow more time for matrix formation before sudden loss of mechanical integrity. This is important for applications where the scaffold has to bear loads for a significant period after implantation.

Poly-lactic-co-glycolic acid (PLGA) is a copolymer composed of PGA and PLA monomers. The material properties of PLGA are dependent on the ratio of each monomer included in the macromolecule. For example, a formulation with a large fraction of PLA will degrade more slowly than one with a large fraction of PGA. Characterization of a 75/25 (PLA/PGA) copolymer showed a degradation time of 4-5 months, whereas a 50/50 copolymer degraded in only 1-2 months (Middleton and Tipton 2000). As with its base components, PLGA degrades into molecules that naturally resorb in the body. General biocompatibility has been investigated in large and small animal models, as well as in clinical trials (Athanasiou et al. 1997; Eid et al. 2001). PLGA has been used extensively as a suture material due to its high tensile strength and controllable degradation rates. It can be fabricated in forms similar to those of PGA and PLA (Zeltinger et al. 2001), with the nonwoven mesh being among the more preferred structures for current cartilage engineering studies.

Another popular synthetic polymer for cartilage engineering is polycaprolactone (PCL). This polymer possesses longer degradation times than PGA, PLA, and PLGA and is generally stronger, making it attractive for many orthopedic applications (Daniels et al. 1990). PCL can be extruded into threads for meshes or felts or formed into porous scaffolds through a salt-leaching process. As with other polyesters, PCL degrades through hydrolytic scission, but this process can take 1-2 years for total degradation of the material (Middleton and Tipton 2000). While this means the scaffold remains at the implant site, it also can help with the mechanical integrity of the construct during early time periods. The resistance of PCL to rapid hydrolysis is an attractive trait. Copolymers including PCL incorporate the strength and elasticity of the material while allowing slightly faster degradation times (Ishaug-Riley et al. 1999).

Poly-L-lactide-ε-caprolactone implanted into mice showed formation of cartilage-like structures after 4 weeks, with minimal degradation (Honda et al. 2000). More recently, a scaffold made of poly-ε-caprolactone hydroxyapatite (PCl-HA) composite with intramedullary stem and microchannels was produced (Figure 4.13) and used to replace the humeral head in the rabbit (Lee et al. 2010).

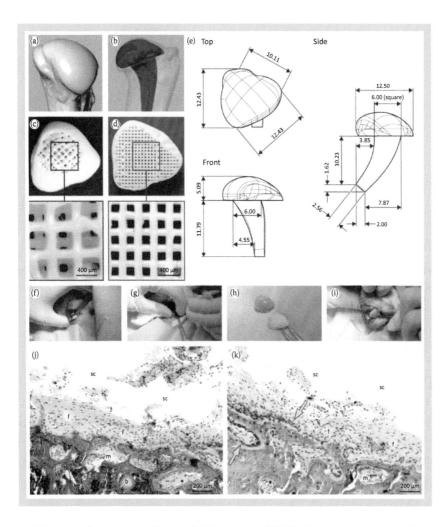

Figure 4.13 A shape-specific scaffold made of PCl-HA with intermedullary stem was designed to replicate the humeral head of the rabbit. (a-e) Design and production of the shape-specific implant with microchannels. (f-i) Implantation and press fit into humerus. Unlike experimental groups, in defect-only animals, H&E (j) and Safranin O (k) staining 4 months after surgery indicated little natural healing. sc, synovial joint cavity; f, fibrous tissue; b, bone; m, marrow. (From Lee, C. H. et al., *Lancet* 376(9739): 440-448, 2010. With permission.)

A more recent trend for synthetic polymers is to fabricate materials that can control the attachment of cells and proteins to the scaffold. The most common method to accomplish this is to modify the hydrophilicity or hydrophobicity of the material (Figure 4.14). Poly-ethylene glycol (PEG) is a polymer that prevents adsorption of proteins and cells due

287

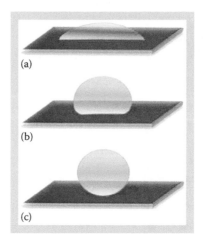

Figure 4.14 A water droplet on substrate figure illustrating the concept of hydrophilic (a), hydrophobic (b), and superhydrophobic (c) materials. (From Latthe, S. et al., *Molecules* 19(4): 4256, 2014. Used under a Creative Commons BY 3.0 License.)

to its high hydrophilicity. PEG can be incorporated into copolymers and thereby modify the cell attachment characteristics of a material. This property can be used to allow cell attachment on only certain portions of an implant or no cell attachment at all. The latter is one reason PEG is often used in copolymers, to improve biocompatibility (Suggs et al. 1999). The incorporation of PEG molecules increases hydrophilicity, which helps to prevent adsorption of antibodies and other proteins, thereby lessening any immune response.

PEG by itself is reported to have mechanical properties similar in compression to those of articular cartilage, with higher modulus values corresponding to higher molecular weights (Zimmermann et al. 2002). It has been copolymerized with a number of different materials to take advantage of its biocompatibility traits to create materials for a variety of applications (Han et al. 1998; Suggs et al. 1998a,b, 1999; Suggs and Mikos 1999; Bryant and Anseth 2001; Anseth et al. 2002; Fisher et al. 2002; Temenoff et al. 2002). Copolymerization is also necessary since PEG does not naturally degrade in the body, an attribute necessary for long-term success of an implanted construct. For articular cartilage engineering, degradation of the scaffold is desired to allow new tissue space to form.

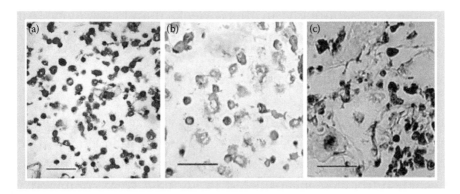

Figure 4.15 Histological section of ELP-chondrocyte constructs after 15 days of culture using H&E (a), toluidine blue (b), and Masson's trichrome (for collagen and ECM) (c) (scale bar 50 µm). (From Betre, H. et al., *Biomacromolecules* 3(5): 910-916, 2002. With permission.)

An alternative approach to synthetic polymers is the creation of macromolecules that imitate natural biomaterials. Researchers have successfully synthesized genetically engineered molecules, such as elastin-like polypeptide (ELP), that are similar to natural proteins found in the body (Figure 4.15) (Betre et al. 2002). Chondrocytes cultured in the gelled form of ELP maintained their phenotype, secreting matrix molecules such as sulfated glycosaminoglycans and collagen.

4.3.3 Composite Scaffolds

Natural and synthetic biomaterials span a large array of options for articular cartilage engineering. However, combining multiple types of materials provides the best solution for some applications. Composite scaffolds consist of two or more of the previously discussed materials incorporated into a single scaffold. This could include a naturally derived hydrogel infused throughout a synthetic mesh (or vice versa) or a fiber scaffold formed from several different natural and synthetic threads. For example, the void fraction of PLGA meshes can be filled with chondrocytes encapsulated in fibrin glue, which allows for a rounded cell phenotype, good cell distribution throughout the scaffold, and tunable degradation characteristics. This approach produced 2.6

times more glycosaminoglycan after 4 weeks than PLGA alone (Ameer et al. 2002). The inclusion of fibrin glue might have helped retain glycosaminoglycan molecules in the construct, whereas glycosaminoglycan simply diffused out of the bare PLGA scaffolds.

Infiltrating a fiber-based scaffold with a hydrogel is a popular form of composite scaffold. However, the cell-material interactions are critically important to the overall success of the construct. In previous studies, chondrocytes encapsulated in alginate were combined with either PLGA or demineralized bone matrix before implantation into mice for 8 weeks (Marijnissen et al. 2000). The PLGA-alginate composite produced type II collagen, a positive indicator of cartilage formation. The demineralized bone matrix-alginate composite, however, did not produce type II collagen. The cell response could be modified by substituting other hydrogels or including growth factors, but the base scaffold materials still play a major role in the type of matrix deposited in the construct.

Another approach to composite materials is to reinforce solid scaffolds with fibers oriented in specific directions. By embedding fibers in a scaffold, the mechanical properties can be modified to improve strength in preferred directions. This is particularly important for anisotropic tissues such as articular cartilage. Fiber-reinforced scaffolds can be fabricated using any combination of materials. Past studies have investigated PGA fiber-reinforced PLGA and found that the compressive modulus and yield strength improved by up to 20% (Slivka et al. 2001). Carbon fibers, while seemingly unadvisable for joint implantation, have been used with satisfactory clinical results for filling defects *in vivo* (Brittberg et al. 1994; Kus et al. 1999). Success rates of 70-80% were achieved based on qualitative measures of pain several years after implantation.

Composite scaffolds that incorporate several types of materials can help replicate the complex structure necessary for providing functional properties appropriate to load-bearing tissues (Moutos and

Guilak 2008). One approach that shows promise is to fabricate three-dimensional structures that exhibit mechanical properties similar to those of articular cartilage immediately after implantation. Woven scaffolds, such as alginate-filled PCL meshes (Moutos et al. 2007), can provide mechanical strength, anisotropy, and a beneficial growth environment (Figure 4.16).

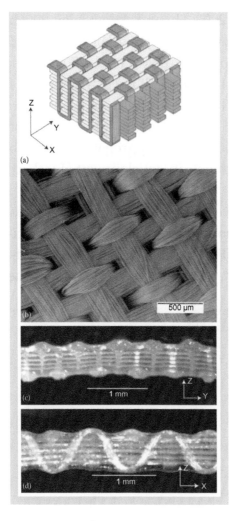

Figure 4.16 Woven composite scaffolds consisting of multiple interlocking layers. Cartoon schematic of woven layers (a), scanning electron micrograph of the surface (b), and cross sections of YZ and XZ planes (c and d). (From Moutos, F. T. et al., *Nat Mater* 6(2): 162-167, 2007. With permission.)

4.3.4 Scaffoldless

Though scaffolds can serve as an additional tool in controlling tissue development (e.g., with the slow release of growth factors or prepatterned to influence organization), they also bring with them issues such as degradation toxicity, stress shielding, and cell signaling hindrance. Techniques have also been developed using chondrocytes to create scaffoldless constructs (Boyle et al. 1995; Adkisson et al. 2001; Grogan et al. 2003; Masuda et al. 2003; Hu and Athanasiou 2006b). Chondrocyte pellets obtained by centrifugation have been cultured *in vitro*. Rotational cultures in bioreactors (Furukawa et al. 2003) and low-density seeding on agarose (Tacchetti et al. 1987) have also formed larger aggregates. It was proposed that the formation of numerous aggregates may serve as a three-dimensional culture methodology for chondrocyte expansion (Furukawa et al. 2003), while aggregates of limb bud cells have been used to examine parallels in development (Tacchetti et al. 1987).

Emerging from developmental studies, scaffoldless culture has been proposed as a method to engineer functional articular cartilage of sufficient dimensions (Figure 4.17). For instance, a self-assembling process has been developed, based on the differential adhesion hypothesis, to

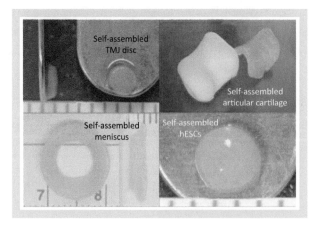

Figure 4.17 Gross appearance of various self-assembled cartilage tissues, indicating shape-specific production. From top left and moving clockwise: temporomandibular joint disc, hyaline articular cartilage, neocartilage using chondro-differentiated human embryonic stem cells, and knee meniscus.

produce robust cartilage constructs that contained two-thirds more glycosaminoglycan than native tissue, and collagen levels that reached one-third the amount of native tissue. Neocartilage, thus, formed contained collagen type II and chondrocytes in lacunae. More importantly, the compressive stiffness of self-assembled cartilage reached more than one-third of the native tissue values (Hu and Athanasiou 2006b).

Within a scaffoldless system, increased N-cadherin expression during neotissue formation suggested that differential adhesion mediated self-assembly (Ofek et al. 2008), while another study has shown that chondrocytes assemble via β1 integrins (Gigout et al. 2008). The biomechanical properties of scaffoldless cartilage have been studied (Graff et al. 2003; Revell et al. 2008), and within scaffoldless cartilage, several biochemical properties have recapitulated cartilage development. An increased proportion of collagen II, a decreased proportion of collagen type VI, a decreased chondroitin 6-to-4 sulfate ratio, and localization of collagen VI to the pericellular matrix (Figure 4.18) (Ofek et al. 2008) are all evidence of maturation in scaffoldless cartilage constructs. These studies showed that the self-assembling process mimics tissue development and maturation, suggesting that a set of exogenous stimuli could then be applied to augment tissue functional properties.

Various growth factors have been applied individually and in combination to self-assembled constructs, with TGF-β1 showing the greatest potency, inducing onefold increases in both aggregate modulus and tensile modulus, and increasing glycosaminoglycan and collagen content (Elder and Athanasiou 2009b). Scaffoldless constructs have also been cultured under various mechanical forces. Hydrostatic pressure stimulation (Elder and Athanasiou 2009c), shear and compression (Stoddart et al. 2006), and other forms of bioreactor culture (Furukawa et al. 2003; Katakai et al. 2009) have shown to be advantageous for scaffoldless constructs. Combined regimens of different classes of stimuli (biochemical and mechanical) have also been examined to show additive and synergistic effects on the functional properties of scaffoldless cartilage (Elder and Athanasiou 2008). Scaffoldless cartilage has also been implanted in goats (Brehm et al. 2006).

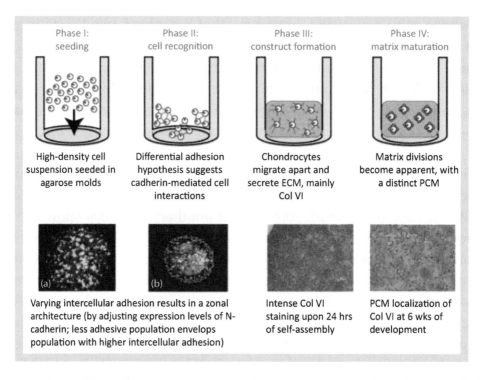

Figure 4.18 The self-assembling process is characterized by distinct phases that are reminiscent of certain developmental processes. Phases include seeding, cell recognition, construct formation, and matrix maturation. Using this scaffold-free approach, milestones in neocartilage formation mimic those seen during articular cartilage development. (Adapted from Ofek, G. et al., *PLoS One* 3(7): e2795, 2008. Used under a *PLoS One* Creative Commons License.)

4.3.5 Mimicking the Zonal Structural of Articular Cartilage

As mentioned previously, scaffolds serve multiple purposes for tissue engineering. The first is structural, providing a framework for cell attachment and arrangement, as well as organization of secreted matrix. Another purpose is stimulation, achieved through cell-substrate binding to cytokines, growth factors, or other functional moieties. The structure of the scaffold can also effectively modulate the stresses and strains experienced by seeded cells. This provides an extra level of complexity to the design of custom scaffolds. Cells seeded in one portion of the construct can be stimulated by intense forces, while other cells are completely shielded. This modulation ability is present in mature articular cartilage (Youn et al. 2006), where the extracellular-pericellular matrix interactions influence the level of strain experienced by individual chondrocytes. The superficial zone of articular cartilage undergoes higher overall strains compared with the middle or deep zones, but the properties of the tissue surrounding chondrocytes are such that these large variations are greatly lessened (Guilak et al. 1995).

The zonal structure of articular cartilage is an important characteristic in the functionality of the tissue. Chapter 1 described this structure in great detail, and it should be no surprise that many researchers have tried to reproduce it in engineered tissues (Sharma et al. 2007; Klein et al. 2009; Ng et al. 2009; Coates and Fisher 2010). While approaches have varied, the goal has typically been to create at least a superficial zone above a middle or deep zone. The superficial zone acts as a bearing surface, protecting the bulk construct from contact shear while also acting as a seal to retain secreted molecules. Other multizone attempts have focused on osteochondral constructs (Figure 4.19), with a cartilaginous region integrated seamlessly with an underlying bone region (Mow et al. 1991; Schreiber et al. 1999).

The materials used to create these scaffold structures range from fibrous polymers to innovative hydrogels (Seidi et al. 2011). An ideal engineered

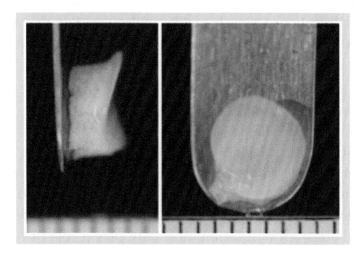

Figure 4.19 Shape-specific osteochondral constructs composed of hydroxapatite (thicker porous white portion) and living self-assembled tissue-engineered cartilage (thinner smooth beige portion). (Courtesy of Dr. Dan Huey.)

construct would reproduce the zonal structure of articular cartilage, particularly because the surrounding tissue also has a zonal structure and would interface better with similar biomechanical properties.

4.4 BIOACTIVE MOLECULES
FOR CARTILAGE ENGINEERING

Growth and development of articular cartilage relies heavily on biochemical signals. The sequence, duration, and intensity of stimulation can all play roles in how cells secrete matrix in a regenerating environment. Bioactive molecules can include growth factors, adhesion proteins, peptide sequences, or any other entity that binds to cells to create a biological response. There are more bioactive molecules present in the body than this chapter can easily encompass, so only a few of the more common growth factors, proteins, and peptides will be highlighted. All have shown proven effects for articular cartilage engineering, and future work will certainly make use of them to accelerate regeneration of functional tissues. Other, less often examined factors can encompass those described in Chapter 2, which discusses cartilage formation during development. Section 4.4.1 focuses initially on growth factors, specifically the TGF-β superfamily, followed by a description of possible scaffold modifications using bioactive molecules. For a more detailed description of growth factors, cytokines, morphogens, adhesion molecules, and mitogens for proliferation, see Chapter 2.

4.4.1 Growth Factors and Combinations

The inclusion of stimulatory growth factors is one of the most common means to accelerate tissue growth in engineered constructs. Many growth factors have been shown to be effective at stimulating cellular proliferation and matrix synthesis in articular cartilage, both *in vitro* and *in vivo*. Since growth factors normally play a role in healing and development, their therapeutic use is intended to replicate this function to promote rapid regeneration of a tissue. Varying amounts of growth factors are constantly present throughout the body, so higher concentrations are typically used in experiments to elicit more dramatic effects. For example, culture medium with 20% fetal bovine serum added was shown to have similar effects on proliferation and protein synthesis as a medium that included the three growth factors (TGF-β1, basic fibroblast growth factor [bFGF], and insulin-like growth factor 1 [IGF-1]) (Chaipinyo et al. 2002). Comparatively, lower concentrations of serum in the medium produced poorer results. The problem with serum, however, is that its composition and the concentrations of its components are generally unknown and can vary widely from source to source and batch to batch (Figure 4.20) (Bilgen et al. 2007).

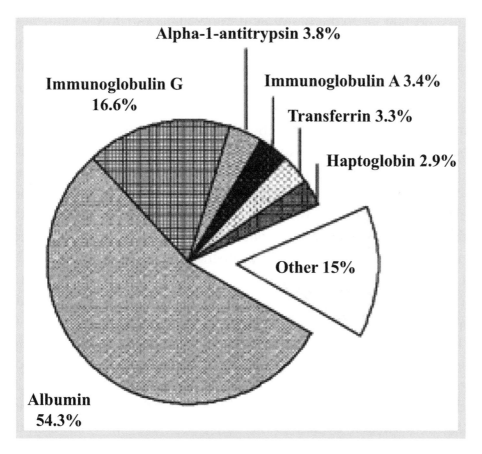

Figure 4.20 Protein composition of human serum by mass abundance. The first six identified proteins account for 85% of the total mass. (From Martosella, J., and N. Zolotarjova, *Methods Mol Biol* 425: 27-39, 2008. With permission.)

Growth factors are a means to stimulate a response using controlled amounts from an external source, which is important for safety concerns. The mechanisms by which growth factor stimulation occurs are discussed in detail in Chapter 2. The following information will focus on the effects of growth factors in terms of cartilage tissue engineering.

Growth factors can have a synergistic relationship with mechanical loading, which is particularly relevant for the engineering tissues that function in load-bearing environments, such as articular cartilage. *In vitro* experiments investigating the effect of growth factors in combination with mechanical stimulation have shown significant increases in matrix production compared with either stimulus alone (Bonassar et al. 2001; Gooch et al. 2001a; Blunk et al. 2002; Elder and Athanasiou 2008). Notably, as demonstrated using scaffoldless constructs formed by the self-assembly process, synergism between growth factors and mechanical stimuli has been observed with respect to improvements in functional properties. That is, the effect of the two stimuli combined is greater than the sum of their separate effects. A 164% increase in the aggregate modulus value (H_A), a 231% increase in the Young's modulus value (E_Y), an 85% increase in glycosaminoglycan/wet weight, and a 173% increase in collagen/wet weight relative to controls can be achieved when combining TGF-β1 and hydrostatic pressure (Elder and Athanasiou 2008). This relationship extends to the *in vivo* environment as well. The effects of soluble stimuli are often context dependent, and an example is GDFs eliciting the formation of either bone-, cartilage-, or tendon-like tissues depending on location and loading environment *in vivo* (Forslund and Aspenberg 2002). Many studies have also been performed with growth factors alone, without interaction with mechanical stimuli. Dramatic effects on proliferation, differentiation, and synthesis have been documented, for example, for IGF-1, bFGF, hepatocyte growth factor (HGF), and platelet-derived growth factor (PDGF) (Darling and Athanasiou 2004). Of particular interest is the TGF-β superfamily, which includes BMPs. This group of bioactive molecules has been shown to significantly stimulate chondrogenesis and bone growth, both of which are important for successful regeneration of osteochondral defects (Reddi 1998).

The TGF-β superfamily is a class of growth factors that is involved in the repair and inflammation response following injury (Frenkel et al. 2000). Numerous studies have shown that these growth factors can also elicit dramatic changes in articular chondrocytes. TGF-β1 is a popular isoform used in articular cartilage engineering studies. Effects are dependent on parameters such as dose, dosing frequency, and duration, and also the cell type and presence of other stimuli, leading to varied results that range from stimulating chondrogenesis and proliferation (Sporn et al. 1986; Guerne et al. 1994; Blunk et al. 2002) to inhibition of matrix formation (van der Kraan et al. 1992; Verschure et al. 1994) to promoting collagen formation (Sporn et al. 1986; Blunk et al. 2002; Elder and Athanasiou 2009b). The effectiveness of the growth factor is also dependent on the differentiation state of the cells. For example, TGF-β1 stimulated proliferation and proteoglycan synthesis in chondrocytes that were cultured for a week *in vitro*, but these effects were not apparent on freshly isolated chondrocytes (van der Kraan et al. 1992). Additionally, arthritic chondrocytes experienced a decrease in proteoglycan synthesis when treated with TGF-β1 (Verschure et al. 1994). Chondrocyte phenotype has been shown to change when placed in *in vitro* culture or in diseased environments, leading to altered responses to not only biochemical but also mechanical stimuli.

BMPs play a major role in endochondral bone formation and show general effects on cellular proliferation and matrix synthesis. As explained above, they are particularly attractive for cartilage engineering studies because they regulate both chondrogenesis and osteogenesis. Osteochondral integration is a critical factor in whether implants succeed or fail *in vivo*, so molecules that can stimulate this response are desirable (Pecina et al. 2002). As with TGF-β, BMPs can act synergistically with mechanical stimuli to accelerate regeneration of joint tissues. Currently, 20 types of BMPs have been identified, but only a subset has been examined for cartilage regeneration (Reddi 2003). BMPs generally have the ability to guide stem cells and immature bone and cartilage cells along the osteochondral pathway (O'Connor et al. 2000). BMP2 upregulated proteoglycan and collagen expression in chondrocytes

(Gooch et al. 2002; Pecina et al. 2002; Valcourt et al. 2002), while also inducing better healing of defects *in vivo* (Frenkel et al. 2000; Pecina et al. 2002). BMP4 showed an ability to stimulate proteoglycan synthesis, bone formation, and cellular proliferation (Luyten et al. 1992; Pecina et al. 2002). BMP7 also showed positive effects on matrix synthesis (Pecina et al. 2002) and proliferation (Mattioli-Belmonte et al. 1999), while also decreasing type I collagen expression and suppressing infiltration of fibroblasts *in vivo* (Kaps et al. 2002). Articular chondrocytes treated with either BMP12 or 13 synthesized elevated levels of glycosaminoglycan, although these increases were less than that observed for cells treated with BMP2 (Gooch et al. 2002). Overall, experimental results have shown that BMPs have a generally positive effect on cartilage differentiation and morphogenesis, whether alone or in combination with other growth factors. For example, BMP2 application with IGF-1 resulted in more than onefold increases in aggregate modulus, accompanied by increases in glycosaminoglycan production, compared with controls (Elder and Athanasiou 2008).

The TGF-β superfamily also includes several other groups of growth factors known to affect cartilage growth and differentiation. Cartilage-derived morphogenetic proteins (CDMPs), osteogenic proteins (OPs), and growth/differentiation factors (GDFs) have all been investigated as possible means to accelerate regeneration of joint tissues *in vitro* and *in vivo*. Some of the growth factors included in these groups are actually the same molecule. For example, the pairs OP-1/BMP7, CDMP1/GDF5, and CDMP2/GDF-6 are the same growth factors with alternate designations (see Chapter 2). All of these molecules can affect chondrocytes in a manner similar to that of other TGF-β superfamily members. OP-1, CDMP1, and CDMP2 all increase proteoglycan synthesis and cellular proliferation (Erlacher et al. 1998), although OP-1 was found to be the more effective stimulus (Gruber et al. 2001). GDF5, which is naturally present in articular cartilage, also increases proteoglycan synthesis (Pacifici et al. 2000).

Growth factors are typically delivered as soluble components in culture media. While this is acceptable for *in vitro* experiments, delivery becomes more complicated once the construct is implanted. An alternative approach is to include polymeric carriers, such as microspheres, in the construct so that growth factors are released over time (Figure 4.21) (Perka et al. 2001). Early approaches found little success since release from most polymers lasted only a few days. Once freed, growth factors can degrade within a week, so long-term treatments using these carriers would be infeasible (Ziegler et al. 2002). However, current research has indicated that alternative polymers, such as ELPs, have the capability to extend the release time of drugs to weeks or months (Betre et al. 2006). These carriers would allow long-term stimulation of the implant with a local source of growth factors, further stimulating matrix growth and possibly helping integration with the surrounding tissue.

Another alternative to long-term growth factor stimulation is to modify the gene expression of implanted cells using either transfection or other forms of exogenous genetic modification (Grimaud et al. 2002; Madry et al. 2002). In this case, growth factors are secreted by the modified cells

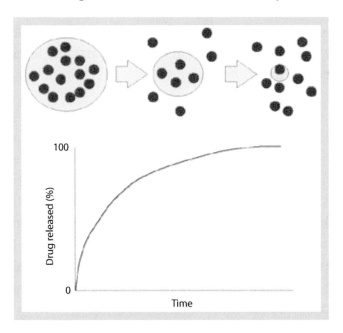

Figure 4.21 Release of drug (dark blue) from microsphere is controlled by the rate the microsphere (light blue) degrades; faster degradation leads to faster drug release. (From Putnam, D., *Nat Mater* 7(11): 836-837, 2008. With permission.)

within the defect site. The defect may be filled completely with modified cells, or only a fraction of the implanted cells may be modified. The modified gene can be conditionally active, which would be advantageous if stimulation is only desired for certain periods during regeneration. Both cost and ease of genetic modification have come down in recent years; commercially available kits allow for a variety of ways to introduce new DNA into cells. The long-term effects of elevated growth factor levels are not known, especially on neighboring tissues that are not involved with the cartilage repair process. However, control of how the new genes are expressed is being improved upon, and guidance is available for researchers on how to demonstrate the safety of altered cells.

Growth factors do not necessarily need to be available as freely diffusible molecules to induce a response from resident cells. Methods have been developed to tether TGF-β, IGF, PDGF, HGF, and FGF onto scaffolds while retaining activity. In contrast to freely diffusing molecules, scaffold-bound molecules can be more uniformly distributed within the scaffold, affecting all regions equally. Growth factor concentration can be sustained longer, and there is also a lower risk for tethered growth factors to elicit systemic effects.

Methods for incorporating growth factors into a construct include mixing the growth factor into the scaffold material or binding the growth factor onto the scaffold. Growth factors can be mixed into various polymers to control their release. For example, a hydrogel consisting of mostly water can enable growth factors to diffuse much faster than a dense polymer with a long degradation time. Incorporating multiple types of materials in a scaffold can allow for finer control of drug release, such as a two-phase PLGA implant loaded with TGF-β, which showed good results when implanted into osteochondral defects (Athanasiou et al. 1997). Microparticles are common for including growth factors in scaffolds with high-porosity and large-pore-size meshes and felts (Elisseeff et al. 2000). Since the degradation characteristics of the carrier polymer can be customized, protein release is more predictable.

302

Binding growth factors to the molecules that make up the scaffolds is another way to incorporate modulatory factors into constructs. The major drawback to this methodology is that immobilizing proteins often decreases their effectiveness. The active regions of a molecule can be obstructed once bound, although this is dependent on the protein being bound and the chemical reaction used to form the covalent bond. An example of how this can be implemented is the covalent binding of TGF-β1 to PEG (Mann et al. 2001b). Tethering of growth factors to the scaffold material is a promising means of retaining activity of the protein while still restricting its movement within a scaffold (Figure 4.22) (Fan et al. 2007).

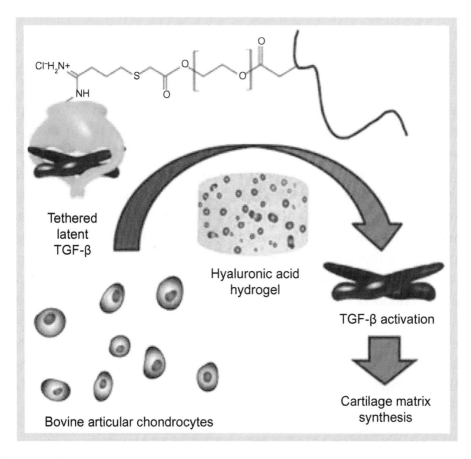

Figure 4.22 Latent TGF-β can be encapsulated within a hydrogel and bound to the material of the scaffold. (From Place, E. S. et al., *Adv Healthc Mater* 1(4): 480-484, 2012. With permission.)

The wide variety of growth factors available creates myriad combinations that could accelerate the growth process, but this must be tempered by knowledge of what additional effects each growth factor has on the construct and surrounding tissues. Combinations of multiple growth factors might be the best approach to creating a functional tissue. For example, IGF-1 has been used to increase glycosaminoglycan synthesis, TGF-β1 for improving collagen content, and interleukin 4 for minimizing glycosaminoglycan-depleted regions in a construct (Blunk et al. 2002). Whether growth factors are applied in a soluble form, encapsulated in polymeric carriers, or chemically bound to a scaffold surface, they are an integral part of the cartilage engineering process and will continue to be a major area of focus for tissue regeneration therapies in the future.

4.4.2 Protein Coating and Peptide Inclusion

In addition to growth factors, scaffolds can also be modified with protein coating, peptide incorporation, or micropatterning to alter cell attachment characteristics. The first two of these approaches capitalize on integrin-receptor relationships between cells and extracellular matrix proteins to direct cell attachment in a controlled manner. Integrins expressed by chondrocytes and the corresponding sequences to which they bind are discussed in Section 2.1.1, and cells have been coaxed into adhering to various structures coated with the appropriate proteins and sequences (LeBaron and Athanasiou 2000). Integrins identified on chondrocytes include $\alpha_1\beta_1$, $\alpha_2\beta_1$, $\alpha_5\beta_1$, $\alpha_V\beta_5$, $\alpha_V\beta_3$, and $\alpha_3\beta_1$, with the latter two being more prevalent on superficial zone chondrocytes than deep zone chondrocytes (Woods et al. 1994; Shimizu et al. 1997). Biomaterials can be modified with proteins that bind to one or more of these integrins to control cell attachment to different regions of the scaffold.

In addition to cell adhesion, extracellular matrix proteins can also promote the haptotactic and chemotactic motility of chondrocytes (Figure 4.23). By modifying the adhesion characteristics of a biomaterial,

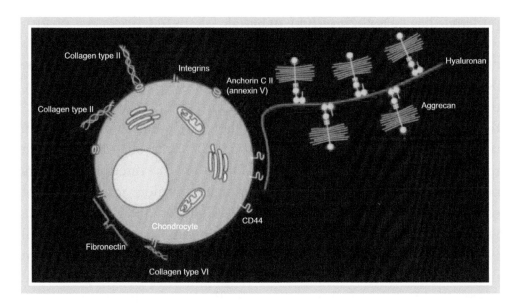

Figure 4.23 Schematic of chondrocyte receptors and their interactions with the extracellular matrix. (From Knudson, W., and R. F. Loeser, *Cell Mol Life Sci* 59(1): 36-44, 2002. With permission.)

cellular migration into a scaffold can be increased or decreased (Shimizu et al. 1997). Adsorption of fibronectin onto a polymer scaffold showed an increase in cell attachment and ingrowth compared with uncoated controls (Bhati et al. 2001). The benefits of increased cell migration have also been observed for *in vivo* experiments. HA scaffolds coated with fibronectin showed increased tissue ingrowth after implantation into osteochondral defects (Solchaga et al. 2002). This ingrowth helped to improve integration with the surrounding bone and cartilage, which is very important for the long-term success of the implant.

One of the more common methods to modify the attachment characteristics of a surface is to coat it with proteins. The hydrophobicity or hydrophilicity of a material determines the degree of surface interaction. Hydrophobic materials in particular allow proteins to readily adsorb to their surfaces, with more hydrophobic materials forming a stronger interaction than less hydrophobic materials (Prime and Whitesides 1991). Following adsorption, cells can then bind to the proteins that coat the scaffold material. Changing the types of proteins adsorbed would bias which cells attach preferentially. Scaffolds not coated with exogenous proteins can by coated by proteins from the body once implanted. Controlling whether proteins such as collagen, thrombospondin, osteopontin, bone sialoprotein, fibronectin, vitronectin, fibrinogen, von Willebrand factor, laminin, entactin, and tenascin (Ruoslahti 1996; LeBaron and Athanasiou 2000) can adsorb helps with the biocompatibility of an implant. Based on the integrin receptors present on chondrocytes, all of these proteins promote adhesion except osteopontin and entactin (Hubbell 1997). Collagen and fibronectin are widely used for cartilage applications, although a large variety of cell types, not just chondrocytes, have shown an affinity for these abundant proteins. In native tissues, extracellular matrix molecules help transmit mechanical and chemical stimuli to cells. Replicating this function in an engineered construct is one of the objectives of using protein coatings. Naturally secreted proteins will likely play a more dominant role as the engineered construct develops, but protein and peptide sequences incorporated into the scaffold can strongly guide the initial formation of an engineered construct.

Collagen has been investigated extensively as a bulk scaffold material for tissue engineering. Since chondrocytes readily attach to collagen surfaces (V. Lee et al. 2000), collagen is a logical choice for coating materials that are otherwise not amenable to cell attachment. The type of collagen used can play an important role in influencing not only attachment, but also phenotype, since the primary collagen in articular cartilage is type II, not type I. Past studies have shown that chondrocytes have a preference for a type II collagen fragment-coated surface over a type I collagen-coated surface, possibly due to the integrin receptors expressed by articular chondrocytes (Jennings et al. 2001). While beneficial for cell adhesion, collagen alone does not appear to help chondrocytes in retaining chondrogenic gene expression when the cells are cultured in monolayer (Darling and Athanasiou 2005b). For cartilage regeneration, collagen is used more often as a scaffold material and less often as a coating.

306

Vitronectin is another protein that has been investigated as a scaffold coating for tissue engineering. Past results showed that vitronectin controls osteoblast attachment and spreading, as opposed to a more abundant protein like fibronectin, when used as a coating *in vitro* (Thomas et al. 1997). While these findings are not directly applicable to chondrocytes, vitronectin could still be important in modulating the attachment of cells in osteochondral constructs. Other experimental studies investigating vitronectin have shown that it competes better than most proteins when adsorbing to surfaces in the presence of serum (Wyre and Downes 2002). Adhesion of chondrocytes to vitronectin may be through the $\alpha_5\beta_1$, $\alpha_V\beta_5$, and $\alpha_V\beta_3$ integrins.

Cartilage matrix protein (CMP), not to be confused with cartilage oligomeric matrix protein (COMP), is expressed almost exclusively in cartilage (Choi et al. 1983). CMP binds to aggrecan and type II collagen, and chondrocytes attach to it via the $\alpha_1\beta_1$ integrin. When used as a coating material, CMP enhanced both cell attachment and spreading on surfaces (Makihira et al. 1999). The addition of type II collagen to the CMP coating showed an improvement in these characteristics. Because CMP is specific to cartilage tissue, it might be a more appropriate protein to target for coating purposes, although issues such as ease of production and cost would certainly be important factors.

Functional cartilage constructs will have to be designed as three-dimensional structures, but preliminary experiments are often conducted in monolayer to investigate questions such as cell-surface interactions. Micro- and nano-technologies now allow for precise control of protein placement on a variety of surfaces (Figure 4.24). Technologies such as soft lithography and self-assembled monolayers allow protein stamping on materials that restrict the attachment of cells to specific regions (Gallant et al. 2002). Custom designs incorporating multiple types of proteins are feasible using these techniques, making possible a wide variety of experiments at the cell, versus the tissue, level. Patterning techniques can be translated to the three-dimensional formation of tissues as an additive manufacturing technique (see Section 6.1.2).

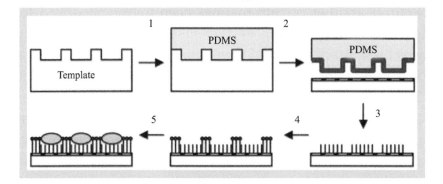

Figure 4.24 Steps involved in microcontact printing using a silicon stamp for micropatterning. (1) A template is used to cast a polydimethylsiloxane (PDMS) stamp. (2) The stamp is coated with alkanethiol and (3) used to transfer the alkanethiol to Au-coated substrate, creating a patterned self-assembled monolayer. (4) The surface is then exposed to a solution containing a different alkanethiol to cover bare Au areas. (5) In this schematic example, proteins adsorb preferentially onto one type of SAM, creating adhesive and nonadhesive domains. (From Gallant, N. D. et al., *Langmuir* 18: 5579-5584, 2002. With permission.)

An attractive alternative to protein coating is to use only the amino acid sequences, or peptides, derived from the larger protein, that are involved in cell-surface binding. The peptides are chemically bound to the scaffold instead of being adsorbed. The number of binding sites and their location can be controlled during fabrication by the density and distribution of the peptides. After modification, materials that are otherwise not amenable to cell attachment can now be successfully seeded and used in tissue engineering applications. In addition to promoting attachment, peptide sequences can also stimulate gene expression and protein synthesis.

Peptides are typically grafted to a material by covalent bonds, which securely attach sequences to a location and prevent their diffusion through the construct or disassociation from the surface. However, as noted previously, chemical binding can have the negative effect of reducing the peptide's biological activity. Tethering the molecules via a linker chain can help prevent this by moving the peptide away from the surface, reducing steric hindrance, and allowing more flexibility in its binding configuration with cells (Figure 4.25) (LeBaron and Athanasiou 2000).

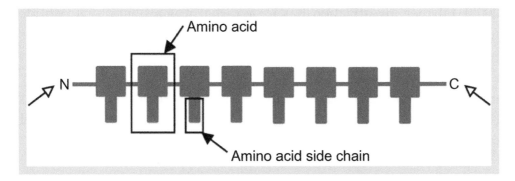

Figure 4.25 An eight-amino-acid peptide is illustrated. Common target sites for immobilization chemistry are noted. Certain amino acid side chains and the amino- and carboxy-terminus are reactive moieties that can be used. (Redrawn from LeBaron, R. G., and K. A. Athanasiou, *Tissue Eng* 6(2): 85-103, 2000. With permission.)

Often, peptides are grafted to biomaterials that, by themselves, do not promote cell attachment. With the addition of different types and concentrations of proteins and peptides at specific locations of the scaffold, scaffolds can be designed with custom attachment characteristics.

The peptide density on a material controls both cell attachment and motility. Increasing the concentration of peptides can increase attachment, but cell migration will eventually be hindered (LeBaron and Athanasiou 2000). Balancing these two parameters is difficult and is highly dependent on cell type and application. For example, if it is desirable for cells to populate the center of a construct, the peptide density cannot be so high as to impede migration. While this might reduce cell attachment during seeding, other parameters, such as the duration of seeding or the total number of cells seeded, might be adjusted to improve seeding efficiency. Alternatively, integrin clustering can be used to help facilitate migration without totally restricting cell motility (Shimizu et al. 1997). This approach is especially important for applications that require ingrowth of surrounding cells into the construct.

The most common peptide sequence used for cell attachment is Arg-Gly-Asp (RGD), which was originally identified as a recognition sequence located on the larger fibronectin molecule (LeBaron and Athanasiou

2000). Further investigation has shown that it is a ubiquitous peptide found in many species of both plants and animals, demonstrating its importance and longevity in evolution (Koivunen et al. 1994). RGD exhibits an ability to bind with 8-12 integrins (out of 20+ currently identified), making it very useful for tissue engineering applications (Ruoslahti 1996). In chondrocytes, RGD binds strongly to $\alpha_5\beta_1$, $\alpha_V\beta_5$, and $\alpha_V\beta_3$ and weakly to $\alpha_3\beta_1$ (Figure 4.26).

Other than RGD, other peptides that have known activities include KGD (αIIbβ3), PECAM ($\alpha_V\beta_3$), KQAGDV ($\alpha_{IIb}\beta_3$), LDV ($\alpha_4\beta_1$ and $\alpha_4\beta_7$), YGYYGDALR and FYFDLR ($\alpha_2\beta_1$), and RLD/KRLDGS ($\alpha_V\beta_3$ and $\alpha_M\beta_2$) (Koivunen et al. 1994; Pasqualini et al. 1996; Ruoslahti 1996).

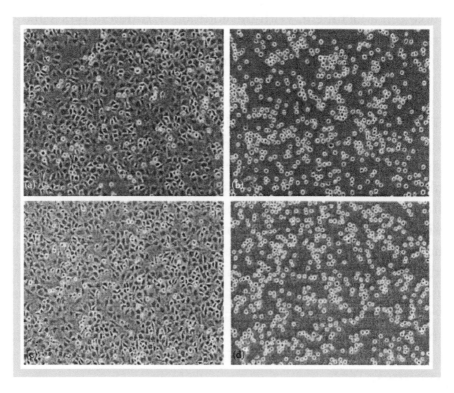

Figure 4.26 Chondrocyte attachment on peptide-coated surfaces is enhanced by RGD-containing peptides. Chondrocytes were incubated on glass coverslips coated with a GRGDSP peptide (a), heparin binding peptide (b), intact fibronectin (c), and ovalbumin (d). (From LeBaron, R. G., and K. A. Athanasiou, *Tissue Eng* 6(2): 85-103, 2000. With permission.)

Chondrocytes have shown a strong binding affinity for RGD, PECAM, YGYYGDALR, FYFDLR, and RLD/KRLDGS with weak binding for KQAGDV and LDV (Ruoslahti 1996).

Short peptide sequences are often preferred because of their versatility. For example, GRGD can be synthesized onto the end of hydrophilic linker chains that are attached to an underlying bulk material, thereby allowing cell seeding on scaffolds that would otherwise not be conducive to cell attachment (Jo et al. 2000). However, functional peptide sequences do not need to be short. Long sequences corresponding to specific attachment proteins have been used successfully to modify scaffold materials. Importantly, the key sequence (e.g., RGD) must be accessible to cells. Sequences such as GRGD (Jo et al. 2000), GRGDSP (Pierschbacher and Ruoslahti 1984), and CGGNGEPRGDTYRAY (Rezania et al. 1997) all use the RGD sequence to facilitate cell binding, but the peptides are modeled on different proteins (e.g., the latter is from bone sialoprotein).

A number of researchers have been investigating how peptides can be incorporated into three-dimensional scaffolds for use in tissue engineering (Mann et al. 2001a; Gobin and West 2002; Petersen et al. 2002). Peptides can be incorporated into hydrogel scaffolds or grafted onto the exposed surfaces of porous scaffolds. As in monolayer, cells are expected to bind to available peptides, thereby altering cellular proliferation, migration, and differentiation. Alginate modified with RGD has been shown to promote cell adhesion, spreading, and chondrocytic differentiation (Alsberg et al. 2001). Other studies using adhesion peptides and PEG hydrogels showed a reduction in proliferation and protein synthesis (Mann et al. 1999; Mann and West 2002). These discrepancies may be caused by differences in peptide density and distribution, which are more difficult to control in three dimension than in two dimensions (monolayer culture).

As with proteins, peptides can be micropatterned to create specific designs on surfaces (Britland et al. 1992; Lom et al. 1993; Chen et al. 1997; Dike et al. 1999). The objective of these types of experiments often focuses on furthering our understanding of how cells attach. Integrin binding reactions can be investigated in a controlled environment using this experimental setup. Additionally, micropatterning can be used to control the geometry of single cells, allowing investigations of cytoskeletal structures. Interactions between different cell populations have also been studied using monolayer micropatterning (Lee et al. 2006). As with protein stamping, peptide-patterned regions allow cell attachment, whereas the rest of the surface does not. Theoretically, if different peptides are patterned in specific regions, then only cells expressing the corresponding integrins will be able to bind to each region. This approach would create a surface with segregated populations based on cell phenotype and would be interesting for coculture experiments.

Micropatterning can control cell morphology by defining where cells are allowed to attach. Cell shape has been shown to influence whether a cell will proliferate, die, or differentiate (Chen et al. 1997). For some cell types, a spread or flat morphology promotes proliferation, while a rounded morphology promotes apoptosis and cell death. Patterned surfaces that fall in between and promote neither growth nor death have been shown to induce cell differentiation (Dike et al. 1999). For each cell type, peptide densities and distributions will need to be optimized to promote proliferation and differentiation. For example, a high density of peptides distributed evenly across a surface may promote cell spreading, whereas a low density of the same peptide might promote a rounded morphology instead. It should be noted that a spherical morphology is highly correlated with the chondrogenic phenotype, and, thus, micropatterning that promotes this morphology may be beneficial in cartilage tissue engineering.

Micropatterning is not limited to stamping peptides and proteins. It can also alter the topography of a surface, which in turn can affect cell attachment, proliferation, and gene or protein expression (Bettinger et al. 2009). By controlling how strongly a cell is bound to the surface, micropatterning affects the migration and proliferation of attached

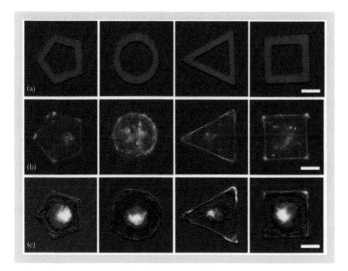

Figure 4.27 Cell adhesion on poly-*N*-isopropylacrylamide (PNIPAM) micropatterns. (a) Various shapes micropatterned with PNIPAM onto glass and coated with fibronectin and fibrinogen-A546 for visualization (red). (b) Mouse embryonic fibroblasts seeded onto the fibronectin-coated micropatterns and stained for F-actin (green). (c) Average distribution of F-actin for cells seeded onto the micropattern. All scale bars are 15 µm. (From Mandal, K. et al., *PLoS One* 7(5): e37548, 2012. With permission.)

cells (Figure 4.27). In general, rough surfaces at the submicron scale allow for weak cell attachment and inhibit extensive spreading, whereas smooth surfaces promote strong attachment and spreading, as well as proliferation and migration. Aligned topographies have also been shown to affect cell morphology and differentiation (Yim et al. 2007).

4.4.3 Catabolic and Other Structure Modifying Factors

While it is counterintuitive to apply catabolic factors to fabricate a piece of tissue, the enzyme chondroitinase ABC (C-ABC) has been applied to cartilage constructs to deplete glycosaminoglycan content and results in improved biomechanical properties (Asanbaeva et al. 2008b; Bian et al. 2009; Natoli et al. 2009a,b; Responte et al. 2012). One hypothesis is that the organization of collagen and other matrix molecules is inhibited by the early presence of glycosaminoglycan in the construct. By removing it, the matrix can become denser, after which glycosaminoglycan can continue to be synthesized and incorporate itself into the newly formed matrix. C-ABC has been shown to increase tensile properties of self-assembled articular cartilage without compromising compressive properties, as glycosaminoglycan levels return posttreatment (Natoli et al. 2009a). Multiple C-ABC treatments further increased tensile properties, reaching values of 3.4 and 1.4 MPa for the tensile modulus and ultimate tensile strength, respectively (Natoli and Athanasiou 2009). C-ABC represents an exciting method for engineering functional articular cartilage by departing from conventional anabolic approaches.

Another structure-modifying agent is lysyl oxidase, which acts to cross-link collagen (Figure 4.28) (Siegel et al. 1970; Makris et al. 2014b). When cartilage explants were treated with β-aminopropionitrile, an inhibitor of lysyl oxidase, both the amount of new cross-links and tensile integrity decreased (Wong et al. 2002; McGowan and Sah 2005; Asanbaeva et al. 2008a). One of the regulatory pathways for lysyl oxidase is through hypoxia-inducible factor (HIF). Hypoxia culture stabilizes HIF-α, leading to the upregulation of lysyl oxidase, resulting in increased cross-links and tensile properties for a variety of native, musculoskeletal soft tissues, including cartilage, fibrocartilage, and ligament (Makris et al. 2014a,b), and also for engineered articular cartilage. Applying lysyl oxidase is also useful in increasing the strength of the interface between engineered and native articular cartilage, leading to its potential use for implant integration (Athens et al. 2013).

Mechanical loading, which will be discussed extensively in the next section, can also have a catabolic effect on articular cartilage matrix. In addition to stimulating anabolic activity from the seeded cells, mechanical forces can upregulate the expression of matrix metalloproteinases (MMPs) 1, 3, and 13, which act to degrade articular cartilage matrix molecules (Nicodemus and Bryant 2010). Once synthesized, these MMPs may help restructure an engineered tissue to better withstand loading. This mimics the natural process that occurs

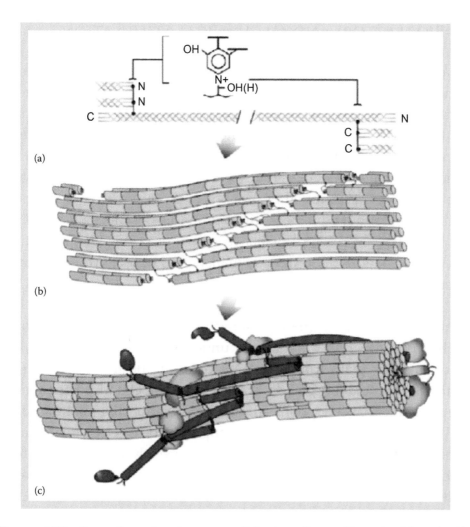

Figure 4.28 Formation of mature cross-links in collagen fibers is driven by the action of lysyl oxidase and subsequent fibril formation. (a) Axial stagger of individual collagen molecules is needed to form pyridinoline (PYR) cross-links between molecules. (b) Fibers group and hydroxylysyl-PYR collagen cross-links form in the large structure, producing the mature (c) heterotypic fibril consisting of type II (yellow), type IX (red), and type XI (blue) collagens. (From Makris, E. A. et al., *Proc Natl Acad Sci USA* 111(45): E4832-4841, 2014. With permission.)

in many tissues throughout the body. Essentially, repairs have to be made to the tissue structure over time, which requires both removing old matrix and adding new matrix. Catabolic activity occurring during remodeling is a critical factor for the eventual functionality of an engineered tissue.

4.5 BIOREACTORS AND MECHANICAL STIMULATION

For articular cartilage, compressive, tensile, and frictional properties are of the utmost importance, and so are the tissue's general wear characteristics. An *in vitro* tissue engineering approach should focus on improving these properties before implantation, and this can be achieved through culture in bioreactors that apply mechanical stimuli. Direct compression and, especially, hydrostatic pressure have been shown to help stimulate the secretion of proteins and other matrix components that contribute to the biomechanical properties of the construct. Low- and high-shear bioreactors also have shown promise in growing functional constructs, perhaps due to the increased nutrient transfer during stimulation.

Although the precise signaling pathways involved in the mediation of mechanostimuli are not completely understood (see Section 1.2.3), evidence suggests that certain types of forces are desirable for cartilage synthesis and modeling. Under static conditions, chondrocytes synthesize a matrix that has poor collagen organization (Dunkelman et al. 1995). Since static culture conditions appear to be inadequate, dynamic culture conditions have been studied extensively for their beneficial effects on articular cartilage synthesis and organization. The creation of cartilaginous material in bioreactors is a promising means to produce tissue constructs (Dunkelman et al. 1995; Freed et al. 1998). In general, the composition, morphology, and biomechanical properties of cartilage synthesized in a bioreactor appear better than those of cartilage grown under static conditions (Vunjak-Novakovic et al. 1999).

Articular cartilage is a mechanically sensitive tissue that can respond favorably or unfavorably to biomechanical stimuli. The results from experimental studies included in this section combine many different approaches for enhancing cartilage regeneration. However, direct comparisons are difficult due to the variety of cell sources, media formulations, and general laboratory practices used from study to study. In general, cell-seeded scaffolds, or constructs, are cultured *in vitro* to produce neotissue with the intent of achieving sufficient mechanical and biochemical properties for implantation.

This section includes descriptions of past and current bioreactors used for stimulating articular cartilage explants or engineered constructs. The categories included in this review of biomechanical stimulation include

- Compression
- Hydrostatic pressure
- High-shear systems (direct fluid perfusion and contact and fluid-surface shearing)
- Low-shear systems (enhanced nutrient transport and "micro-gravity" bioreactors)
- Hybrid bioreactors incorporating multiple loading regimes

4.5.1 Compression

Compressive loading is a major component of normal mechanical stimulation within diarthrodial joints. For example, during standing or walking articular cartilage of the femoral condyle and tibial plateau (and the fibrocartilaginous menisci) experience compression (Figure 4.29). Studies

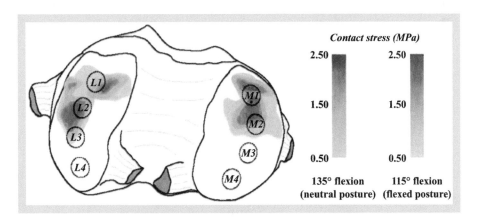

Figure 4.29 Regions of contact stress at the 135° neutral posture and 115° flexed posture in a bovine knee show pressure distributions corresponding to compressive loading in the lateral (L) and medial (M) condyles. (From Neu, C. P. et al., *Arthritis Rheum* 56(11): 3706-3714, 2007. With permission.)

focusing on direct compression typically use platens (Figure 4.30). Static or dynamic loading with these devices mechanically deforms the sample. The mechanism for how direct compression stimulates matrix production in chondrocytes is not fully known, although potential mechanisms are described in Section 1.2.3. While the mechanical stimulus is undoubtedly a major factor, enhanced nutrient transfer and removal of waste products may also be contributing factors (Kim et al. 1994).

Proteoglycan synthesis has often been used in studies as an indicator that a mechanical stimulation is beneficial, although some studies also use DNA synthesis, collagen synthesis, or aggregate modulus as gauges. The incorporation of radioisotopes is one way to measure macromolecule formation, as are the various biochemical assays described in Chapter 7. Synthesis is not necessarily a measure of composition, however, and matrix molecules need to be retained and organized within the construct to impart functional mechanical properties.

Applying direct compression to engineered constructs often consists of moving constructs from static culture to a bioreactor that applies the loading. Bioreactors with medium perfusion may remove the need for manual feeding, allowing the samples to remain in the bioreactor for the study's duration and decreasing the possibility for contamination

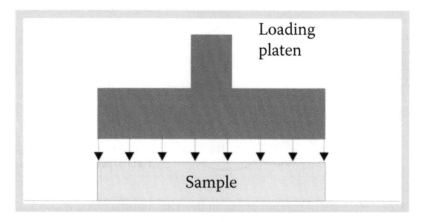

Figure 4.30 Direct compression of a single sample applies a unidirectional force across a uniform area.

(Demarteau et al. 2003; Schulz et al. 2008). Static compression has been shown to inhibit matrix secretion (Kim et al. 1994; Buschmann et al. 1995; Torzilli et al. 1997; Bonassar et al. 2001; Elder et al. 2001; Davisson et al. 2002a), leading to devices designed for dynamic loading (Palmoski and Brandt 1984). However, it has been postulated that it is not necessarily the static mechanical load that is detrimental, but the limited diffusion of wastes and nutrients under static loading, leading possibly to a decrease in the pH of the local environment (Kim et al. 1994).

Dynamic compression, which alternates between loading and unloading the sample, has been shown to be a beneficial stimulus when compared with static compression. The benefits of dynamic compression appear to be uniform throughout the constructs (Kelly et al. 2009). A variety of methods and devices have been constructed to apply compression, and the results for these studies vary widely even under the same testing conditions. The main parameters that are reported are the frequency of the applied load, the duty cycle, the strain or force used, and the duration of the experiment.

Frequencies ranging from 0.0001 to 3 Hz, strains from 0.1% to 25%, loads from 0.1 to 24 MPa, and durations lasting from hours to weeks have been examined for direct compression of cartilage (Sah et al. 1989; Buschmann et al. 1995; D. A. Lee et al. 2000; Mauck et al. 2000, 2006; Bonassar et al. 2001; Kisiday et al. 2004; Campbell et al. 2006; Bougault et al. 2008; Jung et al. 2008; Pelaez et al. 2008; P. Y. Wang et al. 2009; Q. G. Wang et al. 2009). Duty cycle adjustments and alternative loading regimens provide ample areas of investigation, all of which need to be optimized to allow for rapid formation of functional tissue. Challenges prevalent in the application of direct compression include lift-off of the compression platen from the cartilage sample, the changing properties of maturing tissues, and scale-up. As cartilage is compressed, its thickness decreases. With load removal, the rate at which the thickness recovers is dependent on the tissue's viscoelastic properties. The recovery rate is experimentally determined and not known *a priori*, and without knowing this rate, a compression platen may be raised too quickly during the unloading phase of a dynamic compression regimen, causing platen lift-off. As the engineered constructs mature, their mechanical properties change, leading to different rates of recovery. The same amount of strain applied at early culture times may result in much larger stress when applied at later culture times, when the constructs are stiffer. Even at the same time point, variations in the thickness and mechanical properties of each construct can make it difficult to apply the same mechanical stimulus simultaneously to many constructs. Despite these limitations, dynamic compression has shown to be beneficial for improving construct properties over a wide range of loads and frequencies.

Dynamic, direct compression applied to articular cartilage explants or cell-seeded constructs can induce increases in proteoglycan and collagen synthesis, as well as more robust biomechanical properties (Figure 4.31). Dynamic loading increased ³⁵S-sulfate and ³H-proline

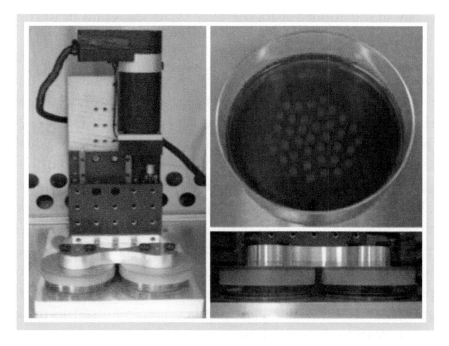

Figure 4.31 Example of a dynamic direct compression loading bioreactor used to apply cyclic compressive loading to two petri dishes simultaneously, each containing cell-seeded agarose constructs (left). (From Mauck, R. L. et al., *Biomech Model Mechanobiol* 6(1-2): 113-125, 2007. With permission.)

incorporation, indicators of proteoglycan and collagen synthesis, respectively, by 15-40% (Sah et al. 1989; Buschmann et al. 1995). More dramatic results were obtained when dynamic compression was applied in conjunction with a growth factor. For example, proteoglycan and collagen synthesis was increased 180% and 290%, respectively, when the growth factor IGF-1 was included during a 0.1 Hz, 3% compression regimen (Bonassar et al. 2001). However, chondrocytes in the tissue were shown to respond differently based on their depth in the tissue. Cells from the deep zone of cartilage explants produced 50% more glycosaminoglycan than static controls under a 1 Hz, 15% strain stimulation, while no significant change was observed for superficial cells. In contrast, superficial zone cells had 40% more ^{3}H-thymidine incorporation than controls, and this was not observed in deep zone cells (D. A. Lee et al. 2000). Direct compression can also affect the magnitude of the aggregate modulus, likely caused by the accumulation of matrix molecules. A peak-to-peak compressive strain amplitude of 10% at a frequency of 1 Hz with three consecutive 1-hour-on/1-hour-off cycles per day, 5 days per week for 4 weeks (Mauck et al. 2000), stimulated 33% higher glycosaminoglycan composition than free-swelling controls and an aggregate modulus of 100 kPa. Strain levels should be monitored carefully when applying direct compression since high deformations have been shown to result in reduced proliferation and matrix synthesis (Meyer et al. 2006).

In addition to IGF-1, TGF-β3 has also been combined with direct compression to improve biomechanical properties and proteoglycan concentrations (Lima et al. 2007). The synergistic effects between physical and biochemical stimuli may require precise timing of when each stimulus is applied (Chowdhury et al. 2003, 2004; Liu et al. 2007). Future work should incorporate knowledge of these time-dependent aspects of the cell response to accelerate the creation of a functional tissue-engineered construct.

The combination of dynamic direct compression, TGF-β1, and C-ABC has been shown to be effective in increasing both biochemical (collagen per weight increased fourfold) and mechanical (compressive and tensile modulus increased three- to fourfold) properties in constructs formed using cocultures of chondrocytes and fibrochondrocytes (Huey and Athanasiou 2011a,b). These results, combined with the results of compression and growth factors, indicate that the combination of mechanical stimulation, growth factors, and catabolic remodeling enzymes is an avenue that should be pursued further in future tissue engineering studies.

For the same strain, mass transfer conditions for a construct under direct compression are slightly better than those under static culture. As with other culture systems, the maximum thickness of an engineered construct is limited by diffusion. Dynamic compression helps alleviate diffusion limitations through creating pressure gradients within the scaffold, as well as through a secondary mixing effect on the surrounding media. The cells still receive their nutrients through diffusion from the culture media, but transport during compression is enhanced by a dynamic pressure gradient created at the surface of the construct (Suh 1996). Compression of the scaffold creates a higher hydrostatic pressure at the center of the construct than at the surface, which causes variations in fluid velocities within the construct as the applied load

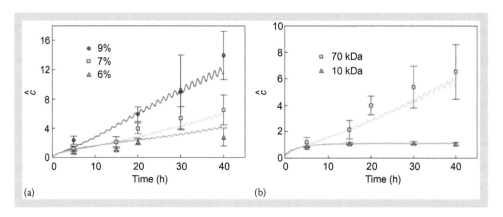

(a) (b)

Figure 4.32 Experimental validation of enhanced solute uptake in dynamically loaded agarose disks. (a) Values for three agarose gels of 6%, 7%, and 9% for solute uptake of 70 kDa dextran. (b) Values for 7% agarose for both 70 and 10 kDa dextran molecular weights. The solid curves represent predicted values. (From Albro, M. B. et al., *J Biomech* 43(12): 2267-2273, 2010. With permission.)

changes. While diffusion of smaller molecules is not affected by the pressure differences created within the scaffold, the movement of larger macromolecules might be hindered (Kim et al. 1994). Dynamic compression may increase the concentration of large solutes within the construct by way of convective transport (Figure 4.32) (Mauck et al. 2003a; Albro et al. 2010).

4.5.2 Hydrostatic Pressure

Chondrocytes in articular cartilage experience hydrostatic pressure during compressive loading of the tissue. The solid matrix of articular cartilage has a small effective pore size, preventing the rapid flow of fluid out of the cartilage and into the joint space. Therefore, pressure within the tissue increases during each instance of compressive loading. While it has been shown that this fluid pressurization has a critical role in bearing loads and in decreasing surface friction, the effect on chondrocytes within the tissue is less clear. The synovial fluid within the joint capsule transmits pressure to the water trapped within the cartilage's matrix, producing a uniform load on chondrocytes in the tissue. Under physiological levels of hydrostatic pressure (7-10 MPa) (Stockwell 1971; Hall et al. 1996), hydrostatic pressure does not stretch or shear cartilage matrix, resulting in minimal tissue deformation (Bachrach et al. 1998) (Figure 4.33). Early attempts at examining hydrostatic pressure applied very low pressure changes in a gas phase (van Kampen et al. 1985; Veldhuijzen et al. 1987). Due to the compressibility of gases, the fluid phase may experience no pressure change at all in these cases, and changes in metabolism may have been due to increases in soluble gases. More recent experiments pressurize the fluid itself, which allows much higher magnitudes.

Application of hydrostatic pressure has, thus, far resulted in tissue-engineered constructs with aggregate modulus values approaching 300 kPa (Elder and Athanasiou 2009c), and its combination with growth factors has shown both additive and synergistic effects in improving construct properties (Elder and Athanasiou 2008).

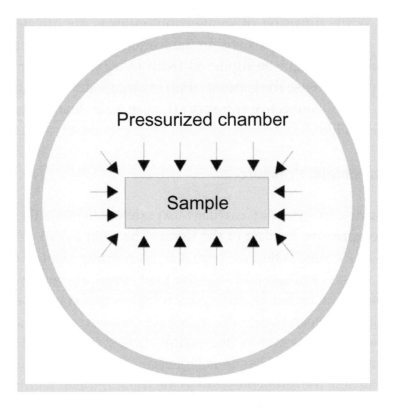

Figure 4.33 Hydrostatic pressure acts perpendicularly from all directions, and, therefore, does not deform a sample under physiological conditions. Secondary effects of this pressurization have been shown to include many positive cellular responses.

As with direct-compression stimulation, researchers can alternate between using a bioreactor to apply hydrostatic pressure and culturing cells under static conditions (Parkkinen et al. 1993a; Smith et al. 1996, 2000a; Hansen et al. 2001) or incorporate a continuous media perfusion approach to minimize handling (Heath and Magari 1996; Carver and Heath 1999c). For the latter, samples do not have to be moved as much, which reduces the possibility of contamination, and the process can be automated to run for long periods of time. Mass transfer is still limited in this setup since fresh media cannot enter the chamber during pressurization (Carver and Heath 1999c), but pressurization cycles are usually short enough that a break in perfusion does not significantly affect nutrient levels.

324

Constant hydrostatic pressure applied for long periods has been shown to have a negative impact on matrix production and cell viability (Parkkinen et al. 1993a; Lammi et al. 1994; Takahashi et al. 1998). As seen with other mechanical stimuli, static loads over long periods are not usually beneficial to tissue formation. Even low-frequency loading can induce a negative response. Application of a 0.0167 Hz stimulus inhibited sulfate incorporation over short and long durations (Parkkinen et al. 1993a). It is possible that low-frequency stimulation is experienced by cells in a manner similar to that of static loading. However, a number of studies have also shown positive effects from constant hydrostatic pressure applied for short durations. An increase of 32% in glycosaminoglycan synthesis was observed when a constant pressure of 10 MPa was applied to a high-density chondrocyte monolayer for 4 hours (Smith et al. 1996). Static pressurization has also yielded engineered articular cartilage that exhibits physiological levels of mechanical and biochemical properties (Elder and Athanasiou 2008, 2009c). Constructs formed using the self-assembly process were exposed to 10 MPa of pressure for 1 hour each day for 5 days, starting at day 10 of a 28-day study. The aggregate and Young's moduli of the constructs were 0.273 and 1.6 MPa, respectively, and glycosaminoglycan and collagen compositions were 6.1% and 10.6% (wet weight), respectively (Elder and Athanasiou 2009c).

It has been shown that a window of pressures and frequencies exists between 0.1 and 15 MPa and 0.05 and 1 Hz, respectively, that produces positive results when culturing chondrocytes (Hall et al. 1991; Heath and Magari 1996; Smith et al. 1996, 2000a; Carver and Heath 1999c; Domm et al. 2000; Hansen et al. 2001). If hydrostatic pressure exceeds the physiological range, negative changes, such as decreased matrix synthesis and increased expression of inflammatory cytokines and heat shock proteins, can be elicited from cells (Hall et al. 1991; Parkkinen et al. 1993b, 1995; Lammi et al. 1994; Kaarniranta et al. 1998; Takahashi et al. 1998; Sironen et al. 2000; Nakamura et al. 2006). High-density chondrocyte monolayers exposed to 10 MPa at 1 Hz for 4 hours a day showed a 9-fold increase in type II collagen mRNA, a 20-fold increase in aggrecan mRNA, and a 65% increase in glycosaminoglycan synthesis (Smith et al. 1996, 2000a). In cell-seeded scaffolds exposed to a 3.5 MPa intermittent force (5/15 seconds on/off for 20 minutes every 4 hours), concentrations of sulfated proteoglycans were twice as high as controls (Carver and Heath 1999c). In general, intermittent hydrostatic pressure that mimics physiological conditions (often 1 Hz) has been shown to be beneficial. However, and quite unexpectedly, studies are now emerging where *statically* applied hydrostatic pressure can also increase the properties of tissue-engineered constructs. For example, when comparing the effects of 1, 5, and 10 MPa under static (0 Hz) and dynamic (0.1 and 1 Hz) conditions, it was found that 10 MPa static hydrostatic pressure significantly increased both construct compressive and tensile properties, while 10 MPa, 1 Hz treatment only resulted in a significant increase in compressive properties (Elder and Athanasiou 2008).

Not all studies using dynamic hydrostatic pressure induce an increase in the expression of extracellular matrix molecules. In two studies using a 345 kPa, 5/30-second on/off regimen, sulfated glycosaminoglycan and collagen secretions decreased when compared with nonloaded controls (Heath and Magari 1996; Carver and Heath 1999c). Hydrostatic pressure has also been shown to increase apoptosis in osteoarthritic chondrocytes (Wenger et al. 2006), as well as cells not surrounded by a pericellular matrix (Nakamura et al. 2006). A protective matrix might be critical to the success of cells exposed to dynamic hydrostatic pressure. Stem cells differentiated in this environment show a rapid accumulation of pericellular matrix in comparison to nonloaded controls (Ogawa et al. 2009). Furthermore, chondrocytic gene expression and cell viability were enhanced. Loading at early time points typically shows negative results, whereas longer culturing times reverse that trend (Heath and Magari 1996; Carver and Heath 1999a). For example, cartilage explants exposed to intermittent pressure showed that proteoglycan synthesis decreased during early loading periods but increased after 20 hours of loading (Parkkinen et al. 1993a). This response could be due to a lack of a pericellular matrix in early cultures and the subsequent formation of the surrounding tissue over time.

Many of the variations in the response of chondrocytes to hydrostatic pressure can be attributed to variations in donors, animal source, and topographical location in the joint (Hall et al. 1991). Additional sources of variation in the response to hydrostatic pressure are likely due to both the loading regimens and the culture conditions (Elder and Athanasiou 2009a). For example, significant differences in marker incorporation rates can exist among donors and across species. The anatomical location of the tissue, as well as the zone from which chondrocytes are isolated, can also be a source of variation.

Response to hydrostatic pressure also varies depending on monolayer versus three-dimensional culture. Chondrocytes dedifferentiate in monolayer culture (Darling and Athanasiou 2005a), and response to hydrostatic pressure is dependent on if dedifferentiation has occurred. It is noteworthy that hydrostatic pressures can induce chondrocyte-specific gene expression even in dedifferentiated chondrocytes; stimulation with hydrostatic pressure can help recover the proper expression profile associated with chondrocytes (Heyland et al. 2006; Kawanishi et al. 2007; Candiani et al. 2008). For example, dedifferentiated chondrocytes in pellet cultures under a 5 MPa, 0.5 Hz pressure regimen showed a fivefold increase in aggrecan gene expression and a fourfold increase in type II collagen gene expression when compared with nonloaded controls (Kawanishi et al. 2007). In a separate study, synthesis of articular cartilage-specific proteins was significantly increased for dedifferentiated cells exposed to intermittent hydrostatic pressure (Heyland et al. 2006). Overall, the results may indicate that hydrostatic pressure, unlike anabolic agents such as IGF-1 and TGF-β, can accelerate the redifferentiation of dedifferentiated chondrocytes.

Since hydrostatic pressure appears to have a positive effect on the chondrocytic phenotype of cells, efforts have used it to help stimulate chondrogenic differentiation in adult stem cells (Miyanishi et al. 2006a,b; Luo and Seedhom 2007; Elder et al. 2008; Sakao et al. 2008; Wagner et al. 2008; Ogawa et al. 2009). Gene and protein expressions for synovium-derived mesenchymal stem cells were enhanced by intermittent pressurization, showing upregulation of proteoglycan core protein, type II collagen, and

Sox9 (Sakao et al. 2008). Adipose-derived stem cells expressed a chondro-cytic phenotype under hydrostatic pressure and accumulated a pericel-lular matrix more rapidly than nonloaded controls (Ogawa et al. 2009). A variety of hydrostatic pressure regimens had chondrogenic effects on bone marrow-derived mesenchymal stem cells (Miyanishi et al. 2006a,b; Luo and Seedhom 2007; Wagner et al. 2008). Furthermore, synergistic effects between growth factors such as TGF-β3 and hydrostatic pressure have been observed for adult stem cells (Miyanishi et al. 2006a). Even in combination with a growth factor, the loading regimen still plays an important role; low-magnitude stimulation has been found to favor Sox9 and aggrecan expression, whereas high magnitudes favor type II colla-gen expression and synthesis (Miyanishi et al. 2006a,b). These findings will undoubtedly guide future experiments for optimizing chondrocyte-specific gene expression in a predictable manner.

As with other mechanical stimuli, hydrostatic pressure might assist in organizing cartilage matrix molecules into a more functional structure. Chondrocytes cultured with exogenous chondroitin sulfate formed an abundant cell-associated matrix when exposed to cyclic pressure. Control samples did not incorporate as much chondroitin sulfate and had a less organized matrix when examined by transmission elec-tron microscopy (Figure 4.34) (Sharma et al. 2008). Self-assembling chondrocyte cultures exhibited higher protein synthesis levels under intermittent hydrostatic pressure and also showed formation of lacu-nae surrounding the cells (Hu and Athanasiou 2006a). This structure is similar to that seen in native cartilage and could be critical to the pro-tection of cells in a mechanically loaded tissue.

In addition to the biochemical and phenotypic effects, hydrostatic pressure has been shown to influence biomechanical properties critical to the func-tion of cartilage constructs. Counterintuitively, the frequency of 0 Hz (i.e., static), 10 MPa, applied for 1 hour on days 10-14 of a 4-week culture, signifi-cantly increased aggregate modulus values by 1.4-fold. This regimen also affected functional properties that seem to be difficult to improve upon, namely, tensile modulus and strength, along with corresponding collagen

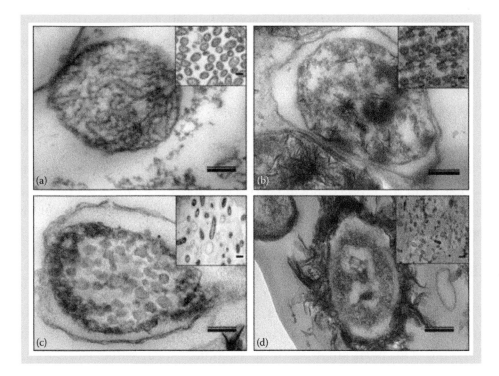

Figure 4.34 Transmission electron micrograph images of goat articular cartilage chondrocytes encapsulated in alginate. (a) Control cell, without cyclic pressure and without addition of chondroitin sulfate (CS) (inset at 4400× showing round cells without pericellular matrix). (b) CS-treated chondrocytes show increased granular matrix. (c) CS- and 1.2 MPa cyclic pressure-treated cells show abundant pericellular matrix. (d) CS- and 2.4 MPa cyclic pressure-treated cells also show abundant pericellular matrix and rounded and oval shapes (inset 1100× showing morphology and matrix). The scale bar is 2 μm. (From Sharma, G. et al., *Osteoarthr Cartil* 16(11): 1387-1394, 2008. With permission.)

content, which increased more than twofold (Elder and Athanasiou 2009c). Thus, it appears that hydrostatic pressure is one of the most potent stimuli toward maintaining chondrogenic phenotype, redifferentiating dedifferentiated chondrocytes, and matrix organization, and increases in biomechanical properties in tissue-engineered articular cartilage.

4.5.3 Shear

Three general categories of high-shear bioreactors have been investigated for tissue engineering studies. The first is a solid-on-solid, contact shear that attempts to replicate the physiological situation where cartilage rubs against another tissue (e.g., cartilage or meniscus), modulated by synovial fluid. The second type, fluid shear, focuses on using fluid flow as a source of shear for monolayer cell populations or cell-seeded constructs. Fluid shear is hypothesized to increase nutrient and waste transfer to increase cell metabolism during culture. Shear can also be applied through direct fluid perfusion. In this case, the stimulus was developed primarily to facilitate nutrient transfer through a three-dimensional scaffold, and the levels of shear can exceed those seen *in vivo*. Low-shear bioreactors have also been developed to increase nutrient transfer at low shear to avoid negative responses that are elicited at high shear.

4.5.3.1 Contact Shear

While solid-on-solid shear loads are minimal because of a pressured fluid film that covers articular cartilage during dynamic loading (Ateshian et al. 1994), small amounts of contact shear still exist. The rubbing of two solid materials can have elements of compression and tension that affect the response of cells within the tissue. As yet, only a few instances of contact or sliding shear bioreactors have been reported in the literature, likely due to the nonuniform stimulation that is applied through the depth of a sheared construct. Future studies might include temporal regimens of contact or sliding shear to enhance functional matrix assembly in the tissue-engineered construct. For example, shear stimulation may commence once significant matrix has been deposited in the construct to withstand the stimulus.

Bioreactors have been designed where shear is applied by fixing a construct's bottom surface while the top surface is moved along one axis (Figure 4.35) (Waldman et al. 2003; Wimmer et al. 2004). Rotational shear devices apply a small amount of compressive strain and then rotate around the z-axis to produce strains in the construct (Frank et al. 2000; Jin et al. 2001, 2003). Attempts have also been made to replicate the physiological mechanical environment through the construction of a bioreactor that rolls a loading shaft across the top of fixed constructs,

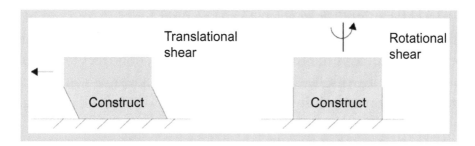

Figure 4.35 Shear forces can be applied to cartilage samples using translational or rotational loading devices. These approaches replicate one aspect of physiological loading in native cartilage.

applying a low level of frictional shear (0.5 N normal force) in a cyclic manner (Stoddart et al. 2006).

As with direct compression and hydrostatic pressure, dynamically applied shear strains have shown more promising results than static conditions. A dynamic shear of 2% at 1 Hz produced constructs with 40% more collagen, 25% more proteoglycan, and a sixfold higher equilibrium modulus (Waldman et al. 2003). Furthermore, stimulation was minimal—only 6 minutes of shear every other day produced impressive increases after 4 weeks. In another experiment, dynamic shear of 1-3% at 0.01-1 Hz increased protein synthesis by 50% and proteoglycan synthesis by 25% (Jin et al. 2001). The addition of IGF-1 to cultures undergoing shear was found to have a synergistic effect on protein and proteoglycan synthesis that was independent of any improvement of convective diffusion (Jin et al. 2003). Applying an interface motion (i.e., sliding shear) to cell-seeded scaffolds has been shown to increase COMP expression (Wimmer et al. 2004). Future research needs to investigate the role of contact shear on extracellular matrix organization in a depth-dependent manner in engineered constructs.

4.5.3.2 Fluid Shear

While the application of fluid shear is more typically associated with vascular tissue engineering, it has been hypothesized that individual chondrocytes might sense shear forces as fluid flows in and out of the cartilage matrix during compression. Cone viscometers have been used extensively to determine the effects of shear on chondrocyte monolayers. More recent work has focused on applying shear as a stimulus in bioreactors or on examining the effects of shear during cell seeding.

A spinner flask uses an impeller to mix oxygen and nutrients throughout the media (Figure 4.36) and, in doing so, applies shear to the cell-seeded scaffolds suspended within the flask, away from the impeller. These constructs benefit from increased nutrient and waste transfer and experience controlled levels of shear. The flask shape and mixing rate can both affect the shear patterns in the culture environment, leading to modifications such as the wavy-walled bioreactor (Gooch et al. 2001b; Bueno et al. 2005). In all of these spinner flasks, cells can be either seeded onto scaffolds before they are inserted into the flask or added as a suspension directly into the media, gradually attaching to scaffolds in the flask (Vunjak-Novakovic et al. 1998). Much work has gone into optimizing cell seeding of scaffolds using spinner flasks, as discussed below. Orbital shakers and rotating plates, which can slowly mix media in a culture without much turbulence (Furukawa et al. 2008), have also been used to apply shear to engineered articular cartilage.

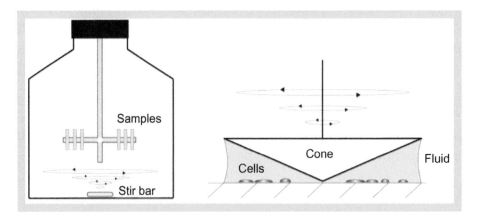

Figure 4.36 Fluid shear is often applied using spinner flasks (left), which have proven to be excellent cell seeding devices. Cone viscometers (right) have been used to study the effects of fluid shear on monolayer cells.

Cell-seeded scaffolds cultured in spinner flasks have shown both positive and negative results, depending on the level of shear applied to the cells. In one study, cartilage constructs experiencing fluid shear (at 50 rpm on an orbital shaker) were more regular in shape and contained up to 70% more cells, 60% more sulfated glycosaminoglycan, and 125% more total collagen (Vunjak-Novakovic et al. 1996). The increase in extracellular matrix is likely due to the increased number of cells. Fluid shear is not always conducive to engineering tissues; undesirable side effects have been seen with high-shear systems. Cell damage has been observed at 150-300 rpm in microcarrier cultures (Cherry and Papoutsakis 1990). Although there is no apparent physical cell damage at 50 rpm, a fibrous capsule forms on the construct surface (Vunjak-Novakovic et al. 1996). A capsule can indicate a protective response to shear forces.

The local shear forces experienced by cells in certain spinner flask configurations are produced by eddies created by the turbulent flow of the impeller. In these cases, cell flattening, proliferation, and formation of an outer capsule may be caused by the pressure and velocity fluctuations associated with turbulent mixing (Vunjak-Novakovic et al. 1996). The mixing rate influences the type, amount, and retention of proteins secreted by cells. Cell-seeded scaffolds exposed to mixing in the range of 80-160 rpm synthesized more collagen and glycosaminoglycan than controls, but actually retained lower fractions of glycosaminoglycan within the scaffold (Gooch et al. 2001b). This loss of glycosaminoglycan from the construct is caused by the continual convective flow in the spinner flask. Fluid shear can also lead to increased total collagen content (Freed et al. 1994b), but a large percentage of this is likely type I collagen from the capsule that surrounds the construct. Despite consisting of type I collagen, the presence of a capsule has been observed to enhance integration of the engineered constructs to native cartilage (Figure 4.37) (Yang et al. 2014).

Spinner flasks and other mechanically driven bioreactors are popular because they increase the mass transfer rate to the cells. However,

333

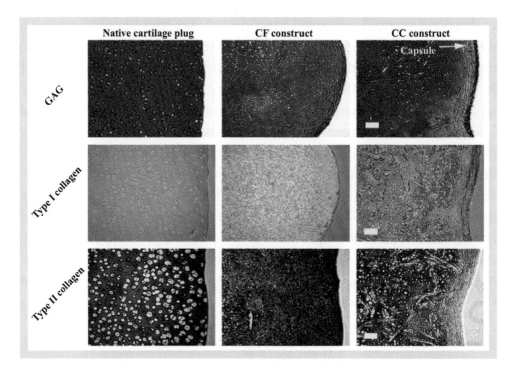

Figure 4.37 Fibrous encapsulation formed on tissue-engineered constructs using a wavy-walled bioreactor showing matrix accumulation of glycosaminoglycans (stained red in the top row) and of type I and II collagen (stained brown in the middle and bottom rows, respectively). The scale bar is 100 μm. Capsule-free (CF, middle column) constructs were formed with IGF-1 stimulation, and capsule-containing (CC, right column) constructs were formed using TGF-β1. (From Yang, Y. H. et al., *Ann Biomed Eng* 42(4): 716-726, 2014. With permission.)

forming articular cartilage using bioreactor with mechanical stirring can face challenges such as nonuniform mass transfer rates, nutrient and pH gradients, and shear gradients, which cause a nonuniform mechanical stimulus over the sample. These issues all contribute to inferior tissue formation compared with other bioreactors (Freed et al. 1993). Shear force at the surface of the impeller is 10 times higher than anywhere else within the bioreactor (Merchuk 1990). Because of this, samples closer to the impeller could experience injurious levels of shear, while samples farther away might not be stimulated at all. If positioned correctly, fibrous encapsulation of the construct will be minimal, and the cells will still benefit from enhanced nutrient transfer. However, low mixing rates or large distances from the mechanical mixer could decrease mass transfer, creating a stagnant environment with increased pH caused by insufficient mixing. For successful use of a stirring bioreactor, a balance has to be obtained between the magnitude of shear and mass transfer.

Some of the limitations mentioned above have been remedied by constructing bioreactors with low shear and a more homogeneous flow environment. A configuration such as the cone-on-plate viscometer (Figure 4.36), which consists of a cone that rotates in media above a flat surface seeded with cells, can achieve a uniform shear distribution with values ranging from 10^{-3} to 10 Pa (Bussolari et al. 1982). This type of device is attractive because it can apply a laminar shear stress at a constant, controllable level. High-density chondrocyte monolayers exposed to a 1.6 Pa shear stress using this configuration showed a 2-fold increase in glycosaminoglycan synthesis, a 10- to 20-fold increase in prostaglandin E_2 release, and a 9-fold increase in tissue inhibitor of metalloproteinase (TIMP) mRNA (Smith et al. 1995). Prostaglandin E_2 is a pro-inflammatory factor with immunosuppressive activity, and TIMPs prevent extracellular matrix degradation. However, interleukin 6 and nitric oxide levels, which are indicators of osteoarthritis, also increased due to this type of mechanical stimulation, and chondrocytic gene expression (aggrecan, type II collagen) decreased significantly (Smith et al. 2000b; Lee et al. 2002). Unidirectional shear chambers have also been developed to investigate the effect of fluid shear on cartilage development. As with the other studies presented above, the formation of a thick type I collagen layer occurs at the surface in response to higher shear forces (Gemmiti and Guldberg 2006, 2009). Taken together, these results show that fluid shear, at least when applied to chondrocytes that are not protected by a scaffold, may not be beneficial to chondrogenesis.

Mechanically stirred bioreactors, such as spinner flasks, have been used effectively for attaching cells to fibrous mesh scaffolds (Vunjak-Novakovic et al. 1998). Mixing provides for rapid, high-yield attachment and a more uniform distribution of cells throughout the scaffold, as well as inducing better overall matrix production in the construct. Static seeding results in cells located primarily in the lower half of the construct, while dynamic seeding distributes cells more evenly through-out the scaffold (Freed et al. 1994b). If the scaffold material is coated with protein (e.g., fibronectin or collagen), then dynamic seeding can result in more attached cells, as well as increased migration of the cells into the scaffold (Bhati et al. 2001). Successful tissue engineering studies rely heavily on well-seeded scaffolds, and dynamic seeding provides a relatively simple approach for obtaining high-cell-density constructs formed using fibrous meshes. In materials such as hydrogels, cells can be distributed evenly at high densities in the absence of a mechanically stirred bioreactor.

4.5.3.3 Perfusion Shear

The last type of shear bioreactor that will be discussed in this section is one that incorporates direct fluid perfusion (Figure 4.38). Devices designed to flow media either around or through a cell construct have both been termed *perfusion bioreactors*. Bioreactors that move medium through the construct are more specifically termed *direct-perfusion bioreactors*. The fluid flow can be controlled to apply a range of shear forces on the construct while enhancing mass transfer. Direct-perfusion systems have been used extensively for bone tissue engineering applications, and experiments conducted for engineering articular cartilage appear promising.

Perfusion bioreactors can be used to feed the cells continuously while applying other mechanical stimuli, like hydrostatic pressure. Perfusion bioreactors can have both positive and negative effects on tissue growth. In one experiment, engineered cartilage constructs in static culture accumulated 300% more sulfated glycosaminoglycans, incorporated 180% more ^{35}S-sulfate, and expressed aggrecan and type II collagen 350% and 240% more, respectively, than perfused constructs (Mizuno et al. 2001). This result could be caused by a loss of newly synthesized matrix molecules to convective flow, which is not present in static conditions. Culture time can also affect the overall response of constructs to direct perfusion. Perfused constructs displaying inhibited glycos-aminoglycan synthesis and retention at early time points nonetheless

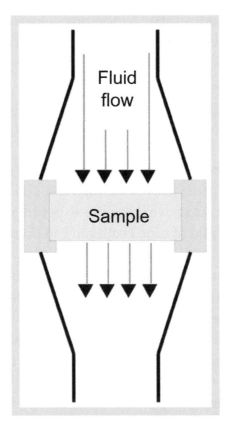

Figure 4.38   Direct fluid perfusion provides mechanical stimulation and increased nutrient availability throughout the entire construct. Directional flow can also induce anisotropy, which may be useful in engineering organized tissues such as articular cartilage.

accumulated more total proteoglycans than nonperfused controls with extended culture (Davisson et al. 2002b).

Continuous media perfusion to a culture dish moves medium around constructs, resulting in increased matrix production by 50-70%, similar to results obtained from direct-perfusion experiments, which are discussed below (Khan et al. 2009). This increase in synthesis could be caused by improved mass transport or stimulation due to shear. If the cells are shielded from the surrounding flow, then the effect of shear is minimalized, and the stimulus would be due to increased nutrient availability. For example, agarose-encapsulated scaffolds placed in a chamber with continuous media perfusion provided cells with nutrients via diffusion, similar to the physiological environment, but also shielded the cells from shear (Sittinger et al. 1994). High flow rates allow for greater mass transfer, but the drawback is increased shear that might result in a deleterious cellular response.

For three-dimensional constructs, a bioreactor that forces media *through* the scaffold allows for the formation of thicker pieces of tissue. In these direct-perfusion bioreactors, cells throughout the construct experience fluid shear as media moves through the construct. Cell response depends on flow rate. As seen in previous experiments with high shear, a fibrous matrix composed of type I collagen can dominate the construct.

Direct-perfusion bioreactors can align cells in the direction of flow, which can be advantageous when producing a tissue with specific cellular orientations like articular cartilage (Pazzano et al. 2000). However, not all cells in native articular cartilage are aligned in the same direction, and it remains to be seen whether this effect can accurately create organization similar to that of native articular cartilage. Variations exist in direct-perfusion designs, but one commonality is a tight fit between the scaffold and walls of the media chamber. If the scaffold has space around it, less fluid is forced through the construct's pores, and uniform mechanical effects are not achieved. A major benefit of direct perfusion is the continuous influx of fresh media to cells throughout the thickness of the construct. Additionally, perfusion removes the need for manual media changes, decreasing labor and reducing the risk of contamination.

Modifications can be made to direct-perfusion bioreactors to alter the growth environment of the samples. For example, medium that has run through the system can be mixed in various proportions with fresh medium. Recycling some of the culture medium keeps beneficial proteins secreted endogenously by the cells (e.g., growth factors and matrix molecules) in the system. Another possible modification to the system involves controlling gas concentrations (e.g., dissolved oxygen) in the fluid (Wendt et al. 2006). If the tissue becomes denser, more oxygen and nutrients can be added to compensate for the increased oxygen usage. Experiments with variable levels of oxygen tension can also be easily controlled in a perfusion system.

Direct perfusion of tissue-engineered constructs can affect cell proliferation and viability, matrix production, and tissue uniformity and is dependent on the cell types used (Figure 4.39). Direct-perfusion bioreactors with limited levels of shear (<0.01 Pa) can stimulate cell proliferation and increase the production of proteoglycans and collagen (Raimondi et al. 2006, 2008). Cell-seeded scaffolds cultured in a direct-perfusion bioreactor running at 1 µm/s (flow rate of 7.6 µL/min) for 4 weeks showed an increase of 184% in glycosaminoglycans, 155% in ^{3}H-proline incorporation, and 118% in DNA content (Pazzano et al. 2000). These increases are promising, although the production of molecules associated with injury response was not measured. Another research group looked at applying direct perfusion at a higher linear velocity of 10.9 µm/s (flow rate of 50 µL/min) (Dunkelman et al. 1995). The resulting constructs were composed of 25% glycosaminoglycans and 15% type II collagen by dry weight (the reminder of the dry weight being accounted for

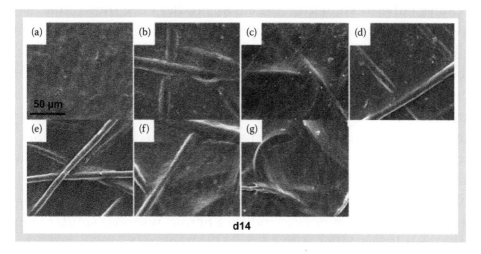

Figure 4.39 Scanning electron microscopy of cell-seeded scaffolds in perfusion bioreactor. Panels (a-g) represent different mixtures of chondrocytes and stem cells, all of which exhibited significant matrix deposition in response to the mechanical stimulus. (Adapted from Levorson, E. J. et al., *Acta Biomater* 10(5): 1824-1835, 2014. With permission.)

by nondegraded polymer, cells, and other proteins). While the collagen composition is still significantly lower than that in native cartilage levels (50-73% by dry weight), the absence of type I collagen indicates that direct perfusion might be a possible option for growing hyaline cartilage. Unfortunately, tissue growth in the scaffold was nonuniform, with more matrix deposition observed for the side of the construct that faced the incoming fluid flow. Increasing the flow rate could mitigate this problem, but the increased shear that comes with greater flow rates can affect the cells negatively. Finding a balance between mass transfer and shear is necessary if direct-perfusion bioreactors are to be used for cartilage tissue engineering. Rotating bioreactors, discussed in Section 4.5.3.4, are a possible solution to this problem.

A challenge in using direct-perfusion bioreactors for cartilage engineering is that matrix production may be nonuniform throughout the thickness of the construct. Since fluid flows from one side of a construct to the other, the side facing the incoming medium tends to lead to a thicker layer of matrix on one side and minimal matrix on the other. Another problem is the induction of molecules associated with injury response rather than matrix formation. Studies have shown that shear levels as low as 0.092 Pa (0.92 dyne/cm^2) can have an adverse effect on cells (Goodwin et al. 1993). While chondrocytes can resist certain types of mechanical stress, turbulence can nonetheless produce deleterious effects (Cherry and Papoutsakis 1990; Freed et al. 1994b; Vunjak-Novakovic et al. 1996). High levels of shear can result in cell death or altered phenotypes, resulting in matrix that is mechanically inferior to native cartilage. In response to high shear, chondrocytes often produce a thick, fibrous matrix composed mainly of type I collagen that helps isolate the cells from the turbulent flow (Tsao and Gonda 1999). High-shear direct-perfusion devices induce a fibrous response similar to that of the capsule formed in some spinner flask cultures, although it is usually restricted to one side of the construct. Given these challenges in the field, it is likely that other novel approaches need to be taken before the zonal organization of native articular cartilage can be duplicated in these bioreactors.

340

4.5.3.4 Low-Shear Microgravity

Flow-based bioreactors are attractive systems for tissue engineering because they improve mass transfer, increasing nutrient concentrations and decreasing waste levels in the constructs. While high-shear perfusion can successfully stimulate matrix production, the resulting tissue is typically fibrous in nature rather than hyaline. Slower fluid flow rates are hypothesized to have a general stimulatory effect on matrix synthesis while still allowing cells to express a chondrocytic phenotype. This is the premise behind low-shear, rotating bioreactors (Figure 4.40).

The origin and evolution of low-shear cartilage bioreactors can be traced back to a modified version of the clinostat, first described in 1872 by Julius von Sachs (Newcombe 1904). Its modern-day representation, the rotating wall bioreactor, provides a culture environment in which constructs are continuously suspended in medium. Sometimes described as a microgravity environment, this device was developed by researchers to investigate the effect of free fall on cell and tissue growth (Briegleb 1983). Subsequently, the rotating wall bioreactor has found success as a low-shear, high-diffusion bioreactor for many cell types. The original design is comprised of a medium-filled, cylindrical vessel that rotates around a central cylinder (also capable of rotation) at 15-30 rpm,

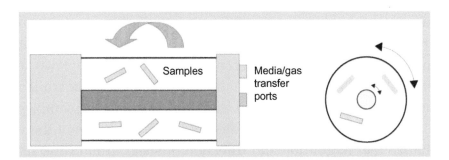

Figure 4.40 Low-shear bioreactors are designed to improve mass transfer over static culture with minimal increases in shear (left). Nutrient and waste transfer are greatly enhanced in these devices that keep constructs "suspended" by balancing gravity with gentle, rotational fluid flow. Constructs are cultured in the chamber formed by two concentric cylinders that can rotate independently. Shear levels can be increased by changing the rotational speed of the outer wall versus the inner cylinder (right).

which keeps constructs or cells floating in suspension. Rotation speed has to be adjusted throughout the culture period to balance any gravity effects as samples mature and change in shape and density. Gas exchange occurs through a gas-permeable membrane that surrounds the hollow, inner cylinder. Dynamic laminar flow in rotating bioreactors provides efficient oxygen supply and allows newly synthesized macromolecules to be retained in the developing constructs (Obradovic et al. 2001). Modifications to this bioreactor include changing the shape of the vessel and the mechanism for gas and media perfusion. The culture environment present in rotating bioreactors makes it attractive for not only tissue engineering studies, but also more basic studies focusing on cartilage healing and cell aggregation (Duke et al. 1993; Tognana et al. 2005). The major difference between rotating bioreactors and past perfusion systems is a reduction in shear force, since high or even moderate levels of shear are undesirable in the formation of hyaline cartilage. A rotating fluid environment was found to be more effective in producing a low-shear, high-mass-transfer bioreactor than many other fluid flow bioreactors (Freed and Vunjak-Novakovic 1995; Martin et al. 1999, 2000; Vunjak-Novakovic et al. 1999; Begley and Kleis 2000).

The rotating bioreactor is capable of adjusting shear levels associated with fluid-construct interaction because of its unique design. Shear forces can induce either positive or negative responses from cultured cells, and a threshold level of 0.092 Pa seems to demarcate that point for rotating bioreactor systems (Goodwin et al. 1993). Constructs cultured in this environment remain suspended in the media by two forces: gravity and fluid flow. Samples "fall" through the media, while rotating fluid flow acts in the upward direction, keeping the samples suspended but also exerting shear. Altering the rotation rate of the vessel can change the magnitude and direction of shear around the sample. Low-shear environments are typically produced by slowly rotating both cylinders at nearly the same rate. Initial experiments used cell-seeded microcarriers to investigate the effect of microgravity on cell growth and development (Goodwin et al. 1993; Tsao et al. 1994; Begley and Kleis 2000). Over the culture period, the microcarriers slowly aggregated to form larger constructs with newly synthesized matrix (Tsao et al. 1997; Tsao and Gonda 1999). Subsequent experiments with larger constructs showed that the samples tended to remain near the ends of the media chamber, not distributing as widely as smaller particles. Because of this, newer versions of the rotating bioreactor (Synthecon, Inc.) have altered the aspect ratio of the media chamber, producing an environment more conducive to culturing large constructs (Tsao et al. 1997). Although the culture environment is not ideal, the flow patterns inside the bioreactor tend to slowly tumble large constructs through the medium, an action that introduces higher shear levels caused by turbulent fluid motion across the construct surface (Tsao et al. 1994). Small-amplitude, long-period oscillations in the fluid wake at this interface may be the source of mechanical stimuli felt by the cells (Freed and Vunjak-Novakovic 1995). Additionally, the magnitude and direction of shear on the construct constantly changes, which might be desirable as a dynamic mechanical stimulus, but also undesirable due to the randomness. The stress exerted on a construct in a bioreactor rotating at 19 rpm was calculated to be ~0.15 Pa (1.5 dyne/cm^2) (Freed and Vunjak-Novakovic 1995), which is significantly higher than the shear level of ~0.0005 Pa (0.005 dyne/cm^2) measured for microcarrier beads in the same environment (Begley and Kleis 2000). However, this shear stress is still significantly lower than that of other fluid flow bioreactors.

Rotating bioreactors, used in articular cartilage tissue engineering, have been reported to produce higher amounts of glycosaminoglycans and collagen than mixed flasks or static culture (Freed et al. 1998; Martin et al. 2000). Constructs cultured for 6 weeks produced tissue that had glycosaminoglycan and total collagen compositions that were 68% and 33%, respectively, of native cartilage levels (Freed et al. 1998). Similar results were obtained in a subsequent study, with engineered constructs accumulating 75% of native glycosaminoglycan and 39% of native type II collagen levels (Martin et al. 2000). Additionally, extending culture to 7 months increased glycosaminoglycan content beyond physiological levels, although collagen remained at 39%. The accumulation of matrix also affected the biomechanical properties, with equilibrium modulus

(950 kPa) and hydraulic permeability (5×10^{-15} m^4/N-s) reaching values comparable to those of healthy cartilage.

Improvements to the engineered tissue are not limited to increased matrix production. The morphology of the constructs shows more uniform deposition of matrix than in other bioreactors (Freed et al. 1998; Martin et al. 1999). Collagen and proteoglycan accumulation occurs in both the peripheral and central regions of the scaffold, and fibrous encapsulation is minimal or even nonexistent (Akmal et al. 2006).

These results indicate that oxygen and nutrients reach the construct center in sufficient amounts, which is important for growing large tissues. While low oxygen concentrations are more representative of the physiological environment in articular cartilage, anaerobic conditions have been shown to cause poor matrix production (Freed et al. 1999; Obradovic et al. 1999). The mass transfer enhancements of the rotating bioreactor are, therefore, critical to its success. Oxygen and nutrients move further into the scaffold, facilitating the growth of constructs as thick as 5 mm after 40 days of *in vitro* culture (Figure 4.41) (Freed et al. 1998). The culture system has also been shown to increase cell proliferation/viability and decrease nitric oxide production (Villanueva et al. 2009).

Bioreactors for cartilage tissue engineering should provide an environment that is conducive to retaining the chondrocytic phenotype. A number of studies have investigated rotating bioreactors, or modified versions of these devices, for their capability to redifferentiate chondrocytes that have nonideal expression patterns (Marlovits et al. 2003a,b; Chen et al. 2008, 2009). Dedifferentiated chondrocytes transfected with BMP2 were cultured in a "rotating shaft" bioreactor to induce chondrogenic gene and protein expression (Chen et al. 2008). Results in static culture were inferior to those in the bioreactor, as were results using nontransfected cells. This indicates a synergistic relationship between biochemical and mechanical stimuli, which can be elicited by combining growth factor use with the rotating bioreactor. Constructs grown

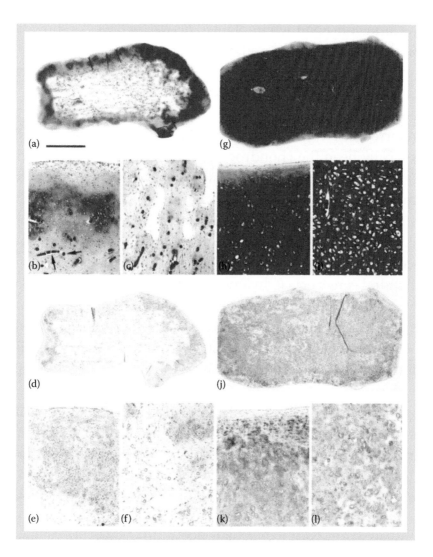

Figure 4.41 Histology and immunohistochemistry of constructs after 12 (a-f) or 40 (g-l) days of *in vitro* culture in the rotating bioreactor. Glycosaminoglycans are stained in panels a-c and g-l, and type II collagen is stained in panels d-f and j-l. The scale bar is 2 mm in panels a, d, g, and j and 300 μm in panels b, c, e, f, h, i, k, and l. (b) Arrows point to polymer fibers of the scaffold. (From Freed, L. E. et al., *Exp Cell Res* 240(1): 58-65, 1998. With permission.)

for 3 weeks *in vitro* and then implanted *in vivo* for 8 weeks showed good histological characteristics and integration with surrounding tissue (Chen et al. 2009). Rotating bioreactors have been reported to stimulate the chondrocytic phenotype (Marlovits et al. 2003a,b).

The preferred cell type for early cartilage tissue engineering studies has classically been the chondrocyte. However, difficulty with obtaining healthy chondrocytes from patients has driven interest toward other cell types, such as stem or progenitor cells. Many different types of cells have been used in the rotating bioreactor because of its apparent conduciveness to the chondrocytic phenotype. Bone marrow-derived mesenchymal cells have been used successfully to create cartilage and osteochondral constructs (Ohyabu et al. 2006; Augst et al. 2008; Sakai et al. 2009). Cells cultured in the rotating bioreactor have been characterized as being more metabolically active than either static or simple perfusion environments (Pound et al. 2006). Another progenitor cell type, synovium-derived stem cells, has shown an ability to secrete matrix rich in glycosaminoglycans and type II collagen after a month in the rotating bioreactor (Pei et al. 2008a,b). Several other cell types, including amniotic mesenchymal cells (Kunisaki et al. 2006), umbilical cord blood cells (Fuchs et al. 2005), and embryonic stem cells (Philp et al. 2005), have all been successfully differentiated down the chondrogenic lineage when cultured in the rotating bioreactor. Numerous researchers are actively investigating how the unique conditions of this culture environment can be used to exploit the multipotentiality of stem and progenitor cells.

Not all bioreactors can accommodate the wide variety of scaffold materials that are present in the field of tissue engineering. The physical, mechanical, and material characteristics of a scaffold can prevent its use in devices that apply large forces or require excessive handling. Rotating bioreactors, however, provide a low-fluid-shear environment that is conducive to many different carriers. Mesh scaffolds, hydrogels, and microcarrier beads can all be cultured with the same ease. Cells can even be cultured without a scaffold, with aggregation occurring within days to weeks. This is not to say that the scaffold-bioreactor compatibility can be ignored. In fact, this interaction is incredibly important when determining the shear forces and nutrient diffusion present in the culture environment (Pei et al. 2002). The effects of the rotating bioreactor have been shown to be dependent on the scaffold used and the culture parameters employed (Hu and Athanasiou 2005). Chondrocyte-seeded poly-D,L-lactic-co-glycolic acid sponges showed formation of hyaline-like tissue when cultured in chondrogenic media for 4 weeks (Emin et al. 2008). Chitosan scaffolds have also been used in a rotating bioreactor, and tissue growth was shown to be strongly influenced by the microstructure of the scaffold (Nettles et al. 2002; Griffon et al. 2006). A chitosan-HA hybrid scaffold was investigated in this culture environment, with results showing near-physiological levels for matrix composition and mechanical properties (Kasahara et al. 2008).

A major concern with rotating bioreactors is the random motion of scaffolds in the culture vessel. Generally, multiple constructs are cultured in a single bioreactor, which results in groups of tumbling samples that can collide into one another or into the walls of the bioreactor. These unpredictable collisions can kill cells or damage the scaffold during early culture periods. Another difficulty is identifying the flow patterns within a bioreactor filled with constructs. One attempt to localize the nutrient flow and keep a more stable culturing environment is the hydrodynamic focusing bioreactor, created by National Aeronautics and Space Administration to simulate a no-gravity cell culture (Figure 4.42) (Tsao et al. 1994, 1997; Tsao and Gonda 1999). As with other rotating bioreactors, the inner and outer walls rotate to produce a range of shear forces. However, instead of having a cylindrical shape, the hydrodynamic focusing bioreactor is a dome. This modification is proposed to focus cells and nutrients together to enhance mass transfer. Another version of the rotating bioreactor is the "rotating shaft" bioreactor (Chen et al. 2004). This device uses the motion of the inner cylinder to move attached samples in a continual rotary motion around the central axis. However, the culture vessel is only half-filled with medium, so samples

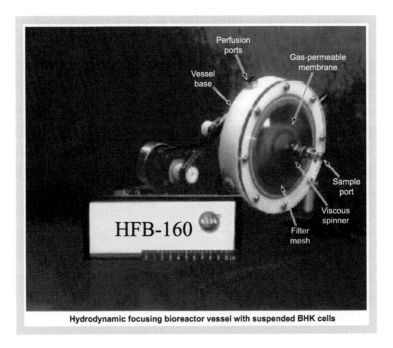

Hydrodynamic focusing bioreactor vessel with suspended BHK cells

Figure 4.42 The hydrodynamic focusing bioreactor utilizes rotation and viscosity to generate hydrodynamic forces for controlling locations of cells and bubbles while maintaining low shear. (Public domain, National Aeronautics and Space Administration.)

move in and out of the liquid. This is proposed to increase oxygenation as well as provide slightly higher levels of shear.

4.5.4 Tension

Tensile strains, inherent in articular cartilage, are a major contributor to the mechanical functionality of the tissue. As described in Chapter 1, the collagen network is in tension to balance outward pressure of the charged fluid phase, providing the basis for cartilage's ability to absorb repeated loading without damage. Despite this, tension-based bioreactors have not been explored extensively for articular cartilage tissue engineering. Investigations have focused mainly on cartilage development or the effects of mechanical strain on the differentiation of stem cells toward the chondrogenic lineage (McMahon et al. 2008; Amos et al. 2009). Results showed that tensile forces have a positive effect on the differentiation of mesenchymal stem cells, increasing the rate of

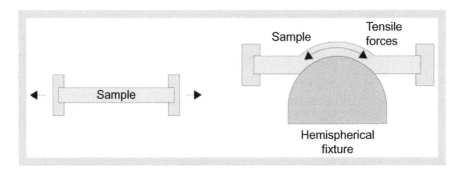

Figure 4.43 Tensile loading is an uncommon technique for cartilage tissue engineering. It can be applied using a simple, uniaxial setup (left) or by stretching the sample biaxially with a hemispherical indenter (right).

glycosaminoglycan production in samples cyclically stretched. While mechanical stimulation of individual cells is postulated as an important factor in this improvement, the increase in nutrient transfer as the cell-seeded scaffold is dynamically strained also likely plays a role. Another application of tensile strain can be found in the use of a biaxial tension device for thin, cell-seeded membranes (Fan and Waldman 2010). A hemispherical loading fixture is used to stretch a membrane with cells in circumferential and radial directions (Figure 4.43).

Many of the bioreactors discussed previously in this section indirectly apply tensile loading. For example, direct compression of a construct can induce strains in cells in the lateral direction. Contact shear has a stretching effect at the scale level of the cell in addition to shear deformation of the tissue. In summary, bioreactors rarely apply only a single type of mechanical stimulation, which may more closely approximate the native environment since articular cartilage experiences multiple types of loading.

4.5.5 Hybrid Bioreactors

As the field of tissue engineering matures, more complex bioreactors have been developed to more faithfully replicate the native environment of target tissues. Each bioreactor reviewed previously has advantages and disadvantages to its design. Some systems appear to have greater effects on collagen production (e.g., direct compression and hydrostatic pressure), while others enhance proteoglycan synthesis (e.g., hydrostatic pressure). More information is continually being accrued that helps elucidate the complicated relationship between mechanical stimuli and cell response. Successfully applying mechanical stimulation can be difficult because each bioreactor has to be optimized to take advantage of its benefits while minimizing its deficiencies. One possible solution is to combine two or more bioreactors that complement each other's strengths and eliminate weaknesses.

Different mechanical stimuli have been integrated into single, hybrid bioreactors. Experiments investigating the combination of small axial compression with rotational shear have shown a stimulatory effect on protein and proteoglycan synthesis (Frank et al. 2000; Jin et al. 2001, 2003). An alternative to this approach is an innovative device that dynamically rolls a cylinder across fixed samples to apply both compressive and frictional shear loading (Stoddart et al. 2006). This stimulus upregulated chondrocytic gene expression and increased protein synthesis in explants after 4 days of culture.

Another hybrid bioreactor reported for cartilage engineering is one that combines hydrostatic pressure and direct fluid perfusion (Lagana et al. 2008; Moretti et al. 2008). This device functions by pressurizing the media as it flows through the interstitial spaces of a cultured construct. Combined effects of these stimuli need to be further elucidated on matrix production and tissue organization. A biaxial tension-compression bioreactor has been used to compress constructs along the z-axis while concurrently stretching them along the x-axis (Wartella and Wayne 2009). Results showed that the combination of both tensile and compressive forces stimulated cellular proliferation and proteoglycan secretion in cell-seeded scaffolds.

Bioreactors do not necessarily need to be combined into one device to be effective. One of the more promising approaches in cartilage engineering is to use a dynamic seeding environment initially, followed by a different type of mechanical bioreactor. For example, scaffolds can be seeded and stabilized for a short period in a spinner flask. Then they can be transferred to another bioreactor, such as intermittent pressurization, to facilitate tissue growth. This approach has been found to achieve better results than either mechanical stimulus alone (Carver and Heath 1999b). When cell-seeded scaffolds were cultured for 2 weeks in a spinner flask and 4 weeks in hydrostatic pressure, constructs had 3.5 times more glycosaminoglycan and 7 times more collagen than static controls. A large field of study is currently open that requires investigation of which specific combinations of mechanical stimuli, as well as their sequences and durations, can elicit the best response from cultured constructs.

Other approaches might include bioreactors that combine the beneficial aspects of several devices into one package. For example, hydrostatic pressure could be combined with a rotating bioreactor to create a stimulating environment that is self-contained. Since the scaffolds are already cultured in a fluid medium, hydrostatic pressure could be applied without compromising the sterile environment. Another possible device would combine direct compression and direct fluid perfusion. This bioreactor could enhance mass transfer while also applying a physiologically relevant strain with cyclic compression. The difficulty with bioreactor design is the extensive testing and validation required before widespread adaptation. While combining two or more established mechanical stimuli seems straightforward, the biological response of an engineered construct could be unpredictable.

4.5.6 Gas-Controlled Bioreactors

Articular cartilage receives its nutrients from the synovial fluid, through diffusion and convective flow (McKibbin and Holdsworth 1966). An important component of these nutrients is oxygen. Scaffold architectures and microenvironment will have a direct bearing on gas and nutrient diffusion in the engineered tissues.

The common approach to regulating oxygen levels in tissue engineering is the use of precisely regulated incubators or bioreactors (Obradovic et al. 1999). These devices allow control of oxygen, carbon dioxide, and nitrogen partial pressures. While standard incubators use ambient air (~20% oxygen), gas-controlled incubators can lower oxygen tension to physiological levels corresponding to those in articular cartilage, estimated to be ~7-10% at the surface and ~1% by the subchondral bone (Silver 1975; Malda et al. 2003; Fermor et al. 2007). Whether high or low oxygen tensions are more beneficial for tissue engineering articular cartilage is under investigation. High oxygen tensions can have a salutatory effect on cell metabolism, but can also result in free radical formation and DNA damage, which is deleterious (Fermor et al. 2005; Cernanec et al. 2007; Davies et al. 2008). Conversely, low tensions provide a more physiological environment but might inhibit robust matrix synthesis and cell proliferation.

In general, tissue engineers strive to reproduce the physiological environment; however, this may not always be beneficial to produce an ideal construct. For example, chondrocytes generally do not proliferate in healthy cartilage. High oxygen tensions promote proliferation and may, thus, be desirable when populating a scaffold (Malda et al. 2003; Schrobback et al. 2012). In contrast, in multiple studies, chondrocytic gene expressions for type II collagen and aggrecan were elevated in 5% oxygen compared with 20% oxygen, whereas expressions for type I and X collagen were decreased (Figure 4.44) (Murphy and Sambanis 2001a; Das et al. 2010; Schrobback et al. 2012). Excessively hypoxic environments can be problematic, however, as shown by decreased glycosaminoglycan synthesis for constructs cultured in 1% oxygen (Murphy and Sambanis 2001b). Results obtained from culturing chondrocytes in hypoxia can appear contradictory, but a recent study hypothesized that different timing may explain these differences. Early hypoxia application suppressed matrix synthesis, but applying hypoxia once collagen has accumulated tends to increase the amount of collagen cross-links, leading to improved tensile properties (Makris et al. 2014a). Future tissue engineering efforts might tailor oxygen tension to construct development by seeding cells and culturing them at a high oxygen tension, and then switching to lower oxygen tensions to promote the chondrocytic

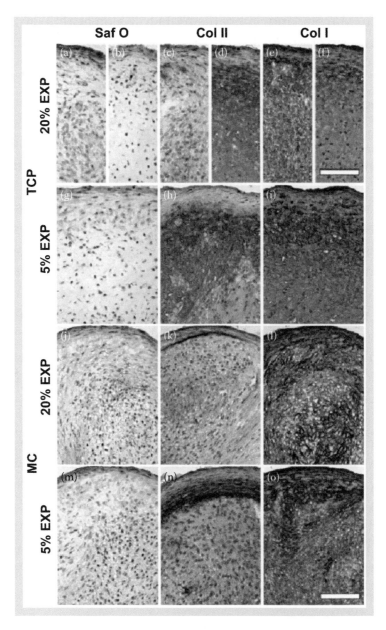

Figure 4.44 Extracellular matrix synthesis and chondrogeneic markers were enhanced by 5% oxygen tension in human osteoarthritic chondrocyte after 28 days of pellet culture. Before pelleting, cells were initially expanded and cultured either on tissue culture plastic (TCP) (a-i) or microcarriers (MC) (j-o) under partial oxygen tensions of 20% (20% EXP) (a-f, j-l) or 5% (5% EXP) (g-i, m-o). Pellets were stained for glycosaminoglycans (red), cell matrix (cyan) (Safranin O/Fast Green), or type I and II collagen (brown) with hematoxylin counterstain (purple). The scale bar is 100 μm. (From Schrobback, K. et al., *Cell Tissue Res* 347(3): 649-663, 2012. With permission.)

phenotype (Murphy and Sambanis 2001a,b; Malda et al. 2004; Saini and Wick 2004; Das et al. 2008, 2010; Wernike et al. 2008; Heywood et al. 2010).

4.5.7 Electrical and Magnetic Stimulation

Efforts to grow and repair articular cartilage have primarily focused on using growth factors, cytokines, and mechanical forces as stimulants. The effects of electric and electromagnetic fields on cartilage regeneration have also been investigated, with particular attention given to clinical applications (Akai and Hayashi 2002; Haddad et al. 2007; Massari et al. 2007). These approaches are based on the hypothesis that electromagnetic pulses can control inflammation (Varani et al. 2002; Ongaro et al. 2012), stimulate anabolic activity, and prevent cartilage degeneration. Additional effects of pulsed electromagnetic fields include increased chondrocyte proliferation (Sakai et al. 1991; Pezzetti et al. 1999), greater matrix synthesis (Aaron and Ciombor 1993; MacGinitie et al. 1994; Boopalan et al. 2010), synergistic responses with anabolic molecules (De Mattei et al. 2004), and inhibition of catabolic cytokines (De Mattei et al. 2003).

Particular attention should be given to how electric and electromagnetic fields might be applied with stem cell or progenitor cell populations, since these fields have been shown to dramatically affect these cell types (Aaron and Ciombor 1996). This effect might be due to the increased synthesis of growth factors that occurs in response to electromagnetic fields (Aaron et al. 2004). Additional investigations are needed to address the mechanism of action of electric and electromagnetic fields on cartilage regeneration and tissue engineering.

4.6 CONVERGENCE OF STIMULI

4.6.1 Synergism versus Additive Effects

Synergy (συνεργία), from Greek *synergos* (συνεργός), meaning "working together," from σύν, meaning "together," and ἔργον, meaning "work"

Synergy is defined as the result of two or more things interacting where the total result is greater than the sum of the parts. When the combined response is equal to the sum of the parts, then the response is additive. Each of the stimuli discussed in the previous sections can act alone or in concert with other stimuli. As described previously, TGF-β1 can synergize with many physical signals, including hydrostatic pressure (Elder and Athanasiou 2008) and direct compression (Huey and Athanasiou 2011a). Growth factors and beneficial cytokines are especially effective when combined with mechanical stimulation (Bonassar et al. 2000; Elder and Athanasiou 2009b; Huey and Athanasiou 2011a,b; Smith et al. 2011). The synergistic response has been shown to produce more matrix than either mechanical stimulation or growth factor alone (Figure 4.45) (Bonassar et al. 2001; Mauck et al. 2003b; Elder and Athanasiou 2008; Ando et al. 2009). One should be aware that the stimulatory environment is not an isolated system, but is an integrated cellular response to both applied and induced factors.

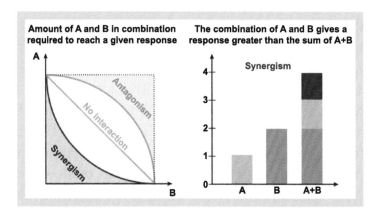

Figure 4.45 Synergy is the interaction or cooperation of two or more organizations, substances, or other agents to produce a combined effect greater than the sum of their separate effects. Left: In drug dosing, this can mean the combination of dose A and dose B requires less of each to produce the same response. Right: If doses A and B are kept constant, synergism can be seen as a response greater than the sum of the responses to A and B separately.

4.6.2 Potential Mechanisms

Mechanotransduction is the phenomenon connecting mechanical stimulation to biological response. The precise mechanisms involved in this process are still not fully understood. However, it is likely that external mechanical signals induce biological signaling through multiple means (see Section 1.2.3). One hypothesized mechanism is physical deformation of the nucleus, which modulates the accessibility of various genes in the chromatin structure of DNA (Figure 4.46).

Membrane-associated signaling is another possible means of transducing mechanical forces via the cytoskeleton or intracellular space. Alterations in ion concentrations are known to occur in response to externally applied forces. Stretch-activated ion channels can open, changing the ionic balance within a cell and setting off a cascade of events to elicit biological changes. Other mechanisms yet to be discovered could further explain how mechanotransduction works.

A seemingly simple act, such as compressing cartilage, can result in complex changes, including matrix and cell deformation, hydrostatic pressure gradients, fluid flow, osmotic pressure changes, and fluctuations in ion concentration and fixed charge density (Urban et al. 1993). Any one of these factors can elicit a biological response from cells, most likely through mechanosensitive ion channels (Martinac 2004) or integrins (Ingber 1991) at the cellular membrane. In the former, mechanical stimulation causes an influx of ions (e.g., calcium) that activate intracellular signaling pathways. Hyperpolarization of the membrane can occur through activation of slow-conductance Ca^{2+}-sensitive K^+ channels (Wright et al. 1996). Alternatively, stretch-activated ion channels can allow an influx of Ca^{2+} to levels that trigger calcium-dependent signaling pathways (Pingguan-Murphy et al. 2005). Membrane-associated integrins also act as intermediaries to external mechanical forces. The integrin receptor has an extracellular domain that binds matrix molecules surrounding the cell and an intracellular region that interacts with cytoplasmic molecules and the

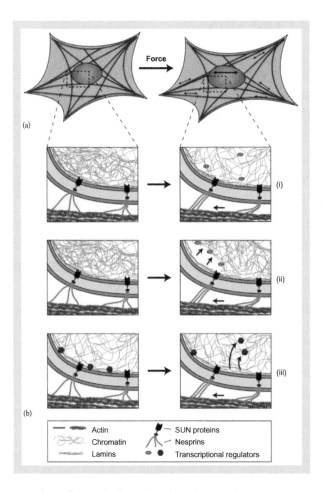

Figure 4.46 Illustration of potential mechanism for mechanosensing by deformation of the nucleus and subsequent gene expression. (a) Schematic of focal adhesion-mediated force transmission through the actin cytoskeleton resulting in nuclear deformation. (b) Various mechanisms and interacting molecules involved in mechanosensing: (i) deformation of chromatin allowing for access and transcription, (ii) change in chromatin localization and detachment from transcriptionally inhibited nuclear lamina, and (iii) conformation or localization changes of lamina allowing nuclear periphery-sequestered transcription factors to have access to chromatin. (From Isermann, P., and J. Lammerding, *Curr Biol* 23(24): R1113-R1121, 2013. With permission.)

cytoskeleton, forming a bridge across the cell membrane. This allows for the transduction of mechanical forces directly to intracellular biochemical responses (Hynes 1992; Martinac 2004; Ramage et al. 2009). See Section 1.2.3 for more detailed discussions of the signaling pathways related to mechanotransduction.

4.7 CHAPTER CONCEPTS

- Though the *in vivo* environment has been thought to contain all the necessary factors (but not necessarily the cells) to effect cartilage repair, *in vitro* tissue engineering is gaining popularity due to the well-controlled environment it offers
- Due to the low availability of differentiated, autologous chondrocytes, alternative cell sources are investigated as the future of articular cartilage tissue engineering.
- There are continuous refinements in the differentiation protocols of various stem cell populations, for example, mesenchymal, induced pluripotent, dermis-derived, adipose-derived, and embryonic stem cells, into chondrocytes
- Combinations of growth factors and environmental conditions, such as three-dimensional culture, can direct stem cell differentiation toward the chondrogenic lineage.
- Desirable characteristics of scaffolds for cartilage repair include biocompatibility, the capacity to bear load, cell attachment, proliferation, and metabolism, and a degradation rate that matches tissue formation.
- Scaffolds can come in several natural or synthetic forms.
- Natural scaffolds that have been studied for cartilage engineering include collagen, alginate, agarose, chitosan, fibrin glue, hyaluronic acid-based materials, and reconstituted tissue matrices.
- Synthetic materials include poly-glycolides, poly-lactides, PCL, and PEG.
- Natural and synthetic materials can be combined to form composite scaffolds. Meshes and hydrogels can be combined to form one construct as well.
- Cartilage tissue engineering has also been accomplished without the use of scaffolds in combination with biochemical and biomechanical stimuli.

- Self-assembly, a scaffoldless tissue engineering approach, has been demonstrated to result in neocartilage of clinically relevant dimensions and with functional properties approaching those of native tissue.
- Bioactive molecules can be soluble or tethered, with intended effects being anabolic or catabolic, or even structural, for improving the functional properties of engineered cartilage.
- TGF-β, BMP, IGF, bFGF, and many other growth factors in their soluble forms have been applied in different concentrations, dosage frequencies, and combinations to engineer cartilage.
- Proteins and peptide coatings and modifications have been used to improve chondrocyte response to biomaterials. These include collagen, vitronectin, CMP, and many amino acid sequences, such as RGD.
- Micropatterning can apply proteins and peptides onto a surface to modulate phenotypical and morphological changes in chondrocytes and other cells.
- Bioreactors can be used to apply chemical and nutrient gradients in the culture of articular cartilage constructs; it can also be used to apply mechanical forces to the developing cartilage.
- Direct compression, hydrostatic pressure, high and low shear, and hybrid bioreactors have all been examined in an effort to replicate physiological loading regimens.
- Cyclic direct compression has been shown to be more beneficial than static compression. For hydrostatic pressure, however, it has been shown that both static and dynamic applications can result in functional improvements.
- In self-assembly of articular cartilage, 10 MPa of hydrostatic pressure, applied statically for 1 hour a day, 5 days total, has been shown to increase both compressive and tensile properties.
- Direct compression applied in combination with growth factors demonstrated enhanced effects.

- Shear can be applied either as contact or as fluid shear in bioreactors.
- Direct fluid perfusion is another way to apply shear to chondrocytes while increasing nutrient and waste transport.
- Since a type I collagen capsule is often seen with the application of shear on chondrocytes, along with upregulations of indicators of osteoarthritis, low-shear bioreactors have been developed to aid in nutrient transfer.
- Tension has been used to stimulate cartilaginous growth, but has been limited in its applications.
- Bioreactors can apply different stimuli simultaneously or in sequence.
- Controlling the concentration of gases in the culture environment can dramatically affect cell proliferation, protein synthesis, and differentiation.
- High oxygen tensions promote cell proliferation, whereas low oxygen levels promote chondrocyte differentiation and collagen cross-linking.
- Electromagnetic field stimulation showed positive effects on the repair of cartilage tissue and is well suited for *in vivo* applications.
- Mechanical, biochemical, and other environmental stimuli can act synergistically to enhance the formation of new cartilage tissue. For example, compression of an engineered construct will increase diffusion throughout the sample, exposing the cells to higher levels of growth factors for longer periods of time.
- Mechanotransduction is the process in which cells respond to mechanical stimuli. This occurs through a combination of membrane-associated proteins, cytoskeletal structures, and physical deformation.

References

Aaron, R. K., B. D. Boyan et al. (2004). Stimulation of growth factor synthesis by electric and electromagnetic fields. *Clin Orthop Relat Res* 419: 30-37.

Aaron, R. K., and D. M. Ciombor. (1993). Therapeutic effects of electromagnetic fields in the stimulation of connective tissue repair. *J Cell Biochem* 52(1): 42-46.

Aaron, R. K., and D. M. Ciombor. (1996). Acceleration of experimental endochondral ossification by biophysical stimulation of the progenitor cell pool. *J Orthop Res* 14(4): 582-589.

Abe, M., M. Takahashi et al. (2004). Cartilage-scaffold composites produced by bioresorbable beta-chitin sponge with cultured rabbit chondrocytes. *Tissue Eng* 10(3-4): 585-594.

Adkisson, H. D., M. P. Gillis et al. (2001). In vitro generation of scaffold independent neocartilage. *Clin Orthop Relat Res* 391(Suppl): S280-S294.

Agrawal, C. M., G. G. Niederauer et al. (1995). Fabrication and characterization of PLA-PGA orthopedic implants. *Tissue Eng* 1(3): 241-252.

Akai, M., and K. Hayashi. (2002). Effect of electrical stimulation on musculoskeletal systems; a meta-analysis of controlled clinical trials. *Bioelectromagnetics* 23(2): 132-143.

Akmal, M., A. Anand et al. (2006). The culture of articular chondrocytes in hydrogel constructs within a bioreactor enhances cell proliferation and matrix synthesis. *J Bone Joint Surg Br* 88(4): 544-553.

Albro, M. B., R. Li et al. (2010). Validation of theoretical framework explaining active solute uptake in dynamically loaded porous media. *J Biomech* 43(12): 2267-2273.

Almqvist, K. F., L. Wang et al. (2001). Culture of chondrocytes in alginate surrounded by fibrin gel: Characteristics of the cells over a period of eight weeks. *Ann Rheum Dis* 60(8): 781-790.

Alsberg, E., K. W. Anderson et al. (2001). Cell-interactive alginate hydrogels for bone tissue engineering. *J Dent Res* 80(11): 2025-2029.

Ameer, G. A., T. A. Mahmood et al. (2002). A biodegradable composite scaffold for cell transplantation. *J Orthop Res* 20(1): 16-19.

Amos, J. R., S. Li et al. (2009). Limb bud mesenchyme cultured under tensile strain remodel collagen type I tubes to produce fibrillar collagen type II. *Biorheology* 46(6): 439-450.

Ando, K., S. Imai et al. (2009). Effect of dynamic compressive loading and its combination with a growth factor on the chondrocytic phenotype of 3-dimensional scaffold-embedded chondrocytes. *Acta Orthop* 80(6): 724-733.

Anseth, K. S., A. T. Metters et al. (2002). In situ forming degradable networks and their application in tissue engineering and drug delivery. *J Control Release* 78(1-3): 199-209.

Asanbaeva, A., K. Masuda et al. (2008a). Cartilage growth and remodeling: Modulation of balance between proteoglycan and collagen network *in vitro* with beta-aminopropionitrile. *Osteoarthr Cartil* 16(1): 1-11.

Asanbaeva, A., J. Tam et al. (2008b). Articular cartilage tensile integrity: Modulation by matrix depletion is maturation-dependent. *Arch Biochem Biophys* 474(1): 175-182.

Ateshian, G. A., W. M. Lai et al. (1994). An asymptotic solution for the contact of two biphasic cartilage layers. *J Biomech* 27(11): 1347-1360.

Athanasiou, K. A., C. M. Agrawal et al. (1998). Orthopaedic applications for PLA-PGA biodegradable polymers. *Arthroscopy* 14(7): 726-737.

Athanasiou, K. A., D. Korvick et al. (1997). Biodegradable implants for the treatment of osteochondral defects in a goat model. *Tissue Eng* 3(4): 363-373.

Athanasiou, K. A., G. G. Niederauer et al. (1995a). Applications of biodegradable lactides and glycolides in podiatry. *Clin Podiatr Med Surg* 12(3): 475-495.

Athanasiou, K. A., G. G. Niederauer et al. (1996). Sterilization, toxicity, biocompatibility and clinical applications of polylactic acid/polyglycolic acid copolymers. *Biomaterials* 17(2): 93-102.

Athanasiou, K. A., A. R. Singhal et al. (1995b). In vitro degradation and release characteristics of biodegradable implants containing trypsin inhibitor. *Clin Orthop* (315): 272-281.

Athens, A. A., E. A. Makris et al. (2013). Induced collagen cross-links enhance cartilage integration. *PLoS One* 8(4): e60719.

Augst, A., D. Marolt et al. (2008). Effects of chondrogenic and osteogenic regulatory factors on composite constructs grown using human mesenchymal stem cells, silk scaffolds and bioreactors. *J R Soc Interface* 5(25): 929-939.

Bachrach, N. M., V. C. Mow et al. (1998). Incompressibility of the solid matrix of articular cartilage under high hydrostatic pressures. *J Biomech* 31(5): 445-451.

Badylak, S. F. (2007). The extracellular matrix as a biologic scaffold material. *Biomaterials* 28(25): 3587-3593.

Banfi, A., G. Bianchi et al. (2002). Replicative aging and gene expression in long-term cultures of human bone marrow stromal cells. *Tissue Eng* 8(6): 901-910.

Barber, F. A., J. Aziz-Jacobo et al. (2010). Anterior cruciate ligament reconstruction using patellar tendon allograft: An age-dependent outcome evaluation. *Arthroscopy* 26(4): 488-493.

Baxter, M. A., R. F. Wynn et al. (2004). Study of telomere length reveals rapid aging of human marrow stromal cells following in vitro expansion. *Stem Cells* 22(5): 675-682.

Beane, O. S., and E. M. Darling. (2012). Isolation, characterization, and differentiation of stem cells for cartilage regeneration. *Ann Biomed Eng* 40(10): 2079-2097.

Bedi, A., B. T. Feeley et al. (2010). Management of articular cartilage defects of the knee. *J Bone Joint Surg Am* 92(4): 994-1009.

Begley, C. M., and S. J. Kleis. (2000). The fluid dynamic and shear environment in the NASA/JSC rotating-wall perfused-vessel bioreactor. *Biotechnol Bioeng* 70(1): 32-40.

Betre, H., W. Liu et al. (2006). A thermally responsive biopolymer for intra-articular drug delivery. *J Control Release* 115(2): 175-182.

Betre, H., L. A. Setton et al. (2002). Characterization of a genetically engineered elastin-like polypeptide for cartilaginous tissue repair. *Biomacromolecules* 3(5): 910-916.

Bettinger, C. J., R. Langer et al. (2009). Engineering substrate topography at the micro- and nanoscale to control cell function. *Angew Chem Int Ed Engl* 48(30): 5406-5415.

Bhardwaj, N., Q. T. Nguyen et al. (2011). Potential of 3-D tissue constructs engineered from bovine chondrocytes/silk fibroin-chitosan for in vitro cartilage tissue engineering. *Biomaterials* 32(25): 5773-5781.

Bhati, R. S., D. P. Mukherjee et al. (2001). The growth of chondrocytes into a fibronectin-coated biodegradable scaffold. *J Biomed Mater Res* 56(1): 74-82.

Bhumiratana, S., R. E. Eton et al. (2014). Large, stratified, and mechanically functional human cartilage grown in vitro by mesenchymal condensation. *Proc Natl Acad Sci USA* 111(19): 6940-6945.

Bian, L., K. M. Crivello et al. (2009). Influence of temporary chondroitinase ABC-induced glycosaminoglycan suppression on maturation of tissue-engineered cartilage. *Tissue Eng Part A* 15(8): 2065-2072.

Bilgen, B., E. Orsini et al. (2007). FBS suppresses TGF-beta1-induced chondrogenesis in synoviocyte pellet cultures while dexamethasone and dynamic stimuli are beneficial. *J Tissue Eng Regen Med* 1(6): 436-442.

Blunk, T., A. L. Sieminski et al. (2002). Differential effects of growth factors on tissue-engineered cartilage. *Tissue Eng* 8(1): 73-84.

Bobick, B. E., F. H. Chen et al. (2009). Regulation of the chondrogenic phenotype in culture. *Birth Defects Res C Embryo Today* 87(4): 351-371.

Bonassar, L. J., A. J. Grodzinsky et al. (2000). Mechanical and physicochemical regulation of the action of insulin-like growth factor-I on articular cartilage. *Arch Biochem Biophys* 379(1): 57-63.

Bonassar, L. J., A. J. Grodzinsky et al. (2001). The effect of dynamic compression on the response of articular cartilage to insulin-like growth factor-I. *J Orthop Res* 19(1): 11-17.

Boopalan, P. R., S. Arumugam et al. (2010). Pulsed electromagnetic field therapy results in healing of full thickness articular cartilage defect. *Int Orthop* 35(1): 143-148.

Bougault, C., A. Paumier et al. (2008). Molecular analysis of chondrocytes cultured in agarose in response to dynamic compression. *BMC Biotechnol* 8: 71.

Boyle, J., B. Luan et al. (1995). Characterization of proteoglycan accumulation during formation of cartilagenous tissue in vitro. *Osteoarthr Cartil* 3(2): 117-125.

Brehm, W., B. Aklin et al. (2006). Repair of superficial osteochondral defects with an autologous scaffold-free cartilage construct in a caprine model: Implantation method and short-term results. *Osteoarthr Cartil* 14(12): 1214-1226.

Briegleb, W. (1983). The clinostat—A tool for analyzing the influence of acceleration on solid-liquid systems. Presented at Workshop on Space Biology, Cologne, Germany.

Britland, S., P. Clark et al. (1992). Micropatterned substratum adhesiveness: A model for morphogenetic cues controlling cell behavior. *Exp Cell Res* 198(1): 124-129.

Brittberg, M., E. Faxen et al. (1994). Carbon fiber scaffolds in the treatment of early knee osteoarthritis. A prospective 4-year followup of 37 patients. *Clin Orthop* (307): 155-164.

Brittberg, M., A. Nilsson et al. (1996). Rabbit articular cartilage defects treated with autologous cultured chondrocytes. *Clin Orthop Relat Res* 326: 270-283.

Bruder, S. P., N. Jaiswal et al. (1997). Growth kinetics, self-renewal, and the osteogenic potential of purified human mesenchymal stem cells during extensive subcultivation and following cryopreservation. *J Cell Biochem* 64(2): 278-294.

Bryant, S. J., and K. S. Anseth. (2001). The effects of scaffold thickness on tissue engineered cartilage in photocrosslinked poly(ethylene oxide) hydrogels. *Biomaterials* 22(6): 619-626.

Bueno, E. M., B. Bilgen et al. (2005). Wavy-walled bioreactor supports increased cell proliferation and matrix deposition in engineered cartilage constructs. *Tissue Eng* 11(11-12): 1699-1709.

Buschmann, M. D., Y. A. Gluzband et al. (1995). Mechanical compression modulates matrix biosynthesis in chondrocyte/agarose culture. *J Cell Sci* 108(Pt 4): 1497-1508.

Bussolari, S., C. Dewey et al. (1982). Apparatus for subjecting living cells to fluid shear stress. *Rev Sci Instrum* 53(12): 1851-1854.

Campbell, J. J., D. A. Lee et al. (2006). Dynamic compressive strain influences chondrogenic gene expression in human mesenchymal stem cells. *Biorheology* 43(3-4): 455-470.

Candiani, G., M. T. Raimondi et al. (2008). Chondrocyte response to high regimens of cyclic hydrostatic pressure in 3-dimensional engineered constructs. *Int J Artif Organs* 31(6): 490-499.

Caplan, A. I. (1991). Mesenchymal stem cells. *J Orthop Res* 9(5): 641-650.

Carver, S. E., and C. A. Heath. (1999a). Increasing extracellular matrix production in regenerating cartilage with intermittent physiological pressure. *Biotechnol Bioeng* 62(2): 166-174.

Carver, S. E., and C. A. Heath. (1999b). Influence of intermittent pressure, fluid flow, and mixing on the regenerative properties of articular chondrocytes. *Biotechnol Bioeng* 65(3): 274-281.

Carver, S. E., and C. A. Heath. (1999c). Semi-continuous perfusion system for delivering intermittent physiological pressure to regenerating cartilage. *Tissue Eng* 5(1): 1-11.

Caterson, E. J., L. J. Nesti et al. (2001). Application of mesenchymal stem cells in the regeneration of musculoskeletal tissues. *MedGenMed* 2001: E1.

Cernanec, J. M., J. B. Weinberg et al. (2007). Influence of oxygen tension on interleukin 1-induced peroxynitrite formation and matrix turnover in articular cartilage. *J Rheumatol* 34(2): 401-407.

Chaipinyo, K., B. W. Oakes et al. (2002). Effects of growth factors on cell proliferation and matrix synthesis of low-density, primary bovine chondrocytes cultured in collagen I gels. *J Orthop Res* 20(5): 1070-1078.

Chang, K. Y., L. H. Hung et al. (2009). The application of type II collagen and chondroitin sulfate grafted PCL porous scaffold in cartilage tissue engineering. *J Biomed Mater Res A* 92(2): 712-723.

Chao, P. H., S. Yodmuang et al. (2010). Silk hydrogel for cartilage tissue engineering. *J Biomed Mater Res B Appl Biomater* 95(1): 84-90.

Chen, C. S., M. Mrksich et al. (1997). Geometric control of cell life and death. *Science* 276(5317): 1425-1428.

Chen, F. H., and R. S. Tuan. (2008). Mesenchymal stem cells in arthritic diseases. *Arthritis Res Ther* 10(5): 223.

Chen, H. C., Y. H. Chang et al. (2009). The repair of osteochondral defects using baculovirus-mediated gene transfer with de-differentiated chondrocytes in bioreactor culture. *Biomaterials* 30(4): 674-681.

Chen, H. C., H. P. Lee et al. (2004). A novel rotating-shaft bioreactor for two-phase cultivation of tissue-engineered cartilage. *Biotechnol Prog* 20(6): 1802-1809.

Chen, H. C., L. Y. Sung et al. (2008). Combination of baculovirus-expressed BMP-2 and rotating-shaft bioreactor culture synergistically enhances cartilage formation. *Gene Ther* 15(4): 309-317.

Cheng, N. C., B. T. Estes et al. (2008). Chondrogenic differentiation of adipose-derived adult stem cells by a porous scaffold derived from native articular cartilage extracellular matrix. *Tissue Eng Part A* 15(2): 231-241.

Cheng, N. C., B. T. Estes et al. (2011). Engineered cartilage using primary chondrocytes cultured in a porous cartilage-derived matrix. *Regen Med* 6(1): 81-93.

Cherry, R. S., and T. Papoutsakis. (1990). Understanding and controlling fluid-mechanical injury of animal cells in bioreactors. In *Animal Cell Biotechnology*, ed. R. E. Spier and J. B. Griffiths. San Diego: Academic Press.

Chesterman, P. J., and A. U. Smith. (1968). Homotransplantation of articular cartilage and isolated chondrocytes. An experimental study in rabbits. *J Bone Joint Surg Br* 50(1): 184-197.

Chlapanidas, T., S. Farago et al. (2011). Regenerated silk fibroin scaffold and infrapatellar adipose stromal vascular fraction as feeder layer: A new product for cartilage advanced therapy. *Tissue Eng Part A* 17(13-14): 1725-1733.

Choi, H. U., L. H. Tang et al. (1983). Isolation and characterization of a 35,000 molecular weight subunit fetal cartilage matrix protein. *J Biol Chem* 258(1): 655-661.

Chou, C. H., W. T. Cheng et al. (2007). Fibrin glue mixed with gelatin/hyaluronic acid/chondroitin-6-sulfate tri-copolymer for articular cartilage tissue engineering: The results of real-time polymerase chain reaction. *J Biomed Mater Res A* 82(3): 757-767.

Chowdhury, T. T., D. L. Bader et al. (2003). Temporal regulation of chondrocyte metabolism in agarose constructs subjected to dynamic compression. *Arch Biochem Biophys* 417(1): 105-111.

Chowdhury, T. T., D. M. Salter et al. (2004). Integrin-mediated mechanotransduction processes in TGFbeta-stimulated monolayer-expanded chondrocytes. *Biochem Biophys Res Commun* 318(4): 873-881.

Chupa, J. M., A. M. Foster et al. (2000). Vascular cell responses to polysaccharide materials: In vitro and in vivo evaluations. *Biomaterials* 21(22): 2315-2322.

Coates, E. E., and J. P. Fisher. (2010). Phenotypic variations in chondrocyte subpopulations and their response to in vitro culture and external stimuli. *Ann Biomed Eng* 38(11): 3371-3388.

Curl, W. W., J. Krome et al. (1997). Cartilage injuries: A review of 31,516 knee arthroscopies. *Arthroscopy* 13(4): 456-460.

Daher, R. J., N. O. Chahine et al. (2009). New methods to diagnose and treat cartilage degeneration. *Nat Rev Rheumatol* 5(11): 599-607.

Daniels, A. U., M. K. Chang et al. (1990). Mechanical properties of biodegradable polymers and composites proposed for internal fixation of bone. *J Appl Biomater* 1(1): 57-78.

Dare, E. V., M. Griffith et al. (2009). Genipin cross-linked fibrin hydrogels for in vitro human articular cartilage tissue-engineered regeneration. *Cells Tissues Organs* 190(6): 313-325.

Darling, E. M., and K. A. Athanasiou. (2003). Articular cartilage bioreactors and bioprocesses. *Tissue Eng* 9(1): 9–26. [Published erratum appears in *Tissue Eng* 9(3): 565, 2003.]

Darling, E. M., and K. A. Athanasiou. (2004). Bioactive scaffold design for articular cartilage engineering. In *Biomedical Technology and Devices Handbook*, ed. J. Moore and G. Zouridakis. Boca Raton, FL: CRC Press, chap. 21.

Darling, E. M., and K. A. Athanasiou. (2005a). Rapid phenotypic changes in passaged articular chondrocyte subpopulations. *J Orthop Res* 23(2): 425-432.

Darling, E. M., and K. A. Athanasiou. (2005b). Retaining zonal chondrocyte phenotype by means of novel growth environments. *Tissue Eng* 11(3-4): 395-403.

Das, R., M. Kreukniet et al. (2008). Control of oxygen tension and pH in a bioreactor for cartilage tissue engineering. *Biomed Mater Eng* 18(4-5): 279-282.

Das, R. H., G. J. van Osch et al. (2010). Effects of individual control of pH and hypoxia in chondrocyte culture. *J Orthop Res* 28(4): 537-545.

Davies, C. M., F. Guilak et al. (2008). Reactive nitrogen and oxygen species in interleukin-1-mediated DNA damage associated with osteoarthritis. *Osteoarthr Cartil* 16(5): 624-630.

Davisson, T., S. Kunig et al. (2002a). Static and dynamic compression modulate matrix metabolism in tissue engineered cartilage. *J Orthop Res* 20(4): 842-848.

Davisson, T., R. L. Sah et al. (2002b). Perfusion increases cell content and matrix synthesis in chondrocyte three-dimensional cultures. *Tissue Eng* 8(5): 807-816.

Demarteau, O., D. Wendt et al. (2003). Dynamic compression of cartilage constructs engineered from expanded human articular chondrocytes. *Biochem Biophys Res Commun* 310(2): 580-588.

De Mattei, M., M. Pasello et al. (2003). Effects of electromagnetic fields on proteoglycan metabolism of bovine articular cartilage explants. *Connect Tissue Res* 44(3-4): 154-159.

De Mattei, M., A. Pellati et al. (2004). Effects of physical stimulation with electromagnetic field and insulin growth factor-I treatment on proteoglycan synthesis of bovine articular cartilage. *Osteoarthr Cartil* 12(10): 793-800.

Deng, Y., J. C. Hu et al. (2007). Isolation and chondroinduction of a dermis-isolated, aggrecan-sensitive subpopulation with high chondrogenic potential. *Arthritis Rheum* 56(1): 168-176.

Diekman, B. O., N. Christoforou et al. (2012). Cartilage tissue engineering using differentiated and purified induced pluripotent stem cells. *Proc Natl Acad Sci USA* 109(47): 19172-19177.

Diekman, B. O., C. R. Rowland et al. (2010). Effects of individual control of pH and hypoxia in chondrocyte culture. *Tissue Eng Part A* 16(2): 523-533.

Dike, L. E., C. S. Chen et al. (1999). Geometric control of switching between growth, apoptosis, and differentiation during angiogenesis using micropatterned substrates. *In Vitro Cell Dev Biol Anim* 35(8): 441-448.

Dobratz, E. J., S. W. Kim et al. (2009). Injectable cartilage: Using alginate and human chondrocytes. *Arch Facial Plast Surg* 11(1): 40-47.

Domm, C., J. Fay et al. (2000). Redifferentiation of dedifferentiated joint cartilage cells in alginate culture. Effect of intermittent hydrostatic pressure and low oxygen partial pressure [in German]. *Orthopade* 29(2): 91-99.

Duke, P. J., E. L. Daane et al. (1993). Studies of chondrogenesis in rotating systems. *J Cell Biochem* 51(3): 274-282.

Dunkelman, N. S., M. P. Zimber et al. (1995). Cartilage production by rabbit articular chondrocytes on polyglycolic acid scaffolds in a closed bioreactor system. *Biotechnol Bioeng* 46: 299-305.

Eid, K., E. Chen et al. (2001). Effect of RGD coating on osteocompatibility of PLGA-polymer disks in a rat tibial wound. *J Biomed Mater Res* 57(2): 224-231.

Elder, B. D., and K. A. Athanasiou. (2008). Synergistic and additive effects of hydrostatic pressure and growth factors on tissue formation. *PLoS One* 3(6): e2341.

Elder, B. D., and K. A. Athanasiou. (2009a). Hydrostatic pressure in articular cartilage tissue engineering: From chondrocytes to tissue regeneration. *Tissue Eng Part B Rev* 15(1): 43-53.

Elder, B. D., and K. A. Athanasiou. (2009b). Systematic assessment of growth factor treatment on biochemical and biomechanical properties of engineered articular cartilage constructs. *Osteoarthr Cartil* 17(1): 114-123.

Elder, B. D., and K. A. Athanasiou. (2009c). Effects of temporal hydrostatic pressure on tissue-engineered bovine articular cartilage constructs. *Tissue Eng Part A* 15(5): 1151-1158.

Elder, S. H., S. A. Goldstein et al. (2001). Chondrocyte differentiation is modulated by frequency and duration of cyclic compressive loading. *Ann Biomed Eng* 29(6): 476-482.

Elder, S. H., J. W. Shim et al. (2008). Influence of hydrostatic and distortional stress on chondroinduction. *Biorheology* 45(3-4): 479-486.

Elisseeff, J., W. McIntosh et al. (2000). Photoencapsulation of chondrocytes in poly(ethylene oxide)-based semi-interpenetrating networks. *J Biomed Mater Res* 51(2): 164-171.

Emans, P. J., M. Hulsbosch et al. (2005). Repair of osteochondral defects in rabbits with ectopically produced cartilage. *Tissue Eng* 11(11-12): 1789-1796.

Emans, P. J., L. W. van Rhijn et al. (2010). Autologous engineering of cartilage. *Proc Natl Acad Sci USA* 107(8): 3418-3423.

Emin, N., A. Koc et al. (2008). Engineering of rat articular cartilage on porous sponges: Effects of tgf-beta 1 and microgravity bioreactor culture. *Artif Cells Blood Substit Immobil Biotechnol* 36(2): 123-137.

Erlacher, L., C. K. Ng et al. (1998). Presence of cartilage-derived morphogenetic proteins in articular cartilage and enhancement of matrix replacement in vitro. *Arthritis Rheum* 41(2): 263-273.

Fan, H., H. Tao et al. (2010). TGF-beta3 immobilized PLGA-gelatin/chondroitin sulfate/hyaluronic acid hybrid scaffold for cartilage regeneration. *J Biomed Mater Res A* 95(4): 982-992.

Fan, J. C., and S. D. Waldman. (2010). The effect of intermittent static biaxial tensile strains on tissue engineered cartilage. *Ann Biomed Eng* 38(4): 1672-1682.

Fan, V. H., K. Tamama et al. (2007). Tethered epidermal growth factor provides a survival advantage to mesenchymal stem cells. *Stem Cells* 25(5): 1241-1251.

Fermor, B., S. E. Christensen et al. (2007). Oxygen, nitric oxide and articular cartilage. *Eur Cell Mater* 13: 56-65; discussion 65.

Fermor, B., J. B. Weinberg et al. (2005). The influence of oxygen tension on the induction of nitric oxide and prostaglandin E2 by mechanical stress in articular cartilage. *Osteoarthr Cartil* 13(10): 935-941.

Finch, J. (2011). The ancient origins of prosthetic medicine. *Lancet* 377(9765): 548-549.

Fisher, J. P., J. W. Vehof et al. (2002). Soft and hard tissue response to photocrosslinked poly(propylene fumarate) scaffolds in a rabbit model. *J Biomed Mater Res* 59(3): 547-556.

Forslund, C., and P. Aspenberg. (2002). CDMP-2 induces bone or tendon-like tissue depending on mechanical stimulation. *J Orthop Res* 20(6): 1170-1174.

Frank, E. H., M. Jin et al. (2000). A versatile shear and compression apparatus for mechanical stimulation of tissue culture explants. *J Biomech* 33(11): 1523-1527.

Freed, L. E., D. A. Grande et al. (1994a). Joint resurfacing using allograft chondrocytes and synthetic biodegradable polymer scaffolds. *J Biomed Mater Res* 28(8): 891-899.

Freed, L. E., A. P. Hollander et al. (1998). Chondrogenesis in a cell-polymer-bioreactor system. *Exp Cell Res* 240(1): 58-65.

Freed, L. E., J. C. Marquis et al. (1994b). Composition of cell-polymer cartilage implants. *Biotechnol Bioeng* 43: 605-614.

Freed, L. E., I. Martin et al. (1999). Frontiers in tissue engineering. In vitro modulation of chondrogenesis. *Clin Orthop* 1999(367 Suppl): S46-S58.

Freed, L. E., and G. Vunjak-Novakovic. (1995). Cultivation of cell-polymer tissue constructs in simulated microgravity. *Biotechnol Bioeng* 46: 306.

Freed, L. E., G. Vunjak-Novakovic et al. (1993). Cultivation of cell-polymer cartilage implants in bioreactors. *J Cell Biochem* 51(3): 257-264.

Frenkel, S. R., P. B. Saadeh et al. (2000). Transforming growth factor beta superfamily members: Role in cartilage modeling. *Plast Reconstr Surg* 105(3): 980-990.

Fuchs, J. R., D. Hannouche et al. (2005). Cartilage engineering from ovine umbilical cord blood mesenchymal progenitor cells. *Stem Cells* 23(7): 958-964.

Furukawa, K. S., K. Imura et al. (2008). Scaffold-free cartilage by rotational culture for tissue engineering. *J Biotechnol* 133(1): 134-145.

Furukawa, K. S., H. Suenaga et al. (2003). Rapid and large-scale formation of chondrocyte aggregates by rotational culture. *Cell Transplant* 12(5): 475-479.

Gallant, N. D., J. R. Capadona et al. (2002). Micropatterned surfaces to engineer focal adhesions for analysis of cell adhesion strengthening. *Langmuir* 18: 5579-5584.

Gemmiti, C. V., and R. E. Guldberg. (2006). Fluid flow increases type II collagen deposition and tensile mechanical properties in bioreactor-grown tissue-engineered cartilage. *Tissue Eng* 12(3): 469-479.

Gemmiti, C. V., and R. E. Guldberg. (2009). Shear stress magnitude and duration modulates matrix composition and tensile mechanical properties in engineered cartilaginous tissue. *Biotechnol Bioeng* 104(4): 809-820.

Gigout, A., M. Jolicoeur et al. (2008). Chondrocyte aggregation in suspension culture is GFOGER-GPP- and beta1 integrin-dependent. *J Biol Chem* 283(46): 31522-31530.

Gobin, A. S., and J. L. West. (2002). Cell migration through defined, synthetic ECM analogs. *FASEB J* 16(7): 751-753.

Gooch, K. J., T. Blunk et al. (2001a). IGF-I and mechanical environment interact to modulate engineered cartilage development. *Biochem Biophys Res Commun* 286(5): 909-915.

Gooch, K. J., T. Blunk et al. (2002). Bone morphogenetic proteins-2, -12, and -13 modulate in vitro development of engineered cartilage. *Tissue Eng* 8(4): 591-601.

Gooch, K. J., J. H. Kwon et al. (2001b). Effects of mixing intensity on tissue-engineered cartilage. *Biotechnol Bioeng* 72(4): 402-407.

Goodwin, T. J., T. L. Prewett et al. (1993). Reduced shear stress: A major component in the ability of mammalian tissues to form three-dimensional assemblies in simulated microgravity. *J Cell Biochem* 51(3): 301-311.

Graff, R. D., S. S. Kelley et al. (2003). Role of pericellular matrix in development of a mechanically functional neocartilage. *Biotechnol Bioeng* 82(4): 457-464.

Grande, D. A., C. Halberstadt et al. (1997). Evaluation of matrix scaffolds for tissue engineering of articular cartilage grafts. *J Biomed Mater Res* 34(2): 211-220.

Griffon, D. J., M. R. Sedighi et al. (2006). Chitosan scaffolds: Interconnective pore size and cartilage engineering. *Acta Biomater* 2(3): 313-320.

Grigolo, B., L. Roseti et al. (2001). Transplantation of chondrocytes seeded on a hyaluronan derivative (hyaff-11) into cartilage defects in rabbits. *Biomaterials* 22(17): 2417-2424.

Grimaud, E., D. Heymann et al. (2002). Recent advances in TGF-beta effects on chondrocyte metabolism. Potential therapeutic roles of TGF-beta in cartilage disorders. *Cytokine Growth Factor Rev* 13(3): 241-257.

Grogan, S. P., F. Rieser et al. (2003). A static, closed and scaffold-free bioreactor system that permits chondrogenesis in vitro. *Osteoarthr Cartil* 11(6): 403-411.

Gruber, R., C. Mayer et al. (2001). Effects of cartilage-derived morphogenetic proteins and osteogenic protein-1 on osteochondrogenic differentiation of periosteum-derived cells. *Endocrinology* 142(5): 2087-2094.

Guerne, P. A., A. Sublet et al. (1994). Growth factor responsiveness of human articular chondrocytes: Distinct profiles in primary chondrocytes, subcultured
chondrocytes, and fibroblasts. *J Cell Physiol* 158(3): 476-484.

Guilak, F. (2002). Functional tissue engineering: The role of biomechanics in reparative medicine. *Ann NY Acad Sci* 961: 193-195.

Guilak, F., B. T. Estes et al. (2010). 2010 Nicolas Andry Award: Multipotent adult stem
cells from adipose tissue for musculoskeletal tissue engineering. *Clin Orthop
Relat Res* 468(9): 2530-2540.

Guilak, F., A. Ratcliffe et al. (1995). Chondrocyte deformation and local tissue strain in
articular cartilage: A confocal microscopy study. *J Orthop Res* 13(3): 410-421.

Guilak, F., L. A. Setton et al. (2000). Structure and function of articular cartilage. In
Principles and Practice of Orthopaedic Sports Medicine, ed. W. E. Garrett,
K. P. Speer, D. T. Kirkendall, and M. D. Kitkowski. Philadelphia: Lippincott
Williams & Wilkins, pp. 53-73.

Haddad, J. B., A. G. Obolensky et al. (2007). The biologic effects and the therapeutic mechanism of action of electric and electromagnetic field stimulation
on bone and cartilage: New findings and a review of earlier work. *J Altern
Complement Med* 13(5): 485-490.

Hall, A. C., E. R. Horwitz et al. (1996). The cellular physiology of articular cartilage.
Exp Physiol 81(3): 535-545.

Hall, A. C., J. P. Urban et al. (1991). The effects of hydrostatic pressure on matrix synthesis in articular cartilage. *J Orthop Res* 9(1): 1-10.

Han, D. K., K. D. Park et al. (1998). Surface characteristics and biocompatibility
of lactide-based poly(ethylene glycol) scaffolds for tissue engineering.
J Biomater Sci Polym Ed 9(7): 667-680.

Hansen, U., M. Schünke et al. (2001). Combination of reduced oxygen tension and
intermittent hydrostatic pressure: A useful tool in articular cartilage tissue
engineering. *J Biomech* 34: 941-949.

Heath, C. A., and S. R. Magari. (1996). Mini-review: Mechanical factors affecting cartilage regeneration in vitro. *Biotechnol Bioeng* 50: 430-437.

Heyland, J., K. Wiegandt et al. (2006). Redifferentiation of chondrocytes and cartilage formation under intermittent hydrostatic pressure. *Biotechnol Lett*
28(20): 1641-1648.

Heywood, H. K., M. M. Knight et al. (2010). Both superficial and deep zone articular
chondrocyte subpopulations exhibit the Crabtree effect but have different
basal oxygen consumption rates. *J Cell Physiol* 223(3): 630-639.

Hoben, G. M., E. J. Koay et al. (2008). Fibrochondrogenesis in two embryonic stem
cell lines: Effects of differentiation timelines. *Stem Cells* 26(2): 422-430.

Homminga, G. N., S. K. Bulstra et al. (1991). Repair of sheep articular cartilage defects
with a rabbit costal perichondrial graft. *Acta Orthop Scand* 62(5): 415-418.

Honda, M., T. Yada et al. (2000). Cartilage formation by cultured chondrocytes in a new scaffold made of poly(L-lactide-epsilon-caprolactone) sponge. *J Oral Maxillofac Surg* 58(7): 767-775.

Hu, J. C., and K. A. Athanasiou. (2005). Low-density cultures of bovine chondrocytes: Effects of scaffold material and culture system. *Biomaterials* 26(14): 2001-2012.

Hu, J. C., and K. A. Athanasiou. (2006a). The effects of intermittent hydrostatic pressure on self-assembled articular cartilage constructs. *Tissue Eng* 12(5): 1337-1344.

Hu, J. C., and K. A. Athanasiou. (2006b). A self-assembling process in articular cartilage tissue engineering. *Tissue Eng* 12(4): 969-979.

Hubbell, J. A. (1997). Matrix effects. In *Principles of Tissue Engineering*, ed. R. Lanza, R. Langer, and W. Chick. Austin, TX: R. G. Landes Company, p. 249.

Huey, D. J., and K. A. Athanasiou. (2011a). Maturational growth of self-assembled, functional menisci as a result of TGF-beta1 and enzymatic chondroitinase-ABC stimulation. *Biomaterials* 32(8): 2052-2058.

Huey, D. J., and K. A. Athanasiou. (2011b). Tension-compression loading with chemical stimulation results in additive increases to functional properties of anatomic meniscal constructs. *PLoS One* 6(11): e27857.

Hung, C. T., R. L. Mauck et al. (2004). A paradigm for functional tissue engineering of articular cartilage via applied physiologic deformational loading. *Ann Biomed Eng* 32(1): 35-49.

Hunter, C. J., S. M. Imler et al. (2002). Mechanical compression alters gene expression and extracellular matrix synthesis by chondrocytes cultured in collagen I gels. *Biomaterials* 23(4): 1249-1259.

Hunziker, E. B. (2002). Articular cartilage repair: Basic science and clinical progress. A review of the current status and prospects. *Osteoarthr Cartil* 10(6): 432-463.

Hunziker, E. B., and L. C. Rosenberg. (1996). Repair of partial-thickness defects in articular cartilage: Cell recruitment from the synovial membrane. *J Bone Joint Surg Am* 78(5): 721-733.

Hutmacher, D. W. (2001). Scaffold design and fabrication technologies for engineering tissues—State of the art and future perspectives. *J Biomater Sci Polym Ed* 12(1): 107-124.

Hutmacher, D. W., J. C. Goh et al. (2001). An introduction to biodegradable materials for tissue engineering applications. *Ann Acad Med Singapore* 30(2): 183-191.

Hwang, N. S., and J. Elisseeff. (2009). Application of stem cells for articular cartilage regeneration. *J Knee Surg* 22(1): 60-71.

Hynes, R. O. (1992). Integrins: Versatility, modulation, and signaling in cell adhesion. *Cell* 69(1): 11-25.

Ingber, D. (1991). Integrins as mechanochemical transducers. *Curr Opin Cell Biol* 3(5): 841-848.

Isermann, P., and J. Lammerding. (2013). Nuclear mechanics and mechanotransduction in health and disease. *Curr Biol* 23(24): R1113-R1121.

Ishaug-Riley, S. L., L. E. Okun et al. (1999). Human articular chondrocyte adhesion and proliferation on synthetic biodegradable polymer films. *Biomaterials* 20(23-24): 2245-2256.

Jennings, L., L. Wu et al. (2001). The effects of collagen fragments on the extracellular matrix metabolism of bovine and human chondrocytes. *Connect Tissue Res* 42(1): 71-86.

Jiang, Y., B. N. Jahagirdar et al. (2002). Pluripotency of mesenchymal stem cells derived from adult marrow. *Nature* 418(6893): 41-49.

Jin, C. Z., J. H. Cho et al. (2011). The maturity of tissue engineered cartilage in vitro affects the repairability for osteochondral defect. *Tissue Eng Part A* 7(23-24): 3057-3065.

Jin, M., G. R. Emkey et al. (2003). Combined effects of dynamic tissue shear deformation and insulin-like growth factor I on chondrocyte biosynthesis in cartilage explants. *Arch Biochem Biophys* 414(2): 223-231.

Jin, M., E. H. Frank et al. (2001). Tissue shear deformation stimulates proteoglycan and protein biosynthesis in bovine cartilage explants. *Arch Biochem Biophys* 395(1): 41-48.

Jo, S., P. S. Engel et al. (2000). Synthesis of poly(ethylene glycol)-tethered poly(propylene fumarate) and its modification with GRGD peptide. *Polymer* 41: 7595-7604.

Jubel, A., J. Andermahr et al. (2008). Transplantation of de novo scaffold-free cartilage implants into sheep knee chondral defects. *Am J Sports Med* 36(8): 1555-1564.

Jung, S. N., J. W. Rhie et al. (2010). In vivo cartilage formation using chondrogenic-differentiated human adipose-derived mesenchymal stem cells mixed with fibrin glue. *J Craniofac Surg* 21(2): 468-472.

Jung, Y., S. H. Kim et al. (2008). Cartilaginous tissue formation using a mechano-active scaffold and dynamic compressive stimulation. *J Biomater Sci Polym Ed* 19(1): 61-74.

Kaarniranta, K., M. Elo et al. (1998). Hsp70 accumulation in chondrocytic cells exposed to high continuous hydrostatic pressure coincides with mRNA stabilization rather than transcriptional activation. *Proc Natl Acad Sci USA* 95(5): 2319-2324.

Kaps, C., C. Bramlage et al. (2002). Bone morphogenetic proteins promote cartilage differentiation and protect engineered artificial cartilage from fibroblast invasion and destruction. *Arthritis Rheum* 46(1): 149-162.

Kasahara, Y., N. Iwasaki et al. (2008). Development of mature cartilage constructs using novel three-dimensional porous scaffolds for enhanced repair of osteochondral defects. *J Biomed Mater Res A* 86(1): 127-136.

Katakai, D., M. Imura et al. (2009). Compressive properties of cartilage-like tissues repaired in vivo with scaffold-free, tissue engineered constructs. *Clin Biomech (Bristol, Avon)* 24(1): 110-116.

Kawakami, M., N. Tomita et al. (2011). Chondrocyte distribution and cartilage regeneration in silk fibroin sponge. *Biomed Mater Eng* 21(1): 53-61.

Kawanishi, M., A. Oura et al. (2007). Redifferentiation of dedifferentiated bovine articular chondrocytes enhanced by cyclic hydrostatic pressure under a gas-controlled system. *Tissue Eng* 13(5): 957-964.

Kelly, T. A., K. W. Ng et al. (2009). Analysis of radial variations in material properties and matrix composition of chondrocyte-seeded agarose hydrogel constructs. *Osteoarthr Cartil* 17(1): 73-82.

Khan, A. A., J. M. Suits et al. (2009). The effect of continuous culture on the growth and structure of tissue-engineered cartilage. *Biotechnol Prog* 25(2): 508-515.

Kim, Y. J., R. L. Sah et al. (1994). Mechanical regulation of cartilage biosynthetic behavior: Physical stimuli. *Arch Biochem Biophys* 311(1): 1-12.

Kisiday, J. D., M. Jin et al. (2004). Effects of dynamic compressive loading on chondrocyte biosynthesis in self-assembling peptide scaffolds. *J Biomech* 37(5): 595-604.

Klein, T. J., J. Malda et al. (2009). Tissue engineering of articular cartilage with biomimetic zones. *Tissue Eng Part B Rev* 15(2): 143-157.

Kleinman, H. K., M. L. McGarvey et al. (1982). Isolation and characterization of type IV procollagen, laminin, and heparan sulfate proteoglycan from the EHS sarcoma. *Biochemistry* 21(24): 6188-6193.

Knudson, W., and R. F. Loeser. (2002). CD44 and integrin matrix receptors participate in cartilage homeostasis. *Cell Mol Life Sci* 59(1): 36-44.

Ko, C. S., J. P. Huang et al. (2009). Type II collagen-chondroitin sulfate-hyaluronan scaffold cross-linked by genipin for cartilage tissue engineering. *J Biosci Bioeng* 107(2): 177-182.

Koay, E. J., and K. A. Athanasiou. (2008). Hypoxic chondrogenic differentiation of human embryonic stem cells enhances cartilage protein synthesis and biomechanical functionality. *Osteoarthr Cartil* 16(12): 1450-1456.

Koay, E. J., and K. A. Athanasiou. (2009). Development of serum-free, chemically defined conditions for human embryonic stem cell-derived fibrochondrogenesis. *Tissue Eng Part A* 15(8): 2249-2257.

Koay, E. J., G. M. Hoben et al. (2007). Tissue engineering with chondrogenically differentiated human embryonic stem cells. *Stem Cells* 25(9): 2183-2190.

Koivunen, E., B. Wang et al. (1994). Peptides in cell adhesion research. *Methods Enzymol* 245: 346-369.

Kunisaki, S. M., R. W. Jennings et al. (2006). Fetal cartilage engineering from amniotic mesenchymal progenitor cells. *Stem Cells Dev* 15(2): 245-253.

Kuo, Y. C., and I. N. Ku. (2008). Cartilage regeneration by novel polyethylene oxide/chitin/chitosan scaffolds. *Biomacromolecules* 9(10): 2662-2669.

Kurth, T., E. Hedbom et al. (2007). Chondrogenic potential of human synovial mesenchymal stem cells in alginate. *Osteoarthr Cartil* 15(10): 1178-1189.

Kus, W. M., A. Gorecki et al. (1999). Carbon fiber scaffolds in the surgical treatment of cartilage lesions. *Ann Transplant* 4(3-4): 101-102.

Lagana, K., M. Moretti et al. (2008). A new bioreactor for the controlled application of complex mechanical stimuli for cartilage tissue engineering. *Proc Inst Mech Eng H* 222(5): 705-715.

Lammi, M. J., R. Inkinen et al. (1994). Expression of reduced amounts of structurally altered aggrecan in articular cartilage chondrocytes exposed to high hydrostatic pressure. *Biochem J* 304(Pt 3): 723-730.

Latthe, S., C. Terashima et al. (2014). Superhydrophobic surfaces developed by mimicking hierarchical surface morphology of lotus leaf. *Molecules* 19(4): 4256.

LeBaron, R. G., and K. A. Athanasiou. (2000). Extracellular matrix cell adhesion peptides: Functional applications in orthopedic materials. *Tissue Eng* 6(2): 85-103.

Lee, C. H., J. L. Cook et al. (2010). Regeneration of the articular surface of the rabbit synovial joint by cell homing: A proof of concept study. *Lancet* 376(9739): 440-448.

Lee, C. R., H. A. Breinan et al. (2000). Articular cartilage chondrocytes in type I and type II collagen-GAG matrices exhibit contractile behavior in vitro. *Tissue Eng* 6(5): 555-565.

Lee, D. A., T. Noguchi et al. (2000). The influence of mechanical loading on isolated chondrocytes seeded in agarose constructs. *Biorheology* 37(1-2): 149-161.

Lee, J. Y., C. Jones et al. (2006). Analysis of local tissue-specific gene expression in cellular micropatterns. *Anal Chem* 78(24): 8305-8312.

Lee, M. S., M. C. Trindade et al. (2002). Effects of shear stress on nitric oxide and matrix protein gene expression in human osteoarthritic chondrocytes in vitro. *J Orthop Res* 20(3): 556-561.

Lee, V., L. Cao et al. (2000). The roles of matrix molecules in mediating chondrocyte aggregation, attachment, and spreading. *J Cell Biochem* 79(2): 322-333.

Levorson, E. J., M. Santoro et al. (2014). Direct and indirect co-culture of chondrocytes and mesenchymal stem cells for the generation of polymer/extracellular matrix hybrid constructs. *Acta Biomater* 10(5): 1824-1835.

Lima, E. G., L. Bian et al. (2007). The beneficial effect of delayed compressive loading on tissue-engineered cartilage constructs cultured with TGF-beta3. *Osteoarthr Cartil* 15(9): 1025-1033.

Liu, T. Y., G. D. Zhou et al. (2007). Influence of transforming growth factor-beta1 inducing time on chondrogenesis of bone marrow stromal cells (BMSCs): In vitro experiment with porcine BMSCs [in Chinese]. *Zhonghua Yi Xue Za Zhi* 87(31): 2218-2222.

Liu, X., H. Sun et al. (2010). In vivo ectopic chondrogenesis of BMSCs directed by mature chondrocytes. *Biomaterials* 31(36): 9406-9414.

Llorens, E., E. Armelin et al. (2013). Nanomembranes and nanofibers from biodegradable conducting polymers. *Polymers* 5(3): 1115-1157.

Lom, B., K. E. Healy et al. (1993). A versatile technique for patterning biomolecules onto glass coverslips. *J Neurosci Methods* 50(3): 385-397.

Luo, Z. J., and B. B. Seedhom. (2007). Light and low-frequency pulsatile hydrostatic pressure enhances extracellular matrix formation by bone marrow mesenchymal cells: An in-vitro study with special reference to cartilage repair. *Proc Inst Mech Eng H* 221(5): 499-507.

Luyten, F. P., Y. M. Yu et al. (1992). Natural bovine osteogenin and recombinant human bone morphogenetic protein-2B are equipotent in the maintenance of proteoglycans in bovine articular cartilage explant cultures. *J Biol Chem* 267(6): 3691-3695.

Macchiarini, P., P. Jungebluth et al. (2008). Clinical transplantation of a tissue-engineered airway. *Lancet* 372(9655): 2023-2030.

MacGinitie, L. A., Y. A. Gluzband et al. (1994). Electric field stimulation can increase protein synthesis in articular cartilage explants. *J Orthop Res* 12(2): 151-160.

Madihally, S. V., and H. W. Matthew. (1999). Porous chitosan scaffolds for tissue engineering. *Biomaterials* 20(12): 1133-1142.

Madry, H., R. Padera et al. (2002). Gene transfer of a human insulin-like growth factor I cDNA enhances tissue engineering of cartilage. *Hum Gene Ther* 13(13): 1621-1630.

Makaya, K., S. Terada et al. (2009). Comparative study of silk fibroin porous scaffolds derived from salt/water and sucrose/hexafluoroisopropanol in cartilage formation. *J Biosci Bioeng* 108(1): 68-75.

Makihira, S., W. Yan et al. (1999). Enhancement of cell adhesion and spreading by a cartilage-specific noncollagenous protein, cartilage matrix protein (CMP/Matrilin-1), via integrin alpha1beta1. *J Biol Chem* 274(16): 11417-11423.

Makris, E. A., J. C. Hu et al. (2014a). Hypoxia-induced collagen crosslinking as a mechanism for enhancing mechanical properties of engineered articular cartilage. *Osteoarthritis Cart* 21(4): 634-641.

Makris, E. A., D. J. Responte et al. (2014b). Developing functional musculoskeletal tissues through hypoxia and lysyl oxidase-induced collagen cross-linking. *Proc Natl Acad Sci USA* 111(45): E4832-E4841.

Malda, J., D. E. Martens et al. (2003). Cartilage tissue engineering: Controversy in the effect of oxygen. *Crit Rev Biotechnol* 23(3): 175-194.

Malda, J., P. van den Brink et al. (2004). Effect of oxygen tension on adult articular chondrocytes in microcarrier bioreactor culture. *Tissue Eng* 10(7-8): 987-994.

Mandal, K., M. Balland et al. (2012). Thermoresponsive micropatterned substrates for single cell studies. *PLoS One* 7(5): e37548.

Mankin, H. J. (1982). The response of articular cartilage to mechanical injury. *J Bone Joint Surg Am* 64(3): 460-466.

Mann, B. K., A. S. Gobin et al. (2001a). Smooth muscle cell growth in photopolymerized hydrogels with cell adhesive and proteolytically degradable domains: Synthetic ECM analogs for tissue engineering. *Biomaterials* 22(22): 3045-3051.

Mann, B. K., R. H. Schmedlen et al. (2001b). Tethered-TGF-beta increases extracellular matrix production of vascular smooth muscle cells. *Biomaterials* 22(5): 439-444.

Mann, B. K., A. T. Tsai et al. (1999). Modification of surfaces with cell adhesion peptides alters extracellular matrix deposition. *Biomaterials* 20(23-24): 2281-2286.

Mann, B. K., and J. L. West. (2002). Cell adhesion peptides alter smooth muscle cell adhesion, proliferation, migration, and matrix protein synthesis on modified surfaces and in polymer scaffolds. *J Biomed Mater Res* 60(1): 86-93.

Marijnissen, W. J., G. J. van Osch et al. (2000). Tissue-engineered cartilage using serially passaged articular chondrocytes. Chondrocytes in alginate, combined in vivo with a synthetic (E210) or biologic biodegradable carrier (DBM). *Biomaterials* 21(6): 571-580.

Marlovits, S., B. Tichy et al. (2003a). Collagen expression in tissue engineered cartilage of aged human articular chondrocytes in a rotating bioreactor. *Int J Artif Organs* 26(4): 319-330.

Marlovits, S., B. Tichy et al. (2003b). Chondrogenesis of aged human articular cartilage in a scaffold-free bioreactor. *Tissue Eng* 9(6): 1215-1226.

Martin, I., B. Obradovic et al. (1999). Method for quantitative analysis of glycosaminoglycan distribution in cultured natural and engineered cartilage. *Ann Biomed Eng* 27(5): 656-662.

Martin, I., B. Obradovic et al. (2000). Modulation of the mechanical properties of tissue engineered cartilage. *Biorheology* 37(1-2): 141-147.

Martinac, B. (2004). Mechanosensitive ion channels: Molecules of mechanotransduction. *J Cell Sci* 117(Pt 12): 2449-2460.

Martosella, J., and N. Zolotarjova. (2008). Multi-component immunoaffinity subtraction and reversed-phase chromatography of human serum. *Methods Mol Biol* 425: 27-39.

Massari, L., F. Benazzo et al. (2007). Effects of electrical physical stimuli on articular cartilage. *J Bone Joint Surg Am* 89(Suppl 3): 152-161.

Masuda, K., R. L. Sah et al. (2003). A novel two-step method for the formation of tissue-engineered cartilage by mature bovine chondrocytes: The alginate-recovered-chondrocyte (ARC) method. *J Orthop Res* 21(1): 139-148.

Mattioli-Belmonte, M., A. Gigante et al. (1999). N,N-Dicarboxymethyl chitosan as delivery agent for bone morphogenetic protein in the repair of articular cartilage. *Med Biol Eng Comput* 37(1): 130-134.

Mauck, R. L., B. A. Byers et al. (2007). Regulation of cartilaginous ECM gene transcription by chondrocytes and MSCs in 3D culture in response to dynamic loading. *Biomech Model Mechanobiol* 6(1-2): 113-125.

Mauck, R. L., C. T. Hung et al. (2003a). Modeling of neutral solute transport in a dynamically loaded porous permeable gel: Implications for articular cartilage biosynthesis and tissue engineering. *J Biomech Eng* 125(5): 602-614.

Mauck, R. L., S. B. Nicoll et al. (2003b). Synergistic action of growth factors and dynamic loading for articular cartilage tissue engineering. *Tissue Eng* 9(4): 597-611.

Mauck, R. L., M. A. Soltz et al. (2000). Functional tissue engineering of articular cartilage through dynamic loading of chondrocyte-seeded agarose gels. *J Biomech Eng* 122(3): 252-260.

Mauck, R. L., X. Yuan et al. (2006). Chondrogenic differentiation and functional maturation of bovine mesenchymal stem cells in long-term agarose culture. *Osteoarthr Cartil* 14(2): 179-189.

McGowan, K. B., and R. L. Sah. (2005). Treatment of cartilage with beta-aminopropionitrile accelerates subsequent collagen maturation and modulates integrative repair. *J Orthop Res* 23(3): 594-601.

McKibbin, B., and F. W. Holdsworth. (1966). The nutrition of immature joint cartilage in the lamb. *J Bone Joint Surg Br* 48(4): 793-803.

McMahon, L. A., A. J. Reid et al. (2008). Regulatory effects of mechanical strain on the chondrogenic differentiation of MSCs in a collagen-GAG scaffold: Experimental and computational analysis. *Ann Biomed Eng* 36(2): 185-194.

Meinel, L., S. Hofmann et al. (2004). Engineering cartilage-like tissue using human mesenchymal stem cells and silk protein scaffolds. *Biotechnol Bioeng* 88(3): 379-391.

Merchuk, J. C. (1990). Why use air-lift bioreactors? *Trends Biotechnol* 8: 66-71.

Meyer, U., A. Buchter et al. (2006). Design and performance of a bioreactor system for mechanically promoted three-dimensional tissue engineering. *Br J Oral Maxillofac Surg* 44(2): 134-140.

Middleton, J. C., and A. J. Tipton. (2000). Synthetic biodegradable polymers as orthopedic devices. *Biomaterials* 21(23): 2335-2346.

Mikos, A. G., S. W. Herring et al. (2006). Engineering complex tissues. *Tissue Eng* 12(12): 3307-3339.

Miyanishi, K., M. C. Trindade et al. (2006a). Dose- and time-dependent effects of cyclic hydrostatic pressure on transforming growth factor-beta3-induced chondrogenesis by adult human mesenchymal stem cells in vitro. *Tissue Eng* 12(8): 2253-2262.

Miyanishi, K., M. C. Trindade et al. (2006b). Effects of hydrostatic pressure and trans-forming growth factor-beta 3 on adult human mesenchymal stem cell chondrogenesis in vitro. *Tissue Eng* 12(6): 1419-1428.

Mizuno, S., F. Allemann et al. (2001). Effects of medium perfusion on matrix production by bovine chondrocytes in three-dimensional collagen sponges. *J Biomed Mater Res* 56(3): 368-375.

Moreno-Arotzena, O., J. G. Meier et al. (2015). Characterization of fibrin and collagen gels for engineering wound healing models. *Materials (Basel)* 8(4): 1636-1651.

Moretti, M., L. E. Freed et al. (2008). An integrated experimental-computational approach for the study of engineered cartilage constructs subjected to combined regimens of hydrostatic pressure and interstitial perfusion. *Biomed Mater Eng* 18(4-5): 273-278.

Moutos, F. T., L. E. Freed et al. (2007). A biomimetic three-dimensional woven composite scaffold for functional tissue engineering of cartilage. *Nat Mater* 6(2): 162-167.

Moutos, F. T., and F. Guilak. (2008). Composite scaffolds for cartilage tissue engineering. *Biorheology* 45(3-4): 501-512.

Mow, V. C., A. Ratcliffe et al. (1991). Experimental studies on repair of large osteochondral defects at a high weight bearing area of the knee joint: A tissue engineering study. *J Biomech Eng* 113(2): 198-207.

Murphy, C. L., and A. Sambanis. (2001a). Effect of oxygen tension and alginate encapsulation on restoration of the differentiated phenotype of passaged chondrocytes. *Tissue Eng* 7(6): 791-803.

Murphy, C. L., and A. Sambanis. (2001b). Effect of oxygen tension on chondrocyte extracellular matrix accumulation. *Connect Tissue Res* 42(2): 87-96.

Nakamura, S., Y. Arai et al. (2006). Hydrostatic pressure induces apoptosis of chondrocytes cultured in alginate beads. *J Orthop Res* 24(4): 733-739.

Natoli, R., C. M. Revell et al. (2009a). Chondroitinase ABC treatment results in increased tensile properties of self-assembled tissue engineered articular cartilage. *Tissue Eng Part A* 15(10): 3119-3128.

Natoli, R. M., and K. A. Athanasiou. (2009). Traumatic loading of articular cartilage: Mechanical and biological responses and post-injury treatment. *Biorheology* 46(6): 451-485.

Natoli, R. M., D. J. Responte et al. (2009b). Effects of multiple chondroitinase ABC applications on tissue engineered articular cartilage. *J Orthop Res* 27(7): 949-956.

Nehrer, S., H. A. Breinan et al. (1997). Canine chondrocytes seeded in type I and type II collagen implants investigated in vitro. *J Biomed Mater Res* 38(2): 95-104. [Published erratum appears in *J Biomed Mater Res* 38(4): 288, 1997.]

Nettles, D. L., S. H. Elder et al. (2002). Potential use of chitosan as a cell scaffold material for cartilage tissue engineering. *Tissue Eng* 8(6): 1009-1016.

Neu, C. P., A. Khalafi et al. (2007). Mechanotransduction of bovine articular cartilage superficial zone protein by transforming growth factor beta signaling. *Arthritis Rheum* 56(11): 3706-3714.

Newcombe, F. C. (1904). Limitations of the klinostat as an instrument for scientific research. *Science* 20(507): 376-379.

Ng, K. W., G. A. Ateshian et al. (2009). Zonal chondrocytes seeded in a layered agarose hydrogel create engineered cartilage with depth-dependent cellular and mechanical inhomogeneity. *Tissue Eng Part A* 15(9): 2315-2324.

Nicodemus, G. D., and S. J. Bryant. (2010). Mechanical loading regimes affect the anabolic and catabolic activities by chondrocytes encapsulated in PEG hydrogels. *Osteoarthr Cartil* 18(1): 126-137.

Obradovic, B., R. L. Carrier et al. (1999). Gas exchange is essential for bioreactor cultivation of tissue engineered cartilage. *Biotechnol Bioeng* 63(2): 197-205.

Obradovic, B., I. Martin et al. (2001). Bioreactor studies of natural and tissue engineered cartilage. *Ortop Traumatol Rehabil* 3(2): 181-189.

O'Connor, W. J., T. Botti et al. (2000). The use of growth factors in cartilage repair. *Orthop Clin North Am* 31(3): 399-410.

Ofek, G., C. M. Revell et al. (2008). Matrix development in self-assembly of articular cartilage. *PLoS One* 3(7): e2795.

Ogawa, R., S. Mizuno et al. (2009). The effect of hydrostatic pressure on 3-D chondroinduction of human adipose-derived stem cells. *Tissue Eng Part A* 15(10): 2937-2945.

Ohyabu, Y., N. Kida et al. (2006). Cartilaginous tissue formation from bone marrow cells using rotating wall vessel (RWV) bioreactor. *Biotechnol Bioeng* 95(5): 1003-1008.

Ongaro, A., K. Varani et al. (2012). Electromagnetic fields (EMFs) and adenosine receptors modulate prostaglandin E(2) and cytokine release in human osteoarthritic synovial fibroblasts. *J Cell Physiol* 227(6): 2461-2469.

Ott, H. C., T. S. Matthiesen et al. (2008). Perfusion-decellularized matrix: Using nature's platform to engineer a bioartificial heart. *Nat Med* 14(2): 213-221.

Pacifici, M., E. Koyama et al. (2000). Development of articular cartilage: What do we know about it and how may it occur? *Connect Tissue Res* 41(3): 175-184.

Palmoski, M. J., and K. D. Brandt. (1984). Effects of static and cyclic compressive loading on articular cartilage plugs in vitro. *Arthritis Rheum* 27(6): 675-681.

Park, K. M., Y. K. Joung et al. (2009). Thermosensitive chitosan-Pluronic hydrogel as an injectable cell delivery carrier for cartilage regeneration. *Acta Biomater* 5(6): 1956-1965.

Parkkinen, J. J., J. Ikonen et al. (1993a). Effects of cyclic hydrostatic pressure on proteoglycan synthesis in cultured chondrocytes and articular cartilage explants. *Arch Biochem Biophys* 300(1): 458-465.

Parkkinen, J. J., M. J. Lammi et al. (1995). Influence of short-term hydrostatic pressure on organization of stress fibers in cultured chondrocytes. *J Orthop Res* 13(4): 495-502.

Parkkinen, J. J., M. J. Lammi et al. (1993b). Altered Golgi apparatus in hydrostatically loaded articular cartilage chondrocytes. *Ann Rheum Dis* 52(3): 192-198.

Parsch, D., J. Fellenberg et al. (2004). Telomere length and telomerase activity during expansion and differentiation of human mesenchymal stem cells and chondrocytes. *J Mol Med* 82(1): 49-55.

Pasqualini, R., E. Koivunen et al. (1996). Peptides in cell adhesion: Powerful tools for the study of integrin-ligand interactions. *Braz J Med Biol Res* 29(9): 1151-1158.

Pazzano, D., K. A. Mercier et al. (2000). Comparison of chondrogensis in static and perfused bioreactor culture. *Biotechnol Prog* 16(5): 893-896.

Pecina, M., M. Jelic et al. (2002). Articular cartilage repair: The role of bone morphogenetic proteins. *Int Orthop* 26(3): 131-136.

Pei, M., F. He et al. (2008a). Repair of full-thickness femoral condyle cartilage defects using allogeneic synovial cell-engineered tissue constructs. *Osteoarthr Cartil* 17(6): 714-722.

Pei, M., F. He et al. (2008b). Engineering of functional cartilage tissue using stem cells from synovial lining: A preliminary study. *Clin Orthop Relat Res* 466(8): 1880-1889.

Pei, M., L. A. Solchaga et al. (2002). Bioreactors mediate the effectiveness of tissue engineering scaffolds. *FASEB J* 16(12): 1691-1694.

Pelaez, D., C. Y. Huang et al. (2008). Cyclic compression maintains viability and induces chondrogenesis of human mesenchymal stem cells in fibrin gel scaffolds. *Stem Cells Dev* 18(1): 93-102.

Perka, C., U. Arnold et al. (2001). The use of fibrin beads for tissue engineering and subsequential transplantation. *Tissue Eng* 7(3): 359-361.

Perka, C., O. Schultz et al. (2000). Joint cartilage repair with transplantation of embryonic chondrocytes embedded in collagen-fibrin matrices. *Clin Exp Rheumatol* 18(1): 13-22.

Petersen, E. F., R. G. Spencer et al. (2002). Microengineering neocartilage scaffolds. *Biotechnol Bioeng* 78(7): 801-804.

Pezzetti, F., M. De Mattei et al. (1999). Effects of pulsed electromagnetic fields on human chondrocytes: An in vitro study. *Calcif Tissue Int* 65(5): 396-401.

Philp, D., S. S. Chen et al. (2005). Complex extracellular matrices promote tissue-specific stem cell differentiation. *Stem Cells* 23(2): 288-296.

Pierschbacher, M. D., and E. Ruoslahti. (1984). Variants of the cell recognition site of fibronectin that retain attachment-promoting activity. *Proc Natl Acad Sci USA* 81(19): 5985-5988.

Pingguan-Murphy, B., D. A. Lee et al. (2005). Activation of chondrocytes calcium signalling by dynamic compression is independent of number of cycles. *Arch Biochem Biophys* 444(1): 45-51.

Place, E. S., R. Nair et al. (2012). Latent TGF-beta hydrogels for cartilage tissue engineering. *Adv Healthc Mater* 1(4): 480-484.

Pound, J. C., D. W. Green et al. (2006). Strategies to promote chondrogenesis and osteogenesis from human bone marrow cells and articular chondrocytes encapsulated in polysaccharide templates. *Tissue Eng* 12(10): 2789-2799.

Pridie, K. H. (1959). A method of resurfacing osteoarthritic knee joints. *J Bone Joint Surg Br* 41: 618-619.

Prime, K. L., and G. M. Whitesides. (1991). Self-assembled organic monolayers: Model systems for studying adsorption of proteins at surfaces. *Science* 252(5010): 1164-1167.

Prockop, D. J. (1997). Marrow stromal cells as stem cells for nonhematopoietic tissues. *Science* 276(5309): 71-74.

Putnam, D. (2008). Drug delivery: The heart of the matter. *Nat Mater* 7(11): 836-837.

Qu, D., J. Li et al. (2011). Ectopic osteochondral formation of biomimetic porous PVA-n-HA/PA6 bilayered scaffold and BMSCs construct in rabbit. *J Biomed Mater Res B Appl Biomater* 96(1): 9-15.

Raimondi, M. T., G. Candiani et al. (2008). Engineered cartilage constructs subject to very low regimens of interstitial perfusion. *Biorheology* 45(3-4): 471-478.

Raimondi, M. T., M. Moretti et al. (2006). The effect of hydrodynamic shear on 3D engineered chondrocyte systems subject to direct perfusion. *Biorheology* 43(3-4): 215-222.

Ramage, L., G. Nuki et al. (2009). Signalling cascades in mechanotransduction: Cell-matrix interactions and mechanical loading. *Scand J Med Sci Sports* 19(4): 457-469.

Reddi, A. H. (1998). Role of morphogenetic proteins in skeletal tissue engineering and regeneration. *Nat Biotechnol* 16(3): 247-252.

Reddi, A. H. (2003). Cartilage morphogenetic proteins: Role in joint development, homoeostasis, and regeneration. *Ann Rheum Dis* 62(Suppl 2): ii73-ii78.

Responte, D. J., B. Arzi et al. (2012). Mechanisms underlying the synergistic enhancement of self-assembled neocartilage treated with chondroitinase-ABC and TGF-beta1. *Biomaterials* 33(11): 3187-3194.

Revell, C. M., and K. A. Athanasiou. (2009). Success rates and immunologic responses of autogenic, allogenic, and xenogenic treatments to repair articular cartilage defects. *Tissue Eng Part B Rev* 15(1): 1-15.

Revell, C. M., C. E. Reynolds et al. (2008). Effects of initial cell seeding in self assembly of articular cartilage. *Ann Biomed Eng* 36(9): 1441-1448.

Rezania, A., C. H. Thomas et al. (1997). The detachment strength and morphology of bone cells contacting materials modified with a peptide sequence found within bone sialoprotein. *J Biomed Mater Res* 37(1): 9-19.

Ruoslahti, E. (1996). RGD and other recognition sequences for integrins. *Annu Rev Cell Dev Biol* 12: 697-715.

Sah, R. L., Y. J. Kim et al. (1989). Biosynthetic response of cartilage explants to dynamic compression. *J Orthop Res* 7(5): 619-636.

Saini, S., and T. M. Wick. (2004). Effect of low oxygen tension on tissue-engineered cartilage construct development in the concentric cylinder bioreactor. *Tissue Eng* 10(5-6): 825-832.

Sakai, A., K. Suzuki et al. (1991). Effects of pulsing electromagnetic fields on cultured cartilage cells. *Int Orthop* 15(4): 341-346.

Sakai, S., H. Mishima et al. (2009). Rotating three-dimensional dynamic culture of adult human bone marrow-derived cells for tissue engineering of hyaline cartilage. *J Orthop Res* 27(4): 517-521.

Sakao, K., K. A. Takahashi et al. (2008). Induction of chondrogenic phenotype in synovium-derived progenitor cells by intermittent hydrostatic pressure. *Osteoarthr Cartil* 16(7): 805-814.

Sanchez-Adams, J., and K. A. Athanasiou. (2012). Dermis isolated adult stem cells for cartilage tissue engineering. *Biomaterials* 33(1): 109-119.

Saris, D. B., N. Mukherjee et al. (2000). Dynamic pressure transmission through agarose gels. *Tissue Eng* 6(5): 531-537.

Schreiber, R. E., B. M. Ilten-Kirby et al. (1999). Repair of osteochondral defects with allogeneic tissue engineered cartilage implants. *Clin Orthop Relat Res* 367(Suppl): S382-S395.

Schrobback, K., T. J. Klein et al. (2012). Effects of oxygen and culture system on in vitro propagation and redifferentiation of osteoarthritic human articular chondrocytes. *Cell Tissue Res* 347(3): 649-663.

Schulz, R. M., N. Wustneck et al. (2008). Development and validation of a novel bioreactor system for load- and perfusion-controlled tissue engineering of chondrocyte-constructs. *Biotechnol Bioeng* 101(4): 714-728.

Scotti, C., L. Mangiavini et al. (2010). Effect of in vitro culture on a chondrocyte-fibrin glue hydrogel for cartilage repair. *Knee Surg Sports Traumatol Arthrosc* 18(10): 1400-1406.

Sechriest, V. F., Y. J. Miao et al. (2000). GAG-augmented polysaccharide hydrogel: A novel biocompatible and biodegradable material to support chondrogenesis. *J Biomed Mater Res* 49(4): 534-541.

Seidi, A., M. Ramalingam et al. (2011). Gradient biomaterials for soft-to-hard interface tissue engineering. *Acta Biomater* 7(4): 1441-1451.

Sekiya, I., J. T. Vuoristo et al. (2002). In vitro cartilage formation by human adult stem cells from bone marrow stroma defines the sequence of cellular and molecular events during chondrogenesis. *Proc Natl Acad Sci USA* 99(7): 4397-4402.

Sharma, B., C. G. Williams et al. (2007). Designing zonal organization into tissue-engineered cartilage. *Tissue Eng* 13(2): 405-414.

Sharma, G., R. K. Saxena et al. (2008). Synergistic effect of chondroitin sulfate and cyclic pressure on biochemical and morphological properties of chondrocytes from articular cartilage. *Osteoarthr Cartil* 16(11): 1387-1394.

Shimizu, M., K. Minakuchi et al. (1997). Chondrocyte migration to fibronectin, type I collagen, and type II collagen. *Cell Struct Funct* 22(3): 309-315.

Siegel, R. C., S. R. Pinnell et al. (1970). Cross-linking of collagen and elastin. Properties of lysyl oxidase. *Biochemistry* 9(23): 4486-4492.

Silver, I. A. (1975). Measurement of pH and ionic composition of pericellular sites. *Philos Trans R Soc Lond B Biol Sci* 271(912): 261-272.

Silverman, R. P., D. Passaretti et al. (1999). Injectable tissue-engineered cartilage using a fibrin glue polymer. *Plast Reconstr Surg* 103(7): 1809-1818.

Singhal, A. R., C. M. Agrawal et al. (1996). Salient degradation features of a 50:50 PLA/PGA scaffold for tissue engineering. *Tissue Eng* 2(3): 197-207.

Sironen, R., M. Elo et al. (2000). Transcriptional activation in chondrocytes submitted to hydrostatic pressure. *Biorheology* 37(1-2): 85-93.

Sittinger, M., J. Bujia et al. (1994). Engineering of cartilage tissue using bioresorbable polymer carriers in perfusion culture. *Biomaterials* 15(6): 451-456.

Slivka, M. A., N. C. Leatherbury et al. (2001). Porous, resorbable, fiber-reinforced scaffolds tailored for articular cartilage repair. *Tissue Eng* 7(6): 767-780.

Smith, G. D., G. Knutsen et al. (2005). A clinical review of cartilage repair techniques. *J Bone Joint Surg Br* 87(4): 445-449.

Smith, R. L., B. S. Donlon et al. (1995). Effects of fluid-induced shear on articular chondrocyte morphology and metabolism in vitro. *J Orthop Res* 13(6): 824-831.

Smith, R. L., J. Lin et al. (2000a). Time-dependent effects of intermittent hydrostatic pressure on articular chondrocyte type II collagen and aggrecan mRNA expression. *J Rehabil Res Dev* 37(2): 153-161.

Smith, R. L., D. P. Lindsey et al. (2011). Effects of intermittent hydrostatic pressure and BMP-2 on osteoarthritic human chondrocyte metabolism in vitro. *J Orthop Res* 29(3): 361-368.

Smith, R. L., S. F. Rusk et al. (1996). In vitro stimulation of articular chondrocyte mRNA and extracellular matrix synthesis by hydrostatic pressure. *J Orthop Res* 14(1): 53-60.

Smith, R. L., M. C. Trindade et al. (2000b). Effects of shear stress on articular chondrocyte metabolism. *Biorheology* 37(1-2): 95-107.

Solchaga, L. A., J. Gao et al. (2002). Treatment of osteochondral defects with autologous bone marrow in a hyaluronan-based delivery vehicle. *Tissue Eng* 8(2): 333-347.

Solchaga, L. A., J. U. Yoo et al. (2000). Hyaluronan-based polymers in the treatment of osteochondral defects. *J Orthop Res* 18(5): 773-780.

Sporn, M. B., A. B. Roberts et al. (1986). Transforming growth factor-beta: Biological function and chemical structure. *Science* 233(4763): 532-534.

Stockwell, R. A. (1971). The interrelationship of cell density and cartilage thickness in mammalian articular cartilage. *J Anat* 109(3): 411-421.

Stoddart, M. J., L. Ettinger et al. (2006). Enhanced matrix synthesis in de novo, scaffold free cartilage-like tissue subjected to compression and shear. *Biotechnol Bioeng* 95(6): 1043-1051.

Suggs, L. J., E. Y. Kao et al. (1998a). Preparation and characterization of poly(propylene fumarate-co-ethylene glycol) hydrogels. *J Biomater Sci Polym Ed* 9(7): 653-666.

Suggs, L. J., R. S. Krishnan et al. (1998b). In vitro and in vivo degradation of poly(propylene fumarate-co-ethylene glycol) hydrogels. *J Biomed Mater Res* 42(2): 312-320.

Suggs, L. J., and A. G. Mikos. (1999). Development of poly(propylene fumarate-co-ethylene glycol) as an injectable carrier for endothelial cells. *Cell Transplant* 8(4): 345-350.

Suggs, L. J., M. S. Shive et al. (1999). In vitro cytotoxicity and in vivo biocompatibility of poly(propylene fumarate-co-ethylene glycol) hydrogels. *J Biomed Mater Res* 46(1): 22-32.

Suh, J. K. (1996). Dynamic unconfined compression of articular cartilage under a cyclic compressive load. *Biorheology* 33(4-5): 289-304.

Tacchetti, C., R. Quarto et al. (1987). In vitro morphogenesis of chick embryo hypertrophic cartilage. *J Cell Biol* 105(2): 999-1006.

Takahashi, K., T. Kubo et al. (1998). Hydrostatic pressure induces expression of interleukin 6 and tumour necrosis factor alpha mRNAs in a chondrocyte-like cell line. *Ann Rheum Dis* 57(4): 231-236.

Takahashi, K., and S. Yamanaka. (2006). Induction of pluripotent stem cells from mouse embryonic and adult fibroblast cultures by defined factors. *Cell* 126(4): 663-676.

Tatebe, M., R. Nakamura et al. (2005). Differentiation of transplanted mesenchymal stem cells in a large osteochondral defect in rabbit. *Cytotherapy* 7(6): 520-530.

Temenoff, J. S., K. A. Athanasiou et al. (2002). Effect of poly(ethylene glycol) molecular weight on tensile and swelling properties of oligo(poly(ethylene glycol) fumarate) hydrogels for cartilage tissue engineering. *J Biomed Mater Res* 59(3): 429-437.

Thomas, C. H., C. D. McFarland et al. (1997). The role of vitronectin in the attachment and spatial distribution of bone-derived cells on materials with patterned surface chemistry. *J Biomed Mater Res* 37(1): 81-93.

Tognana, E., F. Chen et al. (2005). Adjacent tissues (cartilage, bone) affect the functional integration of engineered calf cartilage in vitro. *Osteoarthr Cartil* 13(2): 129-138.

Toolan, B. C., S. R. Frenkel et al. (1998). Development of a novel osteochondral graft for cartilage repair. *J Biomed Mater Res* 41(2): 244-250.

Torzilli, P. A., R. Grigiene et al. (1997). Characterization of cartilage metabolic response to static and dynamic stress using a mechanical explant test system. *J Biomech* 30(1): 1-9.

Tsao, Y. D., and S. R. Gonda. (1999). A new technology for three-dimensional cell culture: The hydrodynamic focusing bioreactor. *Adv Heat Mass Transfer Biotechnol* 44: 37-38.

Tsao, Y.-M. D., E. Boyd et al. (1994). Fluid dynamics within a rotating bioreactor in space and earth environments. *J Spacecr Rockets* 31(6): 937-943.

Tsao, Y.-M. D., S. R. Gonda et al. (1997). Mass transfer characteristics of NASA bioreactors by numerical simulation. *Adv Heat Mass Transfer Biotechnol* 37: 69-73.

Tuan, R. S., G. Boland et al. (2003). Adult mesenchymal stem cells and cell-based tissue engineering. *Arthritis Res Ther* 5(1): 32-45.

U.S. Bone and Joint Initiative (USBJI). (2014). The burden of musculoskeletal diseases in the United States. Rosemont, IL: USBJI.

Urban, J. P., A. C. Hall et al. (1993). Regulation of matrix synthesis rates by the ionic and osmotic environment of articular chondrocytes. *J Cell Physiol* 154(2): 262-270.

Urist, M. R. (1965). Bone: Formation by autoinduction. *Science* 150(698): 893-899.

Vacanti, V., E. Kong et al. (2005). Phenotypic changes of adult porcine mesenchymal stem cells induced by prolonged passaging in culture. *J Cell Physiol* 205(2): 194-201.

Valcourt, U., J. Gouttenoire et al. (2002). Functions of transforming growth factor-beta family type I receptors and Smad proteins in the hypertrophic maturation and osteoblastic differentiation of chondrocytes. *J Biol Chem* 277(37): 33545-33558.

van der Kraan, P., E. Vitters et al. (1992). Differential effect of transforming growth factor beta on freshly isolated and cultured articular chondrocytes. *J Rheumatol* 19(1): 140-145.

van Kampen, G. P., J. P. Veldhuijzen et al. (1985). Cartilage response to mechanical force in high-density chondrocyte cultures. *Arthritis Rheum* 28(4): 419-424.

van Susante, J. L., P. Buma et al. (1999). Resurfacing potential of heterologous chondrocytes suspended in fibrin glue in large full-thickness defects of femoral articular cartilage: An experimental study in the goat. *Biomaterials* 20(13): 1167-1175.

van Susante, J. L. C., J. Pieper et al. (2001). Linkage of chondroitin-sulfate to type I collagen scaffolds stimulates the bioactivity of seeded chondrocytes in vitro. *Biomaterials* 22(17): 2359-2369.

Vanwanseele, B., F. Eckstein et al. (2002). Knee cartilage of spinal cord-injured patients displays progressive thinning in the absence of normal joint loading and movement. *Arthritis Rheum* 46(8): 2073-2078.

Varani, K., S. Gessi et al. (2002). Effect of low frequency electromagnetic fields on A2A adenosine receptors in human neutrophils. *Br J Pharmacol* 136(1): 57-66.

Veldhuijzen, J. P., A. H. Huisman et al. (1987). The growth of cartilage cells in vitro and the effect of intermittent compressive force. A histological evaluation. *Connect Tissue Res* 16(2): 187-196.

Verschure, P. J., L. A. Joosten et al. (1994). Responsiveness of articular cartilage from normal and inflamed mouse knee joints to various growth factors. *Ann Rheum Dis* 53(7): 455-460.

Villanueva, I., B. J. Klement et al. (2009). Cross-linking density alters early metabolic activities in chondrocytes encapsulated in poly(ethylene glycol) hydrogels and cultured in the rotating wall vessel. *Biotechnol Bioeng* 102(4): 1242-1250.

Vo, T. N., A. K. Ekenseair et al. (2014). Synthesis, physicochemical characterization, and cytocompatibility of bioresorbable, dual-gelling injectable hydrogels. *Biomacromolecules* 15(1): 132-142.

Vunjak-Novakovic, G., and L. E. Freed. (1998). Culture of organized cell communities. *Adv Drug Deliv Rev* 33(1-2): 15-30.

Vunjak-Novakovic, G., L. E. Freed et al. (1996). Effects of mixing on the composition and morphology of tissue-engineered cartilage. *AIChE J* 42(3): 850-860.

Vunjak-Novakovic, G., I. Martin et al. (1999). Bioreactor cultivation conditions modulate the composition and mechanical properties of tissue-engineered cartilage. *J Orthop Res* 17(1): 130-138.

Vunjak-Novakovic, G., B. Obradovic et al. (1998). Dynamic cell seeding of polymer scaffolds for cartilage tissue engineering. *Biotechnol Prog* 14(2): 193-202.

Wagner, D. R., D. P. Lindsey et al. (2008). Hydrostatic pressure enhances chondrogenic differentiation of human bone marrow stromal cells in osteochondrogenic medium. *Ann Biomed Eng* 36(5): 813-820.

Waldman, S. D., C. G. Spiteri et al. (2003). Long-term intermittent shear deformation improves the quality of cartilaginous tissue formed in vitro. *J Orthop Res* 21(4): 590-596.

Wang, P. Y., H. H. Chow et al. (2009). Modulation of gene expression of rabbit chondrocytes by dynamic compression in polyurethane scaffolds with collagen gel encapsulation. *J Biomater Appl* 23(4): 347-366.

Wang, Q. G., J. L. Magnay et al. (2009). Gene expression profiles of dynamically compressed single chondrocytes and chondrons. *Biochem Biophys Res Commun* 379(3): 738-742.

Wang, Y., E. Bella et al. (2010). The synergistic effects of 3-D porous silk fibroin matrix scaffold properties and hydrodynamic environment in cartilage tissue regeneration. *Biomaterials* 31(17): 4672-4681.

Wang, Y., H. J. Kim et al. (2006). Stem cell-based tissue engineering with silk biomaterials. *Biomaterials* 27(36): 6064-6082.

Wang, Z. H., X. J. He et al. (2010). Cartilage tissue engineering with demineralized bone matrix gelatin and fibrin glue hybrid scaffold: An in vitro study. *Artif Organs* 34(2): 161-166.

Wartella, K. A., and J. S. Wayne. (2009). Bioreactor for biaxial mechanical stimulation to tissue engineered constructs. *J Biomech Eng* 131(4): 044501.

Wendt, D., S. Stroebel et al. (2006). Uniform tissues engineered by seeding and culturing cells in 3D scaffolds under perfusion at defined oxygen tensions. *Biorheology* 43(3-4): 481-488.

Wenger, R., M. G. Hans et al. (2006). Hydrostatic pressure increases apoptosis in cartilage-constructs produced from human osteoarthritic chondrocytes. *Front Biosci* 11: 1690-1695.

Wernike, E., Z. Li et al. (2008). Effect of reduced oxygen tension and long-term mechanical stimulation on chondrocyte-polymer constructs. *Cell Tissue Res* 331(2): 473-483.

Westreich, R., M. Kaufman et al. (2004). Validating the subcutaneous model of injectable autologous cartilage using a fibrin glue scaffold. *Laryngoscope* 114(12): 2154-2160.

Wimmer, M. A., S. Grad et al. (2004). Tribology approach to the engineering and study of articular cartilage. *Tissue Eng* 10(9–10): 1436-1445.

Wong, M., M. Siegrist et al. (2002). Collagen fibrillogenesis by chondrocytes in alginate. *Tissue Eng* 8(6): 979-987.

Woods, V. L., Jr., P. J. Schreck et al. (1994). Integrin expression by human articular chondrocytes. *Arthritis Rheum* 37(4): 537-544.

Wright, M., P. Jobanputra et al. (1996). Effects of intermittent pressure-induced strain on the electrophysiology of cultured human chondrocytes: Evidence for the presence of stretch-activated membrane ion channels. *Clin Sci (Lond)* 90(1): 61-71.

Wyre, R. M., and S. Downes. (2002). The role of protein adsorption on chondrocyte adhesion to a heterocyclic methacrylate polymer system. *Biomaterials* 23(2): 357-364.

Yamane, S., N. Iwasaki et al. (2005). Feasibility of chitosan-based hyaluronic acid hybrid biomaterial for a novel scaffold in cartilage tissue engineering. *Biomaterials* 26(6): 611-619.

Yang, Y. H., M. B. Ard et al. (2014). Type I collagen-based fibrous capsule enhances integration of tissue-engineered cartilage with native articular cartilage. *Ann Biomed Eng* 42(4): 716-726.

Yim, E. K., S. W. Pang et al. (2007). Synthetic nanostructures inducing differentiation of human mesenchymal stem cells into neuronal lineage. *Exp Cell Res* 313(9): 1820-1829.

Youn, I., J. B. Choi et al. (2006). Zonal variations in the three-dimensional morphology of the chondron measured in situ using confocal microscopy. *Osteoarthr Cartil* 14(9): 889-897.

Yu, J., M. A. Vodyanik et al. (2007). Induced pluripotent stem cell lines derived from human somatic cells. *Science* 318(5858): 1917-1920.

Zaffagnini, S., A. A. Allen et al. (1996). Temperature changes in the knee joint during arthroscopic surgery. *Knee Surg Sports Traumatol Arthrosc* 3(4): 199-201.

Zeltinger, J., J. K. Sherwood et al. (2001). Effect of pore size-and void fraction on cellular adhesion, proliferation, and matrix deposition. *Tissue Eng* 7(5): 557-572.

Ziegler, J., U. Mayr-Wohlfart et al. (2002). Adsorption and release properties of growth factors from biodegradable implants. *J Biomed Mater Res* 59(3): 422-428.

Zimmermann, J., K. Bittner et al. (2002). Novel hydrogels as supports for in vitro cell growth: Poly(ethylene glycol)- and gelatine-based (meth)acrylamidopeptide macromonomers. *Biomaterials* 23(10): 2127-2134.

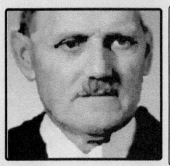

"...fibrils of the cartilage ...from a depth climb in narrow arcades to a tangential course in the upper area [of the tissue]..." "These tangentially-mounted sections of fiber correspond to a connective tissue and connective tissue cells." ...the fibrils deflect and are delivered in the form of arcades at an angle and thereby protect...[the cartilage matrix]." (Form und Bau der Gelenkknorpel in ihren Beziehungen zur Funktion, 1925)
Alfred Benninghoff (1890-1953) was a German anatomist. His main contribution has been the identification and description of the Benninghoff arcades of collagen fibers in articular cartilage.

"Clinical experiences of arthroscopy and an assessment of its value were reported by Michael S. Burman, Harry Finkelstein, and Leo Mater in 1934. In all of these instances the interest in the use of the arthroscope as a means of research and diagnosis was of short duration and in each instance the use of the arthroscope has for practical purposes been abandoned." "...With the special transformer and synchronous exposure attachment to the camera body, this automatic increase in illumination occurs when the shutter release button is pressed. Photography should be done under clear vision and interruption of continuous irrigation with saline..." (Atlas of Arthroscopy)
Masaki Watanabe (1911-1995) was a Japanese orthopedic surgeon, sometimes called the "founder of modern arthroscopy." (Picture taken June 1980, modified from DeMaio [2013].)

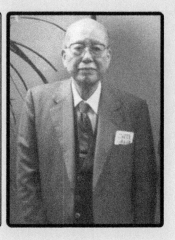

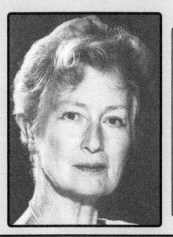

"Connective tissue has generally been regarded as being rather inert with little direct influence on metabolism because its function is mainly a mechanical one..." "In its intial stages osteoarthrosis appears to involve profound changes in the metabolism of cartilage cells set in train by increased hydration of the tissue; only at advanced stages does it become degenerative. At what stage the metabolic changes are reversible is a question of crucial importance in understanding the disease process and in attempting to develop effective therapeutic measures."
Helen Muir (1920-2005) was a British scientist best known for pioneering work into the causes of osteoarthritis. (Image from Wellcome Library, London CC BY 4.0.)

Methods for Evaluating Articular Cartilage Quality

- Imaging techniques
- Ultrastructural techniques
- Quantitative biochemistry
- Biomechanical methods
- Animal models
- Clinical scoring

To evaluate articular cartilage health, pathology, and therapeutic efficacy, it is imperative that appropriate assessment methodologies are developed and used. Assessments can be divided, in general, into qualitative, semiquantitative, and quantitative assays. Qualitative assessments, such as gross morphology and histology, can often provide visual information rapidly and *in toto*. Other qualitative assessments include various imaging modalities, for example, magnetic resonance imaging (MRI) and x-ray computed tomography (CT), which are noninvasive and, therefore, useful for sequential assessment. Features from qualitative assessments can often be used in semiquantitative assessments, such as those employed in standardized cartilage evaluation indices. Finally, quantitative assays include a plethora of biochemical methods that span a wide range of specificity and biomechanical methods based on continuum biome-chanical models of cartilage. Semiquantitative and quantitative results are useful for the statistical comparison of various treatments. Judicious application of these techniques in animal models and in clinical trials is important for the translation of emerging articular cartilage therapies.

A plethora of histological, ultrastructural, and biochemical assessments are available to evaluate articular cartilage, with additional methods continuously being developed. Stains such as Alcian blue, toluidine blue, Safranin O (with Fast Green), and sirius red (in saturated picric acid) are regularly employed, along with combinations such as Movat's penta-chrome and hematoxylin and eosin to histologically demonstrate the location of glycosaminoglycan, collagen, and other extracellular matrix components in articular cartilage. Distribution of specific collagens and glycosaminoglycans can be discerned using immunohistochemistry, and of great interest are the presence and relative distribution of col-lagen type I or II; significant amounts of collagen type I are not seen in hyaline articular cartilage, but in fibrocartilage. Enzyme-linked immu-nosorbent assays (ELISAs) can also achieve a similar purpose by quanti-fying the amount of biochemical components present without showing their distribution. For example, immunohistochemistry and ELISA for superficial zone protein (SZP)/proteoglycan 4 (PRG4) are useful indices for functional cartilage tribology. Noninvasive imaging methods such as MRI, ultrasound, CT, and other modalities are routinely employed to assess joint health and for surgical planning.

The restoration or improvement of joint function will largely depend on the biomechanical properties of repair or regenerated articular cartilage faithfully mimicking native articular cartilage. Accompanying this is the subsidence of pain and inflammation and the management of associated pathologies in adjoining tissues. Functional restoration of tissue exhibit-ing biomechanical properties on par with native tissue may be considered a primary design standard. This has inspired many mechanical testing modalities, accompanied by mathematical models, to describe articular cartilage tissue under conditions of stress or strain. In addition to design standards, evaluation standards are important for both researchers and companies seeking approval from the U.S. Food and Drug Administration (FDA) for the marketing of new therapies. To ensure safety and efficacy, the FDA evaluates scientific data generated by testing potential drugs and devices, both preclinically and clinically. Preclinical data for *devices* can include specific testing protocols such as mechanical and durability testing, while preclinical data for *drugs* can include both *in vitro* and *in vivo* validations of safety and efficacy, and dose response. Certain consensus technical standards, such as those developed by the American Society for Testing and Materials (ASTM) International, are recognized by the FDA, and companies can use these standard test methods in lieu of developing their own. The FDA also encourages the development and validation of computer models to yield preclinical data in the approval process. While consensus standards exist for devices such as implants, no consensus standards exist for cellular therapies such as engineered articular cartilage. Neither do standards exist for evaluating articular cartilage repair tissue that has been induced pharmacologically or surgically. In terms of evaluating the biomechanical properties of articular cartilage, this chapter discusses established procedures, including a description of common modeling approaches used for determining material properties from these tests. It should be kept in mind that not all biomechanical models are the same, and it can be difficult to compare results from different models due to differences in their underlying assumptions.

From the basic science perspective of understanding articular cartilage biology to the clinical perspective of evaluating a new articular cartilage therapy, not all assays carry the same weight. A balance was attempted here, as with Chapter 7, to describe the roles of various assessments important for academia, industry, and therapy. As a result, assays for function, as opposed to metabolism (e.g., the elucidation of various signaling pathways), have a greater representation here because they are useful from the perspectives of basic science (understanding cartilage biology), industrial production (safety, effectiveness, and quality control) and in the clinical setting (therapeutic efficacy and improvements in quality of life). Since articular cartilage regeneration is an interdisciplinary effort, basic information for various classes of assays is presented. This way, scientists, engineers, and physicians who pick up this text will be given a baseline understanding of each other's field. With a rudimentary understanding of the purpose and scope of different assay types, readers may then wish to proceed to Chapter 7, where protocols are presented, or to the list of cited literature that the reader will, by then, be ready to explore with confidence.

5.1 IMAGING TECHNIQUES

Articular cartilage gross morphology has long been used to discern tissue health and pathology. For example, India ink applied to the hyaline surface is a classical method to provide contrast and help identify chondral defects. Figure 5.1 illustrates examples of imaging techniques, ranging from arthroscopy to MRI, that are used clinically to assess cartilage

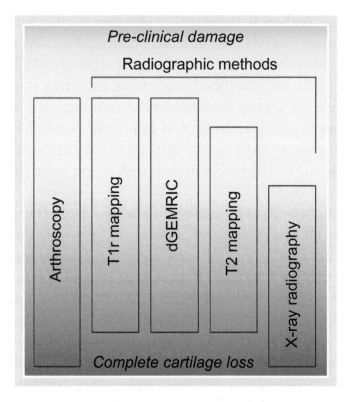

Figure 5.1 Various imaging methods and their usefulness in detecting articular cartilage disease and damage with respect to the severity of pathology.

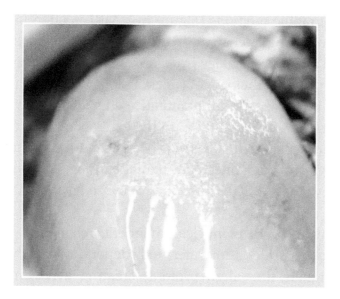

Figure 5.2 Degenerative changes can be observed grossly. In the image, softened osteoarthritic cartilage, which appears to be matted, is surrounded by shiny, smooth, and healthy-looking cartilage. (Courtesy of Jamie White.)

tissue quality with respect to the amount of damage and disease state. Gross morphology can be assessed using arthroscopy, although microscopic or minute changes in cartilage health are oftentimes not visible through gross inspection. *Preclinical damage*, shown in Figure 5.1, is defined as damage that cannot be assessed using the nondestructive methods that are routinely used in the clinical setting.

In the research setting, destructive methods, such as histology, can detect cell death and matrix degradation that occur before changes are grossly visible (e.g., the matted portion shown in Figure 5.2). In the clinical setting, these methods are mostly used on excised diseased tissue. Thus, nondestructive imaging techniques, whether invasive or noninvasive, are part of the first line of assessments of cartilage health and are described in the following sections.

5.1.1 Noninvasive Modalities

MRI is growing in importance as a noninvasive, diagnostic tool to determine early articular cartilage damage that cannot be imaged using routine radiographic methods (Figure 5.3). MRI is often used to assess joint space narrowing or changes in articular cartilage thickness, as well as changes in articular cartilage hydration, features indicative of various stages and types of pathology. Correlations of MRI-based assessment to arthroscopic, histological, and quantitative characteristics vary with the tissues and injuries imaged and with the experience level of the person interpreting the images. MRI has also been used to assess transplants of native cartilage and of engineered articular cartilage in a nondestructive manner (Zalewski et al. 2008; Juras et al. 2009b; Neu et al. 2009).

Based on the property of nuclear magnetic resonance, MRI signals are generated by protons in water and, depending on the tissue, fat. Powerful magnets first align protons, creating a net magnetization parallel to the magnetic field. This net magnetization is called the longitudinal magnetization. In this state, the protons wobble, or precess, around the longitudinal axis with a frequency proportional to the magnetic field strength, called the Larmor frequency. Since the precession

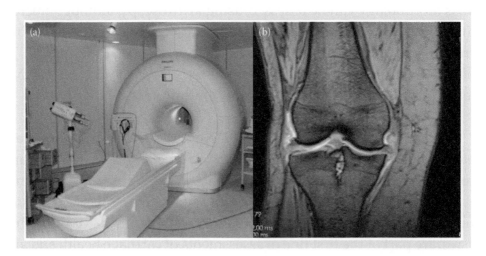

Figure 5.3 The radiofrequency source, a circular coil of the MRI machine (a), generates a strong magnetic field that aligns the axes of the protons in water and, depending on the tissue, fat. When the radiofrequency source is switched off, the axes return to their resting states by releasing a signal that can be detected by the MRI's receiver coils. Using various magnet strengths and radiofrequency pulse sequences, images of the knee can be generated (b). (Image on panel (a) by Jan Ainali, used under CC BY 3.0. Image on panel (b) by Nevit Dilmen, used under CC BY 3.0 Unported.)

of each proton is random, no net transverse magnetization occurs. That is, there is no net magnetization perpendicular to the longitudinal axis. When the protons' alignment is altered by a short-duration secondary magnetic field (radiofrequency pulse, or pulse sequence), a rotating magnetic field is generated by the protons. That is, the longitudinal magnetization of the protons is reduced, and a net transverse magnetization occurs. In different tissues, the protons recover their longitudinal magnetization at different rates. This rate constant is known as the tissue's T1 time and is an inherent property of the tissue. Similarly, the transverse magnetization decays at specific rates for different tissues, and this rate constant is called the tissue's T2 time. The amplitude of the magnetic field generated by the rotating protons is characteristic of the local molecular and magnetic environment around them and the MRI pulse sequence characteristics, creating contrast among different tissue types and pathologic states. Specific pulse sequences can, thus, be developed to accentuate image contrast based on these two properties and also based on proton density. Pulse sequences are the settings on the MRI machine to generate an image. When evaluating MRI images, as a convention, the term *X-weighted* denotes a tissue property. Various pulse sequences yield T1-weighted, T2-weighted, or proton density-weighted images. Although examples of how MRI can provide information on articular cartilage health and pathology are provided below, MRI principles as well as how the various techniques work are beyond the scope of this book. Interested readers are directed to other texts specific to the area (Bowen et al. 2014).

MRI has good penetration depth, and images taken using various pulse sequences, of various planes, and with the joint in extension or flexion allow one to visualize cartilage or associated joint tissues. These settings can vary based on the properties of the tissue one wishes to observe. There is a trade-off between spatial resolution and signal-to-noise. The higher field strengths (i.e., the power of the magnet, measured in tesla, or T) afford better signal-to-noise, which allows better spatial resolution. Since cartilage is a thin tissue, to obtain sufficient resolution, at least 3 T is needed. Higher resolutions at lower T can be

399

obtained, but the acquisition time is so long as to be not feasible in the clinical setting. As illustrated in Figure 5.1, MRI can be used to discern cartilage damage earlier than radiographs, although it is more costly, takes longer, and may not be as accessible as radiographs.

As an example, the anterior cruciate ligament is often imaged using a transverse relaxation time T2-weighted pulse sequence in the sagittal plane for insertion, continuity, and hydration data. Discontinuity or fragmentation seen in any of the imaging planes can indicate anterior cruciate ligament rupture, a condition highly correlated with the development of osteoarthritis (see Chapter 3). Using T2-weighted fast-spin-echo acquisition, fat and water are both hyperintense. To differentiate fat and water, techniques such as chemical fat saturation or a short-tau inversion recovery pulse sequence can be used while maintaining T2 weighting. It has been shown that T2 increases with age, morphologic changes, and importantly, cartilage damage (Keenan et al. 2011; Xu et al. 2011; Caglar et al. 2014; Kim et al. 2014). It is important to note that while T2 is also correlated with clinical scores of pain and function, T2 values are sensitive to the angle and position at which the joint is imaged (Mosher et al. 2001; Wang and Regatte 2015), as well as the pulse sequence and radiofrequency coil used to collect the data (Balamoody et al. 2013; Dardzinski and Schneider 2013; Surowiec et al. 2014).

Also correlated with osteoarthritis are meniscal tears, which can be imaged using T1-weighted images in both the sagittal and coronal imaging planes and with T2-weighted sequences for specific abnormalities (De Smet et al. 1993). T1-weighted images can be acquired using spin-echo and fast-spin-echo sequences. Fat appears brighter and water appears darker graphically. Abnormal hydration can indicate edema for both soft and hard tissues. As with T2-weighted imaging, fast-spin-echo sequences reduce acquisition time. $T_{1\rho}$ mapping has been used to detect cartilage injuries, as verified using the Outerbridge classification through arthroscopy (Lozano et al. 2006; Gupta et al. 2014). Data are acquired by preparing the magnetization with spin-lock pulses prior to image acquisition. $T_{1\rho}$ is the time constant at which the spin-locked magnetization relaxes with respect to the magnetic field in the rotating frame. $T_{1\rho}$ values have been correlated with cartilage damage due to meniscal tears (Matsubara et al. 2015) in patients displaying early stages of osteoarthritis (Kellgren-Lawrence grade of 0-2). Thus, increases in $T_{1\rho}$ values have been observed not only with posttraumatic cases where injuries were acute and observable through arthroscopy, but also for early stage changes. Both $T_{1\rho}$ and T2 values have been observed to increase as osteoarthritis progresses. However, only $T_{1\rho}$ mapping appears to yield differences when comparing normal cartilage to cases of mild osteoarthritis (Nishioka et al. 2015). For example, patients with posterior cruciate ligament injuries who are asymptomatic and display no degenerative changes on plain radiographs or conventional MRI have nonetheless been shown to have significantly increased $T_{1\rho}$ values compared with healthy individuals (Okazaki et al. 2014). As with T2, T1 values are dependent on MRI systems and coils, though careful quality control and cross-calibration can still allow correlations to be drawn (Li et al. 2015).

Arthroscopic evaluations do not typically include biochemical determination, and it is thus important to note that MRI has been used, to a certain extent, to provide biochemical data for articular cartilage. For instance, while glycosaminoglycan content does not appear to change T2, collagen degradation and changes in collagen alignment have both, at times, been observed to result in higher T2 signals (Nieminen et al. 2001; Kretzschmar et al. 2015), while, in other cases, T2 signals were not observed to correlate with collagen as assessed by hydroxyproline (Shiomi et al. 2010). Since cartilage hydration is dependent on glycosaminoglycan content, contrast agents that aim to better visualize this extracellular matrix component have been applied (Burstein et al. 2001; Nieminen et al. 2002). While some studies have shown that signal correlation to collagen content is better than for glycosaminoglycans, this work has seen popular adaptation (Fragonas et al. 1998). For example, delayed gadolinium-enhanced MRI of the cartilage (dGEMRIC) has been shown *in vitro* and *in vivo* to directly correlate with cartilage fixed charge density, and, thus, with glycosaminoglycan content (Williams et al. 2004).

Methods such as diffusion MRI have been used to assess extracellular matrix content and alignment (Nieminen et al. 2001; de Visser et al. 2008). For example, diffusion imaging used to evaluate autologous chondrocyte transplantation was able to discern differences between transplanted and native cartilages (Mamisch et al. 2008). Sodium MRI is another technique that has been correlated with extracellular matrix content in articular cartilage. As proteoglycans are lost during the progression of osteoarthritis, the negative fixed charge density of cartilage is reduced, resulting in a loss of sodium ions, and this can be measured using sodium MRI (Wheaton et al. 2004). Fluid-suppressed sodium MRI signals have also been correlated with Kellgren-Lawrence scores of osteoarthritis (Madelin et al. 2013). Also, collagen is a highly anisotropic matrix component in articular cartilage, and collagen fibers can impose anisotropic translational and rotational motions on sodium ions. For the detection of osteoarthritis, use of sodium MRI appears to depend on subject age and whether the fields assessed include synovial fluid (Newbould et al. 2012, 2013). To summarize, for the evaluation of articular health and disease, techniques to independently assess both glycosaminoglycan content and collagen content must be developed.

dGEMRIC has been used to examine the efficacy of autologous chondrocyte implantation, although in this case, no correlation between the dGEMRIC values and the Knee injury and Osteoarthritis Outcome Score (KOOS) results were observed (Vasiliadis et al. 2010). dGEMRIC has also been used to discern osteoarthritis in a noninvasive manner and for correlation to cartilage biomechanical properties (Juras et al. 2009a) (Figure 5.4).

In general, continuous refinements in imaging techniques need to be made since few assessments are currently available for noninvasive assessment of biomechanical properties. Examples of this include efforts to correlate biomechanical properties directly with MRI data, such as $T_{1\rho}$ signal (Figure 5.5) or using diffusion-weighted imaging (DWI), which yields the apparent diffusion coefficient (ADC). Since the technique displays a map of water mobility, it is postulated that it yields

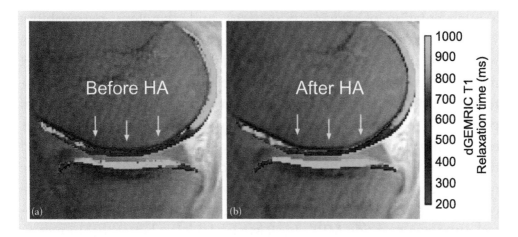

Figure 5.4 dGEMRIC is used here to visualize changes and therapies associated with osteoarthritis. In this case, a region with relatively lower T1 relaxation times, indicative of lower glycosaminoglycan content, is seen in osteoarthritic cartilage (gray arrows in panel a). It appears that injection of hyaluronic acid (HA) does not recover the glycosaminoglycan loss (b). (From van Tiel, J. et al., *PLoS One* 8(11): e79785, 2013. Used under a *PLoS One* Creative Commons License.)

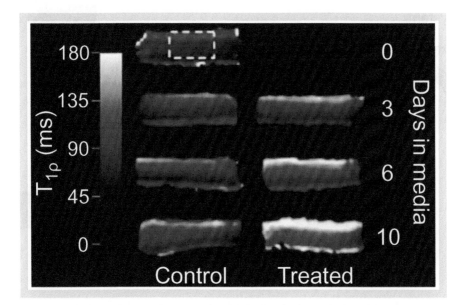

Figure 5.5 $T_{1\rho}$ has been correlated with biomechanical properties. In this case, cartilage explants were cultured in medium or treated with interleukin 1β to mimic cartilage degradation. By day 10, the treated samples had lower aggregate modulus values, higher hydraulic permeability, and higher T_1 signal. (From Wheaton, A. J. et al., *Magn Reson Med* 54(5): 1087-1093, 2005. With permission.)

a representation of average pore sizes, and, therefore, permeability within different areas of the tissue. ADC showed moderate correlation with cartilage viscoelastic properties measured using a Kelvin-Voigt model (Aoki et al. 2012). Due to its correlation with proteoglycan content, dGEMRIC has also been used to assess cartilage mechanical properties. In this case, correlations were made to the instantaneous and equilibrium modulus values and to relaxation time, as collected through indentation with a spherical indenter (Hayes et al. 1972). The many mechanical models that have been developed to describe the viscoelastic properties of articular cartilage (as described later in this chapter) can serve to guide MRI physicists in devising better techniques to noninvasively obtain cartilage biomechanical properties.

As noted earlier, for articular cartilage degeneration, changes in biomechanical properties may precede gross morphological changes (Figure 5.6)

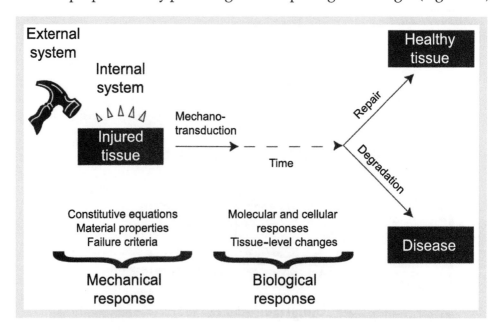

Figure 5.6 In response to injurious loads, microscopic changes take place that are often not visible using current imaging techniques. Molecular- and cellular-level responses in the tissue can lead to either repair or degradation. However, it is not until significant degradative changes have occurred that they become clinically visible. (From Natoli, R. M., and K. A. Athanasiou, *Biorheology* 46(6): 451-485, 2009. With permission.)

(Natoli and Athanasiou 2009). Thus, instead of a soluble marker for early arthritis, advances in imaging techniques may push the threshold of pre-clinical articular damage to eventually become a noninvasive technique for identifying early cartilage degeneration.

In addition to MRI, technological advancements may bring other imaging modalities to the assessment of articular cartilage. For instance, the correlation of ultrasound with physical or biochemical

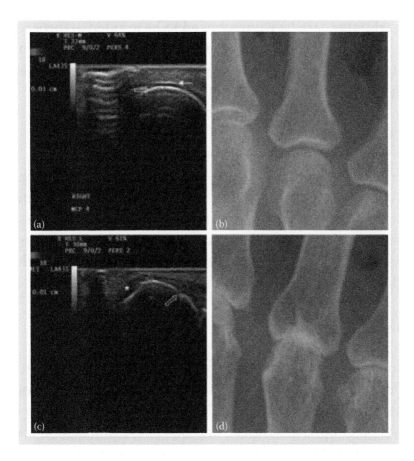

Figure 5.7 Rheumatoid arthritis as imaged with ultrasound and radiographs. The ultrasound images (left column, a and c) are compared with radiographs (right column, b and d) of rheumatoid arthritis of the metacarpal head. The upper row (a and b) images are from healthy cartilage exhibiting normal cartilage thickness and joint spacing. The bottom row (c and d) shows reduced cartilage thickness and joint spacing. (From Moller, B. et al., *Arthritis Rheum* 61(4): 435-441, 2009. With permission.)

properties of normal and damaged articular cartilage has been investigated (Qin et al. 2002; Kuroki et al. 2009a,b). For this technique, image resolution increases with ultrasound frequency, but the trade-off is a decrease in penetration depth and vice versa. As an example, ultrasound can be used in assessing rheumatoid arthritis of the hand (Figure 5.7), which requires relatively small penetration depth. Dense tissues such as bone also interfere with the imaging of soft tissues such as articular cartilage. Thus, while ultrasound is used clinically as a noninvasive imaging technique, for the assessment of articular cartilage it may need to be applied arthroscopically (Huang and Zheng 2009). In general, novel application of imaging techniques for articular cartilage and the application of existing imaging techniques to engineered tissues should first be accompanied by direct biochemical and biomechanical assays to establish robust correlations.

Since articular cartilage damage is associated with incongruous mechanical loading, the success of future cell-based therapies will likely depend on precise implant fitting. Thus, aside from assessing articular cartilage properties, joint contours may be mapped using the noninvasive imaging techniques described here, as well as others, for the production of molds for customized implants.

5.1.2 Invasive Methods

Arthroscopy is the most commonly performed orthopedic procedure in the United States (Figure 5.8). It is minimally invasive, although the joint capsule must be compromised. A small (e.g., 5 mm) port is opened in the joint, and optical, surgical, and other instrumentation are introduced through this port. Arthroscopy can be used not only for imaging but also for a variety of surgical procedures, such as meniscus, anterior cruciate ligament, and articular cartilage repair. Cartilage restoration procedures that can be performed arthroscopically include debridement, various marrow stimulation techniques, and the application of scaffolds intended for cartilage repair.

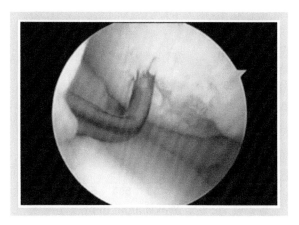

Figure 5.8 Arthroscopy provides a direct portal for more than visual assessment of articular cartilage health and damage. Surgeons can palpate the cartilage to get a qualitative feel of cartilage mechanical integrity and also perform many interventional techniques that range from shaving to reconstruction of the tissues in the joint. (Courtesy of Dr. Nikolaos Paschos.)

Ultrasound and optical methods, such as time-resolved fluorescence spectroscopy, can also be applied arthroscopically in the future to discern cartilage biochemical properties and, by extension, cartilage biomechanical properties based on the characteristics of fluorescence decay.

A probe that combines the light source and detector may be applied directly onto the tissue, and the spectral characteristics of laser-induced autofluorescence would be analyzed to discern cartilage matrix composition (Figure 5.9) (Sun et al. 2012). During its 50 years of usage in the United States, arthroscopy has proved to be a minimally invasive imaging technique for which new, accompanying techniques are continuously emerging to improve outcomes for articular cartilage assessment and therapies.

5.2 HISTOLOGY, IMMUNOHISTOCHEMISTRY, AND OTHER ULTRASTRUCTURAL TECHNIQUES

Histology and histopathology are well-established methods for evaluating native tissues, and readers are directed to excellent texts dedicated

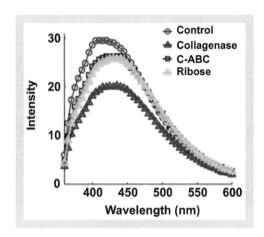

Figure 5.9 Optical techniques can be used to evaluate the mechanical properties of articular cartilage. In this case, changes in signals from laser-induced autofluorescence correspond to changes in mechanical stiffness, altered using collagenase, chondroitinase ABC (C-ABC), and ribose. Collagenase and C-ABC degrade collagen and glycosaminoglycans, respectively, in articular cartilage, leading to reduced stiffness. Ribose cross-links cartilage extracellular matrices, leading to increased stiffness. For example, when the stiffness of cartilage matrix is altered by these agents, the peak intensity resulting from laser-induced autofluorescence shifts to different wavelengths. The nondestructive nature of laser-induced autofluorescence has potential for use in the evaluation of cartilage mechanical properties. (From Sun, Y. et al., *Tissue Eng Part C Methods* 18(3): 215-226, 2012. With permission.)

to this subject, as well as for ultrastructural techniques such as scanning electron microscopy (SEM) and transmission electron microscopy (TEM) (An and Martin 2003; Mescher 2009). These techniques provide information over several scales, from showing the general directions of collagen alignment at the millimeter scale (Figure 5.10a) down to how the collagen molecule is organized around the cells on the nanometer scale (Figure 5.10c).

Of interest here, instead, is the histology of repair and engineered tissues, in which biochemical components may be of different ratios when compared with native tissues, and for which native morphology is absent and, therefore, cannot serve to guide the assessor. Care must be taken not to misinterpret or overstate results based on histological evaluation, and it is important to keep in mind that while a

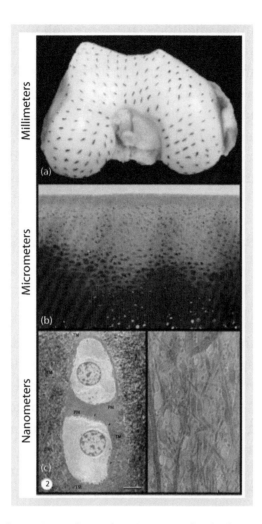

Figure 5.10 Techniques to evaluate the structure of articular cartilage can assess a dimensional range from millimeters (a, showing split lines) to micrometers (b, showing tissue morphology) to nanometers (c, TEM showing cell and collagen structures). (a, image from Below, S. et al., *Arthroscopy* 18(6): 613-617, 2002. b, image courtesy of Dr. Natalia Vapniarsky. c, image from Hunziker, E. B. et al., *Microsc Res Tech* 37(4): 271-284, 1997. With permission.)

few studies have quantitatively correlated biochemical content with histology (Martin et al. 1999), quantitative assessment of engineered tissues should, in general, be accompanied with caution because stains are only specific to certain types of extracellular components and will not discern subspecies from each other. For specificity, immunohistochemical methods are more reliable, although these, too, can suffer from nonspecific binding. In general, histological, immunohistochemistry, and ultrastructural results are qualitative to semiquantitative, providing information such as the absence or presence of extracellular components of interest and their relative distribution. Ultrastructural methods can yield quantitative results, however, such as collagen diameter and degree of alignment; both of these are important contributors to articular cartilage biomechanical properties. Since the solid fraction of articular cartilage is made up of cells, collagen, and glycosaminoglycans, a discussion of some of the methods available for their assessment is presented in the next sections.

5.2.1 Cells

Nuclear stains such as hematoxylin allow cell number and distribution to be assessed. Stages of the cell cycle can also be identified by proliferating cell nuclear antigen (PCNA) and by terminal deoxynucleotidyl transferase (TDT)-mediated dUTP (2′-deoxyuridine 5′-triphosphate) nick end labeling (TUNEL), to assess proliferation and apoptosis, respectively. Figure 5.11 shows an example of how TUNEL staining is used. There are also *in situ* hybridization techniques where cellular mRNA is bound by antisense RNA probes to determine chondrocyte gene expression.

Cell viability assays for cell suspensions and smears typically function by differences in cell membrane permeability (e.g., trypan blue will not enter cells with intact cell membranes) or metabolism. For example, the acetomethoxy derivate of calcein, after entering the cell, is metabolized to calcein after intracellular esterases in live cells remove the acetomethoxy group; calcein is impermeable and retained to yield a signal that fluoresces green (Figure 5.12). Cytoskeletal stains (e.g., rhodamine phalloidin) are important for articular cartilage biology since cell shape and cytoskeletal arrangement are strongly correlated with the chondrocyte and chondrogenic phenotypes.

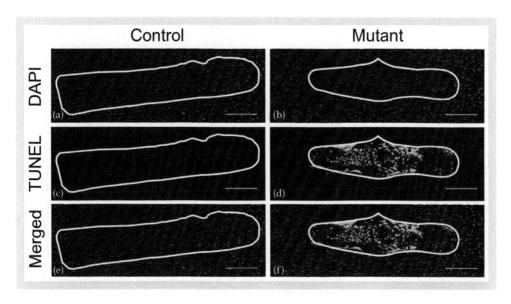

Figure 5.11 TUNEL staining can show DNA fragmentation and cell apoptosis. In this case, TUNEL was used to stain cells of the nucleus pulposus of control (Foxa2^{iCre};HIF-1α$^{f/+}$) (a, c, and e) and mutant (Foxa2^{iCre};HIF-1α$^{f/f}$) (b, d, and f) mice, respectively, at birth. DAPI-stained nuclei fluoresce in blue (a and b). TUNEL staining can be linked to various fluorophores and is green in this case (c and d). The merged image (e and f) shows that the mutant's HIF-1α deletion resulted in cell death in the nucleus pulposus, which led to decreased biomechanical properties of the mouse's intervertebral disc. The bar is 200 μm. (From Merceron, C. et al., *PLoS One* 9(10): e110768, 2014. Used under a *PLoS One* Creative Commons License.)

Cell morphology can also be visualized using cytoplasmic stains or electron microscopy (e.g., SEM and TEM). By using TEM, intracellular features (e.g., Golgi and mitochondria) can be assessed. Visualizing intracellular ion concentration (e.g., using a plethora of Ca^{2+} dyes) is useful for studying chondrocyte signaling and response to chemical and mechanical stimuli (Mizuno 2005; Zhang et al. 2006).

Finally, clusters of differentiation and other cell surface markers or receptors can be used in conjunction with flow cytometry or fluorescence-activated cell sorting (FACS) in determining the cell phenotype. It is worth noting, however, that no definitive set of surface markers have been identified as specific to chondrocytes. This can be particularly problematic for therapies that use stem cells. Where stem cell manipulation

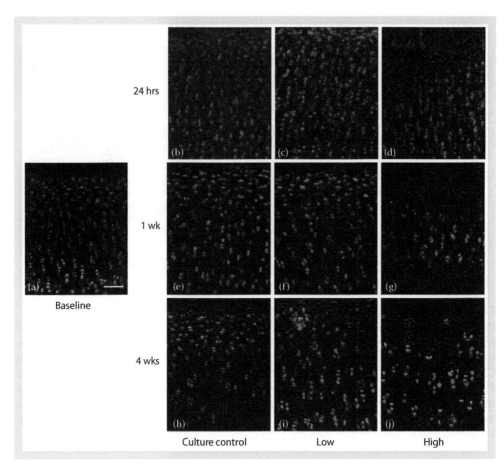

Figure 5.12 Confocal microscopy can be used in combination with live or dead staining to show how cells progressively die in human articular cartilage following impact. Live cells stain green, while dead cells stain red. In this case, cell death is seen immediately after a high level of impact disrupts the cartilage surface (d, g, j). (c, f, i) A low level of impact results in an injury that cannot be observed clinically since there are no aberrations on the cartilage surface. However, as time progresses to 4 weeks (h-j), an increasing number of dead cells can be observed down the middle column. (From Natoli, R. M. et al., *Ann Biomed Eng* 36(5): 780-792, 2008. With permission.)

occurs *in vitro*, flow cytometry data are typically used to verify that the differentiated cells no longer exhibit surface markers associated with stem cells. Even then, it can remain unclear whether the differentiated cells are chondrocytes. For regenerative medicine approaches where stem cells are expected to differentiate *in vivo* into chondrocytes,

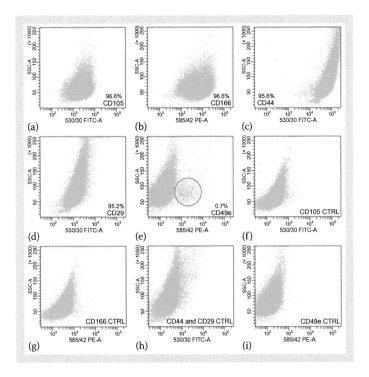

Figure 5.13 Flow cytometry can also be used to analyze cell markers to identify ones useful in isolating cells. In this case, cells were labed with putative stem cell surface markers CD105 (a), CD166 (b), CD44 (c), CD29 (d), and CD49e (e). While only 0.7% of the isolated chondrocytes express CD49e (circled) in this study, 99% of the cells in the clonal cell lines, obtained by adhesion to fibronectin, expressed this marker after expansion. Corresponding immunoglobulin control samples (f-i) are also presented. (From Williams, R. et al., *PLoS One* 5(10): e13246, 2010. Used under a *PLoS One* Creative Commons License.)

phenotypic assessment would likely require biopsies. In addition to surface markers (Figure 5.13), flow cytometry can offer additional information, such as cell size and organelle density.

5.2.2 Collagen

Histologically, general collagen staining can take advantage of the protein's fibril organization, while collagen typing occurs through immunohistochemical staining. For instance, sirius red, used in a saturated solution of picric acid (also known as picrosirius red), stains collagen fibers pink to red as the dye binds to collagen helices (Figure 5.14). Due to the aspect ratio of the dye molecule, trapping accentuates alignment, especially under polarized light (Junqueira et al. 1979), where binding degree can be assessed as lighter-to-heavier staining transitions from yellow to green. Other stains, such as aniline blue, can be used to stain collagen, and, while polarized light microscopy for collagen alignment can also be performed without staining, the effect for observing alignment is not as dramatic as when sirius red is used. SEM and TEM can also be used to visualize collagen fiber thickness and orientation, although these, like histology, are destructive methods.

Second harmonic generation (SHG) microscopy is an optical method that may, in the future, allow for nondestructive quantitative assessment of collagen alignment. Currently, SHG can be combined with various mathematical methods to determine collagen direction on histological sections (Figure 5.15). Collagen alignment is structurally important in native articular cartilage, but despite how simple it can be to visualize, alignment is seldom assessed or reported in engineered or repair cartilage.

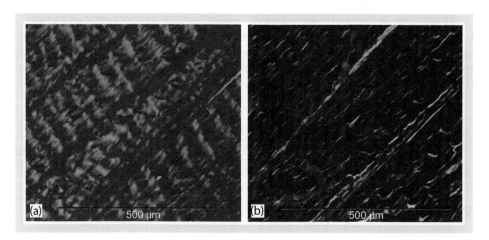

Figure 5.14 The picrosirius red method uses sirius red to stain collagen, as the dye becomes trapped among the collagen fibers (a, tendon). Collagen is often stained in combination with other extracellular matrix components, using for example a Masson's trichrome stain. In this case, aniline blue stains the fibers blue (b). Other stains, such as Light Green SF yellowish, Fast Green FCF, methyl blue, and water blue, are also routinely used for this trichrome stain. (Courtesy of Dr. Natalia Vapniarsky.)

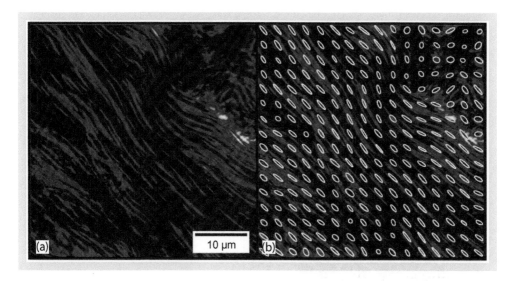

Figure 5.15 SHG can be used to determine collagen organization. In this case, collagen fibers from chicken cartilage have been visualized using SHG and gradient techniques, then pseudocolored (a). By superimposing ellipses over the fibers, one can quickly see the local direction of the fibers (b). The more eccentric (flatter) the ellipses, the more aligned is the collagen. (From Lilledahl, M. B. et al. in *Confocal Laser Microscopy—Principles and Applications in Medicine, Biology, and the Food Sciences*, ed. N. Lagali, Rijeka, Croatia: InTech, 2013, chap. 9. With permission.)

In addition to alignment, collagen fibril diameter and cross-links are both important for articular cartilage biomechanical properties. Fibril diameter can be assessed using electron microscopy (Figure 5.16), but there are currently no widely used ultrastructural assays to evaluate cross-links for type II collagen. Optical methods such as Raman microscopy are useful for discerning autofluorescence signatures of molecules; this and other methods, such as fluorescence lifetime imaging microscopy (Sun et al. 2012), should be adapted to image articular cartilage matrix cross-links in a reliable manner. As with alignment, fibril diameter and the degree of collagen cross-linking are seldom assessed or reported for cartilages generated *in vitro* or as a result of therapeutic interventions; this is despite their structural and functional importance. Ironically, these characteristics are important for cartilage-to-cartilage integration, and their understudied nature may have been a hindrance to advancements in this area.

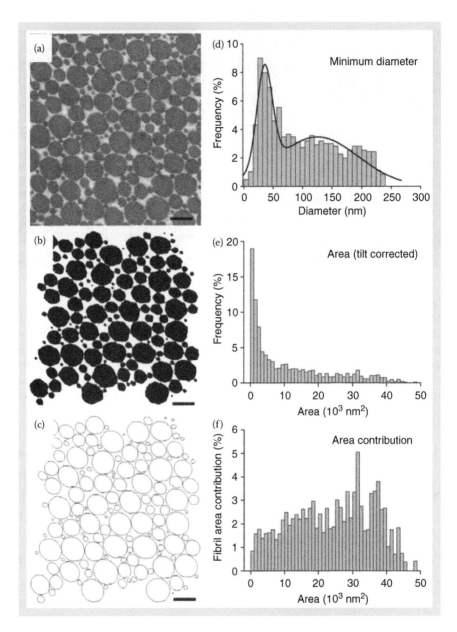

Figure 5.16 Collagen fiber thickness can be quantified using TEM. In this case, the collagen in rat-tail tendon was examined. The TEM image (a) was thresholded to generate a black-and-white image for analysis (b). An algorithm was then used to separate close fibril boundaries (c). From there, fibril diameters (d), area distribution (e), and relative area contribution of fibrils of different sizes (f) can be determined. The scale bars are 200 nm. (From Starborg, T. et al., *Nat Protoc* 8(7): 1433-1448, 2013. With permission.)

5.2.3 Sulfated Glycosaminoglycans

Dyes commonly used for staining cartilage glycosaminoglycans take advantage of the negative charge of molecules, and these include Safranin O, toluidine blue, and Alcian blue (Figure 5.17). Safranin O is a red to orange stain, often used with Fast Green (a neutral dye) as a counterstain. Articular cartilage should first be protonated in an acidic

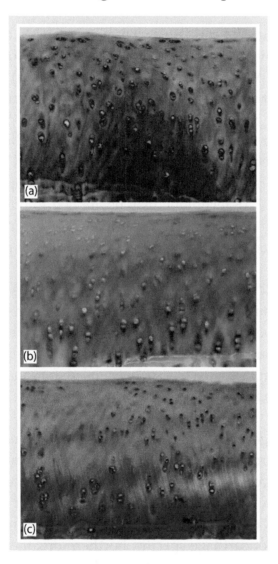

Figure 5.17 Glycosaminoglycans in articular cartilage can be stained using toluidine blue (a), Alcian blue (b), and Safranin O (red, c).

solution before dye binding occurs. Toluidine blue is a metachromatic dye that changes from blue to pink-purple when the sulfated groups of a glycosaminoglycan molecule bring several dye molecules close together. This color change is only visible under aqueous conditions, and dried toluidine blue complexes will appear blue. Toluidine blue has been used in cartilage histology with aqueous mounts to distinguish sulfated glycosaminoglycans from other anionic species.

Alcian blue staining for cartilage is common because it can be used with periodic acid-Schiff (PAS) reagent to specifically stain for cartilage extracellular matrices of various dissociation constant (pKa) values. The pKa of sulfate is lower than that of the carboxyl or phosphate groups, allowing for the sulfate to remain ionized at a lower pH than carboxyl or phosphate groups. For instance, at a pH of 2.5, both the sulfate and carboxyl groups are ionized and will allow Alcian blue to bind to glycosaminoglycans. However, at a pH of 1.0, only the sulfate group will be ionized for staining. The PAS technique may be applied to other cationic dyes besides Alcian blue to stain carboxyl and sulfate groups at a pH of 2.5, while only sulfated glycosaminoglycans will stain at a pH of 1.0.

The ability for Alcian blue to form insoluble complexes with glycosaminoglycans allows it to be combined with Verhoeff-Van Gieson methods (e.g., in Movat's pentachrome) to visualize glycosaminoglycan distribution in relationship to other extracellular matrix components. Soluble Alcian blue complexes have also been used for quantitative assays (Terry et al. 2000; Frazier et al. 2008).

Articular cartilage glycosaminoglycan assays have relied heavily on the anionic nature of these molecules, and caution must be exercised to ensure that glycosaminoglycans, and not other anionic matrices, are measured. As shown with Alcian blue in solutions of pH greater than 1.0, cationic dyes can also be used to bind to acidic, nonsulfated molecules that are not cartilage specific. Furthermore, these cationic dyes, whether used qualitatively or quantitatively, do not give information on which kind of glycosaminoglycan is present (e.g., chondroitin sulfate vs.

dermatan sulfate). As described in Chapter 1, a variety of glycosamino-glycans exist in articular cartilage, each with specific functions; their determination via immunological and enzymatic methods is important for understanding articular cartilage biology and for providing a context for how similar or different repair or engineered tissues are from their native targets.

5.3 TECHNIQUES FOR THE QUANTITATIVE ASSESSMENT OF CARTILAGE TISSUE COMPONENTS

Biochemical techniques are useful in yielding quantitative data for comparison among treatments and across experiments. Solubilized biochemical components are assayed by direct reaction or by binding via dyes or antibodies. For studies on articular cartilage, the lack of standardization may make comparisons among studies difficult. For instance, biochemical data can be represented in a multitude of ways, such as per construct, per dry or wet weight, per cell, based on DNA content, or even as ratios of extracellular matrix components to each other. Unfortunately, individual reports may not provide all data necessary for readers to perform conversions from one normalization method to another, making data difficult to compare. In reviewing the literature on emerging articular cartilage therapies, one should be cognizant of the uses and pitfalls associated with the common assays described below. Examples of some of these biochemical techniques for articular cartilage are discussed in Chapter 7.

5.3.1 Cells

At the cellular level, assessments of gene and protein expression provide information on cellular responses to various stimuli and signals. Toward this end, genomic techniques have been used to answer many basic science questions and to provide direction for identifying specific signaling pathways involved. For instance, immunoblots for intracellular proteins can be used to understand signal transduction. Similarly, single cell biomechanics can be used to determine thresholds of chondrocyte mechanotransduction (Shieh et al. 2006) or to characterize the cells with regard to stiffness (Figure 5.18).

Quantitative reverse transcription polymerase chain reaction (qRT-PCR) is useful for assessing cell phenotype via mRNA expression. qRT-PCR, in conjunction with immunological staining (e.g., flow cytometry and immunohistochemistry) and other biochemical assays (e.g., collagen and glycosaminoglycan), offers a platform for determining the cell phenotype, which is particularly important in directing stem cell differentiation for articular cartilage repair and regeneration strategies. For example, the directed differentiation of mesenchymal stem cells (MSCs) *in situ* in a surgical defect would likely yield longer-term functional restoration if the cells were verified to be of the hyaline phenotype. For emerging therapies where cells are manipulated *in vitro*, stem

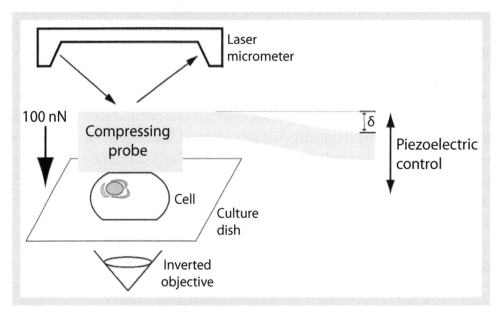

Figure 5.18 Individual cells can be quantitatively assessed using biomechanical techniques. A piezoelectric controller moves the compressing probe at a defined rate and distance, and the deflection of the probe is measured by a laser micrometer. By knowing the stiffness of the probe, the force with which the cell pushes back can be calculated. By compressing or indenting the cells, the cellular response to mechanical stimuli can be quantified. Through the same setup, the biomechanical properties of the cells can also be determined. (From Ofek, G. et al., *J Biomech Eng* 131(6): 061011, 2009. With permission.)

Table 5.1 Markers used for identifying and isolating marrow-derived MSCs

Must express	Must not express
CD105	CD45
CD73	CD34
CD90	CD14 or CD11b
	CD79alpha or CD19
	HLA-DR surface molecules

Source: Dominici, M. et al., *Cytotherapy* 8(4): 315-317, 2006.

cell populations need to be shown to be sufficiently differentiated to the desired chondrocyte phenotype before they can be used clinically. To do so, cellular markers are often assessed using flow cytometry. An example of using markers to quantify, identify, and isolate marrow-derived MSCs is presented in Table 5.1. Cell-based assays are important for the quality control of cells to be used in human therapy; the regulatory requirements for developing therapeutics are discussed in Chapter 6.

5.3.2 Collagen

Collagen is quantified routinely since it plays an important structural role in articular cartilage by conferring tensile properties and by restricting the movement of macromolecules. Collagen has a unique amino acid profile that is high in hydroxyproline content (Section 1.3.3). Collagen hydrolysis releases hydroxyproline, which is then oxidized by chloramine T to form a pyrrole, and the addition of Ehrlich's reagent (*p*-dimethylaminobenzaldehyde) leads to a color change that can be quantified via spectrometry. Since its introduction for quantifying collagens, the hydroxyproline assay has gone through many iterations of improvement (Prockop and Udenfriend 1960; Switzer and Summer 1971), and commercial kits are available.

Care must be taken when mathematically deriving collagen content from the hydroxyproline assay. Conversion factors based on assumptions of hydroxyproline content per collagen are often used, but this ratio may vary among native, repair, and engineered tissues. Collagen content calculated from hydroxyproline analysis of repair and engineered tissues may not be an accurate representation of the tissue's true collagen amount. This assay also makes the assumption that all hydroxyproline assayed is attributable to collagen; results can, thus, be confounded by hydroxyproline from other extracellular matrix components (e.g., elastin) or even by the enzymes used to digest the tissue for assay (i.e., pepsin). For native, articular cartilage, such errors are negligible given the high dry weight percentage of collagen within the tissue. However, for repair or regenerated tissues induced by novel therapies, one should not assume *a priori* that the matrix is composed mostly of collagen. For example, articular cartilage formed using stem cells or cells of elastin-containing tissues may produce elastin at disproportionately high amounts. Alternatively, unwanted collagen types (e.g., collagen type I, which is indicative of fibrocartilage) may contribute to the overall hydroxyproline determination, making immunochemical methods, such as ELISA, particularly important for assessing collagen content in engineered articular cartilage. The lack of specificity in hydroxyproline assays is common for many commercial collagen assays as well. One should familiarize oneself with the limitations of each assay before interpreting and comparing results.

5.3.3 Proteoglycans and Glycosaminoglycans

As described in Section 1.3.4, articular cartilage proteoglycans are largely responsible for imparting compressive stiffness to the tissue. Bound by collagen fibers, the negatively charged proteoglycans cannot leave the matrix, resulting in the Donnan effect. The negative charges are thus important to articular cartilage function and are often assayed through binding assays for quantitative correlation with biomechanical properties.

Many dyes bind to articular cartilage glycosaminoglycans (Figure 5.19) due to their anionic nature that causes the molecule to spread out like tube brushes (Figure 5.20), and these can be used for qualitative and

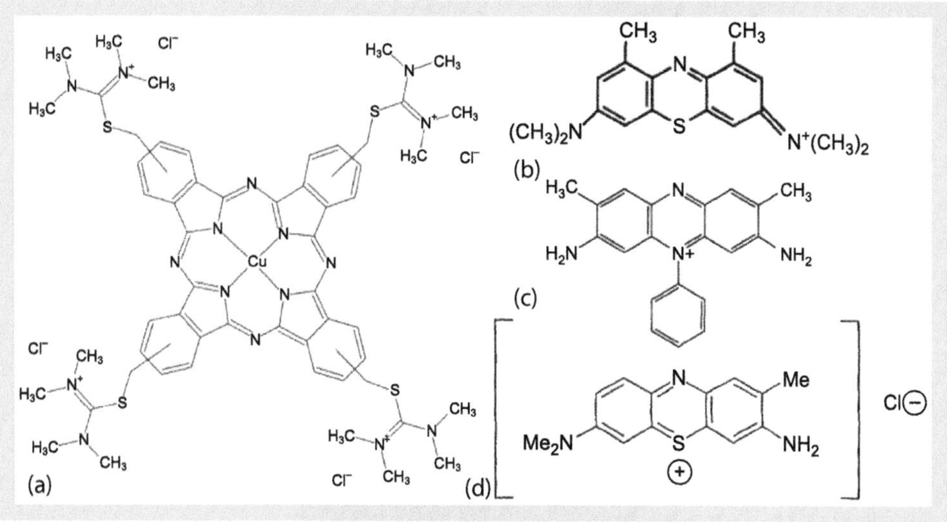

Figure 5.19 Molecular structures of common dyes for glycosaminoglycans include Alcian blue (a), toluidine blue (b), Safranin O (c), and DMMB (d).

quantitative assessment. A classical assay for the sulfated groups of glycosaminoglycans in proteoglycans is colorimetric quantification of 1,9-dimethyl methylene blue (DMMB) dye binding. When the dye is in solution, its peak absorbance is at 590 nm. Sulfated groups of the glycosaminoglycan molecule bring dye molecules together, forming complexes whose peak absorbance is at 530 nm. The color change may be noticeable by eye as solutions change from blue (unbound) to purple (bound), and this change is quantified using a spectrophotometer. Initially described in the early 1980s (Farndale et al. 1982), the DMMB assay has been improved with commercially available products. For instance, a limitation of the original assay is the tendency for DMMB-glycosaminoglycan complexes to flocculate, requiring that data be taken before this occurs; one of the commercially available glycosaminoglycan assay kits collects the precipitated complex and then releases the bound DMMB using a chaotropic salt (e.g., guanidine HCl), leading to a more stable assay.

The immunological determination of glycosaminoglycans is similar to that of other immunological methods and will not be elaborated.

423

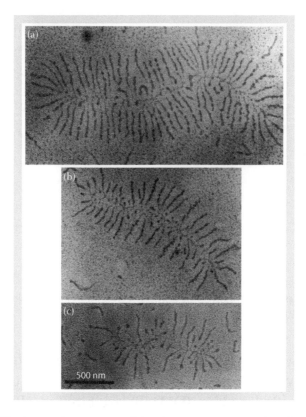

Figure 5.20 Electron microscopy of bovine aggrecan molecules from fetal (a), skeletally immature (b), and skeletally mature (c) animals. The aggrecan molecules not only decrease in size as the animals age, but also display more variations in length. The negative charges give the molecule a brush-like appearance and bind to a variety of dyes, allowing for quantitative assays. (From Buckwalter, J. A. et al., *J Am Acad Orthop Surg* 2(4): 192-201, 1994. With permission.)

Glycosaminoglycan quantification through ELISA and visualization through immunohistochemistry are based on the same principles as ELISAs and immunohistochemistry for other cartilage components, and these widely employed methods for articular cartilage are described in Chapter 7. A useful technique that should warrant more attention in assessing articular cartilage is fluorophore-assisted carbohydrate electrophoresis (FACE) (Ofek et al. 2008). Glycosaminoglycans contain polysaccharide portions that can be cleaved by enzymes specific to certain glycosaminoglycan species, leading to products of lower molecular weights. Based on stoichiometry, quantities of specific glycosaminoglycans can then be determined after gel electrophoresis that separates the digested products. With increasing attention to the mechanical and structural roles that carbohydrates play in cartilage and other mechanical tissues, FACE analysis can be a useful technique for future understanding of cartilage structure-function relationships.

5.4 BIOMECHANICAL TECHNIQUES

The biomechanical properties of articular cartilage can be evaluated using a variety of techniques, most of which involve monitoring the stress and strain in the tissue either over time or at different frequencies of oscillation (Kisiday et al. 2003). The most common analysis techniques consider a material to be elastic, viscoelastic, or multiphasic. These *in vitro* tests require precise experimental setups to account for boundary conditions or edge- or depth-dependent effects.

In vivo testing instruments have also been developed to evaluate cartilage stiffness. The Actaeon probe (Niederauer et al. 2002a,b), the Artscan (Toyras et al. 2001), and Athro-BST™ are handheld devices that can be used arthroscopically. By using the Actaeon, the stiffness of cartilage can be measured easily, and the values are independent of cartilage thickness and degeneration (Niederauer et al. 2002a,b). These devices are particularly useful in combination with other monitors of a patient's health. For example, as was discussed in Chapter 3, changes in cartilage material properties can occur with diabetes and hormonal and steroidal levels. For patients undergoing menopause or injected with anti-inflammatory steroids, such effects are seldom considered. The availability of these handheld devices may aid in promoting better joint health and awareness. However, few biomechanical evaluations are performed clinically, aside from a surgeon's qualitative assessment of gently pressing the cartilage. Most mechanical testing is destructive and performed *in vitro*, as discussed below. For elastic measurements, the relationship between stress and strain is analyzed and then fitted with a suitable mathematical model. Models are often derived that take into account the geometries of the contact region, allowing for a simpler analysis (e.g., force vs. indentation displacement data, directly obtained from the testing device).

Viscoelastic measurements are conducted using time or frequency responses. For time-based tests, the stress or strain is monitored over a set period, and mathematical models are fit to the resulting data. Stress relaxation tests observe the change in stress or force over time in response to an applied constant strain. Creep indentation tests, in contrast, observe the change in strain or deformation due to an applied constant stress. Frequency-dependent tests analyze the relationship between an applied oscillation and its signal response.

More complicated models of cartilage can be applied to experimental data to account for the different phases present in the tissue. These models are typically fit to data obtained from time- or frequency-dependent responses. The most common techniques for evaluating the compressive, tensile, shear, frictional, and fatigue properties of normal, pathological, repair, and engineered articular cartilage, and the mathematical models that accompany them, are described in the next sections. Toward translation of new articular cartilage therapies, test and model selection should be guided by ASTM standards and the FDA. Many of the biomechanical methods discussed below are described in greater detail in Chapter 7, "Experimental Protocols for Generation and Evaluation of Articular Cartilage." For example, compression testing is described in Section 7.6.1.

5.4.1 Compression Testing

A common technique for measuring the compressive properties of cartilage is through indentation (Mak et al. 1987; Mow et al. 1989) (Figure 5.21). For this procedure, a probe of specified geometry (cylindrical, spherical, pyramidal, etc.) is indented into a material. Elastic and viscoelastic properties can be obtained using standard testing approaches (i.e., indentation and creep or stress relaxation). The indentation site should not violate any assumptions in the models. For example, models usually

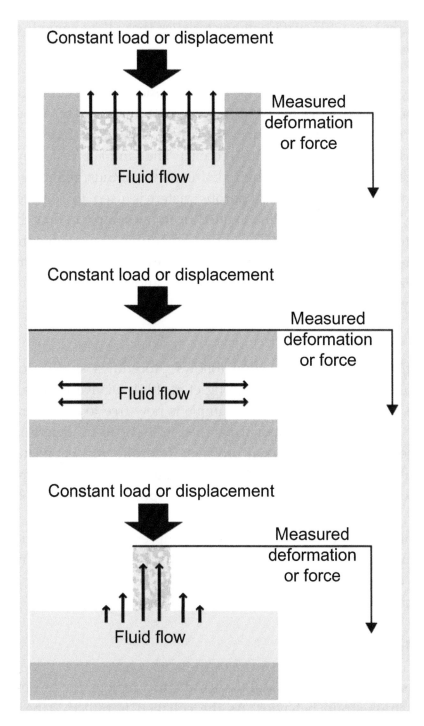

Figure 5.21 Confined compression, unconfined compression, and indentation are three ways to measure compressive properties of articular cartilage.

dictate regions with surface characteristics that allow smooth contact and sites that are sufficiently thick.

Compressive properties can also be determined using a confined compression test (Mow et al. 1980) (Figure 5.21). In this case, the sample geometry is typically a cylindrical disk with parallel surfaces to ensure even load distributions and flush contact. The sample is tested in a confined geometry to prevent any radial expansion, thus, reducing it to a one-dimensional problem. A porous platen is used to compress the sample, which allows for fluid exuded from the sample to flow through the platen-sample interface. The Young's modulus is calculated from the linear region of the equilibrium stress-strain curve, while other material parameters, such as aggregate modulus and permeability, are calculated by fitting an appropriate model to either creep or stress relaxation curves.

Unconfined compression testing follows procedures similar to those of confined compression (Armstrong et al. 1984; DiSilvestro et al. 2001) (Figure 5.21). However, since the sample is now free to expand radially during compression, additional parameters have to be determined to describe this two-dimensional problem. Typically, models include the Poisson's ratio as a determinant of this change. Samples are compressed using solid platens, and the stress or strain response over time is collected.

For confined compression, unconfined compression, or indentation, the mechanical parameters of the tissue can be obtained using testing conditions of stress relaxation or creep (Figure 5.22) and employing appropriate continuum mechanics theories (see Section 5.4.6).

5.4.2 Tensile Testing

For tensile testing of biological tissues, distinct regions can be observed in the stress-strain behavior. As the collagen is pulled, it begins to straighten, resulting in a toe region seen in the stress-strain curve (Figure 5.23). The elastic region represents when the straight collagen

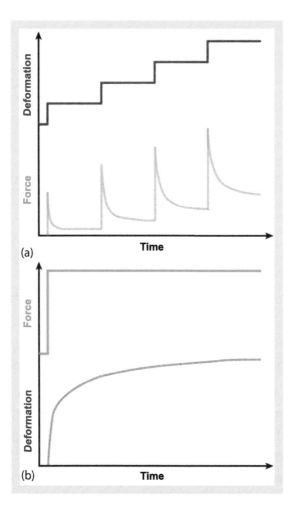

Figure 5.22 Compression tests can be performed under load or displacement control. An example of a displacement-controlled experiment is incremental stress relaxation (a), where, theoretically, deformations are applied instantaneously in a stepwise manner while recording force. An example of simple stress relaxation is shown in Figure 1.29. In creep testing, a force is applied instantaneously and then held constant while displacement data are collected (b).

fibers are pulled. The fibers begin to snap at the yield point and in the plastic region. Failure occurs when all the collagen fibers have broken, leading to separation of the tissue.

The tensile properties of a sample can be determined from both equilibrium stress-strain measurements and time-varying data (Guilak et al. 1994). As with compression data, the Young's modulus can be determined

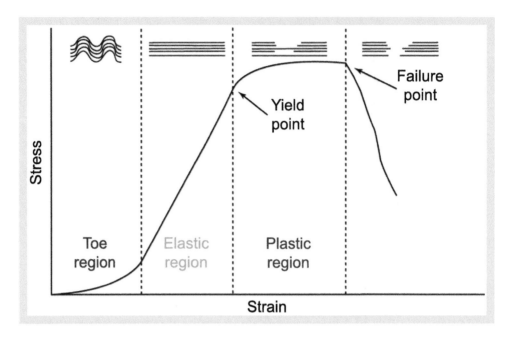

Figure 5.23 A biological specimen under tensile testing displays distinct regions in its stress-strain behavior. These regions are described in more detail in the text.

from the linear region of the equilibrium stress-strain curve obtained from uniaxial tensile testing. The sample should be fixed firmly at the grips such that failure occurs within the working length (i.e., near the center of the sample). Specimen lengths should be significantly greater than their widths to ensure uniform strain through the working length. Extensometers or optical techniques are used to monitor the strain in the region of interest, which is plotted alongside the applied stress for analysis.

5.4.3 Shear Testing

Typically, shear tests are conducted on cylindrical samples in a setup similar to that for unconfined compression tests. A flat platen is placed on the sample, and a small tare load is applied to ensure uniform contact. Shear tests can use either rotational (Stading and Langer 1999; Frank et al. 2000) or translational (Simon et al. 1990; Anderson et al. 1991) displacement strategies. As with the compressive and tensile properties, it is important to characterize both the equilibrium and dynamic responses of the sample under shear. The equilibrium shear modulus,

G, is calculated from the linear region of the stress-strain curve. The dynamic complex shear modulus, G^*, is calculated using the applied and signal response from a series of oscillatory stimuli.

5.4.4 Friction Testing

While many theories exist describing how articular cartilage exhibits such low frictional properties, most tribological studies focus on quantifying the forces present as two surfaces slide across one another (see Figure 5.24 for examples). These studies have examined lubrication

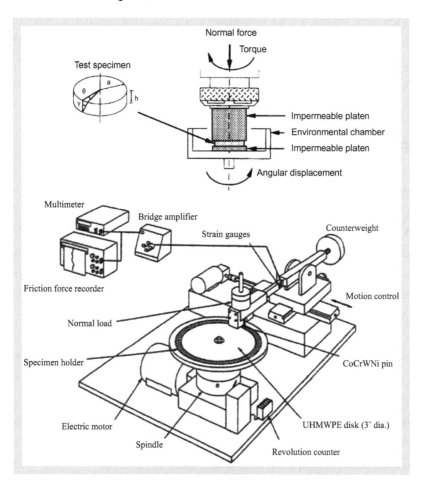

Figure 5.24 Examples of friction testing setups. (Top image from Wang, H., and G. A. Ateshian, *J Biomech* 30(8): 771-776, 1997. With permission. Bottom image from Klapperich, C. et al., *J Tribol* 121(2): 394-402, 1999.)

mechanisms both at the whole joint level (Mow et al. 1993) and at the cartilage tissue level (Katta et al. 2008). A variety of experimental configurations have been used, including pendulums (Walker et al. 1968; Teeple et al. 2007), oscillating arthrotripsometers (McCutchen 1962; Linn 1968; Jay 1992), atomic force microscopy (Park et al. 2004; Coles et al. 2008), and plug-on-plate configurations (DuRaine et al. 2009; Neu et al. 2010). The latter technique is currently the most common approach. This method involves moving a surface or plate translationally or rotationally with respect to a fixed sample. Normal and frictional forces are measured, allowing calculation of the coefficient of friction. Frictional properties are sensitive to variations in bathing solution, sliding rate, and fluid pressurization within the tissue (Forster and Fisher 1996; Krishnan et al. 2004). For more information on cartilage tribology, such as the various modes of lubrication in articular cartilage, as well as coefficients of friction, see Section 1.4.4.

5.4.5 Fatigue Testing

The durability of articular cartilage, such as determined using fatigue testing, is germane to the tissue's overall functionality. Fatigue testing applies repeated loading until the sample fails (Simon et al. 1990; Ker 1999). Usually a specific type of loading is applied, such as compression, tension, or shear, and loading cycles are repeated until the sample is noticeably affected (cracks, fissures, tears, etc.). Fatigue life is defined as the number of cycles necessary until failure.

Fatigue testing of living tissue is inherently different from that of testing nonliving materials because of the capacity of living tissues to adapt and remodel under mechanical stimuli. Special setups are required to keep the tissue hydrated (see Figure 5.25). Accelerated fatigue testing, as commonly described by ASTM standards, results in injurious loading of living tissues and will cause damage not only to the extracellular matrix, but also to the cells, which can release catabolic factors that accelerate matrix destruction. In contrast, repeated loading at physiological frequencies and magnitudes may not fatigue

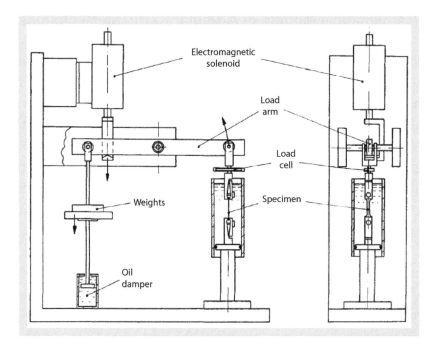

Figure 5.25   An apparatus for fatigue testing of articular cartilage. (From Weightman, B., *Ann Rheum Dis* 34(Suppl 2): 108-110, 1975. With permission.)

the tissue but instead contribute to tissue health and maintenance, as is the case for articular cartilage. Thus, fatigue testing for nonliving tissues has been devised, for example, for vascular applications (Tu et al. 1991), though similar testing for living articular cartilage is not common.

Wear is another measure of fatigue and is defined as the removal of material from a contact surface due to mechanical effects (Katta et al. 2008). Techniques for quantifying wear include characterizing released debris, evaluating surface topography, and imaging the bulk tissue. The severity of a damaging abrasion can be determined by measuring the size of released debris as well as the depth of penetration at the surface (Simon 1971). Cartilage roughness, as determined using a variety of scanning microscope techniques, can indicate how well the material will perform under shear or friction. Other imaging techniques that look at the tissue as a whole can be used to evaluate not only the surface characteristics but also any breakdown of the tissue below the surface.

5.4.6 Mathematical Models of Articular Cartilage Mechanics

Mathematical models are used to interpret results obtained from carefully designed evaluation tests, such as those described in earlier in this section. By fitting a model to experimental data, a quantification of the biomechanical properties can be achieved. Numerical representations of mechanical characteristics are of critical importance for comparison among studies, and researchers typically use similar testing techniques to facilitate this. Properties such as the Young's modulus, coefficient of friction, and streaming potential are just a few of the characteristics that can be used to describe the natural function of articular cartilage.

Some mathematical models are very basic in their description of cartilage, while others are extremely complex. It is important to remember, however, that they are all only representations of how the tissue might function and do not replicate every possible intricacy. Even simple models can provide valuable information, though, and can serve a purpose in evaluating a subset of properties. For example, the elastic components of a material can be described by

$$E = \frac{\sigma}{\varepsilon} \quad (5.1)$$

where E is the Young's modulus, σ is the stress, and ε is the strain. Modeling cartilage just as an elastic material, or as a spring, can provide a measure of its elastic response, but it might not correspond as accurately with experimental data as more complex models. Combinations of elastic and viscous elements can help to describe a material. The viscous components can be modeled by

$$\eta = \frac{\sigma}{\dfrac{d\varepsilon}{dt}} \quad (5.2)$$

where η is the viscosity coefficient and $d\varepsilon/dt$ is the time derivative of strain. By using elastic and viscous (or dashpot) elements, viscoelastic models can be derived.

434

Biological materials are typically considered to be viscoelastic since their deformation characteristics vary with respect to time or frequency. While perhaps also not very appropriate, articular cartilage can be modeled as a viscoelastic material. By fitting to either stress relaxation or creep data, parameters can be extracted that describe the time-dependent response of a material. Simple models of viscoelasticity include Maxwell (spring-dashpot in series) and Kelvin-Voigt (spring-dashpot in parallel). An extension of these models is the Kelvin model, or standard linear solid (spring in parallel with a spring-dashpot), whose deformation response during a creep or relaxation test is represented by

$$\left(1+\tau_\varepsilon \frac{d}{dt}\right)\sigma = E_R\left(1+\tau_\sigma \frac{d}{dt}\right)\varepsilon \quad (5.3)$$

where E_R is the relaxed modulus, τ_ε is the relaxation time for constant strain, and τ_σ is the relaxation time for constant stress. The spring elements in the model describe the stiffness of the tissue, while the dashpot helps describe the time-dependent deformation. The fitted values can be used to calculate the instantaneous modulus and apparent viscosity of the material

$$E_0 = E_R\left(1+\frac{\tau_\sigma - \tau_\varepsilon}{\tau_\varepsilon}\right) \quad (5.4)$$

$$\mu = E_R(\tau_\sigma - \tau_\varepsilon) \quad (5.5)$$

While viscoelastic models are useful for providing a basic description of biological tissue deformation, they are not particularly representative of the actual mechanical characteristics associated with articular cartilage. As discussed previously, cartilage can be described as having two phases: one solid and one fluid. More complex mathematical models of the tissue, such as the biphasic or poroelastic model (Mow et al. 1980; Frank and Grodzinsky 1987), take into account this composition, providing parameters that describe the stiffness, fluid flow, and deformation characteristics of the tissue. One example of this is the following equation that describes confined creep compression of articular carti-lage using the biphasic solution (Mow et al. 1980):

$$\varepsilon_{zz}(t) = \frac{F_0}{H_A}\left[1 - \frac{2}{\pi^2}\sum_{n=0}^{\infty}\left(n + \frac{1}{2}\right)^{-2}\exp\left\{-\pi^2\left(n + \frac{1}{2}\right)^2 H_A kt/[(1 + 2\alpha_0)h^2]\right\}\right] \quad (5.6)$$

where ε_{zz} is the observed strain, F_0 is the applied constant load, H_A is the aggregate modulus, k is the permeability, h is the sample thickness, and α_0 is the solid content ratio. When fit to experimental data, values for H_A and k can be extracted. Other equations exist in the literature for the various geometries and device configurations that are possible for cartilage testing.

More complex models of articular cartilage exist and are useful for identifying particular parameters that might be of interest. For example, an alternative to the biphasic model of cartilage is the poroviscoelastic model, which accounts for the different phases of the tissue, as well as their short and long time responses to loading (Mak 1986). Articular cartilage can be modeled in even more complexity than as just a two-phased tissue. A third phase, the ionic phase, can significantly affect the motion of fluid through the solid matrix, and, hence, the deformation characteristics of the tissue. The triphasic model accounts for contributions from the solid, fluid, and ionic phases of the tissue and results in the same parameters as the biphasic solution, with the addition of fixed charge density (Lai et al. 1991). For a more thorough description of multiphasic materials, poroelasticity, and viscoelasticity, the reader is encouraged to read "Introduction to Continuum Biomechanics" (Athanasiou and Natoli 2008).

Other characteristics that might be of interest include the frictional and torsional properties of the tissue. The coefficient of friction, μ, can be determined using a simple relationship between the normal, N, and friction, F_f, forces measured during friction tests:

$$\mu = \frac{F_f}{N} \quad (5.7)$$

Friction tests are applied by sliding a probe across the cartilage surface and collecting data for the two forces of interest. This can be done at the macroscale (Jay et al. 2004) or microscale (Coles et al. 2008) level of the joint to determine the frictional characteristics of the sample. An alternative approach is to measure friction using a rheometer, which moves two surfaces rotationally. This device can also measure both the simple and dynamic shear properties of cartilage. Simple shear testing can provide a measure of the shear modulus, G.

$$\tau = G\gamma \quad (5.8)$$

where τ is the shear stress and γ is the shear strain. Oscillatory measurements are used to determine the storage and loss moduli, as well as the complex shear modulus, G^*, which is simply the sum of the two.

5.4.7 Cartilage Tribology

As was initially discussed in Section 1.4.4, articular cartilage undergoes multiple modes of lubrication, including hydrodynamic, elastohydrodynamic, squeeze film, and boundary lubrication (Lewis and McCutchen 1959; Radin et al. 1970; Mow and Ateshian 1997; Schwarz and Hills 1998). During the walking cycle, articular cartilage exhibits a mixture of these modes. The minimum film thickness between articulating surfaces, together with the surface roughness (i.e., distance between asperities on opposing surfaces), determines the lubrication mode (Hutchings 1992). An estimation of film thickness between articular cartilage surfaces can be modeled using the formula for loaded-bearing surfaces (Dowson and Higginson 1977):

$$\frac{h_0}{R} = 4.9 \frac{\eta \upsilon}{W} \quad (5.9)$$

where h_0 is the film thickness, R is the radius of the equivalent cylinder, η is the viscosity of the film medium, υ is the sliding speed, and W is the normal load per sample dimension in the travel direction. As can be seen from this formula, altering these parameters, such as normal load or sliding speed can alter the lubrication regime tested.

The ratio λ, given as $\lambda = h_0/\sigma$, provides a measure of how likely, and how severe, asperity interactions will be in lubricated sliding. In this equation, h_0 is the minimum film thickness and σ is the root mean squared roughness of the two surfaces, defined by $\sigma^2 = R_{q1}^2 + R_{q2}^2$, with R_{q1} and R_{q2} as the root mean squared roughness values for each surface. For $\lambda > 3$, a full fluid film separates the two surfaces, asperity contact is negligible, and both the friction and wear should be low, as this defines the hydro-dynamic lubrication regime. The regime $1 < \lambda < 3$ is termed mixed elastohydrodynamic lubrication, and under these conditions some contact between asperities occurs. For $\lambda < 1$, boundary lubrication dominates, surface asperity contact is inevitable, and the presence of surface lubricants (e.g., SZP/PRG4) acts to dissipate shear.

5.5 ANIMAL MODELS

As part of translating new therapeutic approaches in the clinic, safety and efficacy data are often first collected in animals. This is because there are many factors in the living system that cannot be replicated *in vitro*. Selection of the animal model is based on many considerations, including cost and, for articular cartilage, biomechanics. The advantages and disadvantages of small and large animals, as used for studying articular cartilage pathophysiology and regeneration are discussed in the next sections.

5.5.1 Small Animal Models

Rapid maturation and disease progression, coupled with low cost, render mice and rats attractive for elucidating the mechanisms of various disease processes and for providing preliminary data on the safety and efficacy of new articular cartilage therapies. Implantation in heterotopic sites (e.g., subcutaneously, Figure 5.26) permits evaluation of xenogeneic articular cartilage constructs in immunodeficient (e.g., nude) mice and rats.

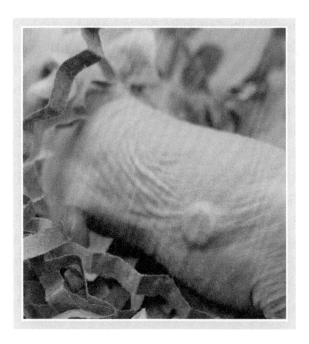

Figure 5.26 A typical small animal model used for articular cartilage studies is the athymic mouse. Here, a piece of engineered cartilage has been implanted subcutaneously to test viability, stability, and integrity of the engineered cartilage.

As the stability of the joint is critical for articular cartilage function, several animal models have been developed in which the anterior cruciate ligament has been transected or in which partial meniscectomy has been performed, resulting in reproducible osteoarthritis. These models are useful in evaluating compounds that can prevent, slow, or reverse osteoarthritis. Implantation in heterotopic sites may subject implants to lower loads than orthotopic sites in the joint, which can be advantageous or disadvantageous, depending on the experiment. For example, if the goal is to assess for toxicity, the implant will not be mechanically destroyed. However, if the goal is to assess for durability, the reduced loading represents an inadequate model. Advantages for choosing these animals include the following:

- Small animals require lower cost for housing, breeding, surgical support, and other related husbandry costs, as well as a smaller footprint and initial capital investment. All studies should conform to Institutional Animal Care and Use Committee (IACUC) guidelines. Rodent models are relatively straightforward, with fewer ethical concerns, when compared with large animals.

- The short lifespan of small animals allows for quick attainment of maturity and breeding age, and disease progression is rapid. Overall, this reduces both time and costs.

- The short breeding cycle of mice has led to the establishment of many genetically modified knockout (KO) and knock-in (KI) mice for the study of articular cartilage pathology. For example, these animals can develop premature cartilage degeneration (Figures 5.27 and 5.28). Animals can also display resistance to degenerative changes; in combination with various osteoarthritis induction models, osteoarthritis-protective models, such as ADAMTS4 and 5 KO mice (Glasson et al. 2004, 2005), have been used to evaluate susceptibility to osteoarthritis. Recently,

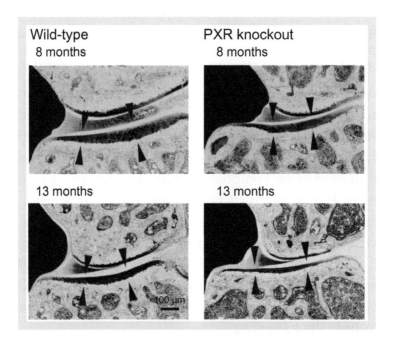

Figure 5.27 A KO mouse model showing age-dependent cartilage wear. Recent evidence has shown that steroid and xenobiotic receptor (SXR) and its murine ortholog, pregnane X receptor (PXR), are expressed in bone. SXR and PXR mediate metabolism, and KO of PXR in the mouse model shows age-dependent, increased cartilage wear by 13 months. (From Azuma, K. et al., *PLoS One* 10(3): e0119177, 2015. With permission.)

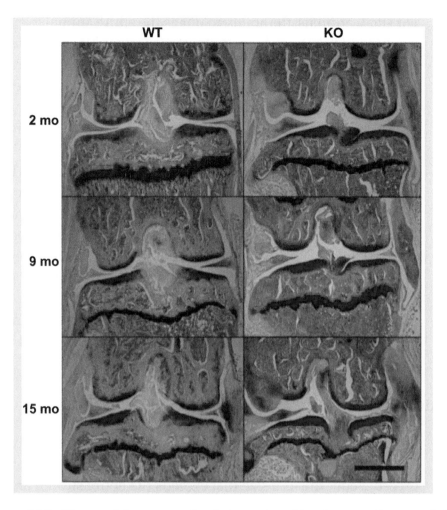

Figure 5.28 There exists a connection between type VI collagen and osteoarthritis. Safranin O and Fast Green histologies of knees from wild-type (WT) mice and type VI collagen KO mice are shown in the left and right columns, respectively. KO mice had thinner subchondral bone and more osteophytes than WT mice. However, with age, KO mice showed delayed or reduced cartilage degradation relative to WT mice. The scale bar is 1 mm. (From Christensen, S. E. et al., *PLoS One* 7(3): e33397, 2012. With permission.)

the inbred murine strains LG/J (healer of ear wounds) and SM/J (nonhealer) have been used to elucidate the heritability of healing in articular cartilage (Rai et al. 2012).

- Immunodeficient rodents permit implantation of allogeneic and xenogeneic materials without the confounding effects of the immune system.

- For small animals, the ability to image the entire animal to examine systemic changes in joint structure is possible, and data are rapidly obtained. This is particularly important for genetic disease models where one wishes to characterize the development of pathology within the musculoskeletal system. Imaging modalities can be applied rapidly and at a lower cost than large animals that have special sedation and equipment requirements. Whole animal fluorescence and positron emission tomography (PET) imaging are also possible for these small animals. Rodent PET imaging has been utilized extensively to study cancer, since the high metabolic rate of cancer cells results in more rapid processing of radiolabeled sugars. Small animal imaging may likewise provide information on the fate (e.g., survival and migration) of implanted cells, as well as implant-induced inflammation.
- Literature describing the use of small animals, especially mice, is extensive, and rodent models are the most versatile and well studied.

Disadvantages of small animal models include the following:

- The small size of small animal joints is not as representative of the human joint, where focal cartilage lesions routinely are at or exceed 2 cm^2; this is a size that exceeds the entire surface area of small animal joints.
- Treatments that have shown efficacy in small animals may not scale up for various reasons, such as diffusion and perfusion limitations.
- Small joints require microsurgery, which, depending on the injury and repair model, can be technically challenging and can limit the utility of these models.
- While one can perform imaging on the entire animal simultaneously, the data obtained for each joint may be limited due to size. Given that commercial ultrasound systems typically have

an accuracy of ~150 μm, imaging rodent cartilage that is typically less than 200 μm thick can be difficult, and the information derived will be limited.

- In mice and rats, articular cartilage is only composed of 5-10 cell layers. Thus, in order to have a reproducible model that mimics higher organisms, but retains some of the advantages of small animal models, intermediate-sized animals such as rabbits are commonly used.

5.5.2 Large Animal Models

Goats, sheep, and horses have been recommended by the FDA as appropriate for evaluating the efficacy and durability of new articular cartilage repair products. While not specified by the FDA, the pig is also a relevant model for temporomandibular joint cartilage because of similarities in biomechanics to humans. Xenotransplant products (although not articular cartilage) from the pig are also currently commercially available. Similar to small animals, various genetic and disease models have been developed in these large animals. Advantages of large animal models include the following:

- Large animal data are specifically described by the FDA's guidance document on the preparation of investigational new drug or device exemptions (INDs/IDEs) for articular cartilage repair products.
- These animals bear similar or more weight than humans and are thus suitable for assessing the efficacy and durability of tissue-engineered implants (Figure 5.29). While similar, the biomechanics of large animal joints are seldom identical to those of humans. Notably, the quadrupedal spine is approximately parallel to the ground, while bipedal, human spines are upright, leading to different loading conditions for the articular cartilage of the facet joints.

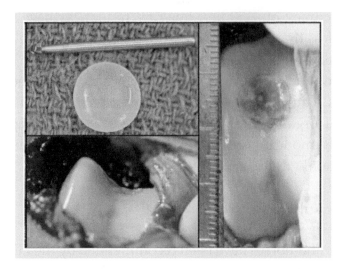

Figure 5.29   Large animal models such as sheep are recommended by the FDA for testing the safety and efficacy of products intended to repair or replace cartilage in the knee. Here, a defect 1 cm in diameter in the sheep trochlea has been covered with a tissue-engineered transplant.

The disadvantages of using large animal models include ethical and logistic issues, such as the following:

- Larger animals are costly since they take longer to reach maturity and require greater resources in husbandry. Similarly, surgical support for larger animals is more expensive and complex.
- For large animals, it is difficult to restrict mobility after surgery, and the newly implanted tissues may be subjected to deleterious compressive and shear loads immediately. Immobilization strategies are complicated and sometimes not possible for large animals. A hammer sling has been utilized for sheep and goats after surgery of the stifle joint (which corresponds to the knee joint of humans). In contrast, postsurgical load bearing in the horse is generally immediate because excessive weight bearing (e.g., loads shifted onto the nonimmobilized leg) can cause laminitis, a serious and debilitating condition.

5.5.3 Genetic and Defect Models

Aside from the KO and KI models cited above, other models that encompass both small and large animals deserve special attention due to their contributions to articular cartilage research. These include animals with compromised immunity and animals designed for xeno-transplants. In combination with these, various injury models have also been employed to induce osteoarthritis and articular defects.

Compromised immunity can be achieved through thymectomy and other models (e.g., nude mice and rats). This model is valuable because it allows for the evaluation of xenogeneic implants (e.g., human cells implanted in livestock) without concerns that the implant may be destroyed by an immune response. Galactose-α-1,3-galactose, or alpha-gal, is a glucose modification that is present in all the animal models discussed but absent in humans and old world primates, and elicits an acute immune response in humans (Oriol et al. 1993; Lin et al. 1997). KO animals without alpha-gal, such as pigs (Dai et al. 2002), have been bred to provide xenogeneic cardiovascular products (Xu et al. 1998; Lai et al. 2002; Tseng et al. 2005), although no articular cartilage products have yet been derived from these animals.

Many defect and injury models have been developed in animals for the examination of relevant pathologies in humans. Reproducible injuries can be induced and verified using quantifiable measures, and in many cases, cartilage degeneration occurs reliably. Trochlear defect models, both chondral and osteochondral (Brehm et al. 2006; Lewis et al. 2009), are often used to assess cartilage repair, while arthritis models generally involve impact, the introduction of foreign materials into the joint, joint immobilization, or joint destabilization. Cartilage impact, as defined under Chapter 3, can be applied to both open (Thompson and Bassett 1970; Trentham et al. 1975, 1977; Dekel and Weissman 1978; Mitchell and Shepard 1980; Haut et al. 1995; Koenders et al. 2005; Plater-Zyberk et al. 2007) or closed (Christiansen et al. 2012) joints. Collagen (Trentham et al.

1977; Joosten et al. 1999), bacteria (Cromartie et al. 1977), and serum (Pettit et al. 2001) have been introduced into the joint to induce osteoarthritis. Immobilization can also induce osteoarthritis (Langenskiold et al. 1979), although it is not as often employed. More prevalent are joint destabilization techniques to induce arthritis, and these include anterior cruciate ligament transection (Figure 5.30) (Brandt et al. 1991a,b; Guilak et al. 1994) and destabilized meniscus (Glasson et al. 2007; Macica et al. 2011) for the knee joint.

While chondral and osteochondral models are useful for providing preclinical data for these indications, it is recognized that osteoarthritis presents a larger and, therefore, more pressing problem. To assess the efficacy and durability of new treatments in the osteoarthritis

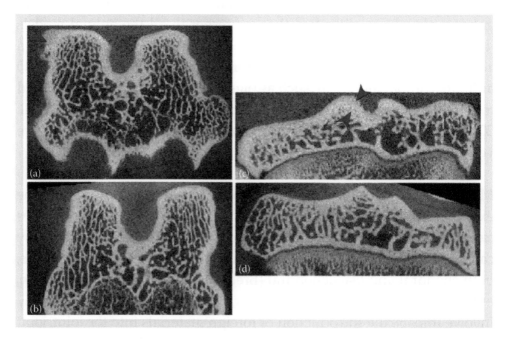

Figure 5.30 ACL transection results in osteoarthritic changes in a rabbit model. Shown are images obtained using *ex vivo* micro-CT from the femur of an ACL-transected rabbit (a), the femur of a sham-operated rabbit (b), the tibia of an ACL-transected rabbit (c), and the tibia of a sham-operated rabbit (d). Osteophytes and thickened, roughened cortical layers (arrowheads) can be seen in the ACL-transected knees. (From Pinney, J. R. et al., *Magn Reson Imaging* 30(2): 271-282, 2012. With permission.)

environment, animal models that faithfully replicate the disease should be used.

To summarize, animal models are used for the advancement of basic cartilage biology and are a critical prerequisite in the translational pathway when combined with the many assays described in this section. These models have been used to study osteoarthritis markers, disease progression, and the therapeutic efficacy of various treatments. Controlling genetic polymorphism and other environmental variables in human populations presents unique challenges. In contrast, pathologies in animals can be induced rapidly with repeatability. Small and large animal models complement each other, although large animals have been specified by the FDA for the assessment of durability and efficacy.

5.6 CLINICAL SCORING SYSTEMS

Many scoring systems have been developed to assess cartilage health, and the choice of which one to use can depend on whether histology can be obtained for the entire defect (e.g., O'Driscoll, Pineda, Wakitani, Sellers, or Fortier score), or if only a biopsy is available (e.g., International Cartilage Repair Society [ICRS] scores). Several morphological scoring systems have been developed for articular cartilage pathology, some originating in the evaluation of other joint maladies. Figure 5.31 shows many scoring systems, including the ones to be discussed below. Parameters can include tissue or synovial fluid coloration, lesion size and depth, and the presence or absence of pathologies in other tissues. An example of this is the Outerbridge classification system, described in Chapter 3. To date, these scoring systems do not include quantitative assessment of articular cartilage biomechanical properties. The advantage of morphological scoring is that it can be and is often applied to animal models to supplement other assessments that have limited reliability or robustness, or are difficult to obtain. For instance, animal activity and behavior, while used as a measure for treatment efficacy,

447

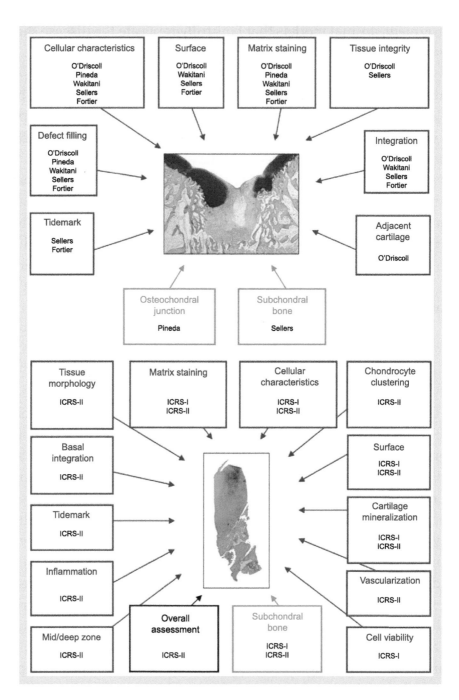

Figure 5.31 Multiple scoring systems exist for evaluating cartilage, and the choice of which one to use typically starts with determining whether the entire defect can be assessed or if only a biopsy is available. (From Orth, P. and H. Madry, *Histol Histopathol* 30(8): 911-919, 2015. With permission.)

vary greatly among animal models and may not correlate well with functional restoration in humans.

Ultimately, the restoration of patient mobility will depend not only on cartilage quality but also on the absence of pain. Scoring systems based on patient feedback offer practical evaluations of treatment efficacy. Such systems include the Cincinnati Knee Rating System (Noyes et al. 1983a,b), the International Knee Documentation Committee (IKDC) subjective scale (Irrgang et al. 2001, 2006), and the KOOS (Roos et al. 1998) and its variants (for the hip, foot and ankle, and rheumatoid and arthritis, HOOS, FAOS, and RAOS, respectively). Often used by the sports medicine community, the Cincinnati Knee Rating System has undergone several modifications (Risberg et al. 1999; Arthur et al. 2007) and was used to assess functional outcomes of Genzyme's Carticel, the first cellular therapy for articular cartilage traumatic defects. This scoring system combines clinical parameters, symptoms, sports activity, and activities of daily living to yield a score between 6 and 100. The IKDC subjective scale evaluates similar parameters and yields a score from 0 to 100.

For both of these scoring systems, a score of 100 represents no limitation in function. The KOOS knee survey uses subscales of 0-4 for pain, other symptoms, function in daily living, function in sports and recreation, and knee-related quality of life. A normalized score is calculated for each subscale, with 100 indicating no symptoms.

5.7 Chapter Concepts

- Common assays for the structural, biochemical, and bio-mechanical properties of articular cartilage can be used both to advance articular cartilage biology and to validate new articular cartilage therapies. This survey of methods for assessing articular cartilage quality prepares the reader for the literature on how current therapies are under continuous evaluation for improving efficacy.

- Engineered articular cartilage can be assessed histologically, immunohistologically, biochemically, via nondestructive imaging, and biomechanically in determining its functionality prior to implantation.

- MRI is a noninvasive technique for observing the morphologies of articular cartilage and other tissues of the joint. Currently, this and other imaging methods have not been shown to correlate fully with salient biomechanical properties, although this is an exciting research area.

- Articular cartilage is anisotropic, a property that can be assessed through polarized microscopy, SEM, and TEM. However, the anisotropy of repair for regenerated tissues is seldom assessed or reported.

- Histological staining for articular cartilage using Alcian blue, Safranin O, and picrosirius red indicates the presence of glycosaminoglycans and collagens but does not identify their specific types.

- Specific collagen typing can be performed using immuno-histochemistry or ELISA.

- There exist multiple protocols in determining biomechanical properties, making inter-study comparisons difficult at times. Establishing consensus standards can facilitate future develop-ment of an engineered cartilage product.

- Among the most important properties of engineered and native articular cartilage are the compressive properties, especially under creep indentation. Compressive characterization, via the derivation of the aggregate modulus, permeability, and Poisson's ratio (or shear modulus), is a necessary biomechanical evaluation for characterization of articular cartilage.
- Tensile characterization via uniaxial testing is important for measuring not only stiffness but also, importantly, the strength of articular cartilage. Tensile properties are indicative of the collagen network in terms of content and cross-linking.
- Critical in the function of articular cartilage is the tissue's ability to exhibit extremely low friction properties. Tribological measurements should be central in any study examining cartilage pathophysiology and regeneration.
- Small animal models are useful to evaluate the initial safety and efficacy of new cartilage therapies. Large animal models should be used to mimic the biomechanical environment of load-bearing joints in humans. Both small and large animal models are recommended by the FDA's guidance documents.

We would like to thank Derek Cissel, VMD, DACVR, PhD, for his careful review and comments during the preparation of this chapter.

REFERENCES

An, Y. H., and K. L. Martin, eds. (2003). *Handbook of Histology Methods for Bone and Cartilage*. New York: Humana Press.

Anderson, D. R., S. L. Woo et al. (1991). Viscoelastic shear properties of the equine medial meniscus. *J Orthop Res* 9(4): 550-558.

Aoki, T., A. Watanabe et al. (2012). Correlation between apparent diffusion coefficient and viscoelasticity of articular cartilage in a porcine model. *Skeletal Radiol* 41(9): 1087-1092.

Armstrong, C. G., W. M. Lai et al. (1984). An analysis of the unconfined compression of articular cartilage. *J Biomech Eng* 106(2): 165-173.

Arthur, A., R. F. LaPrade et al. (2007). Proximal tibial opening wedge osteotomy as the initial treatment for chronic posterolateral corner deficiency in the varus knee: A prospective clinical study. *Am J Sports Med* 35(11): 1844-1850.

Athanasiou, K. A., and R. M. Natoli. (2008). Introduction to continuum biomechanics. *Synth Lect Biomed Eng* 3(1): 1-206.

Azuma, K., S. C. Casey et al. (2015). Pregnane X receptor knockout mice display aging-dependent wearing of articular cartilage. *PLoS One* 10(3): e0119177.

Balamoody, S., T. G. Williams et al. (2013). Magnetic resonance transverse relaxation time T2 of knee cartilage in osteoarthritis at 3-T: A cross-sectional multicentre, multivendor reproducibility study. *Skeletal Radiol* 42(4): 511-520.

Below, S., S. P. Arnoczky et al. (2002). The split-line pattern of the distal femur: A consideration in the orientation of autologous cartilage grafts. *Arthroscopy* 18(6): 613-617.

Bowen, R. W., Y. N. Cheng et al. (2014). *Magnetic Resonance Imaging: Physical Principles and Sequence Design.* Hoboken, NJ: John Wiley & Sons.

Brandt, K. D., E. M. Braunstein et al. (1991a). Anterior (cranial) cruciate ligament transection in the dog: A bona fide model of osteoarthritis, not merely of cartilage injury and repair. *J Rheumatol* 18(3): 436-446.

Brandt, K. D., S. L. Myers et al. (1991b). Osteoarthritic changes in canine articular cartilage, subchondral bone, and synovium fifty-four months after transection of the anterior cruciate ligament. *Arthritis Rheum* 34(12): 1560-1570.

Brehm, W., B. Aklin et al. (2006). Repair of superficial osteochondral defects with an autologous scaffold-free cartilage construct in a caprine model: Implantation method and short-term results. *Osteoarthr Cartil* 14(12): 1214-1226.

Buckwalter, J. A., V. C. Mow et al. (1994). Restoration of injured or degenerated articular cartilage. *J Am Acad Orthop Surg* 2(4): 192-201.

Burstein, D., J. Velyvis et al. (2001). Protocol issues for delayed Gd(DTPA)(2-)-enhanced MRI (dGEMRIC) for clinical evaluation of articular cartilage. *Magn Reson Med* 45(1): 36-41.

Caglar, E., G. Sahin et al. (2014). Quantitative evaluation of hyaline articular cartilage T2 maps of knee and determine the relationship of cartilage T2 values with age, gender, articular changes. *Eur Rev Med Pharmacol Sci* 18(22): 3386-3393.

Christensen, S. E., J. M. Coles et al. (2012). Altered trabecular bone structure and delayed cartilage degeneration in the knees of collagen VI null mice. *PLoS One* 7(3): e33397.

Christiansen, B. A., M. J. Anderson et al. (2012). Musculoskeletal changes following non-invasive knee injury using a novel mouse model of post-traumatic osteoarthritis. *Osteoarthr Cartil* 20(7): 773-782.

Coles, J. M., J. J. Blum et al. (2008). In situ friction measurement on murine cartilage by atomic force microscopy. *J Biomech* 41(3): 541-548.

Cromartie, W. J., J. G. Craddock et al. (1977). Arthritis in rats after systemic injection of streptococcal cells or cell walls. *J Exp Med* 146(6): 1585-1602.

Dai, Y., T. D. Vaught et al. (2002). Targeted disruption of the alpha1,3-galactosyltransferase gene in cloned pigs. *Nat Biotechnol* 20(3): 251-255.

Dardzinski, B. J., and E. Schneider. (2013). Radiofrequency (RF) coil impacts the value and reproducibility of cartilage spin-spin (T2) relaxation time measurements. *Osteoarthr Cartil* 21(5): 710-720.

Dekel, S., and S. L. Weissman. (1978). Joint changes after overuse and peak overloading of rabbit knees in vivo. *Acta Orthop Scand* 49(6): 519-528.

De Smet, A. A., M. A. Norris et al. (1993). MR diagnosis of meniscal tears of the knee: Importance of high signal in the meniscus that extends to the surface. *AJR Am J Roentgenol* 161(1): 101-107.

de Visser, S. K., J. C. Bowden et al. (2008). Anisotropy of collagen fibre alignment in bovine cartilage: Comparison of polarised light microscopy and spatially resolved diffusion-tensor measurements. *Osteoarthr Cartil* 16(6): 689-697.

DiSilvestro, M. R., Q. Zhu et al. (2001). Biphasic poroviscoelastic simulation of the unconfined compression of articular cartilage. I. Simultaneous prediction of reaction force and lateral displacement. *J Biomech Eng* 123(2): 191-197.

Dominici, M., K. Le Blanc et al. (2006). Minimal criteria for defining multipotent mesenchymal stromal cells. The International Society for Cellular Therapy position statement. *Cytotherapy* 8(4): 315-317.

Dowson, D., and G. R. Higginson. (1977). *Elastohydrodynamic Lubrication*. New York: Pergamon Press.

DuRaine, G., C. P. Neu et al. (2009). Regulation of the friction coefficient of articular cartilage by TGF-beta1 and IL-1beta. *J Orthop Res* 27(2): 249-256.

Farndale, R. W., C. A. Sayers et al. (1982). A direct spectrophotometric microassay for sulfated glycosaminoglycans in cartilage cultures. *Connect Tissue Res* 9(4): 247-248.

Forster, H., and J. Fisher. (1996). The influence of loading time and lubricant on the friction of articular cartilage. *Proc Inst Mech Eng H* 210(2): 109-119.

Fragonas, E., V. Mlynarik et al. (1998). Correlation between biochemical composition and magnetic resonance appearance of articular cartilage. *Osteoarthr Cartil* 6(1): 24-32.

Frank, E. H., and A. J. Grodzinsky. (1987). Cartilage electromechanics. II. A continuum model of cartilage electrokinetics and correlation with experiments. *J Biomech* 20(6): 629-639.

Frank, E. H., M. Jin et al. (2000). A versatile shear and compression apparatus for mechanical stimulation of tissue culture explants. *J Biomech* 33(11): 1523-1527.

Frazier, S. B., K. A. Roodhouse et al. (2008). The quantification of glycosaminoglycans: A comparison of HPLC, carbazole, and Alcian blue methods. *Open Glycosci* 1: 31-39.

Glasson, S. S., R. Askew et al. (2004). Characterization of and osteoarthritis susceptibility in ADAMTS-4-knockout mice. *Arthritis Rheum* 50(8): 2547-2558.

Glasson, S. S., R. Askew et al. (2005). Deletion of active ADAMTS5 prevents cartilage
degradation in a murine model of osteoarthritis. *Nature* 434(7033): 644-648.

Glasson, S. S., T. J. Blanchet et al. (2007). The surgical destabilization of the medial
meniscus (DMM) model of osteoarthritis in the 129/SvEv mouse. *Osteoarthr
Cartil* 15(9): 1061-1069.

Guilak, F., A. Ratcliffe et al. (1994). Mechanical and biochemical changes in the
superficial zone of articular cartilage in canine experimental osteoarthritis.
J Orthop Res 12(4): 474-484.

Gupta, R., W. Virayavanich et al. (2014). MR T(1)rho quantification of cartilage focal
lesions in acutely injured knees: Correlation with arthroscopic evaluation.
Magn Reson Imaging 32(10): 1290-1296.

Haut, R. C., T. M. Ide et al. (1995). Mechanical responses of the rabbit patello-femoral
joint to blunt impact. *J Biomech Eng* 117(4): 402-408.

Hayes, W. C., L. M. Keer et al. (1972). A mathematical analysis for indentation tests
of articular cartilage. *J Biomech* 5(5): 541-551.

Huang, Y. P., and Y. P. Zheng. (2009). Intravascular ultrasound (IVUS): A potential
arthroscopic tool for quantitative assessment of articular cartilage. *Open
Biomed Eng J* 3: 13-20.

Hunziker, E. B., M. Michel et al. (1997). Ultrastructure of adult human articular
cartilage matrix after cryotechnical processing. *Microsc Res Tech* 37(4):
271-284.

Hutchings, I. M. (1992). *Tribology, Friction and Wear of Engineering Materials*. Boca
Raton, FL: CRC Press.

Irrgang, J. J., A. F. Anderson et al. (2001). Development and validation of the
International Knee Documentation Committee Subjective Knee Form. *Am J
Sports Med* 29(5): 600-613.

Irrgang, J. J., A. F. Anderson et al. (2006). Responsiveness of the International Knee
Documentation Committee Subjective Knee Form. *Am J Sports Med* 34(10):
1567-1573.

Jay, G. D. (1992). Characterization of a bovine synovial fluid lubricating factor. I.
Chemical, surface activity and lubricating properties. *Connect Tissue Res*
28(1-2): 71-88.

Jay, G. D., K. A. Elsaid et al. (2004). Lubricating ability of aspirated synovial fluid from
emergency department patients with knee joint synovitis. *J Rheumatol*
31(3): 557-564.

Joosten, L. A., M. M. Helsen et al. (1999). IL-1 alpha beta blockade prevents cartilage
and bone destruction in murine type II collagen-induced arthritis, whereas
TNF-alpha blockade only ameliorates joint inflammation. *J Immunol* 163(9):
5049-5055.

Junqueira, L. C., G. Bignolas et al. (1979). Picrosirius staining plus polarization micros-copy, a specific method for collagen detection in tissue sections. *Histochem J* 11(4): 447-455.

Juras, V., M. Bittsansky et al. (2009a). In vitro determination of biomechanical prop-erties of human articular cartilage in osteoarthritis using multi-parametric MRI. *J Magn Reson* 197(1): 40-47.

Juras, V., G. H. Welsch et al. (2009b). Kinematic biomechanical assessment of human articular cartilage transplants in the knee using 3-T MRI: An in vivo reproduc-ibility study. *Eur Radiol* 19(5): 1246-1252.

Katta, J., Z. Jin et al. (2008). Biotribology of articular cartilage—A review of the recent advances. *Med Eng Phys* 30(10): 1349-1363.

Keenan, K. E., T. F. Besier et al. (2011). Prediction of glycosaminoglycan content in human cartilage by age, T1rho and T2 MRI. *Osteoarthr Cartil* 19(2): 171-179.

Ker, R. F. (1999). The design of soft collagenous load-bearing tissues. *J Exp Biol* 202(Pt 23): 3315-3324.

Kim, H. K., S. Shiraj et al. (2014). Age and sex dependency of cartilage T2 relaxation time mapping in MRI of children and adolescents. *AJR Am J Roentgenol* 202(3): 626-632.

Kisiday, J., A. Kerin et al. (2003). Mechanical testing of cell-material constructs: A review. In *Biopolymer Methods in Tissue Engineering*, eds. A. P. Hollander and P. V. Hatton. Totowa, NJ: Humana Press, pp. 239-254.

Klapperich, C., K. Komvopoulos et al. (1999). Tribological properties and microstruc-ture evolution of ultra-high molecular weight polyethylene. *J Tribol* 121(2): 394-402.

Koenders, M. I., E. Lubberts et al. (2005). Blocking of interleukin-17 during reactiva-tion of experimental arthritis prevents joint inflammation and bone erosion by decreasing RANKL and interleukin-1. *Am J Pathol* 167(1): 141-149.

Kretzschmar, M., O. Bieri et al. (2015). Characterization of the collagen component of cartilage repair tissue of the talus with quantitative MRI: Comparison of T2 relaxation time measurements with a diffusion-weighted double-echo steady-state sequence (dwDESS). *Eur Radiol* 25(4): 980-986.

Krishnan, R., M. Kopacz et al. (2004). Experimental verification of the role of intersti-tial fluid pressurization in cartilage lubrication. *J Orthop* Res 22(3): 565-570.

Kuroki, H., Y. Nakagawa et al. (2009a). Ultrasound properties of articular cartilage immediately after osteochondral grafting surgery: In cases of traumatic car-tilage lesions and osteonecrosis. *Knee Surg Sports Traumatol Arthrosc* 17(1): 11-18.

Kuroki, H., Y. Nakagawa et al. (2009b). Ultrasound has the potential to detect degen-eration of articular cartilage clinically, even if the information is obtained from an indirect measurement of intrinsic physical characteristics. *Arthritis Res Ther* 11(3): 408.

Lai, L., D. Kolber-Simonds et al. (2002). Production of alpha-1,3-galactosyltransferase knockout pigs by nuclear transfer cloning. *Science* 295(5557): 1089-1092.

Lai, W. M., J. S. Hou et al. (1991). A triphasic theory for the swelling and deformation behaviors of articular cartilage. *J Biomech Eng* 113(3): 245-258.

Langenskiold, A., J. E. Michelsson et al. (1979). Osteoarthritis of the knee in the rabbit produced by immobilization. Attempts to achieve a reproducible model for studies on pathogenesis and therapy. *Acta Orthop Scand* 50(1): 1-14.

Lewis, P. R., and C. W. McCutchen. (1959). Experimental evidence for weeping lubrication in mammalian joints. *Nature* 184: 1285.

Lewis, P. B., L. P. McCarty 3rd et al. (2009). Fixation of tissue-engineered human neo-cartilage constructs with human fibrin in a caprine model. *J Knee Surg* 22(3): 196-204.

Li, X., V. Pedoia et al. (2015). Cartilage T1ρ and T2 relaxation times: Longitudinal reproducibility and variations using different coils, MR systems and sites. *Osteoarthr Cartil* 23(12): 2214-2223.

Lilledahl, M. B., G. Chinga-Carrasco et al. (2013). Three-dimensional visualization and quantification of structural fibres for biomedical applications. In *Confocal Laser Microscopy—Principles and Applications in Medicine, Biology, and the Food Sciences*, ed. N. Lagali. Rijeka, Croatia: InTech, chap. 9.

Lin, S. S., D. L. Kooyman et al. (1997). The role of natural anti-Gal alpha 1-3Gal antibodies in hyperacute rejection of pig-to-baboon cardiac xenotransplants. *Transpl Immunol* 5(3): 212-218.

Linn, F. C. (1968). Lubrication of animal joints. II. The mechanism. *J Biomech* 1(3): 193-205.

Lozano, J., X. Li et al. (2006). Detection of posttraumatic cartilage injury using quantitative T1rho magnetic resonance imaging. A report of two cases with arthroscopic findings. *J Bone Joint Surg Am* 88(6): 1349-1352.

Macica, C., G. Liang et al. (2011). Genetic evidence of the regulatory role of parathyroid hormone-related protein in articular chondrocyte maintenance in an experimental mouse model. *Arthritis Rheum* 63(11): 3333-3343.

Madelin, G., J. Babb et al. (2013). Articular cartilage: Evaluation with fluid-suppressed 7.0-T sodium MR imaging in subjects with and subjects without osteoarthritis. *Radiology* 268(2): 481-491.

Mak, A. F. (1986). The apparent viscoelastic behavior of articular cartilage—The contributions from the intrinsic matrix viscoelasticity and interstitial fluid flows. *J Biomech Eng* 108(2): 123-130.

Mak, A. F., W. M. Lai et al. (1987). Biphasic indentation of articular cartilage. I. Theoretical analysis. *J Biomech* 20(7): 703-714.

Mamisch, T. C., M. I. Menzel et al. (2008). Steady-state diffusion imaging for MR in-vivo evaluation of reparative cartilage after matrix-associated autologous chondrocyte transplantation at 3 tesla—Preliminary results. *Eur J Radiol* 65(1): 72-79.

Martin, I., B. Obradovic et al. (1999). Method for quantitative analysis of glycos-aminoglycan distribution in cultured natural and engineered cartilage. *Ann Biomed Eng* 27(5): 656-662.

Matsubara, H., K. Okazaki et al. (2015). Detection of early cartilage deterioration associated with meniscal tear using T1rho mapping magnetic resonance imaging. *BMC Musculoskelet Disord* 16: 22.

McCutchen, C. W. (1962). The frictional properties of animal joints. *Wear* 5(1): 1-17.

Merceron, C., L. Mangiavini et al. (2014). Loss of HIF-1alpha in the notochord results in cell death and complete disappearance of the nucleus pulposus. *PLoS One* 9(10): e110768.

Mescher, A. L. (2009). *Junqueira's Basic Histology: Text and Atlas*. 12th ed. Columbus, OH: McGraw-Hill Medical.

Mitchell, N., and N. Shepard. (1980). Healing of articular cartilage in intra-articular fractures in rabbits. *J Bone Joint Surg Am* 62(4): 628-634.

Mizuno, S. (2005). A novel method for assessing effects of hydrostatic fluid pressure on intracellular calcium: A study with bovine articular chondrocytes. *Am J Physiol Cell Physiol* 288(2): C329-337.

Moller, B., H. Bonel et al. (2009). Measuring finger joint cartilage by ultrasound as a promising alternative to conventional radiograph imaging. *Arthritis Rheum* 61(4): 435-441.

Mosher, T. J., H. Smith et al. (2001). MR imaging and T2 mapping of femoral cartilage: In vivo determination of the magic angle effect. *AJR Am J Roentgenol* 177(3): 665-669.

Mow, V. C., and G. A. Ateshian. (1997). Lubrication and wear of diathrodial joints. *Basic Orthopaedic Biomechanics*. V. C. Mow and W. C. Hayes. Philadelphia, PA, Lippincott-Raven Publishers: 275-315.

Mow, V. C., G. A. Ateshian et al. (1993). Biomechanics of diarthrodial joints: A review of twenty years of progress. *J Biomech Eng* 115(4B): 460-467.

Mow, V. C., M. C. Gibbs et al. (1989). Biphasic indentation of articular cartilage. II. A numerical algorithm and an experimental study. *J Biomech* 22(8-9): 853-861.

Mow, V. C., S. C. Kuei et al. (1980). Biphasic creep and stress relaxation of articular cartilage in compression? Theory and experiments. *J Biomech Eng* 102(1): 73-84.

Natoli, R. M., and K. A. Athanasiou. (2009). Traumatic loading of articular cartilage: Mechanical and biological responses and post-injury treatment. *Biorheology* 46(6): 451-485.

Natoli, R. M., C. C. Scott et al. (2008). Temporal effects of impact on articular cartilage cell death, gene expression, matrix biochemistry, and biomechanics. *Ann Biomed Eng* 36(5): 780-792.

Neu, C. P., H. F. Arastu et al. (2009). Characterization of engineered tissue construct mechanical function by magnetic resonance imaging. *J Tissue Eng Regen Med* 3(6): 477-485.

Neu, C. P., A. H. Reddi et al. (2010). Increased friction coefficient and superficial zone protein expression in patients with advanced osteoarthritis. *Arthritis Rheum* 62(9): 2680-2687.

Newbould, R. D., S. R. Miller et al. (2012). Reproducibility of sodium MRI measures of articular cartilage of the knee in osteoarthritis. *Osteoarthr Cartil* 20(1): 29-35.

Newbould, R. D., S. R. Miller et al. (2013). T1-weighted sodium MRI of the articulator cartilage in osteoarthritis: A cross sectional and longitudinal study. *PLoS One* 8(8): e73067.

Niederauer, G. G., G. M. Niederauer et al. (2002a). *Sensitivity of a hand-held indentation probe for measuring the stiffness of articular cartilage.* Presented at Second Joint Meeting of the IEEE Engineering in Medicine and Biology Society and the Biomedical Engineering Society, Houston, TX.

Niederauer, G. G., D. R. Schmidt et al. (2002b). *Applications and advantages of a hand-held indentation device.* Presented at 2002 International Cartilage Repair Society Symposium "Biophysical Diagnosis of Cartilage Degeneration and Repair," Toronto, Canada.

Nieminen, M. T., J. Rieppo et al. (2001). T2 relaxation reveals spatial collagen architecture in articular cartilage: A comparative quantitative MRI and polarized light microscopic study. *Magn Reson Med* 46(3): 487-493.

Nieminen, M. T., J. Rieppo et al. (2002). Spatial assessment of articular cartilage proteoglycans with Gd-DTPA-enhanced T1 imaging. *Magn Reson Med* 48(4): 640-648.

Nishioka, H., J. Hirose et al. (2015). Evaluation of the relationship between T1rho and T2 values and patella cartilage degeneration in patients of the same age group. *Eur J Radiol* 84(3): 463-468.

Noyes, F. R., D. S. Matthews et al. (1983a). The symptomatic anterior cruciate-deficient knee. II. The results of rehabilitation, activity modification, and counseling on functional disability. *J Bone Joint Surg Am* 65(2): 163-174.

Noyes, F. R., P. A. Mooar et al. (1983b). The symptomatic anterior cruciate-deficient knee. I. The long-term functional disability in athletically active individuals. *J Bone Joint Surg Am* 65(2): 154-162.

Ofek, G., C. M. Revell et al. (2008). Matrix development in self-assembly of articular cartilage. *PLoS One* 3(7): e2795.

Ofek, G., V. P. Willard et al. (2009). Mechanical characterization of differentiated human embryonic stem cells. *J Biomech Eng* 131(6): 061011.

Okazaki, K., Y. Takayama et al. (2014). Subclinical cartilage degeneration in young athletes with posterior cruciate ligament injuries detected with T1rho magnetic resonance imaging mapping. *Knee Surg Sports Traumatol Arthrosc* 23(10): 3094-3100.

Oriol, R., Y. Ye et al. (1993). Carbohydrate antigens of pig tissues reacting with human natural antibodies as potential targets for hyperacute vascular rejection in pig-to-man organ xenotransplantation. *Transplantation* 56(6): 1433-1442.

Orth, P., and H. Madry. (2015). Complex and elementary histological scoring systems for articular cartilage repair. *Histol Histopathol* 30(8): 911-919.

Park, S., K. D. Costa et al. (2004). Microscale frictional response of bovine articular cartilage from atomic force microscopy. *J Biomech* 37(11): 1679-1687.

Pettit, A. R., H. Ji et al. (2001). TRANCE/RANKL knockout mice are protected from bone erosion in a serum transfer model of arthritis. *Am J Pathol* 159(5): 1689-1699.

Pinney, J. R., C. Taylor et al. (2012). Imaging longitudinal changes in articular cartilage and bone following doxycycline treatment in a rabbit anterior cruciate ligament transection model of osteoarthritis. *Magn Reson Imaging* 30(2): 271-282.

Plater-Zyberk, C., L. A. Joosten et al. (2007). GM-CSF neutralisation suppresses inflammation and protects cartilage in acute streptococcal cell wall arthritis of mice. *Ann Rheum Dis* 66(4): 452-457.

Prockop, D. J., and S. Udenfriend. (1960). A specific method for the analysis of hydroxyproline in tissues and urine. *Anal Biochem* 1: 228-239.

Qin, L., Y. Zheng et al. (2002). Ultrasound detection of trypsin-treated articular cartilage: Its association with cartilaginous proteoglycans assessed by histological and biochemical methods. *J Bone Miner Metab* 20(5): 281-287.

Rai, M. F., S. Hashimoto et al. (2012). Heritability of articular cartilage regeneration and its association with ear-wound healing. *Arthritis Rheum* 64(7): 2300-2310.

Radin, E. L., D. A. Swann et al. (1970). Separation of a hyaluronate-free lubricating fraction from synovial fluid. *Nature* 228(5269): 377-378.

Risberg, M. A., I. Holm et al. (1999). Sensitivity to changes over time for the IKDC form, the Lysholm score, and the Cincinnati knee score. A prospective study of 120 ACL reconstructed patients with a 2-year follow-up. *Knee Surg Sports Traumatol Arthrosc* 7(3): 152-159.

Roos, E. M., H. P. Roos et al. (1998). Knee Injury and Osteoarthritis Outcome Score (KOOS)—Development of a self-administered outcome measure. *J Orthop Sports Phys Ther* 28(2): 88-96.

Schwarz, I. M. and B. A. Hills. (1998). Surface-active phospholipid as the lubricating component of lubricin. *Br J Rheumatol* 37(1): 21-26.

Shieh, A. C., E. J. Koay et al. (2006). Strain-dependent recovery behavior of single chondrocytes. *Biomech Model Mechanobiol* 5(2-3): 172-179.

Shiomi, T., T. Nishii et al. (2010). Influence of knee positions on T2, T*2, and dGEM-RIC mapping in porcine knee cartilage. *Magn Reson Med* 64(3): 707-714.

Simon, W. H. (1971). Wear properties of articular cartilage in vitro. *J Biomech* 4(5): 379-389.

Simon, W. H., A. Mak et al. (1990). The effect of shear fatigue on bovine articular cartilage. *J Orthop Res* 8(1): 86-93.

Stading, M., and R. Langer. (1999). Mechanical shear properties of cell-polymer cartilage constructs. *Tissue Eng* 5(3): 241-250.

Starborg, T., N. S. Kalson et al. (2013). Using transmission electron microscopy and 3View to determine collagen fibril size and three-dimensional organization. *Nat Protoc* 8(7): 1433-1448.

Sun, Y., D. Responte et al. (2012). Nondestructive evaluation of tissue engineered articular cartilage using time-resolved fluorescence spectroscopy and ultrasound backscatter microscopy. *Tissue Eng Part C Methods* 18(3): 215-226.

Surowiec, R. K., E. P. Lucas et al. (2014). Quantitative MRI in the evaluation of articular cartilage health: Reproducibility and variability with a focus on T2 mapping. *Knee Surg Sports Traumatol Arthrosc* 22(6): 1385-1395.

Switzer, B. R., and G. K. Summer. (1971). Improved method for hydroxyproline analysis in tissue hydrolyzates. *Anal Biochem* 39(2): 487-491.

Teeple, E., B. C. Fleming et al. (2007). Frictional properties of Hartley guinea pig knees with and without proteolytic disruption of the articular surfaces. *Osteoarthr Cartil* 15(3): 309-315.

Terry, D. E., R. K. Chopra et al. (2000). Differential use of Alcian blue and toluidine blue dyes for the quantification and isolation of anionic glycoconjugates from cell cultures: Application to proteoglycans and a high-molecular-weight glycoprotein synthesized by articular chondrocytes. *Anal Biochem* 285(2): 211-219.

Thompson, R. C., Jr., and C. A. Bassett. (1970). Histological observations on experimentally induced degeneration of articular cartilage. *J Bone Joint Surg Am* 52(3): 435-443.

Toyras, J., T. Lyyra-Laitinen et al. (2001). Estimation of the Young's modulus of articular cartilage using an arthroscopic indentation instrument and ultrasonic measurement of tissue thickness. *J Biomech* 34(2): 251-256.

Trentham, D. E., H. A. Silverman et al. (1975). Letter: Cause of adult toxic epidermal necrolysis. *N Engl J Med* 292(16): 870.

Trentham, D. E., A. S. Townes et al. (1977). Autoimmunity to type II collagen: An experimental model of arthritis. *J Exp Med* 146(3): 857-868.

Tseng, Y. L., K. Kuwaki et al. (2005). alpha1,3-Galactosyltransferase gene-knockout pig heart transplantation in baboons with survival approaching 6 months. *Transplantation* 80(10): 1493-1500.

Tu, R., J. McIntyre et al. (1991). Dynamic internal compliance of a vascular prosthesis. *ASAIO Trans* 37(3): M470-M472.

van Tiel, J., M. Reijman et al. (2013). Delayed gadolinium-enhanced MRI of cartilage (dGEMRIC) shows no change in cartilage structural composition after visco-supplementation in patients with early-stage knee osteoarthritis. *PLoS One* 8(11): e79785.

Vasiliadis, H. S., B. Danielson et al. (2010). Autologous chondrocyte implantation in cartilage lesions of the knee: Long-term evaluation with magnetic resonance imaging and delayed gadolinium-enhanced magnetic resonance imaging technique. *Am J Sports Med* 38(5): 943-949.

Walker, P. S., D. Dowson et al. (1968). "Boosted lubrication" in synovial joints by fluid entrapment and enrichment. *Ann Rheum Dis* 27(6): 512-520.

Wang, H., and G. A. Ateshian. (1997). The normal stress effect and equilibrium friction coefficient of articular cartilage under steady frictional shear. *J Biomech* 30(8): 771-776.

Wang, L., and R. R. Regatte. (2015). Investigation of regional influence of magic-angle effect on t2 in human articular cartilage with osteoarthritis at 3 T. *Acad Radiol* 22(1): 87-92.

Weightman, B. (1975). In vitro fatigue testing of articular cartilage. *Ann Rheum Dis* 34(Suppl 2): 108-110.

Wheaton, A. J., A. Borthakur et al. (2004). Proteoglycan loss in human knee cartilage: Quantitation with sodium MR imaging—Feasibility study. *Radiology* 231(3): 900-905.

Wheaton, A. J., G. R. Dodge et al. (2005). Quantification of cartilage biomechanical and biochemical properties via T1rho magnetic resonance imaging. *Magn Reson Med* 54(5): 1087-1093.

Williams, A., A. Gillis et al. (2004). Glycosaminoglycan distribution in cartilage as determined by delayed gadolinium-enhanced MRI of cartilage (dGEMRIC): Potential clinical applications. *AJR Am J Roentgenol* 182(1): 167-172.

Williams, R., I. M. Khan et al. (2010). Identification and clonal characterisation of a progenitor cell sub-population in normal human articular cartilage. *PLoS One* 5(10): e13246.

Xu, J., G. Xie et al. (2011). Value of T2-mapping and DWI in the diagnosis of early knee cartilage injury. *J Radiol Case Rep* 5(2): 13-18.

Xu, Y., T. Lorf et al. (1998). Removal of anti-porcine natural antibodies from human and nonhuman primate plasma in vitro and in vivo by a Galalpha1-3Galbeta1-4betaGlc-X immunoaffinity column. *Transplantation* 65(2): 172-179.

Zalewski, T., P. Lubiatowski et al. (2008). Scaffold-aided repair of articular cartilage studied by MRI. *Magma* 21(3): 177-185.

Zhang, M., J. J. Wang et al. (2006). Effects of mechanical pressure on intracellular calcium release channel and cytoskeletal structure in rabbit mandibular condylar chondrocytes. *Life Sci* 78(21): 2480-2487.

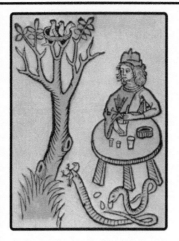

15th-century apothecary, forerunner of the pharmacist, helps treat a poison victim. Woodcut from Ortus Sanitatis, Mainz, 1491 (Museum of the Royal Pharmaceutical Society, London).

1903 patent medicine ad for "snake oil" with claims of treating a multitude of conditions, including rheumatism and stiff joints. These "patent medicines" commonly lacked any form of testing, evidence for effectiveness, or even a list of active ingredient(s). The term *snake oil* would later come to apply to any fraudulent or untested medicine (Oregon state archives).

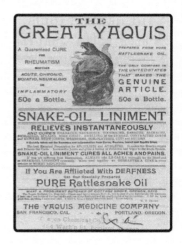

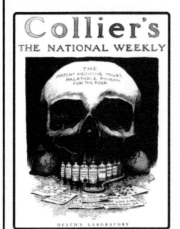

With roots in the mid-19th century, the FDA was founded by the 1906 Pure Food and Drugs Act, led by a series of articles by Samuel Hopkins Adams in Collier's (1905-1906) that exposed the patent medicine fraud.

Perspectives on the Translational Aspects of Articular Cartilage Biology

6

- Challenges and opportunities
- Immunological concerns
- Business and regulatory aspects
- Statutes and guidelines

In the foregoing chapters, we have discussed articular cartilage morphology (Chapter 1), developmental biology and signaling (Chapter 2), pathology (Chapter 3), tissue engineering (Chapter 4), and methods for examining tissue quality (Chapter 5). With this background, we can now consider the challenges and opportunities in the future of articular cartilage biology and therapies. Notable gaps remain in certain specific areas that need to be addressed in order to make inroads into translational aspects of articular cartilage biology. What directions should new therapies take, and how can they be validated and translated to clinical use?

This chapter begins with key questions in cartilage biology that drive the development of new physical therapy, pharmacological, and surgical treatments, as well as considerations that must go into the design of novel therapeutics. Thus, available and emerging therapies for the treatment of cartilage defects are discussed. Emphasis is placed on emerging cellular therapies, since these are also complicated by immunological concerns. An overview of U.S. Food and Drug Administration (FDA) regulations for these products, as well as regulations for devices and pharmaceuticals, closes this chapter.

6.1 CHALLENGES AND OPPORTUNITIES IN ARTICULAR CARTILAGE BIOLOGY AND REGENERATION

Profound voids still exist in the current body of knowledge in articular cartilage biology, despite the considerable progress that has been made in understanding tissue development and maintenance. For example, how is the articular cartilage differentiation program initiated, and what is the biochemical and molecular basis of the stability of the articular cartilage phenotype? For cellular therapies that utilize stem cells, how does one ensure that these cells have differentiated to a stable chondrocytic phenotype and that these cells can be delivered at sufficient purity? An extension of this question relates to how the articular cartilage phenotype is maintained for decades, whereas growth plate cartilage exhibits a relatively ephemeral life. An understanding of how the different layers of cartilage (surface, middle, and deep zones) assemble after the initial differentiation of articular cartilage has also remained elusive. At present, we do not know if the transcription factors in articular cartilage are also responsible for its durable nature. Information gained on this front will be useful for both disease prevention and tissue regeneration.

A major question that has remained unanswered is how physical signals affect articular cartilage phenotype and function. Alternatively, how can the knowledge gained from the effects of mechanical signals (e.g., compression and tension) be integrated into maintaining the cartilage phenotype? Complicating this issue is that articular cartilage is subject to both biomechanical and biochemical signals, and it is a major challenge to determine how these signals are integrated to maintain a stable cartilage phenotype. That is, how are physical signals integrated with morphogens, growth factors, and transcription factors? It is imperative to determine the relationship between cellular and molecular changes with the functional aspects of articular cartilage, including lubrication and resistance to the joint's strenuous biomechanical environment. Solutions to these questions can be derived using different approaches. For instance, genetic dissection of the pathways of morphogenesis, using genetic animal models, may inform new directions for therapy. Concurrently, small-molecule approaches, enabled by combinatorial chemistry, may not only yield information on how physical and biochemical signals are interrelated, but also identify new pharmacological therapies. Considerable progress in untangling the crosstalk among signals needs to be made in the areas of articular cartilage maintenance and regeneration. Progress on this front not only will be useful for the development of pharmaceuticals, but also will improve existing therapies that have a mechanical component, such as continuous passive motion, physical therapy, exercise, and footwear.

The interaction between the subchondral bone and the overlying articular cartilage in both health and pathology must be better defined. Is communication with the subchondral bone through diffusible signals or mechanotransduction? What are the cellular and mechanical interactions between the subchondral bone and articular cartilage, and how do they affect the stability and maintenance of articular cartilage? How does the stiffness of subchondral bone influence the functional phenotype of articular cartilage? More specifically, is focal stiffening of the subchondral bone an etiology for the development of osteoarthritis? Likewise, a better understanding of the interactions between articular cartilage and the other tissues of the joint is also necessary. One must harness the knowledge in morphogenesis of limb development so that some of these pathways can be used for articular cartilage regeneration. As mentioned in the previous paragraph, can a high-throughput, small-molecule approach be employed to optimize agonists for these developmental pathways? Progress in this area will likely be useful as pharmaceuticals or for the engineering of articular cartilage.

There is a gap in the fundamental processes happening in idiopathic osteoarthritis. While some of those gaps have been addressed by

467

genetic models, key questions remain. For instance, what is the deciding factor for progression to osteoarthritis? That is, what triggers the early initiation of osteoarthritis, and are there any approaches to prevent it? Do predictive biomarkers for osteoarthritis exist, and if so, what are they? Similarly, do biomarkers exist for susceptibility to injuries that are strongly associated with osteoarthritis? Novel technologies in imaging and biophotonics need to be developed to predict impending osteoarthritis. With such information, one can then begin to address questions such as, what are the clinical parameters for identifying early stages of pathology, and at what stage should interventions be initiated? What are the ideal targets for pharmacological agents for inhibiting pathology and initiating regeneration? An ability to discern early osteoarthritis will be a powerful tool for all forms of interventions.

Since osteoarthritis is associated with debilitating pain, the origin of pain must be determined. However, as there are no nerves in articular cartilage, where does pain originate? Pain is the dominant motivation for seeking medical care and is the main factor that diminishes quality of life. However, existing therapies often seek to restore mechanical function independently of pain reduction or vice versa. For instance, total knee replacement restores mechanical function and removes the damaged tissue without necessarily addressing the instigator of pain. Likewise, many treatments under development, especially devices and methods for structural modification, do not specifically target pain reduction as an outcome. Destruction of the articulating surface is devastating, but articular cartilage is only one member in the diseased organ system that is the arthritic joint. Nonisolated pain and inflammation must both be addressed for successful therapies of articular cartilage repair.

The properties of native articular cartilage have long been well characterized in different anatomical locations, at various ages and diseased states, and under various hormonal and drug concentrations to provide design criteria for tissue regeneration. As it has been identified that articular cartilage of different anatomical locations can have different properties (Athanasiou et al. 1991, 1994, 1998; Neu et al. 2007), should strategies that target the complete regeneration of articular cartilage be tailored and fine-tuned to specific anatomical locations? At what point does stiffness mismatch result in ill-borne stresses that can lead to tissue damage? It appears obvious that long-term, fully functional regeneration is desirable, but is this to be achieved immediately or at some amount of time after implantation? If the repair or replacement cartilage is initially softer than the native tissue, can functional improvement nonetheless be achieved? Identification of suitable design criteria is critical toward achieving articular cartilage regeneration.

An understanding of the basic biology of articular cartilage differentiation is a prerequisite for any translational aspirations for cartilage regeneration. At the same time, comprehension of biomechanics is also essential. What, then, should be the direction in training for researchers who will integrate articular cartilage biology and biomechanics into translational research? It is apparent that this is a truly multidisciplinary endeavor, but what new avenue(s) should be followed in education and training for the future leaders in this field? The ideal training platform may be through biomedical engineering, where both basic biology and engineering are combined to understand tissue pathophysiology and regeneration.

6.1.1 Complexities of Integrating New Cartilage with Existing Cartilage

An example of how a lack of understanding of basic cartilage biology hinders therapeutic development is the perennial problem of articular cartilage integration. When using implanted grafts or cells, integration between the implanted articular cartilage, be it native tissue allografts or engineered tissues, and the surrounding tissue is of crucial importance for mechanical function. The interface between new and old tissues is often weak, especially on the surface, and failure can occur by stress concentrations unless sufficient healing takes place that helps to integrate the two tissues. Ideally, implants should match the biomechanical properties of the adjacent native tissue or provide a mechanical gradient through the interface. Implants should also account for the native tissue microstructure and create a replacement that has correct alignment of collagen fibers. The alternative is remodeling of the tissue *in vivo*, which, with articular cartilage's naturally limited repair capacity, has been shown not to occur. Various studies have been performed to examine articular cartilage integration, and these can use a variety of methods to assess the mechanical stability of the interface (Figure 6.1). From these, a general consensus regarding the mechanisms that hinder integration has emerged:

- Cell death at the wound edge, even in surgically prepared defects, results in metabolically inactive tissue with antiadhesive properties that prevent cell adhesion and migration to the injury site (Tew et al. 2000; Hunziker et al. 2001; Bos et al. 2002; Peretti et al. 2003; van de Breevaart Bravenboer et al. 2004).

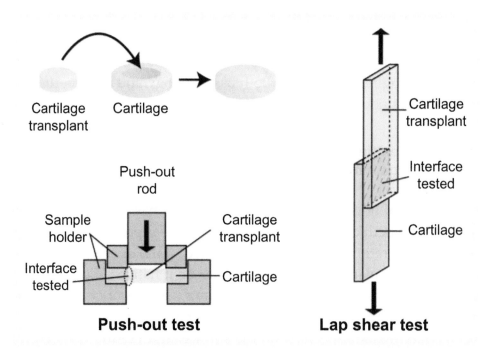

Figure 6.1 Two types of interface testing are shown here. After a piece of cartilage is transplanted into another piece of cartilage, push-out and lap shear tests are two methods to assay the interfacial strength of the integration.

470

- Insufficient numbers of viable cells do not synthesize integrative matrix between the two surfaces to be joined (Reindel et al. 1995; Ahsan and Sah 1999; Tew et al. 2000; Hunziker et al. 2001; Obradovic et al. 2001; Bos et al. 2002).
- Cell migration across metabolically inactive tissue is hindered by dense collagen (Tew et al. 2000; Hunziker et al. 2001; Bos et al. 2002; Peretti et al. 2003; van de Breevaart Bravenboer et al. 2004).
- Cartilage proteoglycans, such as lubricin/proteoglycan 4 (PRG4), can reduce cartilage-to-cartilage integration (Schaefer et al. 2004; Englert et al. 2005).
- Insufficient construct and tissue collagen cross-links do not allow integration (Ahsan et al. 1999; DiMicco et al. 2002; McGowan and Sah 2005).
- Proposed solutions to these obstacles include implanting less mature articular cartilage that contains a large number of metabolically active cells at the construct edge, using enzymes to partially degrade the collagen (Wakitani et al. 1994; Peretti et al. 1999; Yang et al. 2000; Bos et al. 2002; van de Breevaart Bravenboer et al. 2004) and glycosaminoglycans (Hunziker and Rosenberg 1996; Hunziker et al. 2001; Obradovic et al. 2001; Bos et al. 2002; van de Breevaart Bravenboer et al. 2004; Englert et al. 2005; Christensen et al. 2007) of the tissue, and applying agents with the aim of promoting native-to-transplant collagen cross-linking (Arem 1985; Wright et al. 1988; Gerstenfeld et al. 1993; Ahsan et al. 1999; DiMicco et al. 2002; McGowan and Sah 2005).

While these challenges may be daunting, rewards include prolonging or reconstituting articular cartilage function and alleviating the great economic burden related to articular cartilage pathologies. Before these objectives can be accomplished, gaps in our knowledge, examples of which were provided in the previous paragraphs, need to be filled. Structure-function relationships in articular cartilage and how these are influenced by physical and biochemical signals need to be elucidated and used toward developing approaches to restore function or to regenerate the tissue. Indeed, appropriate design criteria need to be developed specific to the different types and stages of pathology encountered. Indications may range from pathology isolated to articular cartilage, such as lesions and tissue softening, to severe osteoarthritis where significant bone remodeling has occurred and the articular surface has been destroyed. Objectives include maintenance or restoration of articular cartilage morphology, phenotype, biochemistry, and biomechanics. Equally important are pain mitigation and inhibition of inflammation or immunological activities (Figure 6.2). Toward developing design criteria and evaluating new therapies, appropriate assessment methodologies need to be standardized and employed.

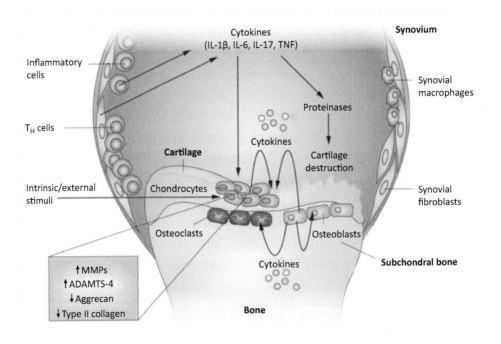

Figure 6.2 Tissue engineering efforts must eventually account for the existing inflammatory processes that are occurring in the pathological joint. Most tissue engineering studies aim to engineer native-like neotissue without considering the neotissue's eventual integration into an inflammatory environment. (From Kapoor, M. et al., *Nat Rev Rheumatol* 7(1): 33-42, 2011. With permission.)

6.1.2 Challenges in Manufacturing Complex Tissue-Engineered Products

In order to address some of the challenges discussed above, such as integration and inflammation, tissue-engineered articular cartilage products in the future may become increasingly more complex. For example, an implant may require the use of multiple cell types or growth factor gradients to promote integration (Figure 6.3). Future implants might

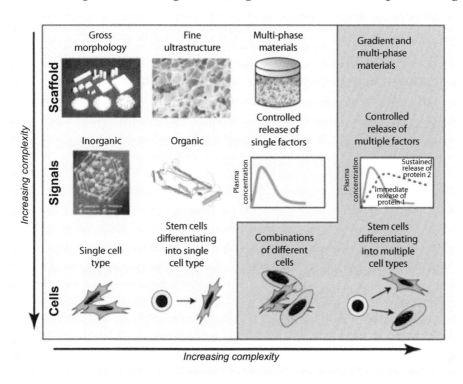

Figure 6.3 The complexity of manufacturing products intended to repair or replace bone and cartilage quickly increases when living cells are introduced as raw materials. Current product categories, illustrated in the blue-shaded area of this figure, consist of scaffolds, signals, and tissues with a single cell type. To address the many challenges discussed in this chapter, such as cartilage integration, products may need to use more than one cell type (e.g., the formation of osteochondral tissues) or manufactured with gradients. Due to their increasing complexity, new product categories (illustrated in the purple-shaded region) may require completely new manufacturing methods. (From Lyles, M. B. et al., in *Regenerative Engineering of Musculoskeletal Tissues and Interfaces*, ed. J. W. F. Syam et al., Cambridge, UK: Woodhead Publishing, 2015, pp. 97-134. With permission.)

contain factors with different release kinetics to target integration on one timescale while defending the implant against inflammation on another timescale. To address large, traumatic defects, implants in the future may consist of not only multiple *cell types*, but also multiple *tissues*. Ways to manufacture products with such complexities have yet to be defined.

One of the new manufacturing methods that may be flexible enough for the processing of the complex, biological products described in Figure 6.3 is additive manufacturing. As defined by the American Society for Testing and Materials (ASTM International 2010), additive manufacturing is "a process of joining materials to make objects from three-dimensional model data, usually layer upon layer, as opposed to subtractive manufacturing methodologies. Synonyms: additive fabrication, additive processes, additive techniques, additive layer manufacturing, layer manufacturing, and freeform fabrication." Examples of additive manufacturing are three-dimensional printing and bioprinting.

Additive manufacturing can potentially address the complexities needed for future cartilage products. Complex internal structures can also be created (Lyles et al. 2015), which may help with engineering articular cartilage with different zones. Multiple materials can be deposited in each layer to generate chemical and mechanical gradients to promote cartilage formation and integration. The same strategy can also result in several tissue types *in vitro* that are finely integrated with each other, such as products that integrate cartilage and bone into one implant. In the future, one can envision the bioprinting of bone, vasculature, and cartilage simultaneously with additive manufacturing (Figure 6.4), as research continues to progress in this area.

In addition to creating more complex implants, additive manufacturing also has the potential to address other important translational issues, such as scaling up. Traditional subtractive manufacturing can be wasteful since it removes and discards raw materials to form the final

474

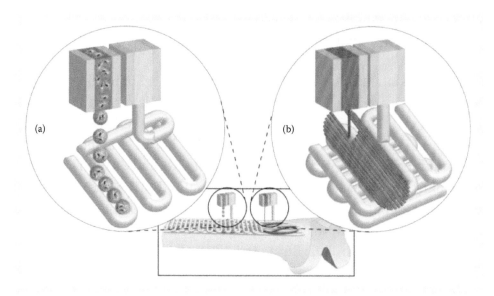

Figure 6.4 Bone, blood vessels, and cartilage can potentially be produced together through additive manufacturing. Cells (a) and blood vessels (b) can be printed in conjunction with scaffold material. (From Lyles, M. B. et al., in *Regenerative Engineering of Musculoskeletal Tissues and Interfaces*, ed. J. W. F. Syam et al., Cambridge, UK: Woodhead Publishing, 2015, pp. 97-134. With permission.)

product. Additive manufacturing can use a lower quantity of raw material (Weber et al. 2013). As related to the production of tissue-engineered cartilage, this manufacturing process can potentially reduce the number of cells required.

Scaling up would require solving challenges such as the automation and standardization of protocols. For example, use of nonsoluble stimuli (e.g., the mechanical stimuli discussed in Chapter 4) on a large scale may be difficult and costly. Quality control and sampling can also be challenging since cell-based articular cartilage products will need to function metabolically and mechanically. To date, it is still unclear what the functional parameters are *in vitro* that will guarantee success *in vivo*. Unintended consequences may arise during scale-up that are as yet undefined. Though not discussed here in detail, scale-up is a common problem for biological products.

6.2 IMMUNE RESPONSE, IMMUNOGENICITY, AND TRANSPLANTS

Being alymphatic and avascular, the tough, extracellular matrix of hyaline articular cartilage prevents easy access to cells embedded within, regardless of the origin of these cells. Cartilage tissue is considered by some to be "immunoprivileged" due to the body's limited ability to detect and reject implanted tissue (Bolano and Kopta 1991). However, cartilage matrix is not itself without rejection issues (Bolano and Kopta 1991; Moskalewski et al. 2002). Collagen types II, IX, and XI and proteoglycan core proteins all have antigenic properties (Yablon et al. 1982; Dayer et al. 1990; Takagi and Jasin 1992; Bujia et al. 1994; Glant et al. 1998). The chondrocytes, too, have been found to contain major histocompatibility complex (MHC) class II antigens, which can elicit a cell-mediated immune response, as described below (Lance 1989; Romaniuk et al. 1995). Natural killer cells can also attack chondrocytes (Malejczyk et al. 1985; Malejczyk 1989; Yamaga et al. 1994). Recently, it was even found that the extent of cartilage immunogenicity is location dependent (Figure 6.5) (Arzi et al. 2015).

Future, clinically applicable treatments for articular cartilage repair or regeneration may encompass treatment of the subchondral bone as well. The basis for the immunoprivileged status of articular cartilage is discussed, and studies involving cartilage or osteochondral transplantation of allogeneic and xenogeneic tissues are presented. These include both cells and tissues transplanted into the joint. To understand the body's reaction, one must first have a basic understanding of the immune rejection process. The sequential steps of rejection are presented, followed by a discussion of immune reactions to articular cartilage grafts.

6.2.1 Humoral and Cellular Responses

The dense, extracellular matrix of cartilage has long been hypothesized to confer immunoprotection to the tissue and its cells. While many studies report qualitative assessments, relatively few

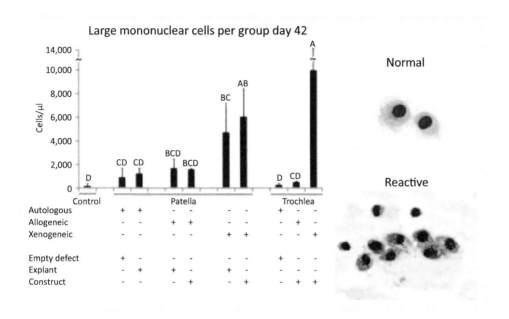

Figure 6.5 Articular cartilage's immunoprivilege is location dependent. As shown here, only the xenogeneic implants elicit immune responses (e.g., as manifested by the presence of large mononuclear cells) at day 42 when the implant is in the trochlea. However, if implanted in the patella, both allogeneic and xenogeneic implants continue to elicit an immune response. Images of normal and reactive large mononuclear cells are shown on the right. (From Arzi, B. et al., *Acta Biomater* 23: 72-81, 2015. With permission.)

studies have quantitatively assayed immune reaction to cartilage implants. To understand the immunological components that may be present in cartilage implants and transplants, it is worthwhile to have a description of the immune system. Thus, this section begins with a brief overview of innate and adaptive immunity. Focus will then be placed on the immune responses during articular cartilage transplantation and repair. The inflammation associated with osteo-arthritis has already been discussed earlier (Chapter 3). It is our goal to introduce the reader to foundations of the immunological basis of tissue rejection, as related to assessment in articular cartilage transplantation strategies.

Allogeneic and xenogeneic cells and matrices can elicit responses from both the innate and adaptive immune systems. Maximal activity of the innate immune system, rapidly reached following the introduction of foreign materials, consists of nonspecific responses by both humoral and cellular components.

The purpose of the innate immune system is to recruit immune cells and promote healing. The complement system is the major component of the humoral response (Figure 6.6). One of the functions of the complement system involves the formation of the membrane attack complex, which causes lysis of foreign cells (e.g., pathogenic bacteria). Complement can also lead to other catabolic cascades. Positive feedback involving protease activity, peptides that recruit immune cells, and increased vascular permeability allow for the destruction of marked, foreign targets.

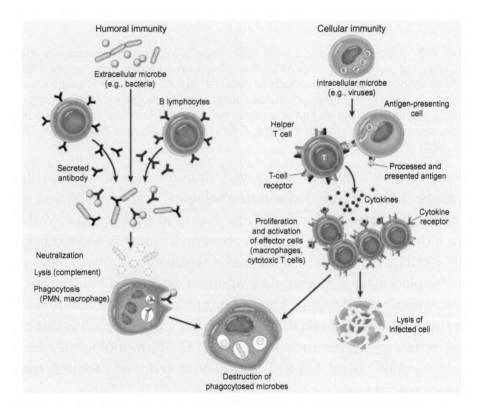

Figure 6.6 Humoral and cellular immunity. (From Kumar, V. et al., *Robbins Basic Pathology*, Philadelphia: Elsevier, Health Sciences Division, 2007. With permission.)

Phagocytic cells that engulf and digest foreign targets include neutrophils, macrophages, and dendritic cells. During the acute phase of immune reactions against implants, the presence, type, and number of these cell types can be quantified, such as through the synovial fluid, in synovial biopsies, and potentially in the implant itself. For a more thorough discussion of the innate immune system, the reader may refer to several publications on this subject (Janeway and Medzhitov 2002; Rus et al. 2005).

Activated by the innate immune system, the adaptive immune system (Figure 6.7) also consists of humoral and cellular components. The humoral response is generally directed against bacteria, though implant rejection can also occur via this response, and is mediated by B lymphocytes. The naïve B cell recognizes the bacteria and presents it to T helper 2 cells. Cytokines then induce B cells to produce antibodies, which can work in several ways to neutralize the antigen. With the antigen defeated, the response is then downregulated, and memory B cells form. Antibodies can inhibit the adhesion of bacteria by surrounding them. Antibodies

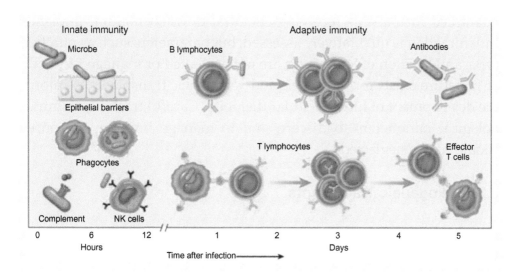

Figure 6.7 The various components of innate and adaptive immunity. (From Kumar, V. et al., *Robbins Basic Pathology*, Philadelphia: Elsevier, Health Sciences Division, 2007. With permission.)

can also promote opsonization. Whereas B lymphocytes mediate the humoral component of the adaptive immune system, the cellular component is mediated by T lymphocytes. First, a sensitization phase occurs whereby an antigen (e.g., a transplant) is recognized by a macrophage and presented to T lymphocytes. Antigen-presenting cells that express appropriate antigenic ligands on their MHC receptors, in addition to required costimulator signals, activate T lymphocytes. Cytokines then initiate the proliferation phase, where cytotoxic T lymphocytes multiply against the antigen. Effector immune responses then proceed to defeat the antigen. Activated T lymphocytes secrete various cytokines (e.g., interleukin 2 [IL-2], interferon γ [IFN-γ], tumor necrosis factor beta [TNF-β]) to recruit a variety of other host immune cells, inducing increased expression of MHC class I and class II molecules by foreign (e.g., donor) cells. Following the destruction of the antigen, the response is downregulated by T suppressor cells, and memory T cells mature for future recurrences (Goldsby et al. 2003; Pietra 2003; Hale 2006; Trivedi 2007).

Both acute and chronic immune responses may be directed toward allogeneic and xenogeneic implants. At present, these responses are seldom quantified for patients receiving chondral or osteochondral implants. Inflammation is qualitatively assessed, but parameters such as number, type, and location of leukocytes are not evaluated or managed. A body of literature exists for allogeneic and xenogeneic transplants to inform the development of future cellular therapies. Careful tracking of immunological parameters to discern and to manage immune responses should not be neglected.

6.2.2 Allogeneic Transplants

As mentioned previously, transplant approaches using autologous chondrocytes and osteochondral plugs are limited by the small amount of available donor tissue. Allogeneic sources provide a larger donor pool. However, the use of allogeneic tissues presents an elevated risk of disease transmission, and testing for diseases such as HIV, hepatitis, and syphilis must first be performed. Immune responses against the cells and tissues also present challenges.

Allogeneic chondrocyte transplantation can be difficult due to the humoral response mounted against these cells (Langer and Gross 1974). Experiments outside of the joint capsule show that allogeneic chondrocytes are not immunoprivileged by themselves. Allogeneic chondrocytes implanted into posterior tibial muscles formed nodules that immediately attracted macrophages, and natural killer and cytotoxic or suppressor T cells were also recruited to destroy the nascent cartilage over time (Romaniuk et al. 1995). This slow destruction of the repair tissue has been shown in several other studies (Kaminski et al. 1980; Ksiazek and Moskalewski 1983; Malejczyk and Moskalewski 1988; Malejczyk et al. 1991). In contrast, cells embedded in matrix were relatively protected. Implantation of chondrocytes alone versus chondrocytes enveloped in matrix has shown that the immune response was greatly diminished in the latter case (Green 1977).

In animal models, when allogeneic chondrocytes were implanted with their extracellular matrices into rat, rabbits, or dogs, neither significant leukocyte migration nor cytotoxic humoral antibodies were observed in several studies (Langer and Gross 1974; Aston and Bentley 1986; Glenn et al. 2006). Another study, however, has shown increased presence of inflammatory mononuclear cells and less repair cartilage for antigen-mismatched transplants in canine articular defects (Stevenson et al. 1989). Due to the potential for immune responses, and due to the lack of availability of fresh cadaveric donor tissue, frozen or pressure-washed osteochondral allografts have been examined. In these cases, the cells are likely dead, reducing the immunogenic response (Elves 1974; Friedlaender 1983), but the grafts are biochemically and histologically inferior to fresh grafts. However, cryopreservation allows for tissues to be banked and greater time in screening the tissues for diseases (Flynn et al. 1994; Bakay et al. 1998).

Allografts have shown considerable success and are often used for defects larger than 2-3 cm². Recent consensus statements indicate that allografts have sufficient evidence for considering their use in lesions greater than 4 cm² (Biant et al. 2015). In long-term follow-ups of up to 15 years of patients receiving fresh osteochondral allografts, allograft survival rates of 75-95% at 5 years, 64-80% at 10 years, and greater than 60% during years 14 and 15 were observed (Beaver et al. 1992; Gross et al. 2005). However, compared to unipolar repairs, clinical trials have demonstrated that allograft implantation is unsuitable for bipolar (replacement of both tibial and femoral condyle in one compartment) lesion repairs, with 50% of grafts surviving after 6 years, compared to 84% in unipolar repairs (Zukor et al. 1989; Chu et al. 1999). Cryopreserved and frozen allografts have yielded good to excellent scores following transplantation in roughly 70% of patients for up to 4 years. It is worth noting that while success has been demonstrated in the treatment of condylar lesions using allografts, the procedure is still considered to be a salvage operation and is currently only suited for young, active patients with isolated patellofemoral articular cartilage disease, for whom previous procedures have failed. Also, a more vigilant effort in identifying the number, type, and location of leukocytes present should be made to observe the time course of immune reactions against the implants. Such studies would determine if allogeneic implants elicit low but chronic immune reactivity and whether this contributes to implant failure.

Live allograft cartilage (De NoVo graft pieces) is currently used as cartilage filler for cartilage defects (Figure 6.8). Alhough not yet available as therapies, emerging technologies employing *in vitro* tissue engineering have shown success when allogeneic cells are combined with scaffolds. Implantation of allogeneic chondrocytes embedded in collagen (Wakitani et al. 1989, 1998; Masuoka et al. 2005), agarose (Rahfoth et al. 1998), and poly-glycolic acid (PGA) (Freed et al. 1994; Schreiber et al. 1999), among other materials, has been examined in various animal models. In general, hyaline histological appearances were found with little to no sign of immunologic reactions. Similarly, the implantation of allogeneic mesenchymal stem cells in a hyaluronic acid-based gel in

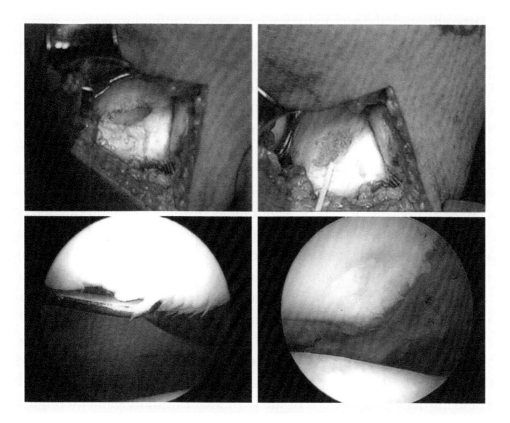

Figure 6.8 Treatment of a patellar chondral defect using juvenile articular cartilage allografts. A second-look arthroscopy at 2 years showed persistent filling of the defect with cartilage. (From Griffin, J. W. et al., *Arthrosc Tech* 2(4): e351-e354, 2013. With permission.)

a goat model has shown only mild immunologic rejection (Butnariu-Ephrat et al. 1996). As seen with the contrast between chondrocytes alone and chondrocytes with associated matrix, *in vitro* seeding and culture of these tissue-engineered constructs allow for the formation of a protective, hyaline-like matrix around the cells prior to implantation.

6.2.3 Xenogeneic Transplants

While allogeneic tissues are more easily procured than autologous tissues, xenogeneic tissues are of even greater abundance. In this case, the source is of a different species, and immunological concerns are heightened. No articular cartilage product using live xenogeneic cells currently exists, although the methodology has been examined in several animal models. Rat chondrocytes implanted in rabbit muscle resulted in the complete destruction of the implant by macrophages and giant foreign body cells (Osiecka-Iwan et al. 2003). However, as articular cartilage is thought to exhibit some immunoprivilege, xeno-implantation into articular defects has been studied, with mixed results. Using fibrin glue as a matrix, rabbit chondrocytes transplanted into the medial femoral condyle of goats resulted in mild synovitis and the formation of fibrous repair tissue (van Susante et al. 1999). Implantation of pig chondrocytes into osteochondral defects of adult rabbits resulted in the production of hyaline-like tissue with the absence of inflammatory cells (Ramallal et al. 2004). The immunogenicity of chondrocytes from transgenic pigs has also been examined *in vitro*. Chondrocytes isolated from H-transferase transgenic pigs have been shown to have lower expression of the Gal alpha(1,3)Gal antigen (alpha-gal) that humans reject (Costa et al. 2002) and, as a result, experience lowered complement deposition and monoblast adhesion (Costa et al. 2008). Knockout animals have been produced that lack α-1, 3-galactosyltransferase and do not produce alpha-gal. These animals can produce tissue with lower immunogenicity (Figure 6.9). Aside from chondrocytes, no immune reaction was found when human mesenchymal stem cells were implanted into a swine model to restore the articular surface (Li et al. 2009). This may be in part because mesenchymal stem cells have been shown to display immune suppressive properties (Ren et al. 2008; Bassi et al. 2011; Kuci et al. 2011; Choi et al. 2012; Han et al. 2012; Yang et al. 2012; Yi et al. 2012).

In addition to cells, xenogeneic tissues have also been examined. In general, the implantation of xenograft tissue results in hyperacute rejection of the implant (Auchincloss 1988; Platt et al. 1990). Typically, joint tissues such as articular cartilage are not subject to hyperacute rejection due to the avascularity of the tissue; thus, cartilage is considered to be relatively nonimmunogenic (Jackson et al. 1992; Revell and Athanasiou 2009). It has been believed that decellularizing xenogeneic tissue will be a viable option for the generation of replacement tissue. Decellularization is a process by which the antigenic intracellular proteins and nucleic acids

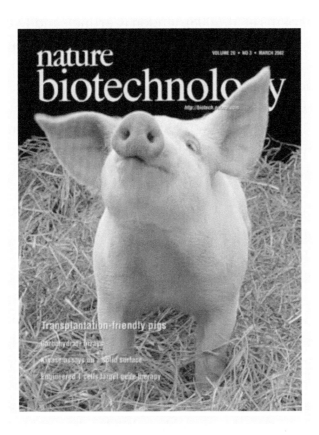

Figure 6.9 Joy is one of five cloned piglets produced with the α-1,3-galactosyl transferase gene knocked out and, therefore, does not produce alpha-gal. (From cover of *Nature Biotechnology*, March 2002, Volume 20, No. 3. Dai, Y. et al., *Nat Biotechnol* 20(3): 251-255, 2002. With permission.)

are removed. It is typically evaluated histologically by the absence of nuclei, and the intent is to preserve the functional properties of the tissue's extracellular matrix. Ideally, the biomechanical properties of the tissue will also be preserved.

Examples of decellularized tissues include an acellular dermal matrix (Chen et al. 2004) that has seen successful use clinically as the FDA-approved Alloderm product or the porcine-derived Strattice product. Experimental investigations into acellular xenogeneic tissues have been conducted for many musculoskeletal applications, including replacements for the knee meniscus (Stapleton et al. 2008), temporomandibular joint disc (Lumpkins et al. 2008), tendon (Cartmell and Dunn 2000), and ACL (Woods and Gratzer 2005). Other tissues, including heart valves (Kasimir et al. 2003; Grauss et al. 2005; Meyer et al. 2005, 2006; Tudorache et al. 2007; Liao et al. 2008; Seebacher et al. 2008), bladder (Rosario et al. 2008), artery (Dahl et al. 2003), and small intestinal submucosa (Hodde and Hiles 2002; Hodde et al. 2007), have also been decellularized. Despite this large body of literature, the absence of cells is not tantamount to the absence of antigens.

The primary assessment method for many decellularization studies is the qualitative or semiquantitative assessment for the presence of cells by histology and nuclear staining. However, it has been shown that (1) residual cells and (2) immunoreactive antigens do not correlate well with the lack of cells (Wong et al. 2011). Decellularization is not tantamount to antigen removal, and residue antigens elicit an immune response. Methods that rupture the cells and degrade the DNA do not necessarily remove the resulting cellular and DNA fragments or debris from the decellularized tissues, especially if the tissues are dense. Nonetheless, short- to mid-term positive effects can be seen with using decellularized tissues. For example, while a photooxidation approach for decellularization of bovine xenografts implanted into sheep femoral condyles reduced monocyte and plasma cell infiltration in the implant after 6 months, the method did not remove DNA or reduce antigens (von Rechenberg et al. 2003). For these implants, however, it is unclear if low-level, chronic immune responses eventually lead to rejection or tissue failure.

Various chemical treatments have been developed for decellularization, such as 1% sodium dodecyl sulfate (SDS), 2% SDS, 2% tributyl phosphate (TnBP), 2% Triton X-100, and hypotonic followed by hypertonic solutions (Cartmell and Dunn 2000; Hodde and Hiles 2002; Kasimir et al. 2003; Grauss et al. 2005; Meyer et al. 2005, 2006; Woods and Gratzer 2005; Hodde et al. 2007; Tudorache et al. 2007; Liao et al. 2008; Lumpkins et al. 2008; Seebacher et al. 2008; Stapleton et al. 2008). Decellularization methods have also been applied to self-assembled tissue-engineered cartilage constructs and cartilage explants (Elder et al. 2009, 2010). All SDS treatments resulted in cell removal histologically, but 2% SDS for 1 hour decreased DNA content by 33%, while maintaining biochemical and biomechanical properties. Additionally, 2% SDS for 8 hours resulted in complete histological decellularization and a 46% reduction in DNA content, although compressive stiffness and glycosaminoglycan content were significantly compromised. There is a dearth of studies demonstrating the effects of tissue decellularization on native as well as engineered articular cartilage constructs. Future work in this area should focus on antigen removal while preserving cartilage biomechanical properties.

Antigen removal should be used as the primary assessment criterion in decellularization processes, and the absence of cell and nuclear materials histologically should serve as an adjunctive but secondary assessment (Figure 6.10). This is because, aside from cell debris that can remain in the tissue after decellularization, the extracellular matrix can also contain antigens that would not appear with nuclear staining,

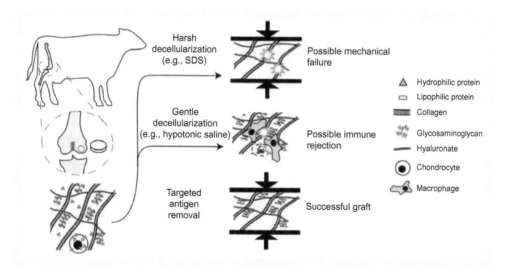

Figure 6.10 For articular cartilage, strategies to remove cells need to balance immunogenicity and mechanical properties because the chemicals used to remove cells can also remove cartilage glycosaminoglycans. Thus, it may be more strategic to remove only the antigens that are responsible for rejection, but no other extracellular component. (From Cissell, D. D. et al., *J Biomech* 47(9): 1987-1996, 2014. With permission.)

a histological technique that is often used as the primary assessment in determining whether a decellularization procedure is successful. An example is alpha-gal, a source of immunogenicity leading to tissue destruction for xenograft implantation in humans and primates (Good et al. 1992; Galili 1993; Sandrin et al. 1993; Collins et al. 1995). Implanted porcine and bovine articular cartilage in cynomolgus monkeys elicited extensive humoral response to the xenografts, leading to chronic graft rejection with fibrous encapsulation and peripheral leukocyte infiltration (Stone et al. 1997). In a follow-up study, implanted porcine or bovine articular cartilage in cynomolgus monkeys resulted in the increase of anti-α-galactosyl IgG by up to 100-fold, accompanied by increased complement-mediated cytotoxicity, indicating a chronic rejection response to the tissue (Galili et al. 1997). Finally, porcine articular cartilage pretreated with α-galactosidase to remove the α-galactosyl epitope resulted in a significant reduction in the inflammatory response to the xenograft and decreased T-lymphocyte infiltration into the tissue in the cynomolgus monkey (Stone et al. 1998). Thus, the α-galactosyl epitope is critical in the immune response to xenogeneic cartilage transplants.

As only humans and primates do not express the α-galactosyl epitope and, therefore, produce anti-α-galactosyl antibodies, α-1,3-galactosyltransferase knockout mice have been developed as a small animal model to study the immune response to this epitope (Tearle et al. 1996). These mice mimic humans and primates in that they do not produce the α-galactosyl epitope, as the α-galactosyl epitope is formed by α-1,3-galactosyltransferase. This model has been used to assess *in vivo* immunogenicity and response to α-galactosyl production of a decellularized vascular graft (Derham et al. 2008) and may be employed to examine xenogeneic cartilage in the future.

6.3 BUSINESS ASPECTS AND REGULATORY AFFAIRS

Depending on the indication, successful articular resurfacing may eventually be achieved using a variety of products and methods. These products might include pharmaceuticals or implants for structural modification, glues and fixatives specifically developed to induce articular cartilage integration, and surgical devices. This brief list represents a few of the potential treatment possibilities that can be marketed. In all cases, safety and efficacy are of paramount importance. The pathway to commercial products is critically dependent on the nature of the product and its intended use. This is an important consideration from a business perspective because some routes take longer and cost more than others. Presented is a brief introduction to the regulatory bodies of the FDA, along with pathways to regulatory approval. Also presented are current and emerging articular cartilage products.

6.3.1 Regulatory Bodies

In the United States, the FDA is charged with protecting the public health by ensuring the safety, efficacy, and security of drugs, biological products, medical devices, radiological products, cosmetics, and domestically produced and imported foods. There are seven product-oriented centers within the FDA to evaluate different classes of products, such as drugs, vaccines, or medical devices. A product that is a combination of more than one class, for example, a medical device that releases drugs, is assigned by the Office of Combination Products to one of the seven centers, where primary jurisdiction over the product will reside. For cartilage therapies, four out of these seven centers are typically involved; these four are described below.

Through the regulation of food, cosmetics, and dietary supplements, the Center for Food Safety and Applied Nutrition (CFSAN) protects the nation's health by ensuring that these products are safe, sanitary, wholesome, and honestly labeled. As described previously, a nonsurgical method that may have potential in relieving joint pain is through dietary supplements, such as chondroitin and glucosamine. These products are specifically labeled as "dietary supplements" because the firms that manufacture or market these products do not claim medical efficacy. Promotional materials are typically vaguely worded with disclaimers that the purported effects have not been evaluated by the FDA. These products are not intended to diagnose, treat, cure, or prevent joint disease and are not drugs. A company that sells glucosamine, chondroitin, and other nutraceuticals (dietary supplements that may exhibit health benefits) may have anecdotal evidence or even peer-reviewed studies linking these products to certain conditions, but may nonetheless lack the rigorous scientific studies required by the FDA to demonstrate significant effects.

As defined by the Federal Food, Drug, and Cosmetic Act, drugs are "articles intended for use in the diagnosis, cure, mitigation, treatment, or prevention of disease" and "articles (other than food) intended to affect the structure or any function of the body." The primary action of drugs is via receptor interactions and chemical pathways. The Center for Drug Evaluation and Research (CDER) ensures that the nation's drugs are safe and effective. This includes over-the-counter, prescription, biological therapeutics, and generic drugs, as well as fluoride toothpaste, antiperspirants, and sunscreens. CDER's Division of Manufacturing and Product Quality ensures that drug manufacturers follow current good manufacturing practices (cGMP), as described by 21 Code of Federal Regulations (CFR) Parts 210 and 211 (FDA 2011a,b). Adverse events are monitored by the Adverse Event Reporting System (AERS), a computerized information database designed to support the FDA's postmarketing safety surveillance program for all approved drug and therapeutic biologic products. For example, analgesics and cyclooxygenase 2 (COX2) inhibitors, useful in relieving joint pain, are regulated by the CDER, as are other structure-modifying pharmaceuticals.

Biological products, such as blood, vaccines, allergenics, tissues, and cellular and gene therapies, are derived from living sources, such as humans, animals, and microorganisms, and are regulated by the Center for Biologics Evaluation and Research (CBER). Similar to drugs, manufacturers of biological products must follow cGMP, as described by 21 CFR 211 (FDA 2011a) and report adverse events to AERS. Considering the tissue engineering methods described in Chapter 4, many potential products can be classified under this category. All autologous, allogeneic, and xenogeneic products are produced by cells and can potentially be regulated by CBER, with some depending on the amount of manipulation that has gone into making the product. For example, autologous chondrocyte implantation (ACI), a procedure that requires external manipulation of the autologous cells that produce tissue *in situ*, is regulated by CBER.

Firms that manufacture, repackage, relabel, or import medical devices sold in the United States are subject to regulation by the Center for Devices and Radiological Health (CDRH). CDRH also regulates radiation-emitting electronic products, including x-ray systems, ultrasound equipment, microwave ovens, and color televisions. A medical device is "an instrument, apparatus, implement, machine, contrivance, implant, *in vitro* reagent, or other similar or related article, including any component, part, or accessory, which is intended for use in the diagnosis of disease or other conditions, or in the cure, mitigation, treatment, or prevention of disease." Implants may be regulated by CDRH even if they contain biologics (e.g., cells) or drugs, depending on the assignment by the Office of Combination Products. The primary mode of effect for devices is mechanical or electrical. Implants whose primary function is to bear mechanical load (e.g., engineered tissues) may have CDRH as their primary regulator. Devices regulated within the CDRH fall into three classes, each with different requirements that the manufacturer must fulfill prior to introducing a product to market. Since CDRH has been assigned jurisdiction over most orthopedic implants, and since CBER regulates cellular products (e.g., tissue engineered products containing cells), pathways to market through these centers will be described in the next section.

6.3.2 Pathways to Market

A medical product intended to promote public health must be both safe and effective. Scientific studies conducted to demonstrate both of these criteria cost time and money. A shorter time to market can potentially result in the earlier realization of benefits to public health, but possibly also a lack of adequate data to ensure safety. On the other hand, excessive burdens in testing can deplete a company's resources and stifle product innovation. In the United States, the FDA balances these concerns and has issued policies and guidelines on demonstrating safety and efficacy.

In Europe, a CE mark is needed to verify that a device meets all regulatory requirements of the Medical Devices Directive (MDD), In Vitro Diagnostic Device Directive (IVDD), or Active Implantable Medical Device Directive (AIMD). Currently, more preclinical and clinical data are often required by the FDA for approval. As a result, this book will focus mainly on the FDA's product approval process.

Through its centers and offices, the FDA performs a balancing act between expediency and assurance of public welfare. To ease the regulatory burden of industry, FDA has established intercenter agreements, for example, between the CBER and the CDRH, and between the CDER and the CDRH. Also, to ensure that adequate effort is expended in evaluating a device, the FDA Modernization Act of 1997 established three classes of devices, each requiring different degrees of rigor in demonstrating efficacy (of course, all devices must be safe). Firms interested in obtaining approval for a device can also meet with the Office of Device Evaluation to determine and facilitate an optimal method that is also the "least burdensome" in demonstrating that a device is effective, through the selection of appropriate pathways for the application.

As discussed in Chapter 5, various animal models are used to assess the safety and efficacy of new drugs and therapies, and these data can be used toward the approval of an investigational new drug (IND) application. With the IND, human clinical trials can begin. Phase I trials screen for safety, Phase II establishes the testing protocol, Phase III assesses both safety and efficacy, and Phase IV consists of postmarket studies (Figure 6.11). Data from Phases I, II, and III, as well as the preclinical data, are submitted to the FDA as a new drug application (NDA). Evaluation of the NDA includes (1) the safety and efficacy for the proposed indications and the drug's risk-to-benefit ratio, (2) whether the drug is appropriately labeled and what it should contain, and (3) whether the drug's production method includes proper controls for the drug's identity, strength, quality, and purity.

A biologics license application (BLA) must be filed for permission to introduce a biologic product into the market. BLA is regulated under

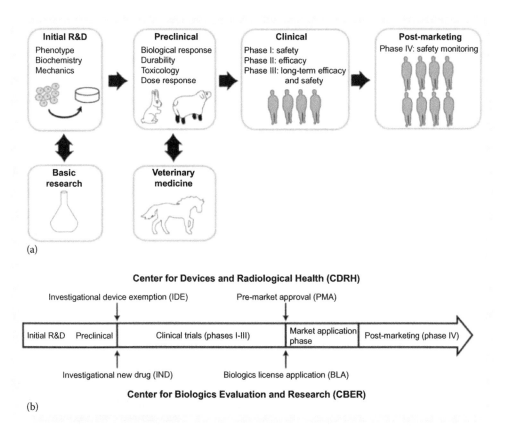

Figure 6.11 The translation of tissue-engineered products is illustrated here using stem cells as an example cell type. (a) Purity, reproducibility, and stability are required by the FDA for stem cell products. Preclinical trials in animals yield data for biological response, durability, toxicology, and dose response. Clinical studies, which evaluate dosage, efficacy, and safety, consist of multiple phases that gradually involve more subjects. (b) For a product intended to replace or repair articular cartilage, two of the most relevant regulatory centers are CDRH (for devices) and CBER (for drugs and biologics). An IND application or IDE application is required before initiating a clinical trial. Market approval allows claims of safety and efficacy to be made. (From Lee, J. K. et al., *Crit Rev Biotechnol* 34(1): 89-100, 2014. With permission.)

21 CFR 600-680. Applicants for a license must comply with requirements set forth by Form 356h, which includes applicant information, product and manufacturing information, preclinical studies, clinical studies, and labeling. Of substantial burden are clinical studies, which can be slow and costly. For implants, the FDA has had a history of classifying most orthopedic implants as medical devices, which are regulated by CDRH. In the case of ACI, the resulting implant is expected to generate

tissue through a cell slurry, which cannot withstand loading immediately as an implant would. Marketing for ACI requires a BLA.

Approval by the CDRH depends on the device's class (Figure 6.12). Class I devices are low risk and pose minimal potential harm. The key regulatory compliance for a Class I device is that a company must demonstrate that it has implemented "general controls." General controls include quality system regulation, as described by 21 CFR 820 (FDA 2011d), to ensure adherence to predefined design controls and cGMP; label requirements to prevent product mislabeling; and the use of Medical Device Reporting (MDR), as the mechanism to maintain records for the reporting of adverse events identified by the user, manufacturer, or distributer of the device. Handheld instruments, elastic bandages, exam gloves, and enema kits are examples of Class I devices. As part of the pathway to market, medical devices must use forms FDA-2891 and FDA-2892 for establishment, registration, and medical device listing.

Class I	Class II	Class III
Protractor for clinical use	Goniometer that uses electrode lead wires and patient cables	Intervertebral body fusion devices that include any therapeutic biologic
Cast removal instrument	Intervertebral body fusion devices with bone grafting material	Knee joint femorotibial metallic constrained cemented prosthesis
Goniometer that does not use electrode lead wires	Knee joint femorotibial metal/polymer constrained cemented prosthesis	Hip joint metal/metal semi-constrained, with a cemented acetabular component, prosthesis
Bandages		
Examination gloves	Hip joint metal/composite semi-constrained cemented prosthesis	
Low risk	Medium risk	High risk

Figure 6.12   Examples of devices in each class.

494

Aside from the requirements listed above for Class I devices, Class II devices, which are of moderate risk, often require a premarket notification 510(k) pathway to market. Prior to proposing to market a device, the manufacturer must notify the FDA 90 days in advance that the device is *substantially equivalent* to a predicate device legally in commercial distribution in the United States before May 28, 1976. Substantially equivalent devices will be labeled as a Class I or II device. Applying for a 510(k) starts with the determination of an appropriate product code for the device and locating a predicate device. The FDA provides guidance documents that a company can review, and either a traditional, special, or abbreviated 510(k) may be filed. A traditional 510(k) takes about 90 days to review. A special 510(k) can be filed when a device is modified. No changes to the intended use of the device can be made, and the manufacturer must declare conformance to design controls. Review for a special 510(k) is faster, generally 30 days. An abbreviated 510(k) also has a reduced review time, but not necessarily down to 30 days. It relies on use of guidance documents or special controls to provide a summary report that describes adherence to the relevant guidance document. After a Class II device goes to market, it may require special controls, such as postmarket surveillance, patient registries, guidances, and standards. Most joint arthroplasty components are approved as Class II devices, as well as other implanted materials, such as pedicle screws and intramedullary nails.

Class III devices support or sustain human life, are of substantial importance in preventing impairment of human health, or present a potential, unreasonable risk of illness or injury. Devices for which substantially equivalent predicates are nonexistent are also classified as Class III devices. If a new device is deemed to be substantially equivalent to a predicate Class III device, then it, too, will be a Class III device. Lastly, if a new device is determined to be substantially equivalent to a Class I or II device that was developed after 1976, it also automatically falls into Class III. A company may petition to have a new device reclassified as Class I or Class II. For a Class III device, a company must submit a premarket approval application (PMA) or product development protocol (PDP) before legal distribution can occur. The PMA process will include both preclinical and clinical data to demonstrate safety and efficacy. To collect clinical data, a new device must first have an investigational device exemption (IDE) before it can be used in humans; see 21 CFR 812 (FDA 2011c). If the device has significant risk, the FDA and institutional review board (IRB) must approve the study before initiation. If the device is of nonsignificant risk, only the IRB needs to approve it.

Due to the combinatorial nature of many tissue repair products, the Office of Combination Products may assign primary jurisdiction to the CDRH if a product's primary mode of effect is not metabolic. For example, Medtronic's InFuse Bone Graft/LT-Cage, consisting of a collagen scaffold with recombinant human bone morphogenetic protein (rhBMP) enclosed within a metallic lumbar fusion device, is regulated as a medical device. In this case, the rhBMP is a recombinant product in combination with a device that provides mechanical support. Similarly, biologic products such as bone void fillers and demineralized bone matrix are classified as Class II devices by the FDA, while BMPs are classified as Class III devices. The FDA has released guidelines for the application of an IND or IDE for products intended to repair or replace knee cartilage. Depending on the nature of a tissue-engineered product, whether it will be assigned to CBER or CDRH is something researchers and companies should consider as they develop the product, because the pathways to market are substantially different for each center.

Additional pathways to market include the humanitarian device exemption (HDE) and the PDP for Class III devices. HDE devices cannot have a profit margin, as this pathway is intended for the development of devices to treat rare (<4,000 patients per year) conditions. To speed the time to approval, regulatory burdens on the manufacturer are lessened for HDE devices; these devices do not have to demonstrate efficacy in large sample sizes since patients may be rare. HDE devices need to be approved by the IRB where they are used, and surgeons must be aware of the dearth of efficacy data for these devices. A PDP is an alternative to the PMA. To pursue this pathway, a company would work with the FDA in designing preclinical and clinical studies, protocols, assessment methods, and acceptance criteria. Few products have been approved through this pathway, though it may be speedier than a PMA, since the FDA would be involved from the initial development of the product all the way to market.

6.4 U.S. STATUTES AND GUIDELINES

The U.S. Federal Food, Drug, and Cosmetic Act of 1938 gives the FDA the authority for regulation and provides definitions for drugs and device classes. Amendments and additional statutes made over the years provide additional regulatory clarifications. It is prudent to engage in a dialogue with the FDA prior to initiating preclinical animal studies, due to their prohibitive costs and time commitment. Pre-IND/IDE and even pre-pre-IND/IDE meetings can be arranged to provide direction for animal studies and to receive updates on the type of data that would be sufficient to demonstrate safety and efficacy. Scientific advancements can necessitate changes in policies, and novel technologies can spur therapeutics that are without precedence and, thus, without clear regulatory pathways. Communications to keep current on the FDA's policies should be based on the published statutes and guidelines, many of which are available for existing and emerging articular cartilage therapies, and some of which are discussed below.

The governing statute for biologic products, Section 351 of 42 USC § 262, defines the requirements for introducing biologics to the market, via a BLA and with proper labeling. Similarly, Sections 501-528 (Chapter V) of 21 USC §§ 351-360dd constitute the governing statute for drugs and devices. Additionally, human cells, tissues, and cell- and tissue-based products (HCT/Ps) are regulated by 21 CFR 1271, biologics are regulated by 21 CFR 600-680, drugs for human use are regulated by 21 CFR 300-460, and devices are regulated by 21 CFR 800-898. Cellular therapies for articular cartilage can serve as an example of how these regulations are applied.

Cellular therapies, where the cell source is from humans, may qualify for regulation as an HCT/P, which is defined as "articles containing or consisting of human cells or tissues that are intended for implantation, transplantation, infusion, or transfer into a human recipient." Regulations include 21 CFR 1271, although not all human-derived materials are regulated under 21 CFR 1271. For instance, "minimally manipulated bone marrow for homologous use and not combined with another article" is not considered an HCT/P. HCT/Ps are regulated solely by 21 CFR 1271 if they are (1) minimally manipulated, (2) for homologous use, (3) not combined with another article (with certain exceptions), and (4) either (i) do not have a systemic effect and are not dependent on metabolic activity of living cells for their primary function or (ii) have a systemic effect or are dependent on metabolic activity for their primary function and for autologous, allogeneic, or reproductive use. Otherwise, additional regulations apply.

Products derived from stem cells will likely be regulated as HCT/Ps because *in vitro* expansion and differentiation would not qualify the cells as "minimally manipulated." In such cases, products must conform to 21 CFR 1271 and other applicable regulations (e.g., 21 CFR 600-680 for biologics, 21 CFR 800-898 for devices, or both 21 CFR 600-680 and 21 CFR 800-898 for a biological device). Additionally, stem cells may not qualify for homologous use, in which case the source and destination tissues and functions will remain the same. Companies seeking to develop new products should consult the FDA since each product differs from the other. Determination of whether the product will be a device, biological, or combination product will be provided by the FDA. Each product can be its own unique case. If the product is a device, one must then determine the classification of a device (Figure 6.13). For biologics, one must determine, for example, if the cells used will be for homologous use. Since marrow mesenchymal stem cells are responsible for the formation of fibrocartilage in humans, should their use in cartilage repair be considered homologous use, or is homologous use restricted to marrow transplants? Scientific progress will necessitate further clarification and changes to these regulations.

To provide clarity and to assist companies in developing new therapies, the FDA has published guidance documents. Those relevant to articular cartilage regeneration include guidance documents for the preparation

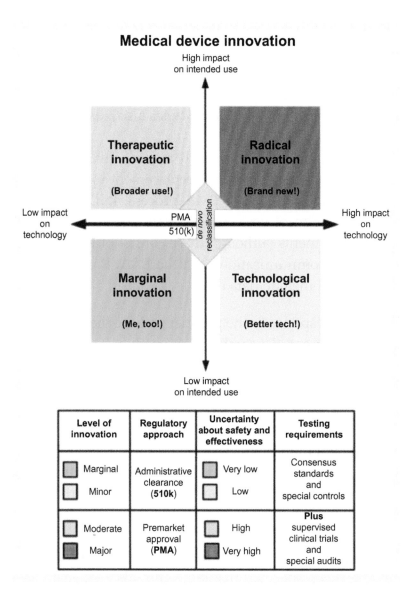

Figure 6.13 Guide for determining in which class a new product for cartilage injuries might be. (From http://www.samaras-assoc.com/regulatory.htm. With permission.)

of IDEs and INDs for products intended to repair or replace knee cartilage (CBER and CDRH 2011); for products comprised of living autologous cells manipulated *ex vivo* and intended for structural repair or reconstruction (CBER 1996); for human somatic cell therapy and gene therapy (CBER 1998); on the chemistry, manufacturing, and control information

499

for human somatic cell therapy INDs (Office of Cellular, Tissue, and Gene Therapies 2008); on the chemistry, manufacturing, and control information for human gene therapy INDs (CBER 2008); and for choice of control group and related issues in clinical trials (CDER and CBER 2001). Other guidance documents for other product types also exist.

It is worth noting that the FDA typically regards investigational devices for knee articular cartilage repair or replacement to be significant risk devices, therefore, requiring the PMA process. IND and IDE applications for the initiation of new clinical trials can be filed by following the guidance documents (although these consist of nonbinding recommendations) and communication with the FDA. Preparation for these applications would include data on

- Biological response to the product and the biological activity of each component of a combination product
- Durability (length of time needed to assess repair of the cartilage lesion, the ability of the product to resist wear and degradation and to withstand physiologically relevant loads over time, etc.)
- Toxicology (potential for local and systemic toxicities due to a component of the product)
- Dose response (e.g., material constituents, cell number, and other characteristics that may affect lesion repair) (CBER and CDRH 2011)

Animal models are recommended for the collection of these preclinical data, and it has been specified that large animals (e.g., goats, sheep, and horses) should be used to assess durability and dose response. Biological responses and toxicology may be related to the chemicals and other materials used to manufacture the cartilage product, as well as the components that will be implanted. Lesion size and location should be scaled and placed to correspond to clinical indications, and study endpoints should mimic clinical endpoints. Arthroscopic and MRI evaluations are encouraged to reduce the number of animals used, but notably, the collection of mechanical data has been specified. Among the models described in Chapter 5, those that yield the aggregate modulus, permeability, and shear modulus should be employed. Also quantified should be the complex shear modulus, as well as indices of strength. Approval of the IND or IDE would allow for clinical studies that are regulated under 21 CFR 812, 21 CFR 312, 21 CFR 50, or 21 CFR 56. Some of the products currently in clinical trials are provided at the end of this chapter.

6.4.1 Currently Available Cartilage Resurfacing Products

Articular cartilage tissue-engineered products are currently not widely available in the United States. Several products undergoing investigation in clinical trials in Europe and in the United States can serve as models to inform those seeking to develop and to market tissue-engineered articular cartilage. Regulatory processes in Europe are different from those of the FDA and are reviewed elsewhere (Brevignon-Dodin and Livesey 2006; Trommelmans et al. 2007). Approval in Europe is granted through the CE mark designation. Engineered cartilage employing allogeneic cells may find commonalities with tissue allografts. For lesions greater than 2 cm^2, Regeneration Technologies has fresh-stored osteochondral allografts that are cleaned, processed, and preserved with maintained chondrocyte viability. A proprietary antibiotic soak and 14 days of culture monitoring, with 28 days of fungal culture monitoring, prepares the allografts for implantation (McCulloch et al. 2007).

Several examples of cartilage treatments using only a biomaterial are available as products to augment marrow stimulation, and Figure 6.14 illustrates many of the strategies that current repair products employ. Trufit (Smith & Nephew) is the first product based on biodegradable polymers introduced to treat focal lesions. Other products in use include Gelrin by Regentis Biomaterials, a fibrin-polyethylene glycol hydrogel that can be cross-linked *in situ* for cartilage defects. BioPoly RS, a subsidiary of Schwartz Biomedical, developed the BioPoly RS (ReSurfacing) device, which is a hydrophilic polymer. SaluMedica has SaluCartilage, which is a hydrogel that can be used for cartilage damage with CE mark approval

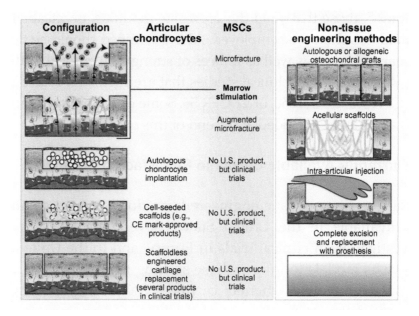

Figure 6.14 Illustrations of cartilage repair or replacement strategies that are currently in use or are on the horizon. (Modified from Huey, D. J. et al., *Science* 338(6109): 917-921, 2012. With permission.)

in Europe but not FDA approval. BST-CarGel, by BioSyntech, is another product with CE mark approval and is used for focal cartilage lesions.

Cell-seeded scaffolds have also been approved for use in Europe. CaReS (Cartilage Regeneration System) by Arthro Kinetics, uses articular chondrocytes for transplantation. Arthro Kinetics also developed CartiPlug, which is an acellular collagen matrix for the same indication, and is currently developing CaReS Plus, which would contain cells for larger cartilage defects. BioTissue Technologies has BioSeed-C, an autologous three-dimensional chondrocyte graft. CellGenix markets CartiGro, which combines autologous chondrocytes with Chondro-Gide collagen membrane (from Geistlick Biomaterials) and is distributed in Europe by Stryker EMEA. Fidia developed Hyalograft C, which uses Hyaff, a hyaluronic acid derivative, and autologous chondrocytes. It is worth noting that the only cell-based product available in the United States does not employ a scaffold, although many products are currently in clinical trials. Genzyme Biosurgery's Carticel consists of the deliverance of a slurry of expanded autologous chondrocytes. Japan Tissue Engineering has an autologous cell transplantation method similar to that of Genzyme.

6.4.2 Emerging Cartilage Products

In addition to the scaffolds currently on the market, many others are in clinical trials, as listed in Table 6.1, along with the countries where the trials are held. Typical among these is the scaffold's use in combination with marrow stimulation, during one single surgical procedure. Scaffolds are made from a variety of natural and synthetic materials in the form of gels, meshes, and osteochondral implants. Please note that not all of the products listed in Table 6.1 are from the United States. Thus, not all of these products conform to U.S. regulations.

6.4.3 Emerging Cellular Therapies

As indicated in Section 6.4.1, there is only one FDA-approved, cell-based articular cartilage repair product available in the United States, Genzyme's Carticel. However, numerous cell-based products are currently in various stages of development. Both chondrocytes and mesenchymal stem cells, manipulated *in vitro*, are used for many cellular therapies in clinical trials (Table 6.2), although, in general, autologous chondrocytes predominate in the approach. Autologous articular cartilage, sometimes removed arthroscopically, yields chondrocytes that are expanded and seeded into a variety of scaffolds for subsequent implantation. Exceptions to this are CellCoTec's Instruct product, which uses both chondrocytes and mesenchymal stem cells; co.DonAG's Chondrosphere, which consists of chondrocyte micromasses; and ISTO/Zimmer's De NoVo ET, which, as an evolution of the De NoVo NT product, consists of allogeneic juvenile cartilage pieces mixed with allogeneic cells.

When the first edition of this book was published in 2012, the therapies listed in Table 6.2 did not include osteochondral products. This remains the case in 2016. While both product types have overlapping indications, articular cartilage resurfacing or regeneration products intended

Table 6.1 Examples of articular cartilage repair products from around the world that do not include cells as part of the product, as of July 2015

Company (product)	Country	Scaffold material	Status
Piramal (CarGel)	Germany	Chitosan Gel	Completed; follow-up by invitation
Kensey Nash (Cartilage Repair Device)	United States	Biphasic collagen and TCP	Terminated (slow enrollment rate)
Geistlich (ChondroGide AMIC)	Switzerland	Biphasic collagen I/III porous and nonporous sides	CE marked; ongoing for Phases II and III but not recruiting
Biomet (Chondux)	United States	PEG/HA photopolymerized	Terminated (enrollment suspended; follow-up continues)
Regentis (GelrinC)	Israel	Polyethylene glycol diacrylate and denatured fibrinogen	Active; not recruiting for Phases I and II
Anika (Hyalofast)	United States	Hydroxyapatite (Hyaff)	CE marked; IDE filed with FDA
Fin-Ceramica (MaioRegen)	Italy	Triphasic collagen, two layers of collagen with magnesium-enriched hydroxyapatite	Phase IV active; not recruiting

(Continued)

Table 6.1 (Continued) Examples of articular cartilage repair products from around the world that do not include cells as part of the product, as of July 2015

Company (product)	Country	Scaffold material	Status
Smith and Nephew (Trufit)	United States	Blend of poly-DL-lactide-co-glycolide, polyglycolide fibers, and calcium sulfate	Completed a Phase IV study
Biomet (Osseofit)	United States	"Osteoconductive scaffold"	Withdrawn prior to enrollment
Cartiheal (Agili-C)	Europe	Aragonite bone phase and aragonite/hyaluronic acid cartilage phase	Phase IV currently recruiting
TRB Chemedica (HYTOP)	Germany	Cartilage phase of purified porcine splint skin and bone phase of collagen fleece/hyaluronan	Study for safety and efficacy of device currently recruiting

Source: http://clinicaltrials.gov/.

Note: This table contains products currently examined in clinical studies, as well as status updates for products that were listed in the first edition of this book. HA, hyaluronic acid; PEG, poly-ethylene glycol; PLGA, poly-lactic-co-glycolic acid; TCP, tricalcium phosphate.

for defects with existing inflammation or osteoarthritis are not available. Nonetheless, progress toward this is being made, for example, in a clinical trial that seeks to determine the immunomodulatory effects of stem cells on osteoarthritis (ClinicalTrials.gov ID NCT01879046). Also, two new products being examined for cartilage repair, listed in Table 6.2, use umbilical cord blood-derived cells, which have also shown immunomodulatory effects *in vitro* (Wang et al. 2009; Shawki et al. 2015).

Table 6.2 Examples of articular cartilage repair products from the United States and around the world with studies that use cells, as of July 2015

Company (product)	Country	Cell source	Scaffold material	Status
CellCoTec (Instruct)	Netherlands	Autologous chondrocytes and mesenchymal stem cells	PEGT/PBT	Completed prospective feasibility study for device
Geistlich (ChondroGide)	Switzerland	Autologous chondrocytes	Biphasic collagen I/III porous and nonporous sides	CE marked; ongoing for Phases II and III but not recruiting
Anika (Hyalograft C)	United States	Autologous chondrocytes	Hydroxyapatite (Hyaff)	Withdrawn from European market
Histogenics (NeoCart)	United States	Autologous chondrocytes	Collagen matrix	Phase II completed; Phase III currently recruiting
co.DonAG (Chondrosphere)	Germany	Autologous chondrocytes	NA	Phases II and III ongoing but not recruiting
TBF Tissue Engineering (Cartipatch)	France	Autologous chondrocytes	Agarose/ alginate gel	One Phase III study completed (2014), but another was terminated in 2015 (manufacturing stopped)
Genzyme (MACI)	United States	Autologous chondrocytes	Biphasic collagen I/III porous and nonporous sides	Phase III completed

(Continued)

506

Table 6.2 (Continued) Examples of articular cartilage repair products from the United States and around the world with studies that use cells, as of July 2015

Company (product)	Country	Cell source	Scaffold material	Status
TeTec (Novocart 3D)	Germany	Autologous chondrocytes	Collagen I and chondroitin sulfate (with protective top membrane)	Phase III ongoing; currently recruiting
ISTO/Zimmer (De NoVo ET)	United States	Allogeneic chondrocytes	NA	Ongoing Phase III trial that is not recruiting
ISTO/Zimmer (De NoVo NT)	United States	Minced cartilage	Juvenile cartilage	Completed; new trial for long-term data is currently recruiting
Medipost (CARTISTEM)	Korea	Allogeneic umbilical cord blood-derived mesenchymal stem cells	NA	Phase III completed; long-term follow-up ongoing but not recruiting
ShenzhenHornetcorn Bio-technology	China	Umbilical cord mesenchymal stem cell transplantation	NA	Phase I currently recruiting

Source: http://clinicaltrials.gov/.

Note: This table contains products currently examined in clinical studies, as well as status updates for products that were listed in the first edition of this book. NA, not applicable; PBT, poly(butylene terephthalate); PEGT, poly(ethylene glycol) terephthalate.

Receiving FDA approval does not mean that the product or service will automatically be approved for reimbursement by various private and public insurers. Since many articular cartilage therapies will be targeted toward the elderly, it is relevant to understand how Medicare approves reimbursement. The Centers for Medicare & Medicaid Services (CMS) makes a decision based on whether a treatment is "reasonable and necessary." While criteria for reasonableness and necessity are open to interpretation, it is clear that the FDA's mandate of "safe and effective" is not sufficient in warranting reimbursement. Criteria for reimbursement by private insurers differ from company to company and add to the complexity of developing business plans for future therapies for articular cartilage repair and regeneration.

6.5 CHAPTER CONCEPTS

- Significant gaps remain in the understanding of basic articular cartilage biology.
- Elucidation of the biochemical and molecular basis of the stability of the articular cartilage phenotype will contribute to both disease prevention and tissue regeneration.
- How mechanical signals are integrated into the chondrocyte phenotype is still unclear.
- Future studies in articular cartilage biology should investigate how the subchondral bone influences the cartilage phenotype.
- The origins of cartilage-associated pain require further investigation.
- Design standards must be identified for tissue-engineered articular cartilage.
- The future of articular cartilage repair and regeneration depends on properly trained scientific personnel. Biomedical engineering may provide a suitable training platform.
- Integration of the engineered cartilage can be a significant hurdle due to the inherent nonadhesive nature of the tissue, the lack of viable cells at the wound edge, and the dense collagen matrix.
- Allogeneic cartilage transplants have been applied with substantial clinical success, and immune reactions are often mild or absent.
- The use of xenografts is predicated not only on decellularization, but also, more importantly, on antigen removal.
- Graft processing should preserve the biomechanical nature of the implant.

- The FDA regulates food, drug, and medical device safety through several centers and offices. As compliance requirements differ with each center, it is important for a company seeking to develop articular cartilage products to consider which regulatory pathway will apply.
- Most orthopedic implants have been classified as devices. Pathways to market for devices include filing for 510(k), PMA, PDP, or HDE applications.
- While several cell and biologic products are available for cartilage resurfacing in Europe, few have been approved in the United States.
- Tissue-engineered articular cartilage products may be regulated by both CBER and CDRH as combination products.

REFERENCES

Ahsan, T., L. M. Lottman et al. (1999). Integrative cartilage repair: Inhibition by beta-aminopropionitrile. *J Orthop Res* 17(6): 850-857.

Ahsan, T., and R. L. Sah. (1999). Biomechanics of integrative cartilage repair. *Osteoarthr Cartil* 7(1): 29-40.

Arem, A. (1985). Collagen modifications. *Clin Plast Surg* 12(2): 209-220.

Arzi, B., G. D. DuRaine et al. (2015). Cartilage immunoprivilege depends on donor source and lesion location. *Acta Biomater* 23: 72-81.

ASTM International. (2010). Standard terminology for additive manufacturing—Coordinate systems and test methodologies. ASTM F29211-11.

Aston, J. E., and G. Bentley. (1986). Repair of articular surfaces by allografts of articular and growth-plate cartilage. *J Bone Joint Surg Br* 68(1): 29-35.

Athanasiou, K. A., A. Agarwal et al. (1994). Comparative study of the intrinsic mechanical properties of the human acetabular and femoral head cartilage. *J Orthop Res* 12(3): 340-349.

Athanasiou, K. A., G. T. Liu et al. (1998). Biomechanical topography of human articular cartilage in the first metatarsophalangeal joint. *Clin Orthop Relat Res* 348: 269-281.

Athanasiou, K. A., M. P. Rosenwasser et al. (1991). Interspecies comparisons of in situ intrinsic mechanical properties of distal femoral cartilage. *J Orthop Res* 9(3): 330-340.

Auchincloss, H., Jr. (1988). Xenogeneic transplantation. A review. *Transplantation* 46(1): 1-20.

Bakay, A., L. Csonge et al. (1998). Osteochondral resurfacing of the knee joint with allograft. Clinical analysis of 33 cases. *Int Orthop* 22(5): 277-281.

Bassi, E. J., D. C. de Almeida et al. (2011). Exploring the role of soluble factors associated with immune regulatory properties of mesenchymal stem cells. *Stem Cell Rev* 8(2): 329-342.

Beaver, R. J., M. Mahomed et al. (1992). Fresh osteochondral allografts for post-traumatic defects in the knee. A survivorship analysis. *J Bone Joint Surg Br* 74(1): 105-110.

Biant, L. C., M. J. McNicholas et al. (2015). The surgical management of symptomatic articular cartilage defects of the knee: Consensus statements from United Kingdom knee surgeons. *Knee* 22(5): 446-449.

Bolano, L., and J. A. Kopta. (1991). The immunology of bone and cartilage transplantation. *Orthopedics* 14(9): 987-996.

Bos, P. K., J. DeGroot et al. (2002). Specific enzymatic treatment of bovine and human articular cartilage: Implications for integrative cartilage repair. *Arthritis Rheum* 46(4): 976-985.

Brevignon-Dodin, L., and F. Livesey. (2006). Regulation of tissue-engineered products in the European Union: Where are we heading? *Regen Med* 1(5): 709-714.

Bujia, J., S. Alsalameh et al. (1994). Humoral immune response against minor collagens type IX and XI in patients with cartilage graft resorption after reconstructive surgery. *Ann Rheum Dis* 53(4): 229-234.

Butnariu-Ephrat, M., D. Robinson et al. (1996). Resurfacing of goat articular cartilage by chondrocytes derived from bone marrow. *Clin Orthop Relat Res* 330: 234-243.

Cartmell, J. S., and M. G. Dunn. (2000). Effect of chemical treatments on tendon cellularity and mechanical properties. *J Biomed Mater Res* 49(1): 134-140.

Center for Biologics Evaluation and Research (CBER) (HFM-591). (1996). Guidance on applications for products comprised of living autologous cells manipulated ex vivo and intended for structural repair or reconstruction. Rockville, MD: Division of Congressional and Public Affairs (HFM-44), Food and Drug Administration.

Center for Biologics Evaluation and Research (CBER). (1998). Guidance for industry: Guidance for human somatic cell therapy and gene therapy. Rockville, MD: CBER, U.S. Department of Health and Human Services.

Center for Biologics Evaluation and Research (CBER). (2008). Guidance for FDA reviewers and sponsors content and review of chemistry, manufacturing, and control (CMC) information for human gene therapy investigational new drug applications (INDs). Rockville, MD: Office of Communication, Training, and Manufacturers Assistance, U.S. Department of Health and Human Services.

Center for Biologics Evaluation and Research (CBER) and Center for Devices and Radiological Health (CDRH). (2011). Preparation of IDEs and INDs for products intended to repair or replace knee cartilage. Rockville, MD: Office of Communication, Outreach and Development, Food and Drug Administration, U.S. Department of Health and Human Services.

Center for Drug Evaluation and Research (CDER) and Center for Biologics Evaluation and Research (CBER). (2001). Guidance for industry—E 10 choice of control group and related issues in clinical trials. Rockville, MD: Office of Training and Communication and Office of Communication, Training and Manufacturers Assistance, U.S. Department of Health and Human Services.

Chen, R. N., H. O. Ho et al. (2004). Process development of an acellular dermal matrix (ADM) for biomedical applications. *Biomaterials* 25(13): 2679-2686.

Choi, Y. S., J. A. Jeong et al. (2012). Mesenchymal stem cell-mediated immature dendritic cells induce regulatory T cell-based immunosuppressive effect. *Immunol Invest* 41(2): 214-229.

Christensen, R., P. K. Kristensen et al. (2007). A meta-analysis of the efficacy and safety of the anti-obesity agent Rimonabant [in Danish]. *Ugeskr Laeger* 169(50): 4360-4363.

Chu, C. R., F. R. Convery et al. (1999). Articular cartilage transplantation. Clinical results in the knee. *Clin Orthop Relat Res* 360: 159-168.

Cissell, D. D., J. C. Hu et al. (2014). Antigen removal for the production of biomechanically functional, xenogeneic tissue grafts. *J Biomech* 47(9): 1987-1996.

Collins, B. H., A. H. Cotterell et al. (1995). Cardiac xenografts between primate species provide evidence for the importance of the alpha-galactosyl determinant in hyperacute rejection. *J Immunol* 154(10): 5500-5510.

Costa, C., J. L. Brokaw et al. (2008). Characterization of cartilage from H-transferase transgenic pigs. *Transplant Proc* 40(2): 554-556.

Costa, C., L. Zhao et al. (2002). Transgenic pigs designed to express human CD59 and H-transferase to avoid humoral xenograft rejection. *Xenotransplantation* 9(1): 45-57.

Dahl, S. L., J. Koh et al. (2003). Decellularized native and engineered arterial scaffolds for transplantation. *Cell Transplant* 12(6): 659-666.

Dai, Y., T. D. Vaught et al. (2002). Targeted disruption of the alpha1,3-galactosyltransferase gene in cloned pigs. *Nat Biotechnol* 20(3): 251-255.

Dayer, E., L. Mathai et al. (1990). Cartilage proteoglycan-induced arthritis in BALB/c mice. Antibodies that recognize human and mouse cartilage proteoglycan and can cause depletion of cartilage proteoglycan with little or no synovitis. *Arthritis Rheum* 33(9): 1394-1405.

Derham, C., H. Yow et al. (2008). Tissue engineering small-diameter vascular grafts: Preparation of a biocompatible porcine ureteric scaffold. *Tissue Eng Part A* 14(11): 1871-1882.

DiMicco, M. A., S. N. Waters et al. (2002). Integrative articular cartilage repair: Dependence on developmental stage and collagen metabolism. *Osteoarthr Cartil* 10(3): 218-225.

Elder, B. D., S. V. Eleswarapu et al. (2009). Extraction techniques for the decellularization of tissue engineered articular cartilage constructs. *Biomaterials* 30(22): 3749-3756.

Elder, B. D., D. H. Kim et al. (2010). Developing an articular cartilage decellularization process toward facet joint cartilage replacement. *Neurosurgery* 66(4): 722-727; discussion 727.

Elves, M. W. (1974). Humoral immune response to allografts of bone. *Int Arch Allergy Appl Immunol* 47(5): 708-715.

Englert, C., K. B. McGowan et al. (2005). Inhibition of integrative cartilage repair by proteoglycan 4 in synovial fluid. *Arthritis Rheum* 52(4): 1091-1099.

FDA. (2011a). Current good manufacturing practice for finished pharmaceuticals. Title 21 Code of Federal Regulations Pt. 211.

FDA. (2011b). Current good manufacturing practice in manufacturing, processing, packing, or holding of drugs. Title 21 Code of Federal Regulations Pt. 210.

FDA. (2011c). Investigational device exemptions. Title 21 Code of Federal Regulations Pt. 812.

FDA. (2011d). Quality system regulation. Title 21 Code of Federal Regulations Pt. 820.

Flynn, J. M., D. S. Springfield et al. (1994). Osteoarticular allografts to treat distal femoral osteonecrosis. *Clin Orthop Relat Res* 303: 38-43.

Freed, L. E., D. A. Grande et al. (1994). Joint resurfacing using allograft chondrocytes and synthetic biodegradable polymer scaffolds. *J Biomed Mater Res* 28(8): 891-899.

Friedlaender, G. E. (1983). Immune responses to osteochondral allografts. Current knowledge and future directions. *Clin Orthop Relat Res* 174: 58-68.

Galili, U. (1993). Interaction of the natural anti-Gal antibody with alpha-galactosyl epitopes: A major obstacle for xenotransplantation in humans. *Immunol Today* 14(10): 480-482.

Galili, U., D. C. LaTemple et al. (1997). Porcine and bovine cartilage transplants in cynomolgus monkey. II. Changes in anti-Gal response during chronic rejection. *Transplantation* 63(5): 646-651.

Gerstenfeld, L. C., A. Riva et al. (1993). Post-translational control of collagen fibrillogenesis in mineralizing cultures of chick osteoblasts. *J Bone Miner Res* 8(9): 1031-1043.

Glant, T. T., E. I. Buzas et al. (1998). Critical roles of glycosaminoglycan side chains of cartilage proteoglycan (aggrecan) in antigen recognition and presentation. *J Immunol* 160(8): 3812-3819.

Glenn, R. E., Jr., E. C. McCarty et al. (2006). Comparison of fresh osteochondral autografts and allografts: A canine model. *Am J Sports Med* 34(7): 1084-1093.

Goldsby, R. A., T. J. Kindt et al. (2003). *Immunology*. New York: W. H. Freeman and Company.

Good, A. H., D. K. Cooper et al. (1992). Identification of carbohydrate structures that bind human antiporcine antibodies: Implications for discordant xenografting in humans. *Transplant Proc* 24(2): 559-562.

Grauss, R. W., M. G. Hazekamp et al. (2005). Histological evaluation of decellularised porcine aortic valves: Matrix changes due to different decellularisation methods. *Eur J Cardiothorac Surg* 27(4): 566-571.

Green, W. T., Jr. (1977). Articular cartilage repair. Behavior of rabbit chondrocytes during tissue culture and subsequent allografting. *Clin Orthop Relat Res* 124: 237-250.

Griffin, J. W., C. J. Gilmore et al. (2013). Treatment of a patellar chondral defect using juvenile articular cartilage allograft implantation. *Arthrosc Tech* 2(4): e351-e354.

Gross, A. E., N. Shasha et al. (2005). Long-term followup of the use of fresh osteochondral allografts for posttraumatic knee defects. *Clin Orthop Relat Res* 435: 79-87.

Hale, D. A. (2006). Basic transplantation immunology. *Surg Clin North Am* 86(5): 1103-1125.

Han, Z., Y. Jing et al. (2012). The role of immunosuppression of mesenchymal stem cells in tissue repair and tumor growth. *Cell Biosci* 2(1): 8.

Hodde, J., and M. Hiles. (2002). Virus safety of a porcine-derived medical device: Evaluation of a viral inactivation method. *Biotechnol Bioeng* 79(2): 211-216.

Hodde, J., A. Janis et al. (2007). Effects of sterilization on an extracellular matrix scaffold. I. Composition and matrix architecture. *J Mater Sci Mater Med* 18(4): 537-543.

Huey, D. J., J. C. Hu et al. (2012). Unlike bone, cartilage regeneration remains elusive. *Science* 338(6109): 917-921.

Hunziker, E. B., I. M. Driesang et al. (2001). Structural barrier principle for growth factor-based articular cartilage repair. *Clin Orthop Relat Res* 391(Suppl): S182-S189.

Hunziker, E. B., and L. C. Rosenberg. (1996). Repair of partial-thickness defects in articular cartilage: Cell recruitment from the synovial membrane. *J Bone Joint Surg Am* 78(5): 721-733.

Jackson, D. W., C. A. McDevitt et al. (1992). Meniscal transplantation using fresh and cryopreserved allografts. An experimental study in goats. *Am J Sports Med* 20(6): 644-656.

Janeway, C. A., Jr., and R. Medzhitov. (2002). Innate immune recognition. *Annu Rev Immunol* 20: 197-216.

Kaminski, M. J., G. Kaminska et al. (1980). Species differences in the ability of isolated epiphyseal chondrocytes to hypertrophy after transplantation into the wall of the Syrian hamster cheek pouch. *Folia Biol (Krakow)* 28(1): 27-36.

Kapoor, M., J. Martel-Pelletier et al. (2011). Role of proinflammatory cytokines in the pathophysiology of osteoarthritis. *Nat Rev Rheumatol* 7(1): 33-42.

Kasimir, M. T., E. Rieder et al. (2003). Comparison of different decellularization procedures of porcine heart valves. *Int J Artif Organs* 26(5): 421-427.

Ksiazek, T., and S. Moskalewski. (1983). Studies on bone formation by cartilage reconstructed by isolated epiphyseal chondrocytes, transplanted syngeneically or across known histocompatibility barriers in mice. *Clin Orthop Relat Res* 172: 233-242.

Kuci, Z., S. Kuci et al. (2011). Mesenchymal stromal cells derived from CD271(+) bone marrow mononuclear cells exert potent allosuppressive properties. *Cytotherapy* 13(10): 1193-1204.

Kumar, V., A. K. Abbas et al. (2007). *Robbins Basic Pathology*. Philadelphia: Elsevier, Health Sciences Division.

Lance, E. M. (1989). Immunological reactivity towards chondrocytes in rat and man: Relevance to autoimmune arthritis. *Immunol Lett* 21(1): 63-73.

Langer, F., and A. E. Gross. (1974). Immunogenicity of allograft articular cartilage. *J Bone Joint Surg Am* 56(2): 297-304.

Lee, J. K., D. J. Responte et al. (2014). Clinical translation of stem cells: Insight for cartilage therapies. *Crit Rev Biotechnol* 34(1): 89-100.

Li, W. J., H. Chiang et al. (2009). Evaluation of articular cartilage repair using biodegradable nanofibrous scaffolds in a swine model: A pilot study. *J Tissue Eng Regen Med* 3(1): 1-10.

Liao, J., E. M. Joyce et al. (2008). Effects of decellularization on the mechanical and structural properties of the porcine aortic valve leaflet. *Biomaterials* 29(8): 1065-1074.

Lumpkins, S. B., N. Pierre et al. (2008). A mechanical evaluation of three decellularization methods in the design of a xenogeneic scaffold for tissue engineering the temporomandibular joint disc. *Acta Biomater* 4(4): 808-816.

Lyles, M. B., J. C. Hu et al. (2015). Bone tissue engineering. In *Regenerative Engineering of Musculoskeletal Tissues and Interfaces*, ed. J. W. F. Syam, P. Nukavarapu, and C. T. Laurencin. Cambridge, UK: Woodhead Publishing, pp. 97-134.

Malejczyk, J. (1989). Natural anti-chondrocyte cytotoxicity of normal human peripheral blood mononuclear cells. *Clin Immunol Immunopathol* 50(1 Pt 1): 42-52.

Malejczyk, J., M. J. Kaminski et al. (1985). Natural cell-mediated cytotoxic activity against isolated chondrocytes in the mouse. *Clin Exp Immunol* 59(1): 110-116.

Malejczyk, J., and S. Moskalewski. (1988). Effect of immunosuppression on survival and growth of cartilage produced by transplanted allogeneic epiphyseal chondrocytes. *Clin Orthop Relat Res* 232: 292-303.

Malejczyk, J., A. Osiecka et al. (1991). Effect of immunosuppression on rejection of cartilage formed by transplanted allogeneic rib chondrocytes in mice. *Clin Orthop Relat Res* 269: 266-273.

Masuoka, K., T. Asazuma et al. (2005). Tissue engineering of articular cartilage using an allograft of cultured chondrocytes in a membrane-sealed atelocollagen honeycomb-shaped scaffold (ACHMS scaffold). *J Biomed Mater Res B Appl Biomater* 75(1): 177-184.

McCulloch, P. C., R. W. Kang et al. (2007). Prospective evaluation of prolonged fresh osteochondral allograft transplantation of the femoral condyle: Minimum 2-year follow-up. *Am J Sports Med* 35(3): 411-420.

McGowan, K. B., and R. L. Sah. (2005). Treatment of cartilage with beta-aminopropionitrile accelerates subsequent collagen maturation and modulates integrative repair. *J Orthop Res* 23(3): 594-601.

Meyer, S. R., B. Chiu et al. (2006). Comparison of aortic valve allograft decellularization techniques in the rat. *J Biomed Mater Res A* 79(2): 254-262.

Meyer, S. R., J. Nagendran et al. (2005). Decellularization reduces the immune response to aortic valve allografts in the rat. *J Thorac Cardiovasc Surg* 130(2): 469-476.

Moskalewski, S., A. Hyc et al. (2002). Immune response by host after allogeneic chondrocyte transplant to the cartilage. *Microsc Res Tech* 58(1): 3-13.

Neu, C. P., A. Khalafi et al. (2007). Mechanotransduction of bovine articular cartilage superficial zone protein by transforming growth factor beta signaling. *Arthritis Rheum* 56(11): 3706-3714.

Obradovic, B., I. Martin et al. (2001). Integration of engineered cartilage. *J Orthop Res* 19(6): 1089-1097.

Office of Cellular, Tissue, and Gene Therapies. (2008). Content and review of chemistry, manufacturing, and control (CMC) information for human somatic cell therapy investigational new drug applications (INDs). Rockville, MD: Office of Communication, Training, and Manufacturers Assistance (HFM-40).

Osiecka-Iwan, A., A. Hyc et al. (2003). Transplants of rat chondrocytes evoke strong humoral response against chondrocyte-associated antigen in rabbits. *Cell Transplant* 12(4): 389-398.

Peretti, G. M., L. J. Bonassar et al. (1999). Biomechanical analysis of a chondrocyte-based repair model of articular cartilage. *Tissue Eng* 5(4): 317-326.

Peretti, G. M., V. Zaporojan et al. (2003). Cell-based bonding of articular cartilage: An extended study. *J Biomed Mater Res A* 64(3): 517-524.

Pietra, B. A. (2003). Transplantation immunology 2003: Simplified approach. *Pediatr Clin North Am* 50(6): 1233-1259.

Platt, J. L., G. M. Vercellotti et al. (1990). Transplantation of discordant xenografts: A review of progress. *Immunol Today* 11(12): 450-456; discussion 456-457.

Rahfoth, B., J. Weisser et al. (1998). Transplantation of allograft chondrocytes embedded in agarose gel into cartilage defects of rabbits. *Osteoarthr Cartil* 6(1): 50-65.

Ramallal, M., E. Maneiro et al. (2004). Xeno-implantation of pig chondrocytes into rabbit to treat localized articular cartilage defects: An animal model. *Wound Repair Regen* 12(3): 337-345.

Reindel, E. S., A. M. Ayroso et al. (1995). Integrative repair of articular cartilage in vitro: Adhesive strength of the interface region. *J Orthop Res* 13(5): 751-760.

Ren, G., L. Zhang et al. (2008). Mesenchymal stem cell-mediated immunosuppression occurs via concerted action of chemokines and nitric oxide. *Cell Stem Cell* 2(2): 141-150.

Revell, C. M., and K. A. Athanasiou. (2009). Success rates and immunologic responses of autogenic, allogenic, and xenogenic treatments to repair articular cartilage defects. *Tissue Eng Part B Rev* 15(1): 1-15.

Romaniuk, A., J. Malejczyk et al. (1995). Rejection of cartilage formed by transplanted allogeneic chondrocytes: Evaluation with monoclonal antibodies. *Transpl Immunol* 3(3): 251-257.

Rosario, D. J., G. C. Reilly et al. (2008). Decellularization and sterilization of porcine urinary bladder matrix for tissue engineering in the lower urinary tract. *Regen Med* 3(2): 145-156.

Rus, H., C. Cudrici et al. (2005). The role of the complement system in innate immunity. *Immunol Res* 33(2): 103-112.

Sandrin, M. S., H. A. Vaughan et al. (1993). Anti-pig IgM antibodies in human serum react predominantly with Gal(alpha 1-3)Gal epitopes. *Proc Natl Acad Sci USA* 90(23): 11391-11395.

Schaefer, D. B., D. Wendt et al. (2004). Lubricin reduces cartilage—Cartilage integration. *Biorheology* 41(3-4): 503-508.

Schreiber, R. E., B. M. Ilten-Kirby et al. (1999). Repair of osteochondral defects with allogeneic tissue engineered cartilage implants. *Clin Orthop Relat Res* 367(Suppl): S382-S395.

Seebacher, G., C. Grasl et al. (2008). Biomechanical properties of decellularized porcine pulmonary valve conduits. *Artif Organs* 32(1): 28-35.

Shawki, S., T. Gaafar et al. (2015). Immunomodulatory effects of umbilical cord-derived mesenchymal stem cells. *Microbiol Immunol* 59(6): 348-356.

Stapleton, T. W., J. Ingram et al. (2008). Development and characterization of an acellular porcine medial meniscus for use in tissue engineering. *Tissue Eng Part A* 14(4): 505-518.

Stevenson, S., G. A. Dannucci et al. (1989). The fate of articular cartilage after transplantation of fresh and cryopreserved tissue-antigen-matched and mismatched osteochondral allografts in dogs. *J Bone Joint Surg Am* 71(9): 1297-1307.

Stone, K. R., G. Ayala et al. (1998). Porcine cartilage transplants in the cynomolgus monkey. III. Transplantation of alpha-galactosidase-treated porcine cartilage. *Transplantation* 65(12): 1577-1583.

Stone, K. R., A. W. Walgenbach et al. (1997). Porcine and bovine cartilage transplants in cynomolgus monkey. I. A model for chronic xenograft rejection. *Transplantation* 63(5): 640-645.

Takagi, T., and H. E. Jasin. (1992). Interactions between anticollagen antibodies and chondrocytes. *Arthritis Rheum* 35(2): 224-230.

Tearle, R. G., M. J. Tange et al. (1996). The alpha-1,3-galactosyltransferase knockout mouse. Implications for xenotransplantation. *Transplantation* 61(1): 13-19.

Tew, S. R., A. P. Kwan et al. (2000). The reactions of articular cartilage to experimental wounding: Role of apoptosis. *Arthritis Rheum* 43(1): 215-225.

Trivedi, H. L. (2007). Immunobiology of rejection and adaptation. *Transplant Proc* 39(3): 647-652.

Trommelmans, L., J. Selling et al. (2007). A critical assessment of the directive on tissue engineering of the European Union. *Tissue Eng* 13(4): 667-672.

Tudorache, I., S. Cebotari et al. (2007). Tissue engineering of heart valves: Biomechanical and morphological properties of decellularized heart valves. *J Heart Valve Dis* 16(5): 567-573; discussion 574.

van de Breevaart Bravenboer, J., C. D. In der Maur et al. (2004). Improved cartilage integration and interfacial strength after enzymatic treatment in a cartilage transplantation model. *Arthritis Res Ther* 6(5): R469-R476.

van Susante, J. L., P. Buma et al. (1999). Resurfacing potential of heterologous chondrocytes suspended in fibrin glue in large full-thickness defects of femoral articular cartilage: An experimental study in the goat. *Biomaterials* 20(13): 1167-1175.

von Rechenberg, B., M. K. Akens et al. (2003). Changes in subchondral bone in cartilage resurfacing—An experimental study in sheep using different types of osteochondral grafts. *Osteoarthr Cartil* 11(4): 265-277.

Wakitani, S., T. Goto et al. (1994). Mesenchymal cell-based repair of large, full-thickness defects of articular cartilage. *J Bone Joint Surg Am* 76(4): 579-592.

Wakitani, S., T. Goto et al. (1998). Repair of large full-thickness articular cartilage defects with allograft articular chondrocytes embedded in a collagen gel. *Tissue Eng* 4(4): 429-444.

Wakitani, S., T. Kimura et al. (1989). Repair of rabbit articular surfaces with allograft chondrocytes embedded in collagen gel. *J Bone Joint Surg Br* 71(1): 74-80.

Wang, M., Y. Yang et al. (2009). The immunomodulatory activity of human umbilical cord blood-derived mesenchymal stem cells in vitro. *Immunology* 126(2): 220-232.

Weber, C. L., V. Peña et al. (2013). The role of the National Science Foundation in the origin and evolution of additive manufacturing in the United States. Washington, DC: IDA Science & Technology Policy Institute.

Wong, M. L., J. K. Leach et al. (2011). The role of protein solubilization in antigen removal from xenogeneic tissue for heart valve tissue engineering. *Biomaterials* 32(32): 8129-8138.

Woods, T., and P. F. Gratzer. (2005). Effectiveness of three extraction techniques in the development of a decellularized bone-anterior cruciate ligament-bone graft. *Biomaterials* 26(35): 7339-7349.

Wright, G. C., Jr., X. Q. Wei et al. (1988). Stimulation of matrix formation in rabbit chondrocyte cultures by ascorbate. 1. Effect of ascorbate analogs and beta-aminopropionitrile. *J Orthop Res* 6(3): 397-407.

Yablon, I. G., S. Cooperband et al. (1982). Matrix antigens in allografts. The humoral response. *Clin Orthop Relat Res* 168: 243-251.

Yamaga, K. M., L. H. Kimura et al. (1994). Differentiation antigens of human articular chondrocytes and their tissue distribution as assessed by monoclonal antibodies. *J Autoimmun* 7(2): 203-217.

Yang, H. M., J. H. Sung et al. (2012). Enhancement of the immunosuppressive effect of human adipose tissue-derived mesenchymal stromal cells through HLA-G1 expression. *Cytotherapy* 14(1): 70-79.

Yang, W. D., S. J. Chen et al. (2000). A study of injectable tissue-engineered autologous cartilage. *Chin J Dent Res* 3(4): 10-15.

Yi, T., D. S. Lee et al. (2012). Gene expression profile reveals that STAT2 is involved in the immunosuppressive function of human bone marrow-derived mesenchymal stem cells. *Gene* 497(2): 131-139.

Zukor, D. J., R. D. Oakeshott et al. (1989). Osteochondral allograft reconstruction of the knee. Part 2: Experience with successful and failed fresh osteochondral allografts. *Am J Knee Surg* 2: 182.

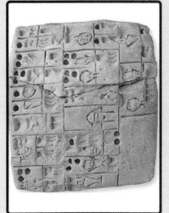

"Ninkasi, you are the one who pours out the filtered beer of the collector vat, it is [like] the onrush of Tigris and Euphrates." (1800 BCE)
Clay tablet detailing the "Hymn to Ninkasi" (Sumerian goddess of brewing and beer), purported to be the oldest known beer brewing recipe, also making it one of the oldest known biological protocols.

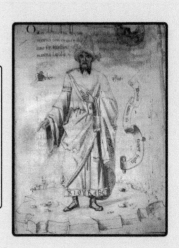

"The first essential in chemistry is that thou shouldest perform practical work and conduct experiments, for he who performs not practical work nor makes experiments will never attain to the least degree of mastery."
Jabir ibn Hayyan (Geber) (721-815 CE), Persian polymath, astronomer, pharmacist, physician, philosopher, and engineer. Considered the "father of chemistry," which grew out of the processes of alchemy, Jabir introduced scientific and experimental approaches or protocols.

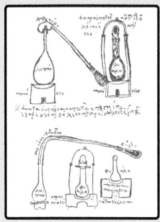

Illustration of ancient Greek alchemical equipment. Ancient equipment and processes, such as reaction vessels and distillation, are recognized as forerunners in the development of modern experimental protocols. From the *Collection des anciens achimistes grecs* (3 vol., Paris, 1887-1888) by Marcelin Berthelot.

Experimental Protocols for Generation and Evaluation of Articular Cartilage

7

- Tissue and cell culture
- Morphological assays
- Biochemical assays
- Mechanical assays

The purpose of this section is to increase understanding of some of the experimental procedures used in cartilage biology and tissue engineering research. It is also intended as a companion to Chapter 5. In this regard, we seek to provide a balance between highly detailed instructions and general conceptual protocols; those included here are not meant to be exhaustive for cartilage biology. It is expected that these protocols will allow for a basic conceptual understanding of the techniques employed in cartilage biology and engineering. These protocols can also serve as a set of "recipes" for investigators and guide them to basic assays related to articular cartilage. It is understood that often multiple variations on a specific assay exist. With these factors in mind, the authors have chosen protocols based on tried-and-true techniques. Often, a generic but detailed version of the protocol has been prepared to accommodate for variations in equipment and supplies available. It should be noted that several other protocol books are available from publishers such as Wiley and Springer. For example, for molecular biology techniques, the *Molecular Cloning: A Laboratory Manual* set, available from Cold Spring Harbor, is quite comprehensive.

Like with any experimental procedure, the reader is cautioned that full consideration should be given to safety procedures. Training and practice are required for both safety and consistency. For example, the tissue and cell culture procedures require previous knowledge and experience with sterile culture techniques. Additionally, many of the assays described in Chapter 5 for mechanical testing may require either custom-built equipment, the modification of commercially available testing machines, or the generation of custom control software. These adaptations will necessitate training beyond what is described in the protocols in this chapter.

Where possible, commercially available kits that simplify and standardize the protocols have been suggested based on the authors' experience. It should be understood that in many cases, multiple vendors offer similar kits; the decision to use any one specific kit does not represent an endorsement by the authors. No company considerations or financial incentives were involved in the choice of any specific, commercially available kit, or choice of materials, and we have no conflicts of interest with any of the companies or products mentioned here.

The inclusion of important safety notes when handling some of the reagents and equipment listed should be in no way taken to be comprehensive. Precautions concerning safety and storage recommendations of reagents should be strictly adhered to at all times.

The authors would like to acknowledge the contribution of Dr. Johannah Sanchez-Adams, in collecting and editing many of the initial versions of the protocols detailed in this section.

7.1 TISSUE AND CELL CULTURE

Each culture technique has advantages, disadvantages, and limitations, and the choice of which to use will depend on the type of hypothesis tested. Chondrocytes in two-dimensional (2D) culture undergo dedifferentiation when plated on tissue culture plastic, marked by changes in the levels of chondrocyte-specific matrix proteins and cell morphology (Vinall et al. 2002). This limitation has led to the development of multiple three-dimensional (3D) culture techniques, which both preserve and restore the chondrocytic phenotype. Several of the more common 3D techniques are described in Section 7.1.5, including reencapsulation of the chondrocyte in a 3D hydrogel, culture at high cell density (micromass or pellet culture), or the use of self-assembly. However, 2D monolayer cultures are valuable for increasing the number of chondrocytes through proliferation, are much easier to extract protein or DNA/RNA from, and generally are more amenable to a variety of other assay techniques.

Due to the short supply of healthy human donor tissues, common sources of human chondrocytes are often from "normal-looking" areas of a diseased joint undergoing total joint replacement. Therefore, obtaining healthy articular cartilage often requires the use of animal sources. However, articular cartilage tissue sources vary by joint and animal species. Sources of commonly used cartilage include cow (bovine), pig (porcine), rabbit (leporine), sheep (ovine), mice and rats (murine), goat (caprine), and horse (equine). Commonly, to have local availability of large amounts of animal tissue may necessitate the use of animals euthanized for other purposes. Due to issues of size and availability, experiments that plan to use large volumes of tissue or high numbers of cells will most likely use either bovine or porcine cartilage due to the ease of obtaining tissue from a local abattoir. Given the authors' extensive experience with bovine tissues, this section will focus on isolation from bovine cartilage, although much of the procedure is fundamentally the same for other species.

7.1.1 Harvesting Cartilage and the Production of Explants

Recent evidence suggests that an explant model system that retains the subchondral bone (i.e., osteochondral model) more closely mimics the *in vivo* system than cartilage explants (de Vries-van Melle et al. 2012). While explant culture requires the least manipulation and is closest to replicating the *in vivo* conditions, extraction of protein, DNA, or RNA may be more difficult than other culture techniques. Explants also have size limitations due to diffusional constraints. Certain experiments, for example, those involving cartilage injury studies, characterizing native properties, or identifying compounds that affect native matrix integrity, are more applicable with tissue explants than other *in vitro* techniques.

Important parameters that influence the success of explant culture include tissue type, explant size, "freshness" (time postmortem), donor age, anatomical location, and whether the explant contains multiple tissue types. Thus, for articular cartilage, explants should ideally be no larger than 1 mm thick due to diffusion limitations. Articular cartilage should be harvested as soon as possible postmortem to ensure the best yield of chondrocytes. If necessary, cells and tissue can be stored at 4°C for multiple days with no large decrease in viability due to the avascular nature of articular cartilage (Shasha et al. 2002).

Though not as common, cartilage explants can also be used to produce an outgrowth 2D culture by depositing a piece of tissue (primary explant) to a tissue culture dish and culturing the cells that migrate out of the tissue onto the culture surface (outgrowth). This allows for production of a subpopulation of cells already predisposed to migrate and likely proliferate. In contrast, enzymatic digestion of the whole tissue may contain populations of cells that may not migrate or proliferate during the subsequent cell culture. The cells that do proliferate will subsequently be selected as they outexpand their nonproliferating counterparts.

The protocol presented here is for extraction of articular cartilage from medium to large animals, for example, sheep or calf (juvenile bovine). Larger joints, especially calf (~1 month), are easily obtainable and provide pristine, relatively thick cartilage (~4 mm). The thickness of the articular cartilage also allows for separation into zonal explants, permitting experimental procedures that would otherwise be difficult in smaller species. The juvenile bovine knee (Figure 7.1) is similar in

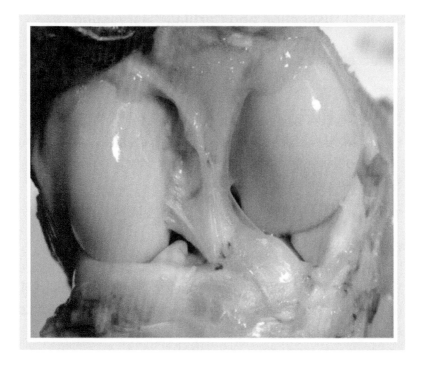

Figure 7.1 Example of pristine articular cartilage of the juvenile bovine knee, from Chapter 1.

size to that of an adult human, although human cartilage is thinner (1-2 mm) depending on anatomical location and age. It should be noted that while the extraction protocol is similar for human tissues, when working with human tissues extra precautions to prevent disease transmission should be taken, and personal protective gear worn at all times.

Adult rabbit articular cartilage is about 0.4 mm thick, and chondrocytes can be isolated similarly to those of bovine cartilage. Though the use of explant culture is possible with rabbit tissue, given the thin nature of its cartilage, zonal separation may be technically challenging.

Directly isolating articular cartilage from the small joints of mouse and rats can be difficult. However, in young animals (less than 35 days in mice and less than 40 days in rats), before the epiphysis of the femur closes, the proximal end of the femur (femoral head) can be easily removed *en bloc* using a prying motion by a spatula.

7.1.1.1 Surgical Dissection and Cartilage Harvesting

A. Materials needed

Equipment
1. Sterile scalpel handles, scalpel blades
2. Clean work surface, such as a stainless steel table or bench
3. Sterile dermal punch or other metal punch
4. Sterile drapes or autoclaved towels
5. 50 ml sterile tube or tissue culture dish

Reagents
1. Tissue source
2. Wash medium: Dulbecco's modified Eagle's medium (DMEM) (Invitrogen 10566) medium containing 1% penicillin-streptomycin-fungizone (PSF)
3. Iodine wash (providine or similar)

Note: Care should be taken to not handle the articular cartilage surface directly unless wearing sterile gloves and to not allow the cartilage surface to dry out. This can be prevented by "wetting" the surface of the cartilage with the wash medium.

B. Procedure

1. Obtain fresh, whole joints within 24 hours of death. Commonly the tibiofemoral articulation (from the "stifle" or knee) is used. For medium to large animals, the metacarpophalangeal joint or other large joints can also be used.
2. Carefully remove skin or hide if present. Examine joint capsule to determine whether it has been breached. If so, tissue should be monitored for contamination.
3. Clean the tissue on the outside of the joint capsule with providine (iodine wash) to remove surface contaminants. Lay on sterile drapes covering the work surface.

4. Dissect and remove unneeded tissue, while taking care to protect the joint capsule. Removing the fascia and extraneous tissue around the capsule will expose a sterile work area before opening the capsule.

5. Using a fresh sterile scalpel blade, open the joint capsule, exposing the condyles. Ideally, this should be done in a sterile tissue culture hood, if possible. For the knee, two approaches can be taken for opening the capsule. Longitudinally, cut parallel to the patellar tendon (dorsal to ventral), or cut across the width of the joint (lateral to medial) at the level just above the meniscus. Bending of the joint to induce tension in the tissues will reduce the effort needed to open the joint capsule.

6. Once the capsule has been entered, transect the patellar tendon and plunge the blade between the condyle to cut the anterior cruciate ligament (ACL) and posterior cruciate ligament (PCL). Continue working around the circumference of the femur, cutting the medial cruciate ligament (MCL) and lateral cruciate ligament (LCL) at the edge of the condyles to separate the tibia from the femur.

7. Continue cutting past the condyles to expose the patellar groove.

8. At this time, explants can be removed using a sterile dermal punch or other tools.

9. Cartilage can also be removed using the scalpel or minced for enzymatic digestion for cell isolation (Section 7.1.2). For mincing, use the scalpel to produce a cross-hatched grid on the cartilage to the desired depth; then, with a shaving motion remove the small slivers of cartilage into a 50 ml tube containing wash medium. A juvenile bovine knee will yield approximately 3-6 ml of cartilage from the femoral condyles and patellar grove, although this will vary based on the depth of cartilage harvested and the person harvesting.

10. Removal of the superficial zone can be achieved either through the use of a dermatome blade or through the use of a specially constructed jig (Figure 7.2). Other zones can be removed in a similar manner.

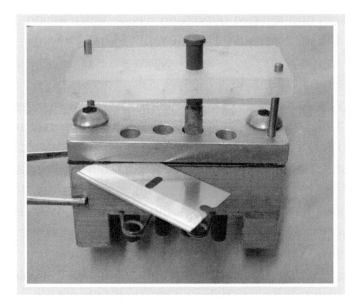

Figure 7.2 Custom jig used for producing reproducible articular cartilage slices. Adjustable spacers inserted between the top and bottom plates (location of razor blade) allow for changes in explant final length and thickness of sections cut. The pictured jig is set for removal of the superficial zone only, using a 0.3 mm thickness plate. (Explant is subchondral bone side up in this picture.)

7.1.2 Cell Isolation

Once harvested, the articular cartilage matrix can be enzymatically digested to release the chondrocytes. The protocol below uses a type II collagenase solution to enzymatically break up the extracellular matrix, with digestion taking place overnight (16 hours) with gentle shaking. An initial digestion for 1 hour with pronase can also be included if desired, as this will accelerate the release of chondrocytes by collagenase digestion from 16 hours to 2-3 hours (Liebman and Goldberg 2001). For nearly complete digestion, cartilage should be minced into approximately 1 mm pieces; however, extremely thin sections of superficial zone or other cartilage may require less digestion time. As this material is harvested from primary tissue sources, contamination of primary cultures should be tested after every manipulation. Cartilage harvested from separate joints should be kept separate until after digestion if possible, and a small amount of the isolated chondrocytes should be cultured separately (assuming the majority are cryopreserved following digestion; see Section 7.1.3).

A. Materials needed

Equipment
1. Sterile scalpel handles, blades
2. Cell culture incubator
3. Orbital shaker that will fit into the incubator
4. Cell strainers, 70 μm
5. 10 mm sterile culture dishes or tall-walled petri dishes
6. 50 ml sterile tubes

Reagents
1. Wash medium: DMEM medium containing 1% PSF
2. Collagenase solution: DMEM (Invitrogen 10566) containing 1% PSF, 3% fetal bovine serum (FBS), and 0.2% type II collagenase, sterile filtered
3. Previously harvested cartilage, minced into pieces approximately 1 mm^3

Note: Care should be taken to not handle the cartilage directly unless wearing sterile gloves and to not allow the cartilage to dry out. This can be prevented by wetting the surface of the cartilage with the wash medium.

B. Procedure

1. Rinse the minced cartilage from each joint twice with wash medium, treat the material from each joint separately, and avoid cross-contamination between containers.
2. In 10 mm sterile culture dishes, add approximately 3-6 ml of cartilage per dish and cover with 30 ml of the collagenase solution.
3. Incubate for 16 hours on the orbital shaker, with gentle shaking. Care should be taken to ensure the shaking does not result in sloshing of the medium out of the dishes.

4. After digestion, monitor dishes for signs of contamination and, if present, discard. Contamination can be detected by observing changes in the medium and, microscopically, microbial growth.

5. After digestion, pipette collagenase-cell solutions through 70 μm cell strainers into sterile 50 ml tubes. Bring the volume of the digest up to 50 ml using wash medium.

6. Centrifuge for 7 minutes at 200 × g.

7. Carefully aspirate the collagenase solution and gently resuspend the cell pellet in 30 ml of wash medium.

8. Repeat steps 6 and 7 to remove residual collagenase.

9. Consolidate the cells into a single 50 ml tube and resuspend cells in 30 ml of wash medium. Note the total volume in the tube and remove a 50 μl aliquot for cell counting. This volume may need to be diluted before counting to stay within the proper count range if using a Coulter Counter or hemocytometer.

10. If cryopreserving, instead of immediately using the cells, remove a small aliquot and culture separately to check for contamination. Otherwise, this cell solution may be used immediately for further protocols.

7.1.3 Cryopreservation of Cells

Cryopreservation allows for the long-term preservation of cells. Cells stored in liquid nitrogen should be viable for a minimum of 10 years. This allows for preservation of modified or interesting cell lines, pooling of cells from multiple isolation steps for large experiments, and staggering isolation procedures that require cells from primary tissue harvested on multiple days. Cryopreservation of cells requires the use of special freezing medium and control of the freezing rate to minimize cell membrane damage due to ice crystal formation. Dimethyl sulfoxide (DMSO), a solvent, is used in the freezing medium as it prevents ice crystal formation that would rupture cell membranes; however, DMSO itself has deleterious effects on the cells and weakens their membrane, making them more sensitive to injury by shear. Harsh manipulation of cells in DMSO, or extended contact with DMSO at elevated temperatures, will reduce cell viability and should be avoided. Glycerol can also be used as a cryo-preservative for certain cell lines sensitive to DMSO; however, as it penetrates cells more slowly, additional care must be taken during freezing.

Ideally, the cells should be frozen at a rate of 1°C per minute until the temperature reaches approximately -80°C. Both passive and active freezing containers are commercially available. Due to cost, passive freezing containers consisting of an isopropanol bath are by far the most common. However, if unavailable, cryovials with cells can be placed into thick-walled polystyrene containers and the outside insulated with paper towels. This method should be avoided, if possible, as it results in decreased cell viability. The initial freezing step occurs at -80°C for at least one overnight period, after which the cryovials can be transferred to long-term storage in a liquid nitrogen chilled Dewar (-196°C). Some loss of viability following thawing is expected; however, chondrocytes appear to handle cryopreservation well, and viability more than 95% is common.

A. Materials needed

Equipment
1. Freezing container (Mr. Frosty)
2. Cryovials

Reagents
1. Wash medium: DMEM medium containing 1% PSF
2. Freezing medium: Prepared as a 2× stock, using 40% DMEM wash medium, 40% FBS, and 20% DMSO; add the DMSO last, mix well, and sterile filter

Note: Wear appropriate gloves and face protection when transferring cells into and out of liquid nitrogen. Cryopreservation tubes or cryovials should always be tightened to prevent liquid nitrogen from entering the containers. Closed containers filled with liquid nitrogen will explode with considerable force as they warm up, resulting in loss of sample or release of biohazardous material.

B. Procedure

Part 1: Freezing cells
1. Disassociate cells as appropriate for tissue or culture conditions and count.
2. Collect cells by gentle centrifugation, aspirate medium, and gently resuspend cells in a half volume of cold wash medium for the total density desired for freezing. For chondrocytes, densities for freezing can be up to 30 million cells per milliliter.
3. Once cells are suspended, add remaining half volume of cold 2× freezing medium to achieve desired cell density, mix gently, and transfer to cryovials.
4. Immediately place cryovials into freezing container and transfer to -80°C for 16 hours or overnight. Cells will remain viable at -80°C for several months.
5. Transfer cryovials to a liquid nitrogen Dewar (-196°C) or cell freezer.

Part 2: Thawing cells
1. Cryovials should be thawed quickly and gently in a 37°C water bath. Once cells have thawed, quickly transfer to a 50 ml tube and dilute out the DMSO with wash medium.
2. Gently centrifuge cells, aspirate medium, and resuspend at the desired density.

7.1.4 2D Cultures

Here, we use 2D culture to describe a single cell layer of cells on tissue culture-treated plastic (i.e., monolayer). The use of 2D cultures is extremely common for multiple cell types, not just chondrocytes. This is due to (1) the ability to expand the number of chondrocytes used, (2) the ability to use treatments and assays not possible or extremely technically difficult for 3D cultures, and (3) the relative ease of extracting protein, DNA, or RNA from 2D culture compared with 3D culture. All procedures outlined here should be done in a sterile tissue culture

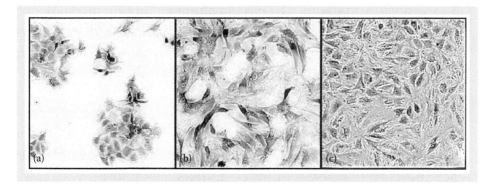

Figure 7.3 Morphological differences of monolayer chondrocytes under different serum (FBS) conditions, and passage numbers. (a) Primary adult rabbit chondrocytes. (b) After three passages (P3) in serum-containing medium. (c) After three passages (P3) in serum-free medium. (Courtesy of Dr. Daniel Huey.)

hood. The use of FBS in continuing cultures should be determined by the experimental design. Generally, the addition of 10% FBS to the medium will enhance proliferation of monolayer chondrocytes (as well as other cells); however, it will also enhance the speed of dedifferentiation (Figure 7.3) and may mask the effects of other culture additives or treatments, such as growth factors or inflammatory cytokines.

7.1.4.1 Monolayer

A. Materials needed

Equipment
1. Tissue culture-treated plastic plates/dishes

Reagents
1. Chondrogenic medium: DMEM (Invitrogen 10566) medium containing 1% PSF, 1% nonessential amino acids (NEAAs), 1% insulin-transferrin-selenium (ITS), 100 nM dexamethasone, 50 μg/ml ascorbate-2-phosphate, 40 μg/ml L-proline, and 100 μg/ml sodium pyruvate
2. Plating medium: Chondrogenic or expansion medium plus 10% FBS

3. Expansion medium: DMEM (Invitrogen 10566) medium containing 1% PSF and 1% NEAA (used primarily for expansion of fibroblasts or other cell types, or when dedifferentiating chondrocytes)—optional
4. Cells in solution

Note: Although multiple medium formulations for cell and tissue culture are available, the DMEM medium formulations presented here have been in use within the authors' laboratories with favorable results when applied to chondrocytes of multiple species; the components are widely commercially available.

B. Procedure

1. Warm all medium reagents to 37°C before use.
2. Determine cell density to be plated; values of 10,000-20,000 cells/cm² work well for initial plating.
3. Resuspend cells to desired density in plating medium and add to tissue culture dishes.
4. Fill tissue culture dishes to the working volume with plating medium.

7.1.4.2 Passaging Cells

Cells grown in monolayer will continue to proliferate until they cover the tissue culture dish and reach confluency. When cells reach confluency, or shortly beforehand, cells must be passaged or otherwise subcultured. Failure to do so will result in reduced proliferation or cell death. To do this, the cells must first be detached from the substrate using a proteolytic enzyme, commonly trypsin, although collagenase and dispase may also be used. This suspension of cells is then counted, fractioned, and used to reseed new tissue culture plates, resulting in a single passage. As discussed before, with increasing culture time and passage, chondrocytes dedifferentiate. It should also be noted that aside from stem cells and immortalized cell lines, most cells can only be passaged a set number of times before reaching senescence.

A. Materials needed

Equipment
1. Tissue culture plates (10 cm)

Reagents
1. Appropriate culture medium (e.g., Section 7.1.4.1)
2. Phosphate-buffered saline (PBS) without calcium or magnesium
3. 0.05% trypsin/EDTA
4. Collagenase solution: DMEM containing 1% PSF, 3% FBS, and 0.2% collagenase type II, sterile filtered; this is optional, but may be required for some chondrocyte cultures, due to the production of trypsin-resistant extracellular matrix components (e.g., collagens)

Note: Monolayer cultures should be washed with calcium- or magnesium-free PBS prior to trypsinizing to remove traces of FBS that contain trypsin inhibitors. While a concentration of 0.05% trypsin is used here, higher working concentrations up to 0.25% are also available; the lowest concentration that removes cells within 5-10 minutes should be used. For many chondrocyte cultures, especially early passages, a 10- to 15-minute pretreatment with collagenase may be necessary before treatment with trypsin to allow for cell isolation. All digestions should be done in the incubator at 37°C with continuous monitoring and with occasional gentle, manual agitation. Long incubation times with trypsin should be avoided and will decrease cell viability. All volumes are for 10 cm tissue culture dishes; larger or smaller dishes and flasks should be adjusted accordingly.

B. Procedure

1. Warm all medium reagents to 37°C before use.
2. Remove old culture medium and gently add 5-8 ml of PBS to the side of the dish to avoid shearing the cells. Gently rock the solution and remove.
3. Add 5 ml of trypsin/EDTA and gently rock the dish to ensure even coverage of the solution.

4. Place dish back in the incubator at 37°C.

5. Check the progress every few minutes, either by eye or by using an inverted microscope to check for detachment of the cells. Gently rock the solution or tap the dish to help dislodge the cells. Return the dish to the incubator if longer digestion time is needed.

6. Once cells have released from the surface, add 5 ml of culture medium containing 10% FBS (e.g., plating medium). The FBS will inhibit further trypsin activity.

7. Remove solution and centrifuge at 200 × g for 5 minutes.

8. Aspirate the supernatant taking care not to disturb the cell pellet; resuspend in plating medium. Repeat steps 7 and 8 to remove residual trypsin.

9. If needed, count cells and determine density desired for subculture or other procedures. Otherwise, a 1:3 or 1:5 dilution can be used for secondary seeding.

10. Plate as described for monolayer culture in Section 7.1.4.1.

7.1.5 3D Cultures

3D cultures aim to recapitulate the 3D environment of the chondrocyte, so as to better retain chondrocyte phenotype. However, as noted before, there are disadvantages to 3D culture. Generally, these cultures are more difficult to assay or extract materials from the sample and usually do not promote chondrocyte proliferation, and so may limit cell number. On the other hand, these cultures are generally easier to handle, and certain experimental techniques, for example, mechanical testing, are more amenable to 3D cultures. Of the 3D culture techniques available, two general methods are used: encapsulation within a hydrogel (see Section 4.3.1) or cell-only techniques. Seeding onto artificial scaffolds, while discussed in Chapter 4, is not presented here.

7.1.5.1 Hydrogel Encapsulation

Agarose is generally stiffer than alginate, and, thus, more amenable to creating shape-specific constructs or for mechanical testing. However, alginate is convenient for situations were recovery of the individual cells (or associated chondrons) is desired due to the ease of dissolution. Both hydrogels are discussed in more detail in Section 4.3.1. While not discussed here, it should be noted that a plethora of other hydrogels are available. Many have novel polymerization strategies or physical properties that may be advantageous to certain types of experiments.

7.1.5.1.1 Agarose

Agarose is commonly employed in applications where constructs will be used for mechanical stimulation due to the favorable compressive properties, compared with other softer hydrogels. A variety of concentrations can be used, although 2-3% agarose will yield a gel with adequate handling, culture, and biomechanical properties. The point at which agarose gels exhibit hysteresis, that is, the point at which the material solidifies, is different than its melting temperature (which is higher). This is beneficial for cell culture, as it means that while the agarose will stay liquid at 37°C, once solidified it can be cultured at 37°C without risk of melting. However, protein, DNA, RNA retrieval from agarose is more difficult than alginate or 2D culture, being on par with native tissue.

A. Materials needed

Equipment
1. Autoclave
2. 12-well tissue culture dish
3. 37°C water bath
4. Sterile spatula
5. Sterile glass plates and spacers, or mold (see note below)—optional

Reagents
1. Low-melt agarose for tissue and cell culture (SeaPlaque®) at twice that of the final, desired concentration (e.g., for a 3% gel, start with a 6% solution)
2. Sterile PBS

3. Chondrogenic medium: DMEM medium containing 1% PSF, 1% NEAA, 1% ITS, 100 nM dexamethasone, 50 µg/ml ascorbate-2-phosphate, 40 µg/ml L-proline, and 100 µg/ml sodium pyruvate
4. Cell suspension

Note: If agarose constructs of predetermined and reproducible dimensions are needed, the agarose-cell mixture can be poured either in molds or between sterile glass plates, and disks of the needed sized punched once the agarose has solidified. These can then be cultured in a manner similar to that of explants. Cell densities of up to 10 million cells per milliliter are commonly used. Also, due to the viscous nature of the agarose-cell mixture, extra volume should be prepared to account for loss (e.g., retention in pipettes).

B. Procedure

1. Autoclave agarose solution to sterilize, and let it set in a 37°C water bath until temperature equilibrates; care must be taken to ensure that the agarose is not hotter than 40°C, as this will significantly reduce cell viability.
2. Gently centrifuge cells at 200 × g, and remove medium.
3. Resuspend desired cells per milliliter in one-half of desired final volume in chondrogenic medium. Add one-half final volume of 6% molten agarose and mix. Work quickly to prevent the agarose from solidifying. Make sure the temperature of the agarose is ~37°C so as to prevent thermal damage to the cells.
4. Pipette liquid agarose into mold or 12-well culture dish to produce constructs. Smaller tissue culture wells (e.g., 24-well dishes) can also be used; volume should be adjusted as necessary.
5. Allow agarose to solidify at room temperature in the tissue culture hood for 30 minutes. Alternatively, it can be transferred to 4°C for shorter gelling times.

6. Agarose constructs can be retrieved from the tissue culture dish or mold using a sterile spatula and transferred to a larger dish containing chondrogenic medium.
7. Wash with chondrogenic medium twice to displace any remaining PBS from the agarose.
8. Constructs can be further cultured similarly to explants.

7.1.5.1.2 Alginate Beads

A. Materials needed

Equipment
1. 10 ml syringe and 22-gauge needle
2. 10 cm tissue culture dish
3. 50 ml sterile tube

Reagents
1. Salt solution: 0.15 M sodium chloride and 25 mM HEPES buffered at pH 7.4, sterile filtered
2. Alginate: 1.25% alginate in salt solution, sterile (can be autoclaved or filtered)
3. 102 mM calcium chloride in water, sterile
4. 55 mM sodium citrate in salt solution, sterile (for cell recovery)
5. Chondrogenic medium: DMEM medium containing 1% PSF, 1% NEAA, 1% ITS, 100 nM dexamethasone, 50 μg/ml ascorbate-2-phosphate, 40 μg/ml L-proline, and 100 μg/ml sodium pyruvate
6. Cells in suspension

Note: Aside from the use of sodium citrate, calcium chelators such as EDTA and EGTA can also be used to recover cells from the alginate beads. Salt solutions, once sterilized, can be stored at room temperature. Cell densities of 1 million cells per milliliter are commonly used, although higher concentrations can be used if desired. Increased calcium concentrations can be used to increase alginate stiffness if desired.

B. Procedure

Part 1: Producing alginate beads
1. Gently centrifuge cells at 200 × g, and remove medium.
2. Resuspend cells in 1.25% alginate solution at desired density.
3. Fill 10 ml syringe with cells and attach 22-gauge needle.
4. Slowly depress syringe allowing cell-alginate mix to drip into a 10 cm tissue culture dish containing 102 mM calcium chloride solution.
5. Beads will appear to polymerize immediately, but should be allowed to fully cure for 5-10 minutes (Figure 7.4).
6. Remove solution and wash beads twice with salt solution.
7. Remove salt solution and wash beads twice with chondrogenic medium.
8. Transfer beads to desired culture container and cover with chondrogenic medium.

Part 2: Release of cells from alginate beads
1. Remove medium and wash beads twice with salt solution.
2. Transfer beads to a 50 ml tube and resuspend in three volumes of 55 mM sodium citrate in salt solution.

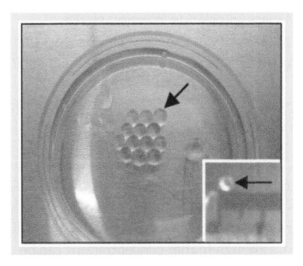

Figure 7.4 Alginate beads, approximately 3 mm (top arrow). Inset, single bead (bottom arrow). (From Bittencourt, R. A. d. C. et al., *Acta Ortop Bras* 17: 242-246, 2009. With permission.)

3. Mix solution with gentle rocking until beads have completely dissolved.

4. Gently centrifuge cells at 200 × g and remove supernatant from cell pellet.

7.1.5.2 Cell-Only Techniques

7.1.5.2.1 Micromass

Micromass is a high-density culture technique; cells are seeded at 100,000 cells in a 10 µl droplet and allowed to attach to tissue culture plastic. Micromass maintains chondrocyte phenotype, promotes chondrodifferentiation, and is easy to use (Figure 7.5).

A. Materials needed

Equipment
1. 24-well tissue culture plastic dish

Reagents
1. Plating medium: Chondrogenic or expansion medium plus 10% FBS (see Section 7.1.4.1 for expansion medium)

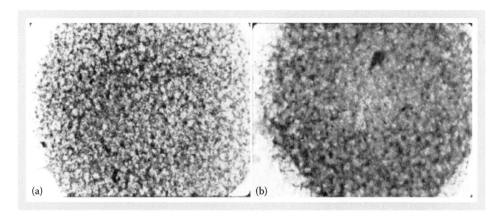

(a)   (b)

Figure 7.5 Bovine articular chondrocytes were grown in micromass culture for 7 days, and either left untreated (a) or treated with transforming growth factor β (TGF-β) (b). Blue color is a result of staining with Alcian blue to detect glycosaminoglycans. (Modified from Ramaswamy, G. et al., *Arthritis Res Ther* 14(2): R49, 2012. With permission.)

2. Chondrogenic medium: DMEM medium containing 1% PSF, 1% NEAA, 1% ITS, 100 nM dexamethasone, 50 µg/ml ascorbate-2-phosphate, 40 µg/ml L-proline, and 100 µg/ml sodium pyruvate
3. Cells in solution

Note: While chondrocytes in the micromass will maintain the chondrocyte phenotype, under certain conditions cells at the periphery may still proliferate and expand across the culture surface to produce a monolayer. Care should be taken to remove the micromass itself if further analysis is wanted, to exclude this monolayer population.

B. Procedure

1. Gently centrifuge cells at 200 × g, and remove medium.
2. Resuspend in final volume of plating medium at a density of 100,000 cells per 10 µl (10 million cells per milliliter).
3. Add 10 µl of cells in a droplet to the center of an empty well. Up to 50 µl can be used if desired.
4. Carefully move the plates into the incubator without disrupting the droplet of cells, and allow the cells to attach for a minimum of 2 hours at 37°C.
5. Add 1 ml of chondrogenic medium to each well, being careful not to disturb the micromass.

7.1.5.2.2 Pellet Culture

A. Materials needed

Equipment
1. 50 ml sterile tubes
2. Sterile spatula
3. Nonadherent petri dish

Reagents
1. Chondrogenic medium: DMEM medium containing 1% PSF, 1% NEAA, 1% ITS, 100 nM dexamethasone, 50 µg/ml ascorbate-2-phosphate, 40 µg/ml L-proline, and 100 µg/ml sodium pyruvate

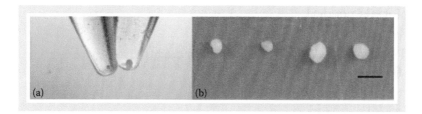

Figure 7.6 Images of pellet culture in 15 ml conical tubes (a) and removed, with 1 mm scale bar (b). In all images, pellets on the left were treated with incomplete chondrogenic medium + 10% FBS, while pellets on the right received complete chondrogenic medium containing TGF-β. (From Estes, B. T. et al., *Nat Protoc* 5(7): 1294-1311, 2010. With permission.)

2. Plating medium: Chondrogenic medium plus 10% FBS
3. Cells in solution, at a concentration of 10 million cells per milliliter

B. Procedure

1. Centrifuge cells at 500 × g for 10 minutes to obtain cell pellets (Figure 7.6).
2. Remove medium and gently replace with sufficient plating or chondrogenic medium to cover the pellet (5-10 ml).
3. Loosen caps of the 50 ml tubes to allow gas exchange and transfer to the incubator (37°C, 5% CO_2).
4. Replace medium daily for the first 3 days of culture.
5. After 3 days of culture, pellets can be transferred to nonadherent petri dishes, and medium replaced every 2-3 days.

7.1.5.2.3 Self-Assembly

Agarose wells are used as a nonadherent culturing environment for self-assembled constructs. Common dimensions for this are 3 or 5 mm wells, formed using custom-made well makers. Preparation of the agarose wells and quality control to discard wells with obvious defects (bubbles or broken agarose) are crucial for good construct formation. Typically, 5 mm wells are seeded with a concentration of 5.5 million chondrocytes in a volume of 100 μl.

A. Materials needed

Equipment
1. 60°C oven
2. Sterile 5 mm well makers
3. Sterile spatulas
4. 48-well plate

Reagents
1. Chondrogenic medium: DMEM medium containing 1% PSF, 1% NEAA, 1% ITS, 100 nM dexamethasone, 50 µg/ml ascorbate-2-phosphate, 40 µg/ml L-proline, and 100 µg/ml sodium pyruvate
2. Agarose 2% in PBS, autoclaved
3. Cells in suspension

Note: Work quickly with the agarose to avoid premature gelling, and return the agarose to the oven after use. Once autoclaved, the agarose remains usable for approximately 1 week and can be microwaved if it solidifies. Agarose that has any changes in color should be discarded. Wells can be made up to 1 week prior to seeding.

B. Procedure

Part 1: Making wells
1. Add 0.8 ml of molten agarose to the center of each of 6 wells in 48 wells and insert well maker (Figure 7.7).

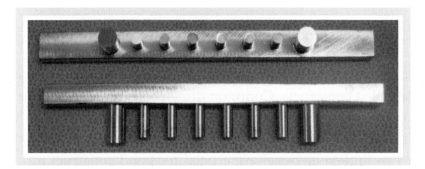

Figure 7.7 Well makers used for producing the 5 mm diameter agarose wells used in self-assembly.

2. Wait ~15-20 minutes until the agarose is set (it will turn slightly opaque).

3. Add >500 μl of chondrogenic medium to each well to displace PBS, allow to set for 5-10 minutes, and remove by aspiration. Refill wells with >500 μl of chondrogenic medium and place in the incubator until needed.

Part 2: Seeding cells

1. Resuspend chondrocytes at a density of 5.5 million per 100 μl. Slowly and carefully pipette into the bottom of the 5 mm diameter agarose wells.

2. Allow seeded chondrocytes to assemble for a minimum of 4 hours before adding 400 μl of chondrogenic medium. Carefully add medium to the top of the well at the edge of the agarose and allow it to gently flow onto the construct, taking care not to disrupt the construct.

3. Replace medium daily (500 μl per well). Take care not to disrupt the construct during medium changes.

4. Prior to day 10 of culture, prepare coated 48-well plates with 500 μl of agarose per well. Replace PBS with medium as described above.

5. After 10 days, using a sterile spatula, transfer the construct to the agarose-coated 48-well plate.

6. Continue culturing as needed. After the time desired (e.g., 4 weeks), constructs can be assayed as needed.

7.2 GROSS MORPHOLOGY, HISTOLOGY, AND IMMUNOHISTOCHEMISTRY

7.2.1 Photodocumentation of Gross Morphology

Gross morphological images provide easy visualization of shape and the measurement of construct dimensions if rulers are included in the images. They can also inform about less easily quantifiable parameters, such as surface texture and translucency. High-quality images should

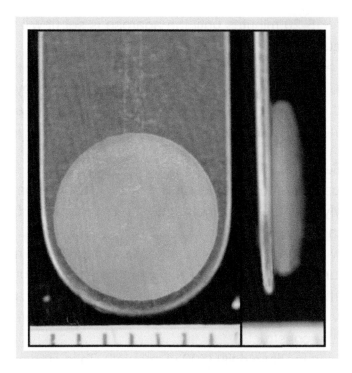

Figure 7.8 Photodocumentation of gross morphology from both top and side views of a bovine self-assembled construct along a ruler (bottom of image) allows for dimensional information to be obtained.

be taken with a stand-mounted digital camera for all pertinent axes of any tissue or tissue-engineered construct prior to mechanical testing or using visualization techniques such as India ink. Thickness, width, or diameter can be extracted from such images if an in-plane ruler is included in the picture (Figure 7.8).

7.2.2 India Ink

Piercing the cartilage surface with a needle dipped in India ink produces a "split" that follows the direction of collagen fibrils. This technique provides a simple way of visualizing fibril orientation at the cartilage surface, that is, via "split lines" (Figure 7.9) (Meachim 1972). A diluted solution of India ink can also be pipetted onto cartilage, and the excess washed off with PBS to increase the contrast of fibrillations or other surface defects.

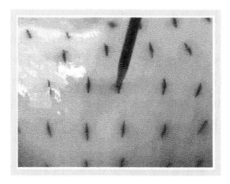

Figure 7.9 Split lines being produced in human cadaveric knee cartilage using a sharpened awl dipped in India ink. (From Below, S. et al., *Arthroscopy* 18(6): 613-617, 2002. With permission.)

A. Materials needed

Equipment
1. 22-gauge needle, sewing needle, or awl

Reagents
1. India ink
2. PBS

Note: Split lines may be difficult to detect in very young cartilage.

B. Procedure

1. Dilute the India ink 1:2 with PBS.
2. Dip the needle or awl into the diluted India ink solution.
3. Lightly poke the cartilage surface with the needle.

7.2.3 Histology

Common stains and their chemistry used for articular cartilage are described in Section 5.2. The general procedure for preparing frozen sections differs from that for fixed paraffin-embedded sections. However, subsequent staining is similar. Fixation involves chemically cross-linking the components of the cells and tissue to preserve morphology. Fixatives for paraffin embedding include neutral buffered formalin, paraformaldehyde, and Bouin's fixative. Frozen sections can be produced with or without prior fixation. After embedding the sample and sectioning, unfixed sections should be fixed prior to staining. The use of a microtome or cryotome for sample sectioning is not described here. It should be noted that sectioning requires a significant amount of "art" to produce quality sections.

Positive and negative controls should be stained along with the samples of interest. Different tissues (native articular cartilage, tissue-engineered articular cartilage, or fibrocartilage) will take up stains differently based on tissue composition. If possible, slides should be fixed, deparaffinized, and stained in a chemical fume hood.

7.2.3.1 Fixing Cryosectioned Slides

Cryosectioned slides should be fixed before staining if not prior to embedding. Slides prepared from frozen sections should be placed on a slide warmer for 10-20 minutes prior to fixation. Fixing directly from the freezer or refrigerator can cause samples to wash off the slide. For immunohistochemistry, slides may be fixed in cold acetone, as per the immunohistochemistry protocol for frozen sections (Section 7.2.3.2).

A. Materials needed

Equipment
1. Glass slides
2. Slide holder and bath
3. Slide warmer

Reagents
1. 10% neutral buffered formalin

Note: If possible, slides should be fixed in a chemical fume hood.

B. Procedure

1. For all histology staining, fix slides in 10% neutral buffered formalin for 10 minutes prior to staining. Slides should go directly from the slide warmer into formalin.
2. After fixing, rinse in deionized water.
3. Slides are ready for further staining.

7.2.3.2 Clearing Paraffin Slides for Staining

Before staining or immunohistochemistry, paraffin-embedded slides need to be cleared of paraffin and rehydrated. Following clearing, paraffin-processed slides can be used for multiple staining protocols.

A. Materials needed

Equipment
1. Glass slides
2. Slide holder and bath

Reagents
1. Paraffin clearing agent, such as Safeclear, Citri-solv, or xylene
2. Ethanol solutions, 70%, 80%, 95%, and 100%, prepared in deionized or ultrapure water

Note: Slides should be cleared of paraffin in a chemical fume hood. While xylene effectively removes paraffin, safer alternatives are available (e.g., Safeclear and Citri-solv).

B. Procedure

1. Place slides in paraffin clearing agent for 5 minutes.
2. Repeat step 1 with a fresh container of clearing agent. Clearing agent from the second step can be reused for the first clearing step for other slides.

3. Place slides in 100% ethanol for 2 minutes.
4. Place slides in 95% ethanol for 2 minutes.
5. Place slides in 80% ethanol for 2 minutes.
6. Place slides in 70% ethanol for 2 minutes.
7. Slides are ready for further staining.

7.2.3.3 Safranin O with Fast Green Counterstain

In articular cartilage, Safranin O dye stains sulfated glycosaminogly-cans (sGAGs) red, while the background counterstains green by the Fast Green, and cell nuclei stain a dark purple (Figure 7.10).

A. Materials needed

Equipment
1. Glass slides
2. Slide holder and bath
3. Coverslips

Reagents
1. Weigart's hematoxylin kit (Sigma HT1079), prepared fresh before use
2. Fast Green, 0.001%, prepared in deionized water

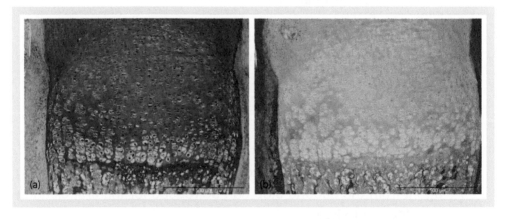

Figure 7.10 Safranin O- and Fast Green-stained (b) and picrosirius red-stained (a) paraffin-embedded section of neonatal canine distal fibula growth plate (10×). (Courtesy of Dr. Natalia Vapniarsky.)

3. Safranin O, 0.1%, prepared in deionized water
4. Acetic acid, 1%, prepared in deionized water
5. Ethanol solutions, 70%, 80%, 90%, 95%, and 100%, prepared in deionized or ultrapure water
6. Permount mounting medium

Note: Safranin O and Fast Green solutions are stable at room temperature for several weeks or longer. Acid solutions should be prepared by adding the concentrated acid solution to the water while mixing.

B. Procedure

1. Place fixed slides in Weigart's hematoxylin for 1 minute.
2. Wash in deionized water until no more dye washes off.
3. Place slides in Fast Green to counterstain for 3 minutes.
4. Wash in deionized water until no more dye washes off.
5. Place in 1% acetic acid for 15 minutes.
6. Place directly from the acetic acid into Safranin O for 1 minute.
7. Wash in deionized water until no more dye washes off.
8. Dehydrate through ascending ethanol in steps of 70%, 80%, 90%, 95%, and 100%; incubate slides 2 minutes per solution.
9. Dry slides for 5 minutes.
10. Mount slides using Permount medium and apply coverslip. Allow to dry for several hours to overnight before imaging.

7.2.3.4 Picrosirius Red

In articular cartilage, picrosirius red stains all collagens red and the background yellow. Stained slides can be viewed using polarized light microscopy to detect collagen fiber alignment. Fibers will appear as brighter regions or "streaks" against a dark background.

A. Materials needed

Equipment
1. Glass slides

2. Slide holder and bath
3. Coverslips

Reagents
1. Picrosirius red, 0.1%, prepared in saturated aqueous picric acid (1.3%)
2. Ethanol solutions, 70%, 80%, 90%, 95%, and 100%, prepared in deionized or ultrapure water
3. Permount mounting medium

Note: Picrosirius red solution is stable at room temperature for several weeks or longer. Dried picric acid is explosive.

B. Procedure

1. Place fixed slides in picrosirius red solution for 1 hour.
2. Wash in deionized water until no more dye washes off.
3. Dehydrate through ascending ethanol in steps of 70%, 80%, 90%, 95%, and 100%; incubate slides 2 minutes per solution.
4. Dry slides for 5 minutes.
5. Mount slides using Permount medium and apply coverslip. Allow to dry for several hours to overnight before imaging.

7.2.3.5 Hematoxylin and Eosin

Hematoxylin and eosin (H&E) is one of the most popular staining methods in histology and pathology. In articular cartilage, H&E will stain glycosaminoglycans dark purple, while nuclei stain blue. Cytoplasm and collagen will stain pink to red (Figure 7.11).

A. Materials needed

Equipment
1. Glass slides
2. Slide holder and bath
3. Coverslips

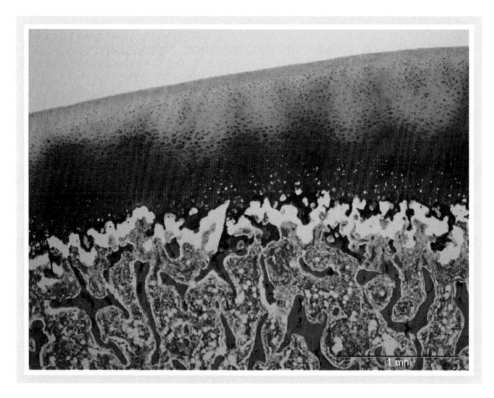

Figure 7.11 H&E-stained and paraffin-embedded section of 5-month-old canine articular cartilage. (Courtesy of Dr. Natalia Vapniarsky.)

Reagents
1. Harris modified hematoxylin, filtered before use
2. Eosin Y solution
3. Acetic acid, 2%, prepared in deionized water
4. Ammonium hydroxide, 1% (NH_4OH), prepared in deionized water
5. Ethanol solutions, 70%, 80%, 90%, 95%, and 100%, prepared in deionized or ultrapure water
6. Permount mounting medium

Note: Both Harris modified hematoxylin and Eosin Y are available commercially as premade solutions from multiple vendors.

B. Procedure

1. Place fixed slides in Harris modified hematoxylin solution for 3 minutes.
2. Wash in deionized water until no more dye washes off.
3. Dip slides in 2% acetic acid eight times.
4. Dip slides in deionized water eight times.
5. Dip slides in 1% ammonium hydroxide solution eight times.
6. Dehydrate through ascending ethanol in steps of 70%, 80%, 90%, and 95%; incubate slides 2 minutes per solution.
7. Place slides in Eosin Y solution for 1 minute.
8. Dehydrate by dipping slides in 95% ethanol three times; repeat with 100% ethanol.
9. Dry slides for 5 minutes.
10. Mount slides using Permount medium and apply coverslip. Allow to dry for several hours to overnight before imaging.

7.2.3.6 Alcian Blue

In articular cartilage, Alcian blue stains glycosaminoglycans (or mucins) blue. This dye should be maintained at a pH of 1.0 to detect sGAGs, or at a pH of 2.5 to detect other glycosaminoglycans. See Figure 7.5 for an example of Alcian blue staining of a micromass culture.

A. Materials needed

Equipment
1. Glass slides
2. Slide holder and bath
3. Coverslips

Reagents
1. Alcian Blue 8GX, 0.05%, pH 2.5, in 3% acetic acid, or pH 1.0 in 0.1 M hydrochloric acid
2. Ethanol solutions, 70%, 80%, 90%, 95%, and 100%, prepared in deionized or ultrapure water
3. Permount mounting medium

Note: Alcian blue solution is stable at room temperature for several weeks or longer.

B. Procedure

1. Place fixed slides in Alcian blue solution for 1 hour.
2. Wash in deionized water until no more dye washes off.
3. Dehydrate through ascending ethanol in steps of 70%, 80%, 90%, 95%, and 100%; incubate slides 2 minutes per solution.
4. Dry slides for 5 minutes.
5. Mount slides using Permount medium and apply coverslip. Allow to dry for several hours to overnight before imaging.

7.2.4 Immunohistochemistry

Similar to antibody detection methods employed for Western blot and enzyme-linked immunosorbent assay (ELISA), described in Section 7.3.3, immunohistochemistry uses antibodies to detect specific antigens, commonly proteins, on slides of tissues or cells. This allows for detection and localization information to be determined for a specific antigen. For example, this is commonly used to determine if type I collagen is present in tissue-engineered articular cartilage. Some antigens may be more favorably detected by immunohistochemistry from frozen sections as opposed to paraffin-embedded sections. Also, individual antibodies will likely need to be tested on positive controls to determine optimum dilutions and staining conditions. Species variability may require different antibody conditions to be used per species tested due to differences in antibody binding and substrate specificity.

Following fixation and embedding (especially with paraffin), insufficient signal may be seen with immunostaining, as epitopes may be obscured. Formalin or other aldehyde fixation forms protein cross-links that mask the antigenic sites in tissue specimens, thereby giving weak or false negative staining for immunohistochemical detection of certain proteins. To overcome this limitation, several methods of "antigen retrieval" have been developed. The choice of which specific method to use is dependent on both the antibody used andthe epitope being analyzed.

7.2.4.1 Antigen Retrieval

A citric acid buffer-EDTA-based solution is used to break the protein cross-links produced during fixation, unmasking the antigens and epitopes and enhancing antibody staining intensity. This antigen retrieval protocol is relatively gentle and works well with articular cartilage tissue samples that have been paraffin embedded. Slides should be deparaffinized (Section 7.2.3.2) before undertaking antigen retrieval.

   A. Materials needed

      Equipment
      1. Slide holder
      2. Staining dish or other heat-resistant container
      3. Hot plate

      Reagents
      1. Citric acid buffer: 10 mM citric acid, 2 mM EDTA, and 0.05% Tween-20, pH 6.2

Note: Citric acid buffer can be stored at room temperature for up to 3 months or at 4°C for up to 6 months. Incubation time in the citric acid buffer may need to be optimized depending on sample type, but should be kept consistent within a group of samples to reduce artifactual staining intensity differences.

   B. Procedure

      1. Rinse deparaffinized slides (see Section 7.2.3.2) in deionized water.

2. Preheat water bath with staining dish containing citric acid buffer until almost boiling (~95°C).
3. Place slides in slide holder in the staining dish or other container. Cover container loosely and heat for 15 minutes.
4. Remove slides and allow to cool for 20 minutes before proceeding with immunohistochemistry.

7.2.4.2 Antibody Detection for Immunohistochemistry

Unfixed sections that have been cryosectioned should be fixed prior to immunohistochemistry, as described below in Part 1 of the protocol. Paraffin-embedded sections should be cleared of paraffin prior to immunohistochemistry. This protocol starts at Part 2 and is modified from the Vectastain manufacturer's instructions.

A. Materials needed

Equipment
1. Slides with specimens
2. Slide holder and baths
3. Humidified slide box
4. PapPen, or other hydrophobic marker (e.g., grease pen)

Reagents
1. Primary antibody, diluted in PBS according to specific antibody, commonly 1:50-1:1000
2. Vectastain kit, including secondary antibody, blocking solution, and visualization agent, 3,3′-diaminobenzidine (DAB)
3. PBS-Tween: PBS with 0.025% Tween-20
4. Blocking buffer: PBS with 0.025% Tween-20 and 5% normal serum
5. Wash/incubation buffer: PBS with 0.025% Tween-20 and 0.2% normal serum
6. Harris hematoxylin for counterstaining nuclei—optional
7. 2% acetic acid (used with hematoxylin counterstaining)

8. Bluing solution: Five drops of concentrated ammonium hydroxide (NH_4OH) in 100 ml of water
9. Ethanol solutions, 70%, 80%, 90%, 95%, and 100%, prepared in deionized or ultrapure water
10. 3% hydrogen peroxide (H_2O_2) in methanol (MeOH)

Note: Never allow sections to dry out; keep sections moist at all times.

B. Procedure

Part 1: Fixing cryosectioned slides for immunohistochemistry
1. Place on slide warmer at <37°C for at least 6 hours.
2. For frozen slides that have not previously been fixed, fix in chilled acetone at 4°C for 20 minutes.
3. Allow to air-dry, and then outline samples on the slides with a PapPen.
4. Rehydrate through descending ethanol in steps of 100%, 95%, 90%, 80%, and 70%, ending with water; incubate slides 2 minutes per solution.

Part 2: Antibody staining for immunohistochemistry (e.g., Figure 7.12)
1. Wash slides for 5 minutes with PBS-Tween.
2. Incubate slides in 3% hydrogen peroxide in methanol for 30 minutes to quench native peroxidases.
3. Wash slides three times with PBS-Tween.
4. Incubate slides with normal serum block for 20 minutes at room temperature.
5. Incubate slides with primary antibody for 1 hour at room temperature.
6. Wash slides three times with PBS-Tween.
7. Make ABC solution 30 minutes prior to use.
8. Incubate slides with secondary antibody from Vectastain kit for 30 minutes.
9. Wash slides three times with PBS-Tween.

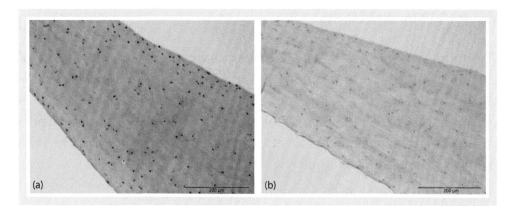

Figure 7.12 H&E staining (a) and type II collagen immunohistochemistry (IHC) of juvenile bovine meniscus (b). The IHC section (a) indicates the presence of type II collagen (brown); dark blue nuclei are also visible due to counterstaining with hematoxylin. (Courtesy of Dr. Natalia Vapniarsky.)

10. Incubate slides with ABC solution for 30 minutes.
11. Wash slides three times with PBS-Tween.
12. Incubate slides with DAB for 4-8 minutes, or until color develops.
13. Wash slides three times in deionized water, until dye no longer runs off.

Part 3: Counterstaining nuclei with Harris hematoxylin (optional)
1. Incubate slides in Harris hematoxylin for less than 10 seconds.
2. Rinse slides in water.
3. If stain is too dark, destain slides with 2% acetic acid for 1.5-3 minutes.
4. Rinse slides in water.
5. Place slides in bluing solution for 30 seconds.
6. Rinse slides in water.

Part 4: Dehydration and coverslipping
1. Dehydrate through ascending ethanol in steps of 70%, 80%, 90%, 95%, and 100%; incubate slides 2 minutes per solution.
2. Dry slides for 5 minutes.
3. Mount slides using Permount medium and apply coverslip. Allow to dry for several hours to overnight before imaging.

7.3 PROTEIN ANALYSIS

The following protocols deal with both extraction and processing of protein from samples for qualitative and quantitative detection of protein presence, quantity, and posttranslational modifications such as phosphorylation. These techniques can be applied to determine important signaling events and their effect on protein expression within the pathway analysis paradigm.

The pathway analysis paradigm includes several steps: applying a stimulus, determining a measurable output, detecting changes in the signaling of target pathway components (usually changes in phosphorylation), and then altering that signaling via inhibition or activation (commonly by pharmacological means) to determine changes in the previously determined output. Through systematic probing, it can be determined if pathway components are sufficient or necessary for a specific stimulus to result in a specific output.

7.3.1 Protein Extraction

Extraction of proteins from 2D cultures is relatively simple, while extraction from 3D cultures or tissue requires mechanical dissociation, such as pulverization in liquid nitrogen (Section 7.3.1.2). The extraction protocols listed below are generalized for extracting cellular or cytoplasmic proteins using a lysis buffer based on a gentle detergent. For many of the insoluble or less soluble matrix proteins, this procedure may be inadequate, and guanidine or other strong extraction methods may be required. The lysis buffer presented here, NP40 buffer, is suitable for most whole cell extractions; however, for proteins known to form insoluble aggregates, or for nuclear proteins, radioimmunoprecipitation assay (RIPA) buffer may be preferred. Both are commercially available and are mildly denaturing buffers (RIPA more so than NP40). However, for determination of signaling events and other forms of pathway analysis, these lysis buffers will result in satisfactory material for further detection procedures, such as ELISA and Western blot. It should be noted that for conditions where native conformations or other protein-protein interactions are needed, a mild 50 mM Tris buffer can be used with mechanical lysis. However, this will not solubilize membrane-bound or cytoskeletal proteins. Following lysis, cellular proteins begin to degrade through the processes of proteolysis, denaturation, and dephosphorylation. This can be inhibited by keeping the samples on ice (4°C) and through the use of protease and phosphatase inhibitors in the lysis buffer. Premade cocktails of these inhibitors are commercially available from Roche, Pierce, or Sigma.

7.3.1.1 Protein Extraction for 2D Cultures

A. Materials needed

Equipment
1. Cell scraper, placed on ice
2. Ice bucket
3. Tissue or cell culture dish with cells in monolayer
4. 1.5 ml microcentrifuge tubes (on ice)
5. Refrigerated microcentrifuge

Reagents
1. Lysis buffer (NP40 buffer): 150 mM sodium chloride, 1.0% NP40 (or Triton X-100), and 50 mM Tris, pH 8.0; to produce RIPA buffer instead, add 0.5% sodium deoxycholate and 0.1% sodium dodecyl sulfate (SDS); keep on ice at all times
2. Protease inhibitor (Roche cOmplete ULTRA tablets) or phosphatase inhibitor cocktail (Roche PhosSTOP, phosphatase inhibitor cocktail tablets)
3. PBS, placed on ice

Note: Lysis buffer is stable at 4°C for greater than 1 month, and aliquots can be stored at -20°C for up to 1 year. Protease or phosphatase inhibitors should be added to the lysis buffer just prior to use. All reagents and samples should be kept on ice at all times.

B. Procedure

1. Place the culture dish on ice and remove medium. Gently wash cells with cold PBS.
2. Remove PBS and cold lysis buffer. For confluent (~10 million cells) 10 cm dishes, add 1 ml; for smaller dishes, reduce lysis buffer volume. Approximately 100 µl of lysis buffer should be used per 1 million cells.
3. Scrape cells off dish and transfer to a cold 1.5 ml microcentrifuge tube.
4. Keep on ice for 15 minutes and vortex every 2-3 minutes.
5. Centrifuge at 4°C on maximum speed in a refrigerated microcentrifuge.
6. Transfer the tubes onto ice gently, making sure not to disrupt the cell pellet.
7. Transfer the supernatant to fresh 1.5 ml tubes and keep on ice. Discard the cell pellet.

7.3.1.2 Liquid Nitrogen Pulverization and Protein Extraction for Tissues and 3D Cultures

Extraction of protein from tissues and 3D cultures of cartilage is hindered by the extensive extracellular matrix. Review 2D culture protein extraction (Section 7.3.1.1) for determination of appropriate amounts of lysis buffer to use and other instructions.

A. Materials needed

Equipment
1. Dewar flask to store liquid nitrogen; for temporary storage, Styrofoam containers can be used
2. Styrofoam container (disposable); check the bottom for leaks following this protocol and replace as necessary
3. Cryo gloves, goggles, and other needed personal protective equipment

4. Aluminum foil, two squares (5-7 cm) for each sample
5. Pulverizer, or mortar and pestle

Reagents
1. Liquid nitrogen
2. Lysis buffer (NP40 buffer): 150 mM sodium chloride, 1.0% NP40 (or Triton X-100), and 50 mM Tris, pH 8.0; to produce RIPA buffer instead, add 0.5% sodium deoxycholate and 0.1% SDS; keep on ice at all times
3. Protease inhibitor (Roche cOmplete ULTRA tablets) or phosphatase inhibitor cocktail (Roche PhosSTOP, phosphatase inhibitor cocktail tablets)

Note: Tissues or 3D cultures can also be disrupted by using an electric homogenizer if liquid nitrogen is not available. However, care should be taken to thoroughly clean between samples, and always homogenize samples on ice to prevent heating. Although the protocol described here uses a custom-built metal pulverizer (Figure 7.13), these are also commercially available. The use of aluminum foil surrounding the sample eases cleanup between samples and

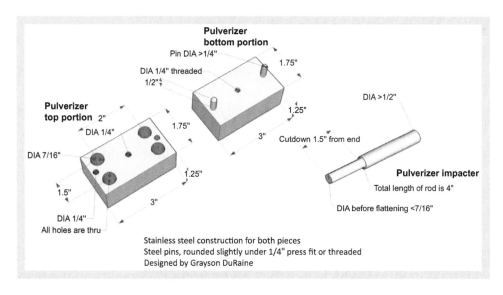

Figure 7.13 Dimensioned drawing of a custom-built metal pulverizer for protein and RNA extraction.

reduces the loss of the powdered sample. Generally, the aluminum foil should not interfere with protein extraction. Alternatively, a mortar and pestle can also be used. As this protocol uses liquid nitrogen, personal protective equipment should be worn at all times.

B. Procedure

1. In a Styrofoam container, place the pulverizer and add liquid nitrogen to a level about 1 cm above the top of the pulverizer. The addition of a flat metal plate below the pulverizer will extend the life of the Styrofoam container.
2. After the liquid nitrogen evaporates below the top of the pulverizer base, push a piece of foil over the well, push the pulverizer piston down into the well, and tap it to create an aluminum foil disk to place the sample on.
3. Place sample on aluminum foil.
4. Place second piece of aluminum foil over hole and push down gently to sandwich the sample between the foil.
5. Using the pulverizer piston, pulverize the sample between the pieces of aluminum foil.
6. Disassemble the pulverizer, remove the aluminum foil and sample, and place in lysis buffer.
7. Keep on ice for 15 minutes and vortex every 2-3 minutes.
8. Centrifuge at 4°C on maximum speed in a refrigerated microcentrifuge.
9. Transfer the tubes onto ice gently, making sure not to disrupt the cell pellet.
10. Transfer the supernatant to fresh 1.5 ml tubes and keep on ice. Discard the cell pellet.

7.3.2 Protein Quantification

The most common method for quantifying proteins is the bicinchoninic acid (BCA) method, which, like the Lowry method, depends on the reaction being under alkaline conditions of Cu^{2+} with specific amino acid residues converting to the Cu^+ form. This is detectable as a colorimetric change from green to purple (562 nm); however, this suffers from sensitivity to the presence of reducing agents. This method is also dependent on the amino acid sequence of the assayed proteins themselves, as this conversion varies based on the presence of cysteine, cystine, tyrosine, or tryptophan groups. As these groups are in low abundance in collagen, this may not be suitable for protein solutions of cartilage that contain abundant collagen. An alternate technique, the Bradford assay, is based on the binding of Coomassie blue and absorbance shift to 595 nm of the blue dye. Preferentially, this binding is to the side groups on the arginine, phenylalanine, proline, and tryptophan residues, but this assay suffers from sensitivity to detergents (such as SDS). Other techniques are also available for protein quantification; however, the ease of use of the BCA and Bradford techniques has made them extremely common. In practical use, these limitations in detection are rarely important, as most quantification is relative. Commonly, quantification is between sample treatment groups, which are rarely different enough in total protein profile to cause problems using these techniques. As with any protein quantification technique, the preparation of an appropriate standard curve within the linear range of the particular assay is paramount. Generally, bovine serum album (BSA) will give satisfactory results as a protein standard, especially where determination of relative protein quantification is more important, for example, to standardize gel loading on a Western blot.

7.3.2.1 Bicinchoninic Acid

A. Materials needed

Equipment
1. Spectrophotometer and cuvettes; alternatively, plate reader and 96-well plates
2. 15 ml tubes
3. Water bath at 60°C

Reagents
1. Pierce Micro BCA Protein Assay Kit

2. Protein standard, BSA, is provided in the kit and is suitable for most proteins
3. Working solution: BCA reagents; 1 ml working solution is needed per sample or standard; to produce this solution, add 25 parts reagent "MA" to 24 parts reagent "MB" and 1 part reagent "MC" and mix; the working solution is stable for several days at room temperature if kept away from light

Note: This method is modified from the manufacturer's instructions; the detection range is 0.5-20 µg/ml. Volumes can be reduced to one-fifth of stated values for a plate reader using a 96-well format.

B. Procedure

1. Prepare a standard curve using 2 mg/ml BSA stock solution (provided in 1 ml ampules) spanning the estimated concentration of your samples. If possible, standards should be made with the same diluent as the sample.
2. Pipet 1 ml of each standard and sample into 15 ml centrifuge tubes. Blank tubes should consist of 1 ml of diluents.
3. Add 1 ml of the working solution to each 15 ml centrifuge tube containing samples or standards.
4. Incubate the tubes for 1 hour at 60°C.
5. Allow tubes to cool to room temperature; agitate occasionally as they cool.
6. Measure the absorbance at 562 nm; samples should be read as soon as possible as color will continue to develop.

7.3.2.2 Coomassie Blue Assay (Bradford)

A. Materials needed

Equipment
1. Spectrophotometer and cuvettes; alternatively, plate reader and 96-well plates

Reagents
1. Coomassie® Plus Protein Assay Reagent (Pierce 23237, 100 ml)
2. BSA protein standard

Note: The standards should be diluted in the same solution as that of the samples (if possible). Protein concentrations outside of the detection range may require dilution or use of the low-protein-concentration protocol (Part 2). This protocol is modified from the manufacturer's instructions. Volumes can be reduced to one-fifth of stated values for a plate reader using a 96-well format.

B. Procedure

Part 1: Protocol for protein concentrations in the range of 75-1,500 µg/ml
1. Mix reagent in bottle prior to use by gentle inversion.
2. Prepare a known protein concentration series of BSA or other protein standard in concentrations between 75 and 1,500 µg/ml. Concentrations of 75, 150, 300, 450, 900, and 1,500 µg/ml work well.
3. Add 0.05 ml of standard or sample into a cuvette.
4. Add 1.5 ml of Coomassie Plus Protein Assay Reagent; mix well.
5. Read absorbance at 595 nm of standards and samples. Subtract absorbance of a blank filled with the same solution as that used for the standards.
6. Determine the protein concentration for each sample based on the standard curve.

Part 2: Protocol for protein concentrations in the range of 1-25 µg/ml (microassay)
1. Mix reagent in bottle prior to use by gentle inversion.
2. Prepare a known protein concentration series of BSA or other protein standard in concentrations between 1 and 25 µg/ml. Concentrations of 1, 5, 10, 15, and 25 µg/ml work well.
3. Add 1.0 ml of dilute standard or sample into a cuvette.
4. Add 1.0 ml of Coomassie Plus Protein Assay Reagent; mix well.

5. Read absorbance at 595 nm of standards and samples. Subtract absorbance of a blank filled with the same solution as that used for the standards.

6. Determine the protein concentration for each sample based on the standard curve.

7.3.3 Antibody-Based Detection Methods

Antibody-based detection methods take advantage of the high substrate specificity of antibodies. Both ELISA (Figure 7.14) and Western blot (also known as immunoblot) work on similar principles. Fundamentally, a primary antibody against the protein or antigenic epitope of interest is incubated with a bound sample containing the target. A secondary antibody specific to the nonvariable heavy-chain region of the primary antibody is then added; commonly, this will be conjugated with an enzyme to allow visualization by changing a chemical substrate.

Protein extracted for Western blot use may also be used for ELISA; however, detection of proteins poorly solubilized by detergents, such as collagen, may be poor. Ideally, ELISA should be used where quantification of proteins, for example, quantification of signaling components, or phosphorylation events is wanted. Protein preparations for Western blot make use of a gentle detergent lysis buffer and exclude enzymatic digest. Western blot allows for separation of proteins based on

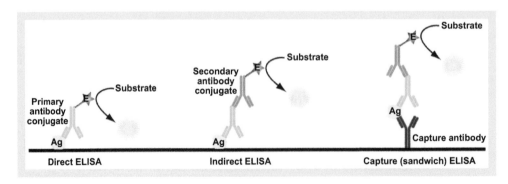

Figure 7.14 Diagram of several common types of ELISA assays in use. Ag, antigen; E, enzyme.

molecular weight through a polyacrylamide gel and is a qualitative to semiquantitative procedure. However, the gel-based separation by size allows for detection of components with similar antigenic sites that may vary in size, for example, determining if a specific protein is cleaved by enzymatic activity, or where the specificity of the antibody is poor.

It should be noted that for collagens, which are largely insoluble, enzymatically digested samples may be recommended for ELISA over those extracted using detergent-based lysis buffers. However, the choice of digestion enzyme and time and temperature of digestion may alter results from the ELISA, and digested samples are usually not suitable for Western blot. The sandwich ELISA presented here is commonly used for type I and type II collagen detection using a pepsin-elastase digestion. However, this may have compatibility issues with hydroxyproline-based, total collagen assays. The use of papain-digested samples for ELISA may render lower protein concentrations, so every assurance should be made that the standards used for detection accurately correspond to the samples tested.

7.3.3.1 Enzyme-Linked Immunosorbent Assay

Multiple types of ELISA are available, including standard, sandwich, and competitive. Presented in this protocol are the classic standard ELISA and the sandwich ELISA. While the sandwich ELISA has better substrate specificity and sensitivity, it requires multiple primary antibodies directed against the target, which may not be readily available for all targets.

7.3.3.1.1 Standard ELISA

A. Materials needed

   Equipment
   1. Clear 96-well ELISA protein binding plate
   2. Foil for covering plates during incubation steps

3. Squirt bottle or multiwell pipette
4. Plate reader

Reagents
1. ELISA coating buffer: 50 mM sodium carbonate, Na_2CO_3 (15 mM), and $NaHCO_3$ (35 mM); pH should be 9.80-9.95; do not adjust
2. PBS-Tween
3. PBS-Tween with 1% BSA
4. Primary and secondary antibodies; secondary antibody should be enzyme conjugated
5. TMB solution: Tetramethyl benzidine (Pierce N301)
6. 1 N HCl
7. Protein of interest, or samples
8. Protein standard matched to primary antibody

Note: Proteins in medium or samples in lysis buffer may need to be diluted before adding to coating buffer to prevent inhibition of subsequent steps. Visualization steps will depend on the specific substrate chosen. While horseradish peroxidase (HRP)/TMB chemistry is described in this protocol, HRP/enhanced chemiluminescence (ECL) chemistry also works well.

B. Procedure

1. Dissolve protein or samples in ELISA coating buffer at 1 μg/ml; add coating buffer to samples, not vice versa. At a minimum, plate duplicate wells per sample.
2. Coat wells with 60 μl at room temperature for 16 hours, or for 2 hours at 37°C, in a humidified chamber. Do not allow wells to dry out.
3. Wash plate three times with PBS-Tween by gently filling all wells with a squirt bottle; invert plate and tap to empty.
4. Block plate with PBS-Tween with 1% BSA for 30 minutes at room temperature.
5. Incubate with primary antibody in PBS-Tween at 4°C overnight.

6. Wash plate three times with PBS-Tween by gently filling all wells with a squirt bottle; invert plate and tap to empty.
7. Add 100 µl of secondary antibody for 1 hour at room temperature.
8. Wash five times with PBS-Tween.
9. Add 100 µl of TMB and incubate at room temperature for 5-30 minutes, until standards begin to show a gradation of blue color.
10. Add 100 µl of 1 N HCl to stop reaction; solution color will change to yellow.
11. Read plate at 450 nm absorbance.

7.3.3.1.2 Sandwich ELISA

The sandwich ELISA allows for the quantification of different types of proteins, including collagens much like the standard ELISA. In this assay, an antibody against the target (capture) is first adsorbed onto the surface of the plate, after which the sample of interest is added. The capture antibody then binds to the epitope of interest in the solution, and the other materials in the solution are washed away. A second antibody (detection/primary), which binds to a different portion of the same protein of interest, is then added to detect the captured protein of interest. A secondary antibody with conjugated enzyme is then added that is specific to the primary antibody. Finally, a substrate (here TMB) is added to the well, and the enzyme conjugated to the secondary acts on the substrate, changing its color proportional to the amount of enzyme present, which corresponds to the amount of captured protein of interest. The reaction is then finally terminated with a strong acid, and the absorbance values are measured using a plate reader.

A. Materials needed

Equipment
1. Clear 96-well ELISA protein binding plate
2. Foil for covering plates during incubation steps
3. Squirt bottle or multiwell pipette
4. Plate reader

Reagents

1. ELISA coating buffer: 50 mM sodium carbonate, Na_2CO_3 (15 mM), and $NaHCO_3$ (35 mM); pH should be 9.80-9.95; do not adjust
2. PBS-Tween: PBS with 0.025% Tween-20
3. PBS with 2% BSA
4. Capture antibody, detection/primary and secondary antibodies; secondary antibody should be HRP conjugated
5. TMB solution: Tetramethyl benzidine (Pierce N301), 1 N HCl solution
6. Protein of interest, or samples
7. Protein standard matched to primary antibody

Note: Proteins in medium, or samples in lysis buffer, may need to be diluted before adding to coating buffer, to prevent inhibition of subsequent steps. Visualization steps will depend on the specific substrate chosen. While HRP/TMB chemistry is described in this protocol, HRP/ECL chemistry also works well.

B. Procedure

1. Plate samples or standards in duplicate in 96-well ELISA plate.
2. Add 100 μl of capture antibody in coating buffer.
3. Incubate plates overnight at 4°C.
4. Wash twice with PBS-Tween.
5. Add 200 μl of PBS with 2% BSA to block for 2 hours at room temperature or overnight at 4°C.
6. Wash three times with PBS-Tween.
7. Add 100 μl of standard diluted in PBS with 2% BSA.
8. Determine how much sample is needed to fall within the mid-point of the standard curve (1-100 μl) and add to 96-well plate.
9. Incubate for 2 hours at room temperature or overnight at 4°C.
10. Wash three times with PBS-Tween.
11. Add 100 μl of detection/primary antibody diluted in PBS with 2% BSA; incubate for 2 hours at room temperature or overnight at 4°C.

12. Wash twice with PBS-Tween.
13. Add 100 µl of secondary antibody diluted in PBS with 2% BSA for 1 hour at room temperature.
14. Wash five times with PBS-Tween.
15. Add 100 µl of TMB; incubate at room temperature for 5-30 minutes until standards begin to show a gradation of blue color.
16. Add 100 µl of 1 N HCl to stop reaction; solution color will change to yellow.
17. Read plate at 450 nm absorbance.

7.3.3.2 Western Blot/Immunoblot

The general assembly of a Western or immunoblot (Figure 7.15) will necessarily be determined by which manufacturer's blot apparatus is used. Membrane selection will be dependent on the charge of the proteins being investigated; commonly, polyvinylidene difluoride (PVDF) or nylon membranes will cover most cytosolic and other proteins of interest.

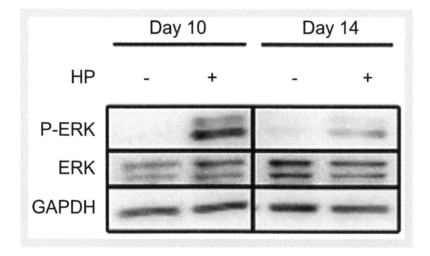

Figure 7.15 Example of immunoblot imaged with chemiluminescence (ECL) reagent. The immunoblot was initially probed with the antibody against phosphorylated extracellular signal-regulated kinase (P-ERK) and then stripped and reprobed for total ERK and GAPDH as loading control. (From DuRaine, G. D., and K. A. Athanasiou, *J Tissue Eng Regen Med* 9(4): 368-374, 2015. With permission.)

Several of the chemicals used are toxic; SDS is a very fine powder that is extremely irritating to the lungs, eyes, and skin. Always wear dust mask, glasses, and gloves. Acrylamide is a neurotoxic material; wear gloves, glasses, and a dust mask. Liquid solutions should be used when possible to reduce the risk of exposure. If possible, use of a fume hood is recommended when weighing out or initially mixing these reagents into solution.

A. Materials needed

Equipment
1. Western blot gel box and transfer apparatus
2. Power supply
3. Hot plate, with beaker full of water
4. Rocker or shaker
5. 1.5 ml microcentrifuge tubes
6. PVDF membrane
7. Filter paper and transfer sponges
8. Gel loading pipette tips
9. X-ray film or gel documentation system

Reagents (see note below)
1. 4× sample buffer
2. 10× Tris-glycine running buffer; make 1× before use with ultra-pure water
3. Transfer buffer: Towbin's 1× buffer
4. PBS-Tween: PBS with 0.025% Tween-20
5. Dried milk powder or BSA (used for blocking the membrane)
6. Blocking solution: PBS-Tween with 5% dried milk powder or 1% BSA
7. Methanol
8. β-Mercaptaethanol (BME)
9. Stripping buffer: 2% SDS and 70 mM, Tris pH 7 (strict)
10. 0.2 M sodium hydroxide (NaOH), used for stripping gels (gentle)

11. Premade Tris-glycine gel; 15% or 5-20% gradient gels will resolve most cytoplasmic proteins of interest; the brand of premade or precast gels should match that of the gel box
12. ECL reagent (Pierce)
13. Protein ladder

Note: Due to the large number of buffers and solutions, they are listed separately along with their needed reagents. Ponceau S or other stains can also be used to stain the membrane as an alternative to Coomassie blue.

4× sample buffer (makes 10 ml)

1.6 g	SDS
4.8 g	urea (8 M) (optional, deionize before use)
0.60 g	Tris (hydroxymethyl) aminomethane (0.5 M)
10 ml	ultrapure water

pH to 6.8

Add bromophenol blue until deep blue in color; the amount <1 g covering the tip of a spatula is sufficient

10× Tris-glycine running buffer (makes 1 L)

30 g	Tris (hydroxymethyl) aminomethane (0.25 M)
144 g	glycine (1.92 M)
10 g	SDS
1,000 ml	ultrapure water

pH 1× solution to 8.3 before use

20× Towbin's buffer (makes 1 L)

30 g	Tris (hydroxymethyl) aminomethane (0.25 M)
144 g	glycine (1.92 M)
1,000 ml	ultrapure water

1× Towbin's buffer (makes 4 L)

200 ml	20× Towbin's buffer
800 ml	methanol
3,000 ml	ultrapure water

Coomassie blue stain (makes 1 L)
- 400 ml   methanol (40%)
- 100 ml   isopropanol (10%)
- 100 ml   glacial acetic acid (10%)
- 400 ml   ultrapure water
- 8 g   Coomassie blue

B. Procedure

Part 1: Sample preparation and SDS-polyacrylamide gel electrophoresis (PAGE) gel loading
1. Mix 200 μl of 4× sample buffer with 20 μl of BME. BME will reduce disulfide bonds in the proteins.
2. Add 3.33 μl of sample buffer and BME to 10 μl of sample in a 1.5 ml microcentrifuge tube.
3. Heat at 95°C for 5 minutes in a beaker of water on a hot plate; tubes can be placed in a foam "floaty" upright. Do not fully immerse samples as tube tops may open.
4. Set up electrophoresis apparatus with premade gel.
5. Fill electrophoresis apparatus with Tris-glycine running buffer; approximately 600 ml is required for most small gel boxes.
6. Add 5 μl of marker to wells on each side of gel using a gel loading tip.
7. Add 10 μl of sample to each well.
8. Run gel at 160 V for 75 minutes.

Part 2: Transfer of the blot to membrane
1. Remove gel from electrophoresis apparatus.
2. Carefully open plastic gel cast and cut away the top and bottom edges of the gel.
3. Place blotting cassette in container filled with Towbin's buffer 1×.
4. Add two sponges into the submerged cassette, and ensure removal of all bubbles.
5. Add filter paper on top of sponges in submerged cassette.
6. Carefully place gel on top of filter paper in Towbin's buffer 1×.

7. Soak PVDF membrane in methanol, and then in Towbin's buffer 1×, and then place membrane on top of gel.
8. Add filter paper on top of PVDF membrane.
9. Add three sponges soaked in Towbin's buffer 1× into the cassette, and ensure the removal of all bubbles.
10. Close cassette and assemble blotting apparatus.
11. Fill electrophoresis apparatus with Towbin's buffer 1×; approximately 600 ml is required for most small gel boxes.
12. Blot gel at 25 V for 90 minutes.

Part 3: Coomassie staining
1. Once transferred, disassemble and check blot for transfer efficiency. Blot can now be Coomassie stained or blocked.
2. For Coomassie staining, place in dish with stain for 5 minutes on rocker.
3. Place in 40% methanol and 10% acetic acid in ultrapure water and wash, observing background. Watch until background appears light, but be careful not to destain too much; then wash off in deionized water.
4. For further use, place in methanol and wash two or three times on the rocker until staining disappears, or until solution is clear; wash off methanol in water.
5. Block blot for 1 hour in blocking solution.
6. Prepare primary antibody in blocking solution depending on concentration.
7. Place blot into small dish, add primary antibody solution (1-2 ml usually), and place on rocker for 1 hour.
8. Wash blot in PBS-Tween three times for 5 minutes each on rocker.
9. Prepare secondary antibody in 1-5 ml of PBS, cover blot similar to primary antibody, and place on rocker for 1 hour.
10. Wash blot in PBS-Tween three times for 5 minutes each on rocker.
11. If using ECL, mix chemiluminescence reagents and incubate on blot for 1 minute; seal blot in plastic film and image either by film or via gel documentation system suitable for ECL.

Part 4: Blot stripping (strict)
1. Heat stripping buffer to 70°C.
2. Add BME to 100 mM (stock is ~14 M).
3. Then pour onto blot and allow to cool.
4. Wash with PBS to remove stripping buffer.
5. Block and reprobe as usual.

Part 5: Blot stripping (gentle, easier, quicker protocol; may retain some prior signal)
1. Place blot in 0.2 M NaOH at room temperature for 5 minutes.
2. Wash with PBS to remove NaOH.
3. Block and reprobe as previously described.

7.3.3.3 Cell Labeling for Flow Cytometry

Flow cytometry (Figure 7.16) assays can identify the presence or absence of cell surface markers using the same concepts as other antibody

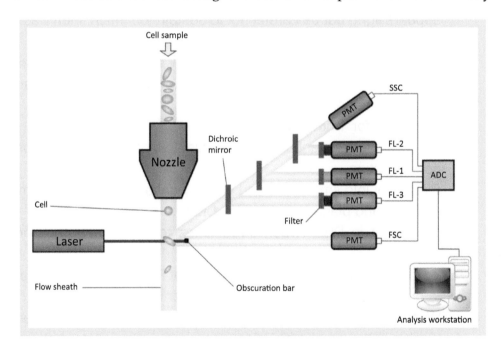

Figure 7.16 Schematic diagram of a flow cytometer. (Image created by Kierano. Used under a Creative Commons Attribution 3.0 Unported License.)

detection methods, such as ELISA. To accomplish this, cells are blocked with a normal serum and then probed with primary and secondary antibodies analogous to ELISA. However, instead of an enzyme-conjugated secondary antibody, a fluorescent dye-tagged secondary antibody is used. Also, to prevent nonspecific interactions, an isotype control primary antibody is used to ensure that the primary antibody binds specifically to the protein of interest. This isotype control antibody will be determined based on the type of primary antibody used. To detect the bound secondary antibody with fluorescent marker, the labeled cells will then be run through the flow cytometer. The detected amount of the fluorescent marker, relative to the isotype antibody control, is used to determine the number of cells expressing the surface marker of interest. As the gain settings on the flow cytometer can vary between groups, unstained control cells are used to determine the group-specific gain.

A. Materials needed

Equipment
1. Flow cytometer
2. Microcentrifuge
3. 1.5 ml microcentrifuge tubes

Reagents
1. 50,000-100,000 cells in a 1.5 ml tube; for each type of stain, at least three tubes of cells are needed per experimental group:
   Unstained control
   Isotype control
   Stained cells
2. Paraformaldehyde 1% solution for fixation
3. PBS
4. PBS with 1% BSA + 1% sodium azide (used to prevent internalization of antibody)
5. Normal serum block (species matched to secondary antibody)
6. Primary antibodies and isotype control antibodies
7. Secondary antibody

Note: The procedures for setting up and gating the flow cytometer are not discussed here, as these are both machine and antibody specific.

B. Procedure

1. Centrifuge cells at 800 × g for 3.5 minutes to make a pellet.
2. Wash one time with 200 µl per tube of cells with PBS, vortexing gently to resuspend pellet.
3. Centrifuge as in step 1.
4. Fix or block according to type of sample.
5. Isotype controls and stained samples: Add 100 µl of normal serum block, gently vortex, and let sit for 30 minutes.
6. Unstained controls: Resuspend in 300 µl of 1% paraformaldehyde, gently vortex immediately to resuspend pellet, and place at 4°C or on ice for storage.
7. Centrifuge isotype and stained samples as in step 1.
8. Resuspend samples in 100 µl of isotype control or primary antibody as appropriate.
9. Incubate at room temperature for 30 minutes (this should be done *in the dark* if the primary antibody is conjugated to a fluorophore).
10. Wash once with PBS with 1% BSA and 1% sodium azide, 200 µl per tube.
11. Centrifuge as in step 1.
12. If primary or isotype controls are not already conjugated to a fluorophore, resuspend in secondary antibody (100 µl per tube); otherwise, proceed to the next step.
13. Incubate with secondary antibody for 20 minutes at room temperature *in the dark.*
14. Centrifuge as in step 1 and wash twice with PBS with 1% BSA and 1% sodium azide.
15. Centrifuge as in step 1 and resuspend in 300 µl of 1% paraformaldehyde, vortexing gently and immediately for even suspension.
16. Run on flow cytometer.

7.4 INSOLUBLE MATRIX COMPONENT EXTRACTION AND ASSAYING

Extraction or dissolution techniques are dependent on the type of assay to be performed. To solubilize collagens or glycosaminoglycans, enzymatic digestion of the tissue or construct is common. However, other protocols are necessary for sample disruption for more sensitive materials, such as protein (Section 7.3.1) and RNA (Section 7.5).

7.4.1 Sample Dehydration by Lyophilization

A. Materials needed

Equipment
1. Lyophilizer
2. Microbalance
3. 1.5 ml microcentrifuge tube
4. Parafilm

Reagents

1. Liquid nitrogen—optional

Note: The wet weight of samples should be taken either at the time of collection or prior to lyophilization. This can be compared with the postlyophilized sample to determine percent water content.

B. Procedure

1. Measure the wet weight of each sample and then place in a 1.5 ml microcentrifuge tube.
2. Cover tube opening with parafilm and poke two or three holes in the parafilm.
3. Flash-freeze samples in liquid nitrogen or -80°C freezer.
4. Place tubes in lyophilizer beaker; if other samples are on the lyophilizer, shut their valves. Hook your beaker to the lyophilizer

and slowly open your valve, allowing the pressure to drop. Once the pressure reaches 50-200 mTorr, open valves of other samples to return them to vacuum.

5. Leave on lyophilizer (at 50-200 mTorr and -80°C) for at least 48 hours.
6. To remove samples, again shut valves of any other samples on the machine.
7. Vent sample of interest; remove sample and shut valve.
8. Open valves of other samples on machine to return them to vacuum.
9. Take dry weights of each sample.

7.4.2 Papain Digestion

A. Materials needed

Equipment
1. 60°C water bath
2. 1.5 ml microcentrifuge tubes
3. Parafilm

Reagents
1. Phosphate buffer: 0.44% monobasic potassium phosphate and 0.29% dibasic potassium phosphate, pH 6.5
2. Papain solution: 125 µg/ml papain, 5 mM *N*-acetyl-L-cysteine, and 5 mM EDTA, in phosphate buffer

Note: Label tubes with tape, as marker may come off during incubation in the water bath.

B. Procedure

1. Set hot water bath to 60°C.
2. Prepare papain solution; approximately 1 µl of solution should be used per microgram of dry sample weight.

3. Add papain solution to each sample in 1.5 ml tubes, close tubes, and seal over the top with parafilm.
4. Digest samples at 60°C for 18 hours.
5. Remove tubes from water bath and allow to cool to room temperature.
6. Vortex samples for several minutes to ensure complete breakup of the samples.
7. Freeze digested samples at -80°C until needed.

7.4.3 Assaying Glycosaminoglycan Content

Other alternatives for this assay involve the commercially available kit for detection of sGAGs produced by Biocolor (Blyscan GAG assay), which is based on the initial dimethyl methylene blue (DMMB) assay (Farndale et al. 1986). The protocols for the original DMMB assay and a commercially available modified form of the Blyscan GAG assay for a microplate format are provided here.

7.4.3.1 Simple DMMB Assay for the Detection of sGAGs

A. Materials needed

Equipment
1. Spectrophotometer and cuvettes

Reagents
1. Glycine/NaCl solution: 0.3% glycine, 0.24% sodium chloride (NaCl), and 0.01 M HCl
2. DMMB solution: 16 µg of DMMB per milliliter in glycine-NaCl solution, pH 3
3. Phosphate-buffered EDTA: 100 mM sodium phosphate(Na_2HPO_4) and 10 mM EDTA, pH 6.5
4. Chondroitin sulfate standard: Prepared as a 0.1 mg/ml solution in phosphate-buffered EDTA; at 4°C, this is stable for more than 3 months

Note: Samples should be read immediately, as absorbance will change with time. This assay can also be prepared in a microplate format, by adjusting the volumes as required. Section 7.4.3.2 describes a commercially available version of this assay that is more robust and easier to use for large numbers of samples.

B. Procedure

1. Prepare chondroitin sulfate standard curve at concentrations of 0, 1, 2, 3, 4, and 5 µg. The DMMB assay is linear up to 5 µg. For sample concentrations higher than this, dilute until within this range.
2. In a cuvette, add 50 µL of standards or sample to 1.25 ml of DMMB solution. Each sample should be read before preparing the next sample.
3. Read absorbance at 525 nm immediately.

7.4.3.2 Biocolor Assay

The Blyscan GAG assay by Biocolor is a commercially available kit that measures the amount of sGAGs in a sample. It uses DMMB to bind and precipitate sGAGs, and, therefore, will not detect non-sGAGs such as hyaluronan. This precipitate is resuspended in a dye dissociation reagent that releases the bound dye. The absorbance of the dye can then be measured on a plate reader. This protocol is modified from the manufacturer's instructions.

A. Materials needed

Equipment
1. Microcentrifuge
2. Plate reader for absorbance measurement
3. 1.5 ml microcentrifuge tubes
4. Clear 96-well plate

Reagents
1. Blyscan GAG assay kit (dye and dissociation reagents)

584

2. Blyscan sGAG standard (chondroitin sulfate)
3. Digest solution used to digest samples (e.g., papain) for making standards and diluting samples

Note: Samples should be protected from light and measured immediately.

B. Procedure

1. Determine the scale of the standard curve (0-5 µg); increments of 1, 2, 3, 4, and 5 µg work well. Make standards, and bring total volume to 100 µl with digest solution.
2. Estimate how much sample digest solution is needed (1-100 µl) to fall within the linear midportion of the standard curve.
3. Label tubes and make up sample preparations; add digested sample to a 1.5 ml tube, and bring total volume to 100 µl with digest solution.
4. Add 500 µl of dye reagent to each sample or microcentrifuge tube.
5. Vortex every 5 minutes for 30 minutes; protect tubes from light.
6. Centrifuge tubes for 10 minutes at max speed, >10,000 × g.
7. Pour off supernatant, taking care not to disturb pellet; remove excess liquid with a pipette or tissue.
8. Resuspend pellet in 500 µl of dissociation reagent.
9. Vortex every 5 minutes for 30 minutes or until pellets completely dissolve (Figure 7.17). Protect tubes from light.
10. In a clear, 96-well absorbance plate, aliquot 100 µl of sample or standard per well in triplicate.
11. Read absorbance on the plate reader at 650 nm.

7.4.4 Assaying for Total Collagen Content

The hydroxyproline collagen assay measures the amount of hydroxyproline in a sample. Since collagen is a hydroxyproline-rich molecule, this assay can be used to correlate how much total collagen is in a sample by using a collagen standard curve. However, this assumes the

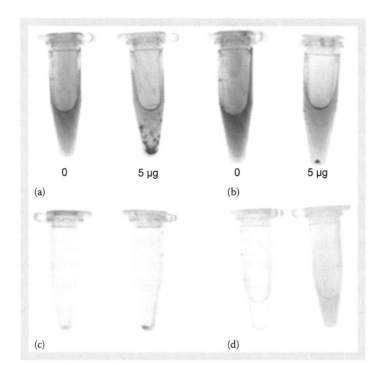

Figure 7.17 Steps in the Biocolor assay. (a) 0 and 5 μg of sGAG and Blyscan Dye after 15 minutes mixing. (b) Formation of the sGAG Dye pellet after continued mixing and high-speed centrifugation (c). Remaining supernatant or unbound non-sGAG Dye is drained from the tubes with care to ensure retention of the pellet. (d) Dye dissociation reagent used to release bound sGAG Dye for colorimetric quantification. (From Biocolor Life Science Assays. With permission.)

amount of hydroxyproline per collagen molecule is constant between the standard and the sample tested. This technique also does not discriminate between types of collagen, and will detect both elastin and pepsin, which both contain hydroxyproline. For this reason, papain digestion (see Section 7.4.2) is suggested.

A. Materials needed

Equipment
1. 5 ml Cryule vials with screw tops (Wheaton)
2. Autoclave with liquid setting
3. Water bath at 65°C

4. Plate reader for absorbance measurement
5. Clear 96-well plate

Reagents
1. Collagen standard
2. Extra papain digest solution; standards should be prepared in diluents similar to the digest
3. 4 N NaOH and 4 N HCl; make sure that these solutions neutralize when equal amounts are combined
4. Stock Chloramine T buffer: 27.3 g of citric acid (monohydrate), 35 g of sodium acetate, 17 g of NaOH, and 6 ml of acetic acid; bring to 500 ml of solution with deionized water
5. Chloramine T solution: 1.41% Chloramine T, 20.7% water, 26% isopropanol, and 53.3% stock Chloramine T buffer
6. 4-(Dimethyl-amino)benzaldehyde (a.k.a. Ehrlich's): 15% Erlich's, 60% isopropanol, and 26% perchloric acid
7. Isopropanol
8. Perchloric acid

Note: Perchloric acid is very dangerous. Use only in a chemical wash-down hood with glass pipettes, and wear appropriate personal protective equipment at all times. Make sure tubes used to contain the solutions are autoclavable.

B. Procedure

1. After lyophilization, take dry weight of each sample.
2. Determine the scale of your standard curve (0-50 µg); typically values of 0, 2.5, 5, 10, 25, and 50 µg work well.
3. Estimate how much sample digest solution is needed (1-200 µl) to fall within the midportion of your standard curve.
4. Label 5 ml tubes and make up standards.
5. Label 5 ml tubes and make up sample preparations.
6. Add amount of digest solution determined in step 2 to 5 ml Cryule vial.

7. Add papain digest solution, pepsin-elastase digest solution, and deionized water to a final volume of 200 μl.
8. Add 200 μl of 4 N NaOH to each vial and vortex gently.
9. Loosen all caps and put in autoclave tray with a few centimeters of water covering only the bottom part of the tubes.
10. Autoclave on the liquid cycle with the shortest time.
11. Warm water bath to 65°C.
12. Prepare Erlich's and Chloramine T solutions based on the number of sample or standards; add 10% more to account for pipetting errors.
13. When samples are done autoclaving, let cool for 10 minutes.
14. Add 200 μl of 4 N HCl to each tube and vortex gently.
15. Add 1.25 ml of Chloramine T solution to each tube and vortex gently.
16. Let samples stand at room temperature for 20 minutes.
17. Add 1.25 ml of Erlich's solution to each tube and vortex immediately; this is crucial to avoid phase separation.
18. Place samples in a 65°C water bath for 20 minutes.
19. Cool samples to room temperature by placing in a tap water bath.
20. Using a clear 96-well plate, plate 200 μl of each sample or standard in triplicate.
21. Read plate on plate reader at 550 nm.

7.4.5 DNA Quantification by PicoGreen

PicoGreen (Figure 7.18) is a fluorescent dye that binds double-stranded DNA. As most mammalian cells contain approximately 7.7 pg of DNA per cell, the total cell number can be calculated. This protocol can be used with papain or other enzyme-digested samples. While this assay assumes dye binding is equivalent between a lambda phage DNA standard and the target sample, for best results a species-matched DNA sample should be used and the concentration of DNA standard remeasured prior to the assay (Forsey and Chaudhuri 2009).

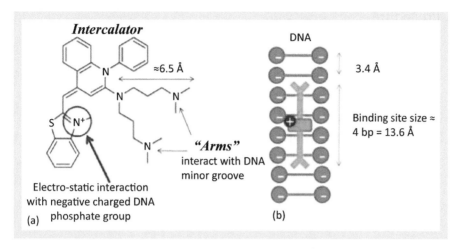

Figure 7.18 Molecular structure of PicoGreen (a) and associated model of the PicoGreen-DNA complex (b). (From Dragan, A. I. et al., *Biophys J* 99(9): 3010-3019, 2010. With permission.)

A. Materials needed

Equipment
1. 1.5 ml microcentrifuge tubes
2. 15 or 50 ml tube for fluorescent dye mix
3. Aluminum foil
4. Black or white (opaque, for fluorescence) 96-well plate
5. Plate reader for fluorescence measurement
6. Spectrophotometer (to determine DNA standard concentration) —optional

Reagents
1. PicoGreen fluorescent dye
2. 1× Tris-EDTA (TE) buffer
3. DNA standard (commonly lambda phage DNA)

Note: Thaw the PicoGreen dye in the dark prior to use. To account for pipetting errors, the amount of solutions produced should be the number of samples and standards in triplicate plus 10%.

B. Procedure

1. Determine the scale of your standard curve; values of 0, 4, 16, 64, 128, and 200 ng of DNA, are commonly used. Make up dilutions in 1× TE buffer.
2. Plate all standards in triplicate in an opaque 96-well plate.
3. Estimate the number of cells per sample. To calculate the amount of sample digest solution that is needed (1-100 µl) to fall within the midportion of the standard curve, assume 7.7 pg of DNA/cell.
4. Using the estimation from step 3, plate all samples in triplicate, adding 1× TE buffer to reach a final volume of 100 µl per well.
5. Dilute PicoGreen stock 1:200 in 1× TE buffer and keep light protected.
6. Add 100 µl of diluted PicoGreen mix to each well containing sample or standard. Protect plate from light by covering with aluminum foil.
7. Read plate on a plate reader using excitation/emission wavelengths of 485/528 nm. Ensure the standard curve is linear and that all samples fall within the standard curve.

7.5 RNA EXTRACTION AND GENE EXPRESSION

This section consists of techniques for extracting RNA from different culture conditions or tissues (e.g., 2D vs. 3D) and the manipulation and detection of changes in gene expression. It is important to note that for extraction and handling of RNA, it may be advisable to have a small section of the lab bench cordoned off with reagents and pipettes only used for RNA handling. RNA is extremely sensitive to degradation, and RNAses are ubiquitous and very stable. Care should also be taken to prevent DNA contamination, especially from polymerase chain reaction (PCR) products, which may give false signal during quantitative reverse transcription (qRT) PCR measures of gene expression. The following protocols are separated by RNA extraction from 2D culture via lysis buffer and RNA extraction from 3D culture following liquid nitrogen pulverization. The procedure for the column cleanup is identical for both. Depending on the size of columns used, the amount of starting material should be adjusted to ensure the column is not overloaded. It should be noted that extraction of good-quality RNA is also possible without the use of columns by using TRI-reagent-based chemistry (such as TRIzol). However, on-column DNA removal may still be necessary for some applications.

Most spin columns work by preferential nucleotide binding to silica columns, and removal of contaminants through the process of several washes with alcohol-based solutions that render the nucleotides insoluble. To remove contaminating DNA, a DNase treatment is used, and the final RNA is eluted using a Tris buffer or RNase-free water. The following protocol is based on the manufacturer's protocol used for the RNeasy brand columns by Qiagen. Multiple other companies provide RNA extraction and cleanup columns. The choice of this brand of columns is based on the authors' familiarity and success when using this manufacturer's columns.

RNA quality and concentration can be determined by absorbance measurements. Quality RNA will have 260/280 and 260/230 ratios from 1.8 to 2.0. Care should be taken to prevent carryover phenol (used in the 3D culture or tissue extraction), as it will alter absorbance. Typical concentrations of extracted RNA range from 50 to 200 ng/μl, but this will depend on the number of cells or size and type of tissue or sample used.

7.5.1 RNAse/DNAse-Free DEPC Water

Diethyl pyrocarbonate (DEPC) reacts with the amines of proteins, such as RNAses and DNAses, rendering them inert. Following autoclaving, DEPC degrades harmlessly, leaving an RNAase- and DNAse-free solution. However, due to the reaction with amines, DEPC should not be used to treat amine-containing buffers such as Tris.

A. Materials needed

Equipment
1. Autoclave

Reagents
1. DEPC
2. Ultrapure water or other solutions

Note: DEPC is a noted carcinogen and should be handled with care.

B. Procedure

1. Add DEPC to a solution at a concentration of 0.1%.
2. Incubate solution at 37°C for 2 hours or at room temperature overnight.
3. Autoclave solution on liquid cycle.

7.5.2 RNA Extraction from 2D Cultures

The extraction of RNA from 2D monolayer cultures is much easier than that from 3D culture and tissues. Many common manufacturers' protocols exist for extracting RNA from monolayer, and most follow a straightforward approach of applying a lysis buffer, commonly guanidine based, to cells, followed by scraping and column cleanup. TRI-reagent, TRIzol, or QIAzol-based lysis or separation buffers also work and allow for potential separation of RNA, DNA, and protein from the same sample. The following protocol is based on the Qiagen RNeasy column kit, although many others are available.

A. Materials needed

Equipment
1. Microcentrifuge
2. Qiagen RNeasy mini kit; contains buffers RLT, RW1, and RPE and columns

3. RNase-free area, including RNase-free pipette tips and RNase-free pipettes
4. Spectrophotometer or NanoDrop (for evaluating RNA quality and quantity)
5. -80°C freezer
6. 1.5 ml microcentrifuge tubes
7. 20-gauge needle and 3 ml syringe to shear DNA
8. Cell scraper
9. DNAse I kit (Qiagen)—optional

Reagents
1. Monolayer cells or samples prepared according to kit instructions
2. RNase Away or 3% hydrogen peroxide solution

Note: Prepare the RNA isolation area by spraying liberally with RNase Away or 3% hydrogen peroxide solution. Wipe down all pipettes, centrifuges, tube racks, and other equipment in the area with the same solution. The use of good benchtop "sterile technique" is important due to the ubiquitous nature of contaminating RNases, especially on human skin. Extra care should be taken when opening and closing microcentrifuge tubes to avoid contamination. After eluting the RNA, measure the absorbance to determine quality and quantity. This protocol is based on the manufacturer's instructions.

B. Procedure

1. Remove medium from monolayer cultures.
2. Add 700 μl of RLT lysis buffer per 5 million cells or 10 cm dish.
3. Scrap cells in RLT lysis buffer.
4. Using a 20-gauge needle, pipet the lysis buffer plus cells up and down several times to shear genomic DNA.
5. Add 700 μl of sample in lysis buffer into an RNeasy spin column; centrifuge at >8,000 × g for 15 seconds at room temperature.

6. Discard the flow-through and reuse the 2 ml collection tube on the column.

7. Repeat previous two steps for the remainder of the sample. If the volume is extremely large, consider splitting into two RNeasy spin columns.

8. If doing the on-column DNase digestion, go to the next step. If not, add 700 µl of RW1 and centrifuge at >8,000 × g for 15 seconds at room temperature. Discard flow-through and 2 ml collection tube and go to step 12.

9. Add 350 µl of RW1 and centrifuge at >8,000 × g for 15 seconds at room temperature and discard the flow-through.

10. Add 10 µl of DNase I stock solution to 70 µl of Buffer RDD. Mix by gently inverting the tube. Do not vortex. DNase is extremely sensitive to physical denaturation.

11. Pipet 80 µl of DNase I incubation mix directly onto the RNeasy membrane and allow to sit at room temperature for 15 minutes.

12. Add 350 µl of RW1, centrifuge at >8,000 × g for 15 seconds at room temperature, and discard the flow-through.

13. Transfer to a new 2 ml collection tube, add 500 µl of RPE, centrifuge at >8,000 × g for 15 seconds at room temperature, and discard the flow-through.

14. Add 500 µl of RPE again, centrifuge at >8,000 × g for 2 minutes at room temperature, and discard the flow-through.

15. Centrifuge dry at >8,000 × g for 1 minute at room temperature and discard flow-through and 2 ml collection tube.

16. Transfer RNeasy spin column to a new 1.5 ml microcentrifuge tube, and add 50 µl of RNase-free water to the membrane. Centrifuge at >8,000 × g for 1 minute at room temperature to elute the RNA. For smaller samples, extract with 30 µl of RNase-free water.

7.5.3 RNA Extraction from 3D Cultures and Tissue

This extraction protocol is similar to that of the protocol in Section 7.3.1.2 for liquid nitrogen pulverization for protein extraction, although the lysis buffer is different.

A. Materials needed

Equipment
1. Dewar flask to store liquid nitrogen; for temporary storage, Styrofoam containers can be used
2. Styrofoam container (disposable); check the bottom for leaks following this protocol and replace as necessary
3. Cryo gloves, goggles, and other needed personal protective equipment
4. Aluminum foil, one square (5-7 cm) for each sample
5. Pulverizer or mortar and pestle
6. RNeasy lipid tissue mini kit—QIAzol lysis reagent
7. Centrifuge and compatible tubes of approximately 14 ml

Reagents
1. Liquid nitrogen
2. 70% ethanol in DEPC or RNAse-free water
3. Chloroform

Note: QIAzol is a lysis reagent from Qiagen based on the classical phenol-chloroform-guanidine trireagent for DNA, RNA, and protein extraction. This protocol has been modified from that of the manufacturer's original protocol to include mechanical pulverization. Care should be taken to never mix guanidine-containing solutions with bleach.

B. Procedure

1. In a Styrofoam container, place the pulverizer and add liquid nitrogen to a level about 1 cm above the top of the pulverizer. The addition of a flat metal plate below the pulverizer will extend the life of the Styrofoam container.
2. After the liquid nitrogen evaporates below the top of the pulverizer base, push a piece of foil over the well and push the pulverizer piston down into the well and tap it to create an aluminum foil disk to place your sample on.
3. Place sample on aluminum foil.
4. Add 1 ml of QIAzol on top of sample.
5. Place second piece of aluminum foil over hole and push down gently to sandwich the sample and QIAzol between the pieces of foil.
6. Using the pulverizer piston, pulverize the sample between the pieces of aluminum foil.
7. Disassemble pulverizer, remove aluminum foil and sample, and place in additional lysis buffer. Add tissue and 3 ml of QIAzol as you add in tissue. Make sure to wash the walls of the tube and vortex as you do this.
8. Incubate at room temperature for 5 minutes.
9. Add 200 µl of chloroform per 1 ml of QIAzol used (600 µl) and shake by hand for 15 seconds.
10. Incubate at room temperature for 2-3 minutes.
11. Centrifuge at 12,000 × g for 15 minutes at 4°C; solution will separate into an upper aqueous phase (RNA), a white interphase (DNA), and a red organic phase (protein and other materials).
12. Transfer the upper aqueous phase containing the RNA to a new 1.5 ml tube.
13. Continue RNA extraction as previously described under the protocol described in Section 7.5.2 (step 5).

7.5.4 Gel Electrophoresis for DNA and RNA

The procedure used for running DNA and RNA agarose gels is very similar. The agarose gel, much like an SDS-PAGE gel, separates molecules based on molecular size, allowing for visualization of different molecular weight bands. For RNA, this provides a simple method for determining RNA quality by determining the 28S/18S ribosomal RNA ratio. Ideally, this should be a ratio of 2 for nondegraded RNA. While newer equipment such as the Agilent Bioanalyzer allows this to be done without the need for agarose gels, gels are still in widespread use due to their ease of use. For applications using DNA, agarose concentration and gel run time will need to be adjusted depending on the size (base pairs) of the DNA, although fragments larger than 10 kb are not amenable to agarose separation. Gels can be imaged to collect semiquantitative information (Figure 7.19).

A. Materials needed

Equipment
1. Gel box with combined casting tray

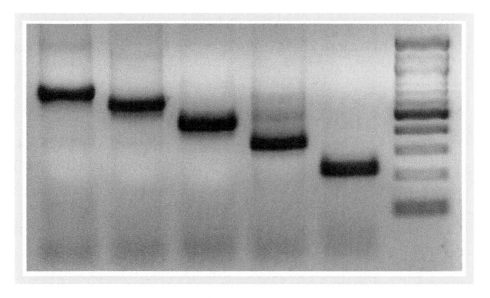

Figure 7.19 DNA gel of PCR products imaged using ethidium bromide (first five lanes). Far left lane featuring a series of bands is the DNA ladder. Note that the image is color inverted for better viewing.

2. Power supply
3. UV source or light box, such as a blue light-emitting diode (LED) light source and orange filter; a gel documentation system with camera is preferred
4. Gel loading tips—optional

Reagents
1. 1% agarose prepared in 0.5× TAE buffer; microwave 1.5-2 minutes until all agarose has dissolved, taking care not to boil over
2. Running buffer: 0.5× TAE buffer
3. Loading buffer, can be purchased commercially or prepared as a 30% glycerol and 0.25% bromophenol blue solution in deionized water
4. RNA or DNA ladder

Note: Avoid contact with your skin. Melted agarose is hot and may cause burns; care should be taken when pouring gels. Running voltages that are too high will cause overheating and melting of the agarose. Reduced voltages will increase size resolution on the gel, but increase running time. Care must be taken not to run smaller DNA fragments off the end of the gel. Gel concentrations can be increased from 1% to 3% for smaller DNA fragments. RNA and DNA are negatively charged and will travel toward the positive side of the gel.

B. Procedure

1. Prepare gel box by placing gel carrier perpendicular (with gaskets on box walls) in the gel box and placing sample comb in position to make loading wells.
2. Pour agarose to fill gel box without pausing.
3. Allow agarose to cool for approximately 20-30 minutes; the agarose will become more opaque as it sets.
4. Pull gel carrier out of gel box, and carefully remove comb.
5. Replace carrier with wells aligned to the black lead (-); samples will run toward the red lead (+).
6. Fill gel box to fill line with 0.5× TAE buffer.

7. Prepare samples for loading into gel by adding 2 µl of loading buffer to 10 µl of sample. The loading buffer will make the sample easier to see, and increases the density so it settles to the bottom of the well.
8. Carefully load samples into gel, avoiding spilling sample or puncturing the bottom of the well.
9. Load 3-5 µl of RNA or DNA ladder into empty wells at the sides of the gel.
10. To ensure that samples run straight in the gel, load 12 µl of deionized water mixed with loading buffer into each unused well.
11. Attach leads to gel box and turn on power source.
12. Make sure bubbles form in the running buffer on each side of the gel box.
13. The gel should take about 1 hour to run for a medium-sized gel at 150 V; check progress every 15 minutes. The loading buffer dyes will indicate progress: the yellow dye will run faster and separate from the blue dye. When the yellow dye front has almost run to the end of the gel, turn off the power supply.
14. Carefully remove gel from the buffer box and gel carrier.
15. Place gel on the blue LED light source and visualize using the orange filter.
16. Take a picture of your gel, noting the exposure time and other camera parameters (if applicable).

7.5.5 Polymerase Chain Reaction

PCR allows for the easy amplification of a DNA sequence provided primers flanking the desired sequence are available. As the amplification is exponential, with each cycle doubling the DNA quantity, minimal sample is required to produce large amounts of PCR product (Figure 7.20).

A. Materials needed

Equipment
1. Thermocycler or other PCR machine

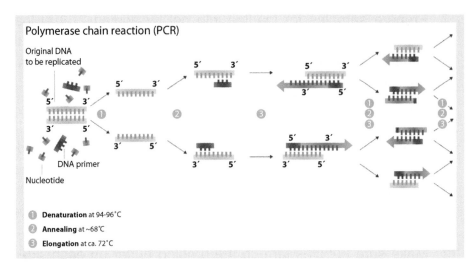

Figure 7.20 Illustration of the PCR process. (Image created by Enzoklop. Used under the Creative Commons Attribution-Share Alike 3.0 Unported License.)

Reagents
1. Platinum PCR SuperMix (Invitrogen 11306-016) or similar
2. DEPC or RNAse-free water
3. Forward and reverse primers for the gene of interest
4. Template or sample DNA source (e.g., complementary DNA [cDNA], plasmid, or extracted DNA)

B. Procedure

1. Calculate the volume of DNA solution you will use for each sample and the amount of forward and reverse primers to add to the PCR SuperMix.
2. If your DNA is highly concentrated, you may need to dilute with DEPC water.
3. Typical concentrations of primers in the final PCR solution are 200-900 nM.
4. The Platinum PCR SuperMix is provided at 1.1× concentration so that the final 10% of the solution is made up of some combination of primers, template (DNA), and DEPC water.
5. For a 50 μl reaction volume, use 45 μl of SuperMix and 5 μl of primers, DNA, and DEPC water.

6. Make up the reaction volumes in RNase-free or DNase-free microcentrifuge tubes (0.2-0.6 ml) depending on PCR machine.
7. Keep chilled (on ice) during this process.
8. Vortex gently and centrifuge briefly to collect solutions at the bottom of the tube.
9. Place in PCR machine and run your thermal cycling protocol, which is dependent on the PCR mix and the primers used.
10. For Platinum PCR SuperMix, cycles of 94°C, 2 minutes, and 40 cycles of 94°C, 15 seconds; annealing temperature, 30 seconds; and 72°C, 60 seconds work well. Running 40 cycles ensures that maximum amplification is achieved.
11. Annealing temperature will be determined by the primers used. Using an annealing temp that is too high will restrict binding, whereas one that is too low will encourage nonspecific binding.
12. Once thermal cycling is finished, chill on ice.
13. If desired, place samples at -20°C and run on an agarose gel later.

7.5.6 Quantitative Reverse Transcription PCR

The protocol describes a method for two-step qRT-PCR. Other methods exist that combine these into a single application, with RNA being directly added to the solution for RT-PCR. However, given the rapid degradation and sensitive nature of RNA, the two-step method allows for easier storage of cDNA produced from RNA; as DNA is inherently more stable, it also reduces the amount of handling of the initial RNA if a long-term archival storage is desired.

Quantitative reverse transcription PCR (qRT-PCR) allows for detection of relative amounts of mRNA for genes of interest compared with an internal housekeeping gene or control, such as glyceraldehyde-3-phosphate dehydrogenase (GAPDH), actin, or 18S ribosomal RNA. The concept of qRT-PCR is the same as regular PCR, except the amount of PCR product amplified during each cycle is measured quantitatively.

This is termed real-time PCR, which is often also somewhat confusingly abbreviated as RT-PCR or rtPCR. This allows for detection of relative amplification differences during the linear phase of PCR amplification. This detection and quantitative measurement is made using a fluorescent dye that either (1) binds to double-stranded DNA (SYBR Green) or (2) binds to a specific region in your gene of interest between the forward and reverse primers (probe). There are benefits and drawbacks to using either SYBR Green or a probe. SYBR Green is typically less expensive than probes and can work for all gene amplifications. On the other hand, SYBR Green binds to double-stranded DNA nonspecifically, so DNA product due to unwanted reactions will also be measured. Probes are sequence specific, and, therefore, ameliorate detection of off-target reactions and have the advantage that they can be designed with various fluorophores such that multiple genes can be amplified in the same reaction tube (multiplexing). However, probes are more expensive and more time-consuming to design, and using probes to multiplex requires significant optimization. The particular type of detection technique used will depend on the available primers for the gene of interest.

The resultant data from a real-time PCR are a graph showing fluorescence versus cycle number for the various PCRs. From this graph, the cycle at which the fluorescence starts to increase rapidly is called the takeoff point or cycle at takeoff (C_t). Usually, a smaller C_t value indicates more abundant mRNA for that gene. Comparing the difference in C_t for the gene of interest compared with the housekeeping gene generates the ΔC_t. By comparing between treatment groups ($\Delta \Delta C_t$), it can be determined if a specific treatment up- or downregulates relative gene expression. Primers and probes for qRT-PCR can be designed using the NCBI Primer Designing tool or are commercially available as preoptimized primer-probe combinations for a variety of genes and species from several companies, such as Applied Biosystems.

7.5.6.1 cDNA Creation

Reverse transcription is the process of taking mRNA and transcribing a cDNA from the RNA sequence using a reverse transcriptase enzyme. This is needed as PCR requires a DNA sequence. To complete this process, a commercially available kit containing all of the necessary materials to reverse transcribe the RNA is used. Steps to perform the reverse transcription should be followed based on the manufacturer's instructions. Since these vary by vendor, they are not described here.

The use of random hexamers avoids the problems of 3′ bias seen with oligoDT primers during cDNA creation. OligoDT primers only create cDNA from mRNA species with 3′ poly A tails. This has limitations in that the processivity of reverse transcriptase may limit the length of cDNA created from long-sequence mRNAs. Generally, sequences exceeding 2 kb may have reduced representation in the final cDNA. Primers for RT-PCR that are used with OligoDT-generated cDNA should take this into account and preferably not be more than 1.5-2 kb from the 3′ end of the sequence. Furthermore, internal standards, such as 18S RNA, will not be produced unless random hexamers are used, as 18S RNA lacks the poly A tail.

A. Materials needed

Equipment
1. PCR machine (RotorGene) or other thermal cycling equipment
2. Ice bucket
3. Metal tube rack or 96-well cooler
4. 0.2 ml RNase- and DNase-free microcentrifuge tubes

Reagents
1. Reverse transcription kit, Superscript III First-Strand Synthesis System for RT-PCR (Invitrogen 18080-051) or similar
2. DEPC water
3. -80°C freezer

Note: For standardization, either the amount of RNA converted to cDNA should be kept the same for each sample, or the amount of cDNA for each PCR should be kept the same. Extra care should be taken with the technique used here, as often tubes will need to be manipulated multiple times to add reagents.

B. Procedure

1. Defrost kit reagents and RNA on ice.
2. According to the cDNA kit protocol, calculate the amount of RNA you will reverse transcribe for each sample. Usually, amounts in the 8-10 ng range will yield material sufficient for several other assays.
3. Return RNA to -80°C as soon as possible after use.
4. Follow all manufacturers' instructions included with the RT kit.
5. Chill reagents and tubes on ice in between steps or during addition of reagents, where applicable.
6. Store cDNA at -80°C.

7.5.6.2 Quantitative Real-Time PCR

While multiple chemistries are available for quantitative real-time PCR, SYBR Green and probe-based primer chemistries are the most common. SYBR Green binds to double-stranded DNA and has the advantage of requiring only forward and reverse primers, without needing a probe (reduced cost). However, significant primer optimization is required to prevent primer dimers and other false signals. Given the commercial availability of many primer-probe combinations, these are often the preferred choice.

A. Materials needed

Equipment
1. 100 μl PCR tubes, RNase- and DNase-free
2. RotorGene with small rotor (72 wells) or other thermocycler capable of real-time detection

Reagents
1. Primers: Forward and reverse for housekeeping gene and each gene of interest
2. SYBR Green mastermix or probe with PCR mastermix
3. DEPC water

Note: Although the protocol below uses the RotorGene, multiple other real-time-capable thermocyclers are available in both 96-well and 384-well formats. These all use similar chemistry. Care should be taken to avoid contamination of cDNA with PCR product. If possible, separate pipettes should be used from those used for RNA work. Before starting, the work area should be wiped down with RNase-Away or 3% hydrogen peroxide.

B. Procedure

1. Make up reaction volumes according to mastermix instructions. Be extremely careful with the pipetting technique here; small errors in volume at this stage can result in large errors in the amplification process.
2. Mastermixes are available as concentrated mix to allow for dilution by the primers and cDNA to the correct concentration.
3. Once all reagents have been added to the tube, centrifuge gently for 30 seconds to ensure all reagents are at the bottom of the tube. If using a RotorGene, run a 30-second cycle.
4. In the thermocycler software, choose SYBR Green or other fluorescent program based on the type of fluorescent dye you are using.
5. Label the positions of the tube or plates in the software and set up a thermal cycle protocol. This should be based on the manufacturer's recommendation for the type of mastermix used and the prescribed annealing temperature for the primers used.
6. After every cycle, a fluorescent reading will be taken and graphed as fluorescence versus cycle.

7. Once the protocol has finished running, you can calculate the C_t (cycle threshold) for each sample.
8. Use the C_t values to quantify the relative abundance of your genes of interest relative to your control group.

7.6 ASSAYING TISSUE BIOMECHANICAL PROPERTIES

Multiple assays can be deployed to determine relevant compressive and tensile properties of native articular cartilage or engineered tissue. This is important in not only developing baseline biomechanical properties for native tissue, but also determining if engineered tissue replicates these properties. The protocols described below define testing parameters that measure both compressive and tensile properties by fitting the collected data to the appropriate mathematical model (see Section 5.4.6).

7.6.1 Compression

7.6.1.1 Load-Controlled Testing via the Creep Indentation Apparatus Compression Test

Creep indentation of biological tissues is performed by applying a constant force (load) to a tissue sample and recording the displacement of the probe over time as the material deforms (Mow et al. 1989). A platen of known dimension and size is used to indent the sample under constant stress, and deformation is measured over time. A porous platen is used to allow for fluid to exude from the sample at the platen contact site. By fitting the stress versus time data with finite element analysis using the biphasic model, the aggregate modulus, Poisson ratio, and permeability of the sample can be determined. The porous indenter on the end of the probe is counterbalanced to a neutral position in the PBS fluid the sample is bathed in. Prior to this loading, a tare load is first applied, and the tissue is allowed to equilibrate, and then a test load is dropped and the displacement data are recorded. As a creep test requires an instantaneous application of load to the sample, the load is applied by dropping a known weight (test load), held above the probe by vacuum.

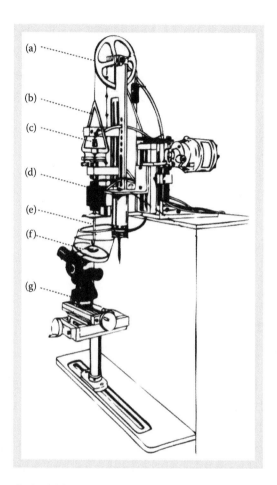

Figure 7.21   Creep indentation apparatus. (a) Pivot point for counterbalance and air bearings. (b) Adjustment platform/triangle, supported by micrometer from beneath (not shown) to allow for fine adjustment. (c) Test load held by vacuum valve. This will drop onto the platform/triangle to apply the test load. (d) LVDT to measure displacement. The tare weight sits on top of the movable section of the LVDT, with the (e) indenter probe screwed into the bottom of the LVDT. (f) Bottom platen and dish filled with PBS, with sample mounted and indenter probe in contact with the sample. (g) Ball-and-socket camera mount for angle adjustment, mounted on an x-y-z adjustable mount. (Modified from Mow, V. C. et al., *J Biomech* 22(8-9): 853-861, 1989. With permission.)

A. Materials needed

Equipment

1. Creep indentation apparatus (CIA); see Figure 7.21.
2. Tare and test weights: For self-assembled articular cartilage constructs, usually 0.2 g tare and 0.7 g test weights are used; stiffer

materials, such as native tissue, will require higher tare and test weights; maximum strain should not exceed 15%.

3. Probe of appropriate diameter (probe diameter must be less than one-third the diameter of the sample and composed of a porous material such as sintered stainless steel); a probe of 0.8 mm is used for most tests.
4. 30 ml syringe
5. Ultrasonic cleaner
6. Forceps
7. Spatula to position sample
8. Data analysis software (e.g., MATLAB®)

Reagents
1. PBS
2. Superglue
3. Sample with thickness greater than 0.4 mm

Note: Due to the small displacement values measured during this procedure, the device is extremely sensitive to vibration. Testing equipment should be placed appropriately to minimize vibration, and the use of passive dampening is preferred. Specimens should be allowed to equilibrate 5 minutes in the bath solution before testing to allow for samples to regain fluid loss during the gluing procedure; typically, this time is achieved while proceeding to the other adjustment steps for the machine. The porous indenter tips should be ultrasonically cleaned to ensure fluid flows easily into the tip.

B. Procedure

1. Make sure air and vacuum are turned on for the air bearings and test load release valve.
2. Measure sample thickness.
3. Superglue sample onto bottom platen and cover with PBS.
4. Screw platen into place on creep indentation apparatus.

5. Screw in the probe with indenter tip.
6. Apply the tare weight to the platform/triangle connected to the indenter tip. This will stabilize minor vibrations of the tip, making it easier to adjust the position.
7. Level sample with respect to the indenter tip. A small flat metal cylinder may be positioned on the sample to achieve this; remove before raising the platen.
8. Use syringe to submerge platen and sample in PBS.
9. Align probe and sample in the x-y plane; raise the platen until the sample is within 1-2 mm of the probe tip.
10. Load software to read the linear variable differential transformer (LVDT) output.
11. Adjust or raise the platform/triangle with the micrometer until the LVDT reads at approximately within the middle of the linear range.
12. Move sample as close to tip as possible without touching; align sample and tip.
13. Remove tare weight.
14. Stabilize pendulum.
15. Add PBS until neutral buoyancy is achieved with respect to the probe tip. Usually, this will be detected as a minor fluctuation in the LVDT reading.
16. Put tare weight back on the probe.
17. Bring sample up until it bumps the probe; the LVDT readout will increase.
18. Quickly raise the platform/triangle using the micrometer off the sample a small distance; 50-100 µm is sufficient.
19. Raise the platform/triangle by hand off the micrometer until it touches the test load suspended above. Lower the test load while holding the platform/triangle against the test load until it is within 50-100 µm of the value achieved when resting on the micrometer tip.
20. Load computer test program and run; release the micrometer simultaneously, allowing the probe to come in contact with the sample.
21. Data are analyzed using the biphasic model.

7.6.1.2 Stress Relaxation Compression Test

The protocol described here utilizes stress relaxation testing at 10%, 20%, and 30% strain of the cartilage tissue or construct, with 15 cycles of 5% strain preconditioning, but these values can easily be adjusted for the type of tissue being tested. The stress-relaxation curves generated are fitted to a standard linear solid model. For this specific protocol, an Instron electromechanical testing device (model 5565) is used to apply the unconfined compression via a nonporous stainless steel or polysulfone platen or indenter (Figure 7.22). The sample is attached to a bottom platen with raised edges and submerged in PBS.

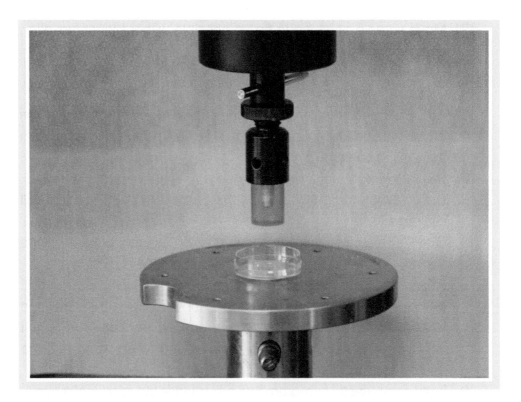

Figure 7.22 Platen setup for stress relaxation test. Sample is immersed in the culture dish in the center, while the nonporous platen is raised above the dish, awaiting loading of the sample.

A. Materials needed

Equipment
1. Blades and punches, to cut samples to cylindrical shape
2. Instron electromechanical tester or equivalent
3. 48-well plate
4. Data analysis software (e.g., MATLAB)

Reagents
1. PBS

Note: The use of protease inhibitors in the PBS is suggested to prevent sample degradation; however, it is not required. A load cell should be chosen with a range appropriate to the estimated sample properties.

B. Procedure

1. Remove sample from well and measure final diameter using the calipers.
2. Place in small petri dish with 3 ml of PBS.
3. Measure sample height using the height detection program on the Instron. This requires knowing the starting position of the inside of the dish and the point at which the platen just touches the sample.
4. Make sure that the preconditioning is turned off.
5. Open appropriate testing protocol for the software.
6. Turn on preconditioning with cycles of 5% strain.
7. Complete stress relaxation testing of the sample at 10%, 20%, and 30% strain.
8. Save the resulting data set.
9. Remove sample from Instron, pat dry, and measure wet weight on the microbalance.
10. Place sample in 1.5 ml tube and freeze at -20°C.
11. Copy data file and analyze using data analysis software such as MATLAB with the Curve-Fitting Toolbox.

7.6.2 Strain-to-Failure Tensile Test

This protocol is for testing native tissue or engineered constructs in tension, using an elastic strain-to-failure test. The tensile test presented here has been developed to deduce two critical parameters of a material, the Young's modulus and the ultimate tensile strength at failure. To measure tensile modulus, a set of grips are fixed to apply a constant strain rate of 1% to the tissue and pull the sample apart until failure. The tensile modulus can then be calculated from the linear region of the stress-strain curve, and the ultimate tensile stress from the maximum point at failure. Samples should always be cut into a reproducibly sized dog bone shape, so that failure result will occur across a well-defined area of the sample. Small samples may need to be attached to a carrier test strip of paper via gluing of the sample across a cutout in the paper. The test strip can then be at the center to allow for testing of the central portion of the material, while both ends attached to the paper can more easily be positioned in the grips.

A. Materials needed

Equipment
1. Scalpel blade and 3 mm dermal punch, used to cut sample to dog bone shape
2. Instron electromechanical tester or equivalent
3. Calipers or camera setup with ruler
4. Small petri dishes
5. Paper tensile mounting strips
6. Data analysis software (e.g., MATLAB or Excel)

Reagents
1. Superglue

Note: The cross-sectional area of the dog bone sample should always be measured to calculate the area of material being tested. Samples must break at the dog bone portion of the sample to be considered a valid test.

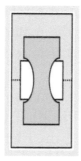

Figure 7.23 Schematic of dog bone sample glued to a paper test strip. Once loaded in the grips, the paper can be cut on either side (dotted lines) to allow testing of the sample.

B. Procedure

1. Cut dog bone shape (Figure 7.23) from tissue of interest using dermal punches or straight utility blades. Smaller samples may need to be glued to a paper test strip to aid in gripping.
2. Measure width and depth of smallest portion of dog bone shape with calipers or by taking front- and side-view pictures with camera.
3. From the measurements, determine the gauge length and enter 1% of this value into the software of the testing machine.
4. Zero the displacement of the grips on the testing machine.
5. Carefully load sample into grips.
6. Ensure that grips are lined up, and that no slipping should occur during the test.
7. Open appropriate testing protocol for the software.
8. Complete testing protocol.
9. Ensure that sample fails in the middle of the dog bone and does not slip or tear at grips.
10. Save the resulting data set.
11. Remove sample from the grips and dispose.
12. Copy data file and analyze using data analysis software, such as MATLAB with the Curve-Fitting Toolbox.

7.6.3 Measuring the Friction Coefficient

Determination of the friction coefficient can be achieved using a variety of methods. Here we present the use of a tribometer, which utilizes a pin-on-disk method consisting of a rotating disk and cantilever arm design, with a pin containing the material to test contacting the disk (reminiscent of a record player). The coefficient of friction (μ) is determined using the calibrated loads to deflect the cantilever arm and calculated from the ratio of the frictional force to the loading force on the pin (μ = friction force/normal load). This protocol has been adapted primarily for use in measuring the friction coefficient during boundary lubrication (see Section 1.4.4) but is capable, by changing speed and load, of measuring multiple different modes of lubrication. While not discussed here, it should be noted that due to the design of this tribometer, wear of a material can also be measured with minor modifications to the testing procedure.

A. Materials needed

Equipment
1. Tribometer
2. Ultrasonic cleaner
3. Glass cleaner: 0.1% SDS in 50 mM Tris pH 7.4

Reagents
1. PBS
2. Superglue

Note: For boundary mode lubrication, a pin-on-disk tribometer can be used in reciprocating mode. This will avoid wedge film buildup. Also, as samples may lose material that is transferred to the glass disk, this surface should be rotated to a clean portion after each sample and ultrasonically cleaned after every four samples.

B. Procedure

Part 1: Loading sample and running test (for boundary lubricating conditions)
1. Calibrate the tribometer strain gauges using a set of weights from 0 to 500 g.

2. Ensure glass is clean before every test. Ultrasonically clean glass in glass cleaner for 5 minutes.
3. Place sample against opposing surface, such as glass, and apply load (~0.1 MPa).
4. Let sample sit for at least 2 minutes to allow time for interstitial fluid depressurization.
5. Turn on motor and slide sample against glass at a reciprocal, linear sliding speed of 0.5 mm/s for 5 minutes.

Part 2: Data analysis

1. Record data points at changes in direction, including 1 second before and after (i.e., -1, 0, and 1 at direction changes).
2. Convert voltage readings from strain gauges to forces using calibration curve obtained in step 1.
3. Calculate coefficient of friction based on these values (μ = friction force/normal load) over time.

7.7 ANIMAL PROTOCOLS

Surgical procedures involving animal models will require both special training in the humane handling of animals and the participation of trained veterinary staff for surgical procedures and other animal care issues. Given this complexity, the choice of a specific animal model, the special considerations of different species, and the ethical and regulatory considerations of using animal models are described in Chapter 5. We also refer the reader to the international manual of the Association for Assessment and Accreditation of Laboratory Animal Care (AAALAC) for further details.

REFERENCES

Below, S., S. P. Arnoczky et al. (2002). The split-line pattern of the distal femur: A consideration in the orientation of autologous cartilage grafts. *Arthroscopy* 18(6): 613-617.

Bittencourt, R. A. d. C., H. R. Pereira et al. (2009). Cultura de condrócitos em arcabouço tridimensional: Hidrogel de alginato. *Acta Ortop Bras* 17: 242-246.

de Vries-van Melle, M. L., E. W. Mandl et al. (2012). An osteochondral culture model to study mechanisms involved in articular cartilage repair. *Tissue Eng Part C Methods* 18(1): 45-53.

Dragan, A. I., J. R. Casas-Finet et al. (2010). Characterization of PicoGreen interaction with dsDNA and the origin of its fluorescence enhancement upon binding. *Biophys J* 99(9): 3010-3019.

DuRaine, G. D., and K. A. Athanasiou. (2015). ERK activation is required for hydrostatic pressure-induced tensile changes in engineered articular cartilage. *J Tissue Eng Regen Med* 9(4): 368-374.

Estes, B. T., B. O. Diekman et al. (2010). Isolation of adipose-derived stem cells and their induction to a chondrogenic phenotype. *Nat Protoc* 5(7): 1294-1311.

Farndale, R. W., D. J. Buttle, and A. J. Barrett. (1986). Improved quantitation and discrimination of sulphated glycosaminoglycans by use of dimethylmethylene blue. *Biochim Biophys Acta* 883(2): 173-177.

Forsey, R. W., and J. B. Chaudhuri. (2009). Validity of DNA analysis to determine cell numbers in tissue engineering scaffolds. *Biotechnol Lett* 31(6): 819-823.

Liebman, J., and R. L. Goldberg. (2001). Chondrocyte culture and assay. *Curr Protoc Pharmacol* 12: Unit 12.

Meachim, G. (1972). Light microscopy of Indian ink preparations of fibrillated cartilage. *Ann Rheum Dis* 31(6): 457-464.

Mow, V. C., M. C. Gibbs et al. (1989). Biphasic indentation of articular cartilage. II. A numerical algorithm and an experimental study. *J Biomech* 22(8-9): 853-861.

Ramaswamy, G., P. Sohn et al. (2012). Altered responsiveness to TGF-beta results in reduced Papss2 expression and alterations in the biomechanical properties of mouse articular cartilage. *Arthritis Res Ther* 14(2): R49.

Shasha, N., P. P. Aubin et al. (2002). Long-term clinical experience with fresh osteochondral allografts for articular knee defects in high demand patients. *Cell Tissue Bank* 3(3): 175-182.

Vinall, R. L., S. H. Lo et al. (2002). Regulation of articular chondrocyte phenotype by bone morphogenetic protein 7, interleukin 1, and cellular context is dependent on the cytoskeleton. *Exp Cell Res* 272(1): 32-44.

GLOSSARY

Allograft: Donor tissue coming from a genetically different individual than the recipient, but of the same species.

Anabolic: Pertaining to the set of factors or metabolic pathways that produce larger molecules from smaller units.

Anchorage dependence: Need of cells to attach to a solid surface for proliferation or survival.

Anlage: Initial rudimentary structure of a particular organ or tissue, especially during embryogenesis. For example, during fetal development the skeleton is initially made of cartilage.

Apparent diffusion coefficient (ADC): Measure of how freely water molecules diffuse within a tissue measured using diffusion-weighted MRI and typically expressed in units of mm^2/s; the word *apparent* is included to indicate that other processes (e.g., flow) may influence the observed movement of water *in vivo*.

Appendicular skeleton: Portions of the skeleton that include the upper and lower limbs, clavicle, scapula, and pelvic girdle, but not the skull, vertebral column, or ribs and sternum.

Appositional growth: Increase in cartilage thickness of the cartilage anlage by the addition of extracellular matrix to the cartilage peripheral surface. Chondroblasts differentiating from the surrounding perichondrium also contribute to this growth.

Arg-Gly-Asp (RGD) sequence: Highly conserved tripeptide sequence in proteins capable of binding to integrin.

Arthritides: Plural form of arthritis (see Chapter 3), denoting types of arthritis.

Arthropathy: Disease of the joints, for example, arthritis, an inflammation of the joints.

Atrophy: Process of regressing or degenerating in tissues and organs.

Basal lamina: Layer of extracellular matrix on which the epithelium lies, secreted by the epithelial cells, containing the glycoprotein laminin and type IV collagen.

Bilateral symmetry: Referring to having symmetrical halves across the sagittal plane; the plane that divides the body into left and right.

Biocompatibility: Property of a material that allows it to function in a host with an appropriate response without eliciting harmful effects.

Biomaterial: Any material of synthetic or natural origins that interacts with living systems in a directed manner. Commonly, a biomaterial can be used to engineer replacement tissues or organs.

Biomimesis (biomimicry): Process of imitating models, systems, and elements of nature toward solving biological problems. In the case of tissue engineering, this term refers to engineering a replacement tissue or organ with properties mimicking those of the native tissue or organ.

Bioreactor: Any device that supports a biologically active environment. Commonly, this takes the form of a vessel used to carry out a biological or chemical process or reaction using either living organisms or organism-derived biochemically active molecules. In tissue engineering, a bioreactor may be used to apply biochemical or biomechanical stimuli or simulate the *in vivo* physiological environment.

Bioresorbable: Pertaining to a material that can be broken down and absorbed by the body; commonly used in sutures, scaffolds, or surgical implants where mechanical removal is not desired. Frequently used bioresorbable materials are made of polylactides, polyglycolides, and their copolymers.

Birefringence: Property of an optically anisotropic material due to it possessing a refractive index dependent on the light polarization and propagation direction. For example, using a polarized light source in combination with a polarizing filter, ordered structures within a material can be detected, such as collagen fibers and gout crystals.

Cadherins: Class of type 1 transmembrane proteins that participate in cell adhesion and are dependent on calcium (Ca^{2+}) ions. The term is derived from *calcium-dependent adhesion*.

Canonical (pathway): Common, generalized signaling pathway for a specific stimulus (within a specific cell or tissue context). This is in contrast to a noncanonical pathway, which may be a lesser known or alternative signaling pathway.

Capitellum: Small, rounded eminence at the extremity of a bone.

Catabolic: Pertaining to the set of factors or metabolic pathways that produce smaller molecules from larger units.

Cavitation: Formation of an empty space within a solid or liquid (e.g., bubble).

Cell migration: Act of cell movement commonly toward or away from a stimulus.

Chemical fat saturation: Technique for suppressing signal from fat in an MR image based on modifying a pulse sequence to exploit the slight difference of precessional frequencies exhibited by protons in fat compared with protons in water to yield an MR image in which fat appears black; this is an alternative to short-tau inversion recovery imaging.

Chemotaxis: Movement of an organism or cell in response to a chemical stimulus. Can be either toward or away from the chemical substance.

Chondromalacia patellae: Softening and inflammation of the cartilage of the patella.

Cognate: Describing the specific interaction of two molecules, for example, a receptor and its specific ligand, or an enzyme and its preferred substrate.

Compressive (loading): Load applied to a material or tissue by pushing on it.

Copolymer: Polymer formed from monomers of different chemical species. This is accomplished via the process of polymerization that involves the reaction of monomer molecules to form polymer chains or three-dimensional networks.

Covalent bonding: Chemical bond formed between atoms due to the sharing of a pair of valence electrons.

Creep: Viscoelastic response of a material denoting deformation with time in response to a constant stress or load. In general, this is the tendency of a material to deform as a function of time under the influence of stress.

Crepitus: Popping, cracking, or grating sounds of the joint. In pathology, this sound may be due to two rough surfaces, for example, ends of a fracture or arthritic cartilage, coming into contact.

Cytodifferentiation: Differentiation of specialized cells from precursor cells. *See* differentiation.

Deacetylation: Process by which an acetyl group is removed from a molecule.

Debride: Removal of dead or damaged tissue to improve healing of the remaining tissue.

Demineralize: Removing mineral, commonly the removal of calcium from tissue or bone.

Dermatome: Somite lateral wall during embryonic development that becomes the connective tissue of the skin.

dGEMRIC: Delayed gadolinium-enhanced MRI of cartilage. A technique that allows for evaluation of cartilage glycosaminoglycan content by measuring the T1 time of cartilage after administration of a gadolinium-based MRI contrast medium; absorption of gadolinium shortens a tissue's T1 time, but gadolinium is excluded from healthy cartilage with normal glycosaminoglycan content.

Diarthrodial: Any freely movable joint, for example, shoulder, hip, or knee.

Differentiation: Process by which cells change from one cell type to another, for example, commonly a less specialized cell becoming a more specialized type, such as a stem cell becoming a somatic cell.

Diffusion MRI: *See* diffusion-weighted imaging.

Diffusion-weighted imaging (DWI): Technique that produces MR images with signal intensities that depend on diffusion of water within a tissue; two or more images with varying diffusion weighting can be used to calculate and map the apparent diffusion coefficients of tissues.

Discontinuity or fragmentation: In MRI, a region of the tissue or structure with abnormal change in signal indicating a change in the material.

Dynamic compression: Compression that cycles between two (or more) load conditions.

Eburnated: Degenerative changes to the subchondral bone found in osteoarthritis patients, resulting in exposed bone that appears dense and ivory-like.

Echo time (TE): Important MRI pulse sequence characteristic defining the amount of time (typically milliseconds) between proton excitation and signal (i.e., echo) acquisition during which decay of transverse magnetization can occur.

Ectoderm: Most exterior of the three primary germ layers in the developing embryo. The epidermis and nerve tissue form from this layer.

Elastic (properties): Properties of a material that determine the deformation when an external load is applied. The corresponding stress and strain are linearly related and independent of time.

Elastic energy: Form of energy stored in a material due to its volume or shape distortion. It is a potential energy that develops when materials are deformed, for example, via compression or stretching.

Elastin: Protein found in many tissues that allows them to resume their shape following stretching and bending.

ELISA: Enzyme-linked immunosorbent assay. This is a plate-based immunoassay making use of antibody specificity for an antigen to detect various biological molecules, such as hormones, peptides, proteins, and antibodies. Detection is based on the use of an enzyme bonded to either one of the antibodies used in the assay or the antigen itself. See Section 7.3.3.1 for further details.

Endochondral bone formation: During fetal development, this process, along with intramembranous ossification, forms the bones of the skeleton. However, unlike intramembranous ossification, a cartilage precursor is required.

Endocytosis: Energy-dependent process by which cells engulf molecules via invagination of the membrane and vacuole formation.

Epiphyseal plate: Area of growing cartilage found at the ends of the long bones, commonly in juvenile organisms. Also known as the growth plate or physis.

Equilibrium modulus: Intrinsic property of the material denoting stiffness at equilibrium. In articular cartilage, this is commonly determined once the interstitial fluid of the tissue stops flowing. This corresponds to when the tissue has ceased straining under stress or its stress has relaxed under strain.

Etiology: Cause or causes of a disease.

Ex vivo: "Outside of life." It refers to a process or procedure that takes place outside of a living organism. Commonly used to refer to the use of tissue removed from an organism for experimentation.

Exocytosis: Energy-dependent process by which the cell releases molecules to the extracellular space through fusion of a secretory or exocytotic vesicle (a type of cell vacuole) to the cell membrane.

Exogenous: Originating from outside an organism or cell.

Fast spin echo: Type of MRI pulse sequence; following excitation of protons in a tissue, multiple 180° radiofrequency pulses are used to generate signal "echoes" from which an MR image can be reconstructed with shorter acquisition time compared with a single spin-echo pulse sequence. *See also* spin echo.

Fibrillation: One of the initial degenerative changes in osteoarthritis, denoted by cartilage softening and formation of linear marks on the cartilage surface.

Focal adhesion: Large macromolecular assembly at the cell membrane that regulates interactions and transmits signals between the extracellular matrix and the internal processes of the cell.

Friction: Resistance to movement, or intended movement, of one surface upon another surface.

G protein (guanine nucleotide binding protein): Family of intracellular proteins that act as molecular switches based on their ability to bind to and hydrolyze guanosine triphosphate (GTP) to guanosine diphosphate (GDP).

G protein-coupled receptors: Part of a large family of transmembrane receptors that sense molecules or ligands in the extracellular space and activate intracellular signaling pathways.

Genetic linkage: Tendency of alleles of a gene to be inherited together due to their physical proximity on a chromosome. Being physically close to each other on a chromosome means the genes are less likely to be separated onto different chromatids during chromosomal crossover of meiosis.

Gradient echo: T type of MRI pulse sequence; following excitation of protons in a tissue, magnetic field gradients are used to generate a signal "echo" from which the MR image is reconstructed. *See also* spin echo.

Guanidine: Colorless strong base soluble in polar solvents, found in urine as a product of protein metabolism.

Guanine nucleotide exchange factor (GEF): Family of proteins involved in the activation of small GTPases. Mechanistically, this occurs by inducing the release of guanosine diphosphate (GDP) from the small GTPase to allow binding of guanosine triphosphate (GTP) to the small GTPase, which causes activation. This activation of the small GTPase allows for further downstream intercellular signaling.

Haptotaxis: Directional movement of cells in contact with a surface-bound gradient. Commonly, this gradient is due to bound chemoattractants or matrix proteins expressing cellular adhesion sites.

Hemopexin (domain): Propeller-shaped protein domain that facilitates binding to a variety of molecules and proteins, such as collagen.

Heparin affinity chromatography: Column consisting of immobilized heparin used for purification of a variety of biomolecules based on their binding to heparin.

Heterotrimer: Trimer of two or more different monomers, such as type I collagen.

Histology: Study of the microscopic anatomy of tissues.

Histomorphology: Histological study of cell morphology.

Histopathology: Histological study of tissues to observe disease.

Homeostasis: Ability to adjust the physiological processes of an organism or cell to maintain internal equilibrium.

Hydrolytic scission: Process by which addition of water to a chemical bond causes it to break.

Hydrophilicity/hydrophobicity: Terms used to describe solubility in water. Hydrophilicity is a property of molecules that are polar ("water loving"). Hydrophobicity is a property of molecules that are nonpolar ("water fearing").

Hydrostatic pressure: Stress experienced by any point within a fluid at equilibrium due to the force of gravity. As a result, an object immersed in fluid experiences equal forces that are perpendicular to all surfaces. In tissue engineering, hydrostatic pressure is employed as an anabolic stimulus to which chondrocytes appear to be responsive. This can be accomplished by compressing fluid within a confined space.

Hydroxylation: Introduction of a hydroxyl group (-OH) into an organic compound; biologically, this is commonly facilitated by hydroxylase enzymes.

Hyperplasia: Enlargement of an organ or tissue due to increased cell proliferation rate.

Hysteresis: In mechanical systems, it denotes the energy loss or dissipation in a material during loading and unloading due to friction of its internal constituents.

Idiopathic: Disease that arises spontaneously or by an unknown cause.

Immunohistochemistry: Histological technique using the antigen binding specificity of antibodies to detect antigens, commonly proteins, in tissue sections.

Indication: Symptom or particular circumstance that suggests certain medical treatment is necessary.

Integrins: Protein superfamily made up of transmembrane cell adhesion receptors that participate in cell-cell, cell-matrix, and cell-ligand interactions.

Interstitial fluid: Extracellular fluid that surrounds cells and extracellular matrix components.

In utero: "Inside the womb." It is used to describe phenomena with reference to the embryo.

In vitro: "In glass." It refers to a process or procedure that takes place outside of a living organism. Commonly used to refer to the use of cells or biological molecules in a test tube or cell culture dish.

In vivo: "In life." It refers to a process or procedure that occurs inside of a living organism.

Isoforms: Any of two or more proteins that have a similar but not an identical amino acid sequence. These may arise from different genes, or from the same gene by alternative splicing.

Isomers: Molecules with the same chemical formula but different arrangements of atoms.

Isotropic organization: Uniform organization in all directions of a material. In biomechanics, isotropy denotes the same mechanical properties irrespective of direction.

Kellgren-Lawrence grade: Tool for scoring a knee radiograph for the severity of osteoarthritis, consisting of a 0-4 scale, with higher numbers indicating increasing severity.

Kinase: Group of enzymes that catalyze the transfer of a phosphate group (e.g., from ATP) to a substrate protein or molecule. This transfer is used to regulate a variety of important cellular processes.

Larmor frequency: Frequency of precession of protons in a magnetic field, which depends on magnetic field strength; for a 1.5 T MRI system, the Larmor frequency, typically denoted by ω_o, equals 63.9 MHz.

Limb bud: Initial bulge-like structure formed in the limb field during limb development. This is a result of proliferation of mesenchymal cells, mesodermally derived from the lateral plate.

Limb field: Region specified by the expression of homeobox and other transcription factor genes that will become the developing limb.

Longitudinal magnetization: Net magnetization occurring parallel to the MRI primary magnetic field representing the summed magnetic moments of all protons in a given volume; longitudinal magnetization is positive for a sample at equilibrium and is typically reduced following a radiofrequency pulse.

Lyophilize: Process utilizing high vacuum and low temperatures to remove water from a material, also known as freeze-drying. This process depends on sublimation to allow water to go from a frozen state to a gas without going through the liquid state.

Mechanobiological: Regarding the interplay of mechanical forces or mechanical properties and coupled biological processes. It is usually viewed as how cell or tissue biomechanics impacts cellular function.

Mechanoregulated: Referring to regulation of biological processes by mechanical (physical) stimuli, especially at the cellular or subcellular level.

Mechanosensing: Ability to sense and respond to mechanical stimuli, especially at the cellular or subcellular level.

Mechanotransduction: Mechanisms used by cells to translate mechanical stimuli into biochemical signal transduction.

Meckel's cartilage: Structure typically present during fetal development. This is the bilaterally paired, rod-like, cartilaginous ventral precursor component of the lower jaw, or ventral mandibular arch.

Meniscectomy: Surgical removal of the meniscus, usually that of the knee.

Mesoderm: Middle germ layer during early embryonic development, situated between the endoderm and ectoderm. This germ layer gives rise to multiple tissues, including, but not limited to, muscle, bone, cartilage, and connective tissues.

MH2 domain: "Mad-homology 2" is a c-terminal domain that contains a conserved loop-helix region that can bind phosphoserine residues. This domain is conserved across different members of the Smad family of proteins.

Micropatterning: Process for producing miniature patterns, commonly of a protein or other biological molecules, upon a substrate.

Mitosis: Normal cell division, resulting in two daughter cells with the same number of chromosomes as the parent cell.

Moiety: Part of a molecule. It commonly refers to a functional group that has similar chemical reactivity across different molecules that contain that group.

Molecular pore space: Nonsolid space within a material on the molecular scale.

Morphogenesis: Process by which cell, tissue, and organ development is regulated to produce the shape of an organism.

Morphogens: Molecules that regulate the pattern of cell and tissue development during morphogenesis.

Mosaicplasty: Surgical procedure used to fill focal cartilage defects through the transplantation of many smaller osteochondral grafts into a larger defect.

Multipotency: Ability of undifferentiated cells to differentiate into a limited range of more than one cell type, for example, adult stem cells.

Myotome: During embryonic development, the dorsal part of the somite that will give rise to portions of the musculature of the skeleton.

Neocartilage: Tissue-engineered cartilage construct; literally "new cartilage."

Neoplastic: Tissue changes that are cancerous. *Nonneoplastic* refers to tissue changes that are pathological but not cancerous.

Neural crest: During embryonic development, a group of ectodermally derived migratory and multipotent cells from the most dorsal region of the neural tube. These cells migrate extensively and give rise to the craniofacial cartilage and bone; melanocytes; smooth muscle; sensory, sympathetic, and parasympathetic neurons and glial cells; and adrenal medulla cells.

Newtonian (fluid): Fluid whose shear stress is linearly related to the strain rate via a constant coefficient (coefficient of viscosity). In contrast, in a non-Newtonian fluid the constitutive equations are nonlinear such that the relationship between the shear stress and the strain rate is not constant and may depend on the rate of applied stress or stress history, for example, synovial fluid.

Orthopedics: Medical specialty that focuses on injuries and diseases of the bones and joints.

Osteogenesis: Process by which bone is formed.

Osteolysis: Loss or destruction of bone in pathological conditions.

Oxidative stress: Level of damage caused by reactive oxygen species at the cell, tissue, or organ level.

Palmitoylated: Posttranslational modification consisting of the covalent binding of fatty acids to a protein, for example, palmitic acid attached to cysteine in a membrane protein.

Perichondrium: Dense connective tissue surrounding the cartilage in developing bone. It can also be found at the perimeter of elastic and hyaline cartilage, but is not found at the articulating cartilages of the synovial joints. In developing bone, once perichondrium is vascularized, it will become the periosteum.

Periosteal flap: Tissue flap produced from the periosteum, the dense vascular connective tissue that covers the bones. It was often used to cover a cell-filled defect in articular cartilage during autologous chondrocyte implantation.

Permeability (hydraulic): Mechanical property describing the rate of flow of a liquid or gas through a material. In articular cartilage, permeability denotes the ease or difficulty with which interstitial fluid moves past the pores of the solid extracellular matrix.

Phagophore: Double-membrane structure that can enclose cytoplasmic organelles or other components and transport them to the lysosome.

Phenotype: Set of observable traits of an organism due to the combination of genetic and environmental factors. These include, but are not limited to, such traits as an organism's morphology, development, or physiological properties.

Phorbol esters: Group of tetracyclic diterpenoid molecules that are able to activate protein kinase C, a regulator of multiple signal transduction pathways.

Phosphorylation: Process of adding a phosphate group to a substrate, commonly a protein. This process can activate or inactivate enzymes or other molecules and is heavily involved in signal transduction.

Phosphorylation activation loop: Loop-shaped region of a protein, commonly an enzyme, that activates the protein when phosphorylated.

PI-3K pathway: Intracellular signal transduction pathway that regulates the cell cycle (see Figure 2.22).

Pluripotent: Ability of undifferentiated cells to differentiate into all cell types that make up the body, for example, embryonic stem cells.

Polysaccharide: Large carbohydrate molecule composed of smaller simple sugar molecules. Examples include starch and cellulose.

Precocious arthropathy: Joint pathology that develops at an earlier age than usually observed.

Preparative electrophoresis: Fractionation technique based on the motion of particles under the influence of an electric field. This process is used to purify or enrich for low-abundance proteins or nucleic acids.

Prestrain: Strain applied to a material before loading or testing.

Proprioceptive: Relating to internal stimuli, especially those involved with position and movement of the body or limbs.

Pulse sequence: Specific combination of radiofrequency pulses, magnetic field gradients, and timed data acquisition to create an MR image; characteristics of a pulse sequence partly determine the appearance of tissues in an MR image.

Radiofrequency pulse: Oscillating magnetic field with frequency equal to the Larmor frequency used to excite protons for the purposes of MRI.

Repetition time (TR): Important MRI pulse sequence characteristic describing the amount of time between sequential excitation pulses, thus, determining the amount of time during which longitudinal recovery can occur in a tissue.

Scaffold: In tissue engineering, a biomaterial or structure produced to aid in forming a 3D tissue.

Sclerotic: Pertaining to the abnormal hardening of tissues or anatomic structures.

Sclerotome: During embryonic development, this is the portion of the somite that gives rise to some of the skeletal tissues.

Self-assembling process: Scaffoldless tissue engineering technology that produces tissues that demonstrate spontaneous organization without external forces; this occurs via the minimization of free energy through cell-to-cell interactions.

Self-assembly: Process by which order spontaneously results from disorder without the use of external input. For tissue engineering, this is the mechanism driving the self-assembling process.

Semicrystalline: Describing the structure of a solid that possesses areas of highly ordered regions (termed crystalline) and regions that lack organization (termed amorphous). As an example, one can consider polylactic acid polymerized with different monomeric forms and used in sutures, scaffolds, or biodegradable fixation devices.

Serological: Relating to the characteristics of sera. Primarily used with reference to blood serum drawn for diagnostic tests.

Shearing: Loading environment that results in deformation in a material such that parallel internal surfaces slide in relationship to each other. It is a product of a force applied parallel to the surface of the material.

Short-tau inversion recovery (STIR): Technique for suppressing signal from fat in an MR image involving a pulse sequence that utilizes the difference in recovery of longitudinal magnetization by protons in fat compared with other tissues in order to yield an MR image in which fat appears black; this is an alternative to chemical fat saturation.

Soft lithography: Process of using elastomeric materials in the production of various structures. For micropatterning, this commonly uses stamps or molds to produce desired patterns on a substrate.

Somatomedin (domain): Protein domain of vitronectin and proteoglycan 4. In vitronectin, this domain regulates cell adhesion.

Somite: Structure found during embryonic development, consisting of repeating bilateral units of paraxial mesoderm that forms along the length of the neural tube. Somites give rise to vertebrae, the rib cage, dermal layers of the skin, skeletal muscle, cartilage, and tendons.

Spin echo: Type of MRI pulse sequence; following excitation of protons in a tissue, a 180° radiofrequency pulse is used to generate a signal "echo" from which the MR image is reconstructed. *See also* fast spin echo, gradient echo.

Stereoelectronic effect: Changes in the properties of a molecule that are due to overlap of the electronic orbitals of the constituent atoms making up the molecule.

Stereoisomers: Isomeric molecules with the same sequence of atomic bonding and differing only by the 3D orientation of the atoms in the molecule. For example, enantiomers are two stereoisomers that are related to each other by a reflection, such that they are mirror images of each other.

Sterically hinder: When the 3D shape or size of a molecule interferes in a chemical reaction that would be seen with smaller groups.

Stress relaxation: Viscoelastic response of a material denoting changes in stress with time in response to a constant strain or deformation. Initially, stress peaks to a maximum value and then relaxes to an equilibrium or asymptotic value. Unlike in solids, in viscoelastic fluids stress relaxes to zero since fluids cannot sustain stress.

Synchondrosis: Slightly mobile joint characterized by bones joined with a layer of either hyaline cartilage or fibrocartilage. Commonly, this is a developmental structure, such as the epiphyseal growth plate, which mineralizes into bone with skeletal maturity. An exception to this is the synchondroses of the vertebral column.

Syndesmosis: Slightly mobile fibrous joint characterized by bones joined by connective tissue. Examples include the tibiofibular and radioulnar sydesmoses.

Synergistic/synergism: When the combined interaction of two or more terms with respect to a control is larger than the sum of the differences of each term with respect to the control. In other words, the effect of the interaction is larger than the sum of the effects of each term.

T1: Inherent tissue or material property expressed as a time constant (typically in units of milliseconds) that characterizes the rate of recovery of longitudinal magnetization by a tissue in an external magnetic field following excitation of the tissue's protons by a radiofrequency pulse; a tissue's T1 time largely depends on the frequency of molecular motion within the tissue relative to the Larmor frequency. *See also* T2.

T2: Inherent tissue or material property expressed as a time constant (typically in units of milliseconds) that characterizes the rate of decay of transverse magnetization by a tissue in an external magnetic field following excitation of the tissue's protons by a radiofrequency pulse; a tissue's T2 time largely depends on local variations in the magnetic field experienced by protons due to the presence of large molecules. *See also* T1.

Telomeres: Repetitive sacrificial nucleotide sequence at the end of the chromosome that is truncated during cell division. This sequence protects the genes on the chromosome from being truncated during cell division and inhibits chromosomal fusion.

Tensile (loading): Load applied to a material or tissue by pulling on it.

Teratoma: Tumor composed of cell types or tissues derived from more than one germ layer. A teratoma often contains tissues not normally present at the site.

Time constant: Quantity of time necessary for some defined process to occur; time constants are often used to characterize time-dependent processes that exhibit exponential behavior, for example, half-life of a radioactive material or the T1/T2 time of a tissue in a magnetic field.

Transverse magnetization: Net magnetization occurring perpendicular to the MRI primary magnetic field representing the summed magnetic moments of all protons in a given volume; transverse magnetization is induced by a radiofrequency pulse and subsequently decays to zero at equilibrium.

Tubercle: Small rounded eminence especially on a bone. Examples include the tibial tuberosity, greater and lesser tubercles of the humerus, radial tuberosity, and Lister's tubercle of the radius.

Ultrafiltrate: Solution that contains only low-molecular weight solutes as a consequence of passing through membrane with small molecular size pores.

Vascularization: Formation of blood vessels.

Viscoelastic: Pertaining to materials that exhibit time-dependent mechanical behaviors, such as hysteresis, creep, and stress relaxation. The behaviors of these materials are due to a combination of elastic and viscous responses.

Wear: Damage to an object's surface via the removal and deformation of material on the surface due to movement and commonly caused by friction.

Xenogeneic: Transplanted tissue or organ from a donor species different from the host.

We would like to thank Derek Cissel, VMD, DACVR, PhD, for his assistance with the glossary.

Index

Page numbers with f and t refer to figures and tables, respectively.

Printed and bound by CPI Group (UK) Ltd, Croydon, CR0 4YY

01/11/2024

01782603-0015